Natural Substances for Cancer Prevention

Natural Substances for Cancer Prevention

by

Jun-Ping Xu

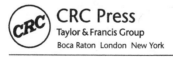

CRC Press
Taylor & Francis Group
Boca Raton London New York

CRC Press is an imprint of the
Taylor & Francis Group, an **informa** business

CRC Press
Taylor & Francis Group
6000 Broken Sound Parkway NW, Suite 300
Boca Raton, FL 33487-2742

First issued in paperback 2022

ISBN-13: 978-0-815-36538-9 (hbk)
ISBN-13: 978-1-03-233924-5 (pbk)
DOI: 10.1201/9781351261005

Library of Congress Cataloging-in-Publication Data

Names: Xu, Jun-Ping, author.
Title: Natural substances for cancer prevention / Jun-Ping Xu.
Description: Boca Raton : CRC Press, [2018] | Includes bibliographical
references and indexes.
Identifiers: LCCN 2017040848 | ISBN 9780815365389 (hardback : alk. paper) |
ISBN 9781351261005 (ebook)
Subjects: LCSH: Cancer--Prevention--Nutritional aspects. | Bioactive
compounds.
Classification: LCC RC268 .X85 2018 | DDC 616.99/4052--dc23
LC record available at https://lccn.loc.gov/2017040848

**Visit the Taylor & Francis Web site at
http://www.taylorandfrancis.com**

**and the CRC Press Web site at
http://www.crcpress.com**

Contents

Preface

The goals of cancer research are not only to hamper cancer cell growth, metastasis, and drug resistance and to promote tumor cell death but also to stimulate the immune defense and to eliminate carcinogenesis-related factors. With the exception of basic studies in cancer treatment, food studies involved in cancer prevention have largely ascended to favor today. There has been a prominent progression in cancer prevention by foods during the recent decade. Hence, when the work of publishing a book titled *Cancer Inhibitors from Chinese Medicines* in 2016 was complete, I immediately started to reorganizing and replenishing the manuscript of my new book *Natural Substances for Cancer Prevention*. Hopefully, this book will help people to understand the possibility of preventing cancer through daily diet.

Actually, owing to the era of food nutritional recognition that preceded the development of current pharmacological bioassays, it is necessary to reexamine the medicinal potential of foods. In recent years, the emphases on food studies have expanded from food's nutritional value to exploration of its functional bioactive ingredients. Thus, foods are frequently the subject of investigation for cancer prevention. On the more positive side, one of the most striking aspects of this field is its interdisciplinary nature; natural product chemists, biochemists, and food nutritionists collaborating with pharmacologists and oncologists, whose interest and involvement are essential for meaningful progress to advocate the prominence of functional foods in lowering cancer incidences. The comprehensive investigations show that natural substances have significant potential in the functional foods that can be used to prevent cancer and other chronic diseases.

This book shows a great value in viewing the latest advances in science. It highlights 93 functional foods that are widely commercialized in western and/or eastern food markets, providing interesting and useful results for cancer prevention. The functional comestibles described in this book include vegetables, fruits, beans, grains, flavorings, beverages, mushrooms, seaweeds, microalgae, and animal-based foods. The frequent combination of these foods and similar functional foods in the diet should be highly encouraged. The effort is definitely believed to be beneficial to our body protection and health promotion if the dietary habit is followed for years. By the way, this is an academic book without any pictures; however, when reading this book, it is suggested that you use Google to search for various photos of foods and their sources. From the abundant gallery, you can effortlessly get intuitive images that will help you read and understand this book and make it easier to use in your life.

Finally, I dedicate this book to my dear parents, Bingheng Xu and Tingying Li, for their appreciation, deep love, and full understanding; to my wife, Wendy, and son, Alex, for their strong support for many years; and to my sister's family, Junfang Xu and Yanming Zhu, for taking care of our parents for a long time. In addition, thanks to Lucas Johnson, a student at Arizona State University, Tempe, Arizona, for his assistance in preparing the abstracts and introductions for each chapter of this book.

Jun-Ping Xu

Author

Jun-Ping Xu, a research professor at the School of Molecular Science of Arizona State University, Tempe, Arizona, received his undergraduate training in pharmaceutical science at the Shanghai University of Traditional Chinese Medicine, Shanghai, China, and pursued advanced professional studies at the Shanghai Institute for Drug Control, China. He started his academic career in Chinese natural medicines at the Shanghai Institute of Pharmaceutical Industry, China, and then studied in Japan. After earning his PhD from Tokyo University of Pharmacy, Japan, he returned to Shanghai to join Professor Rensheng Xu's group at the Shanghai Institute of Materia Medica (SIMM), Chinese Academy of Science, for researching biologically active and functional agents from Chinese herbs. During the 2 years at SIMM (1989–1990), he submitted 9 papers and 1 review article to international science journals. In 1991, he came to the U.S. to join the Cancer Research Institute at the Arizona State University as a postdoctoral research fellow, working with the Director and Professor G. R. Pettit on the discovery and development of novel cancer inhibitors from marine organisms and microorganisms. He has published more than 100 scientific papers related to these interests. From 2008 to 2013, he taught a class on the history of Chinese medicine to introduce the origination and development of Chinese medicine and also to explain the basic concepts of Chinese medicine theoretical system and practice skills, and Chinese ancient philosophy for university students in the Chinese Flagship Program. Jun-Ping Xu is author of *Cancer Inhibitors from Chinese Medicines*, published by the CRC Press/Taylor & Francis Group in 2016.

Introduction

There is nothing in today's daily existence that cancer doesn't touch. The seriousness of cancer causes stress in people's mind and body and in the relationships with their friends and family. As reported by the World Health Organization (WHO) in 2012, more than 14 million new cases of cancer occurred that led to more than 8.2 million deaths worldwide. The numbers will be whoppingly amplified by 70% globally in the next 20 years. These shocking facts exhibit that cancer has endangered the safety of human life and that conquering cancer is the scientist's greatest wish in this generation and the next. Cancer, nevertheless, stands proudly in front of mankind, like the Himalayas, relentlessly blocking the journey of scientists. In more than six decades, every step of the battle against cancer has been tough and hard, but it is possible to believe that humanity will eventually climb this peak. The future development of cancer therapies and prevention should still follow the knowledge and discoveries gained in cancer basic studies to advance new strategies and challenges. The hope is coming again since 2016, because of the passage of the 21st Century Cure Act in the Congress of the United States by an overwhelming majority and securing U.S.$4.8 billion in federal research funding, including the Cancer Moonshot and the Precision Medicine Initiative. Several approvals from the FDA include explorations and advances in precision medicine, immunotherapy, targeted therapy, combination therapy, and development of better immune checkpoint inhibitors and better refining predictive biomarkers of cancer, which will contour the future of cancer diagnosis and treatment. With the convergence of incredible technical advances, there is a lot to look forward to in the field of cancer care.

1. CANCER PREVENTION IS FEASIBLE AND NECESSARY

In spite of cancer diagnosis and therapies that are developing and improving recently, cancer is still a major cause of morbidity and mortality on this globe. This foremost public health issues involve not only the developed countries but also the developing countries. It is apparent today that changes in cancer-prevalence patterns are extensively influenced by rapid industrialization and urbanization, lifestyle alteration, and environmental pollution. The cause of cancer generally comes down to mutations in gene and DNA. Chemicals (such as carcinogens), radiation, hormones, smoking, chronic inflammation, obesity, viruses, and a number of other factors have been proven as being able to provoke cancer-related mutations. Principally, owing to their anarchic characteristics, cancer cells have extraordinary capabilities, resulting in their growth without any limitations by neglecting inhibitory signals in cell proliferation and replication, escaping immune systemic monitors, dodging apoptosis, and eliciting invasion and angiogenesis. Even so, oncologists have proven that carcinogenic process occurs through multistages of multiple genetic alterations and aberrant signaling, which need an extended period of time. This time gap may give people plenty of opportunity to eliminate the hidden dangers of tiny cancerous foci. For successful cancer prevention, removing the substantial factors of cancerous formation from human daily life as soon as possible should be the best strategy. Definitely, human societies have to eradicate the pollution of water, air, and comestibles and constrain the pollution that comes from radiation, and individuals and families ought to improve diet patterns and lifestyle habits. If done so, in accordance with WHO reports, 35% of all cancer cases can be defused. Hence, regardless of the enormous difficulties in cancer therapy, currently there is an overall agreement that it is preferable to prevent the disease than cure its end stage. Chemoprevention is regarded as one of the most promising and realistic approaches in the prevention of human cancer.

2. THE BEST CANCER PREVENTION IS THE DIETARY CONSUMPTION OF FUNCTIONAL FOODS

With the growing recognition of dietary benefits for health in recent years, functional foods are now being highlighted for their positive properties of controlling various disorders such as neoplastic, cardiovascular, neurological, and immunological diseases. In this field, chemoprevention is gaining a lot of attention. Emerging evidences indicate that healthy diets are closely associated with the decline of cancer threat and carcinogenesis in human populations. After the evaluation of colon cancer, prostate cancer, mammary cancer, liver cancer, and other cancers, the epidemiological and preclinical investigations have disclosed an inverse relationship between the consumption of functional food and incidences of carcinoma. In the past three decades, numerous studies in chemical biology and molecular biology have established strong scientific evidences, demonstrating the properties of naturally occurring bioactive chemicals to hamper all stages of cancers (from initiation to metastasis). A variety of biologically active food and chemical compounds are found to be integral components of human diet, which are commonly present as food constituents of flowering plants, mushrooms, seaweeds, some animal foods, and particularly plant foods.

Likewise, large numbers of population-based and case-controlled surveys and statistical analyses have concluded that individuals frequently adding natural functional foods such as green plant-based foods, benignant mushrooms, and seafood into their diet menu would dramatically increase considerable safeguards to maintain lifetime health and to diminish the risk of cancer initiation. Accordingly, it is clear that the major concern for cancer prevention is the modification of dietary habits and frequent intake of more anticancer-related natural substances. More significantly, these bioactive chemicals presented in the functional foods are readily available, inexpensive, nontoxic, and nutritional. Therefore, healthy food-related programs should be carried out worldwide to educate the population on the importance of eating a variety of functional foods habitually for health promotion and to advocate dietary strategies to effectively resist cancer initiation, proliferation, and progression.

3. THE ANTIOXIDANT SUBSTANCES IN FUNCTIONAL FOODS CONTRIBUTE TO CANCER PREVENTION

As we all now know, oxidation is a critical process for all living organisms to produce energy necessary for biological processes. Free radicals are the main factor of oxidative damage in animals and humans. Reactive oxygen species (ROS) are formed by hydrogen peroxide or superoxide anions and the ROS production in a higher level can lead to oxidative stress. When there is accumulation of oxidative stress to excess, DNA is damaged and cells and tissues are harmfully attacked. Therefore, a variety of diseases, including mutagenesis, carcinogenesis, cellular aging, neurodegeneration, coronary heart disease, diabetes, and so on, would be elicited by the oxygen-centered free radicals, ROS production, and oxidative stress. Despite most organisms holding self-protective capacities through antioxidant defense and system-repairing capacities against oxidative damage, the body systems are sometimes insufficient to eliminate these damages entirely, especially in the weak and ill. Nowadays, extensive attention has been paid to consuming natural bioactive foods that contain abundant and safe antioxidant chemicals. Vitamins can be obtained from a dietary supplement intake of nutritional and functional foods and vitamins A, C, and E are capable of resisting ROS production. More important, these foods and their by-products concurrently provide rich nonvitamin antioxidants, such as polyphenols (such as flavonoids, phenylpropanoids, stilbenes, carotenoids, tannins, flavonoids, proanthocyanidin, anthocyanidin, and catechin) and polysaccharides, which effectively exert strong hindrance against ROS production through free-radical scavenging, thereby defusing carcinogenesis and mutation.

4. THE IMMUNOMODULATING SUBSTANCES IN FUNCTIONAL FOODS CONTRIBUTE TO BODY DEFENSE

In addition to correlation of oxidation with cancer, immune-system dysfunction would also cause various diseases, including cancer and infectious diseases. As important immune organs, the indexes of spleen and thymus reflect the immune function of organisms owing to the secretion of diverse immune cells and immune factors to compose an immune system for human body defense. The responsibility of the immune system is to detect and destroy abnormal and mutant cells either spontaneous or enthetic. Many of the immune cell types belonging to both innate (NK cells and macrophages) and adaptive (T-cells and B-cells) immune systems participate in the immune functions in the control of cancer and tumorigenesis. In normal cases, the functional immune system is capable of resisting cancer initiation and development. However, cancer cells sometimes escape the detection and attacks of immune cells and immune factors. On the other hand, cancer can weaken the immune system by spreading into the bone marrow and then stopping the bone marrow from producing enough blood cells to exert immunity. Similarly, chemotherapy, biological therapies, and radiotherapy can temporarily weaken systemic immunity by causing a drop in the number of white blood cells generated in the bone marrow. Consequently, critically important in cancer prevention and therapy is exerting the immunity in a healthy level and/or reversing the immune defense up to a healthy level by rebuilding the weakened immune function.

Most science reports have confirmed that various natural substances in functional foods and herbs possess remarkable abilities in the activation of the host's immune system and anticancer immunity, subsequently leading to the suppression of cancer-cell viability. These natural substances also attenuate the toxicity/side effects caused by chemo- and radiotherapies owing to their significant immunoregulative functions. The human immune response is a highly complex and extraordinarily sophisticated system that involves mechanisms both innate and adaptive. Numerous bioactivity-guided chemistry studies demonstrated that a variety of natural immunoenhancing substances can be gained from a diet of functional foods. Among the substances, the macromolecules such as polysaccharides, glycoproteins, and lectins usually play a key role in potentiating immune responses in host organisms, whereas the natural polyphenolics are also excellent antioxidants, and some types of flavonoids, stilbenes, and phenylpropanoids also showed immunomodulating activities. The field of study of immunoenhancing compounds, of course, is not new, but natural products from functional foods represent a rich and promising source of bioactive ingredients with immunomodulating properties. In most cases, these components integrate with beneficial compounds from other sources that effectively augment the body's defense and immunity.

5. THE BIOACTIVE SUBSTANCES IN FUNCTIONAL FOODS CONTRIBUTE TO CANCER INHIBITION

It is now well known that a dietary habit of rich functional food is significantly associated with reducing risk of various types of carcinoma and chronic degenerative disorders (such as cardiovascular diseases and neurodegenerative disorders). According to plentiful findings from biology connected bioorganic chemistry studies, vegetables, fruits, seaweeds, flavorings, beverage materials, and microalgae are great sources of antioxidant micromolecules (e.g., phenolics, flavonoids, terpenoids, carotenoids, proanthocyanidin, anthocyanidin, catechin, and tannins), whereas grains, beans, fruits, mushrooms, and animal-based foods are rich sources of macromolecules (e.g., polysaccharides, glycoproteins, proteins, lectins, and/or enzymes). Moreover, lab experiments have further revealed the direct and indirect anticancer potentials of natural substances with micromolecules or macromolecules, which are obtained from the isolation of natural functional foods and their by-products. Though they showed only a weak-to-moderate range of suppression against cancer viability, proliferation, invasion, metastasis, and angiogenesis, these bioactive substances presented high safety and reliability and showed other health-improving benefits. In most of the cases, their direct cancer-growth inhibitory effects primarily resulted from the induction of cell apoptosis and cell-cycle arrest and the obstruction of inflammatory factors, whereas indirect suppressive effects are attributed to the anticancer immunity power of the functional foods, particularly these bioactive macromolecular substances that are capable of prompting the cytotoxicity of natural killer (NK) cells and lymphocytes and boosting the phagocytosis of macrophages, leading these defensive cells to attack and kill the cancer cells. Moreover, these capacities in immunoregulation remarkably led these macromolecules to reverse the immunosuppression caused by neoplastic growth and conventional cancer therapies and to reduce radiotherapeutic irradiation and chemotherapeutic drugs that caused toxicities to bone marrow, liver, kidney, and heart. Overall, these positive characteristics, that is, weak-to-moderate degrees of direct anticancer activity, indirect anticancer immunity, and immunostimulation, make functional foods suitable for cancer prevention and supplementary cancer therapy. The body protecting and health-promoting benefits can be easily acquired habitually from our daily diet if the right menu with the right functional food is selected.

6. THE PROFILE AND CHARACTERISTICS OF THIS REFERENCE BOOK

The functional foods and their bioactive molecules are becoming popular as promising demulcents against various ailments, including cancer and carcinogenesis. This book, *Natural Substances for Cancer Prevention*, is an effort to sum up the health-promoting information regarding functional foods with special references and claims to cancer prevention and associated body protection (literature search to 2016). To help people understand the characteristics of functional food in cancer prevention, this reference book has comprehensively summarized the scientific evidences of 93 common dietary natural comestibles in western and/or eastern countries. From the point of view of bioorganic chemistry and molecular biology, this book focuses on the anticancer properties of natural foods in six main aspects: (i) the cancer-inhibitory and growth-arresting substances (included extracts and components) from the foodstuffs and their potentials in cancer prevention; (ii) the activity spectrum in a diversity of neoplastic cells, such as antiproliferative, antiviability, anti-growth, antimetastatic, antiangiogenic, and antitumorigenic effects; (iii) the potent antioxidant, anticancer immunity, and immunoenhancing functions; (iv) the exploration of mechanisms of cancer growth-deterring proapoptotic and immunomodulatory activities in natural comestibles; (v) the synergetic activities and detoxification of functional foods in combination with conventional chemotherapy or radiotherapy; (vi) the formulation approaches for nano- and microcapsules (techniques of which may have promising potential in food manufacturing); and (vii) other health-promoting benefits. Therefore, this professional reference book highlights the potentials of natural foods in cancer prevention and provides more scientific reasons for efficient use of these dietary foods in body protection. In addition to affording much clear scientific information and many useful suggestions, this book advocates cancer prevention at initiation stages to be feasible and effective and encourages readers to widely spread the advanced and helpful knowledge for application of natural functional foods, leading to make it more available and more accurate to minimize the incidence of cancer.

7. IMPORTANT ADVICE THAT IS HELPFUL FOR CANCER PREVENTION

Besides these recommendable 93 health foods for cancer prevention, some important advice has to be shown here for more effective anticarcinogenesis. Similar to cancer-preventive foods, there are some foods that are often consumed by people, but are classified as cancer-causing foods because of the possibility of producing and increasing some carcinogens in food processing and preservation, such as grilled red meat and fish (containing benzpyrene), smoked foods (containing polyaromatic hydrocarbon), salted and pickled foods (containing nitrates and nitrites), fried foods (containing polyaromatic hydrocarbon and benzpyrene), farmed fishes (that have been treated with antibiotics and pesticides), hydrogenated oils (containing unhealthy omega-6 fats), and moldy foods (containing aflatoxins). According to scientifically proven facts, these cancer-causing foods would largely augment the chance of carcinoma diagnosed in the human lifetime. These processed foods and food materials provide unique and delicious taste, but frequent consumption can accumulate potential carcinogens in the body over time. Eventually, such toxins cause damage at the cellular level and lead to diseases such as cancer. Therefore, such dietary processed foods ought to be limited in their intake sizes and frequencies, whereas moldy foods must be discarded. To lower cancer risk, it is unwise not to limit consumption of cancer-causing foods while being enthusiastic about cancer-preventive foods. Similarly, eating only functional foods at the same time significantly reduces or abandons other healthy and nutritious foods, which is also not good for maintaining overall health. On the other hand, physical exercise is also important for cancer prevention in addition to consuming functional foods and nutritional foods. Integration with appropriate exercises should be conducive to absorbing both functional and nutritional foods and playing a more effective cancer-preventive role against carcinogenesis.

Finally, I dedicate this book to all those who have a responsibility for taking care of his or her family members and himself or herself in the hope that the information gathered in this book might provide some helpful references and guidance to protect our body from cancer risk and to give some assistance to cancer patients in treatment.

Jun-Ping Xu

1 Cancer-Preventive Substances in Green Vegetables

1. Amaranth/*Amaranthus* plants

2. Asparagus/*Asparagus officinalis*

3. Brassicaceae Vegetables/*Brassica oleracea* and its cultivars

4. Celery/*Apium graveolens*

5. Chive/*Allium tuberosum*

6. Chinese Garlic and Scallion (Green onion)/*Allium macrostemon, A. chinense*

7. Leek/*Allium ampeloprasum* var. *porrum, A. porrum*

8. Spinach/*Spinacia oleracea*

The vegetable kingdom is a plentiful source of vitamins, minerals, and dietary fibers that play an important role in human nutrition. It is absolutely true that the vegetables are an essential dietary component for a healthy human life. Hence, nutritionists and doctors always encourage people to consume plenty of vegetables and often suggest at least five servings per day. Demands for vegetables have increased substantially worldwide, especially in countries that still practice traditional animal husbandry. Being well known for nutritional value, the functional abilities of vegetables have also received increasing attention.

Owing to the immense diversity of vegetables, it is best to divide them into three groups according to the main edible portion: (1) green vegetables (including whole plants and leaves with/without stem), (2) fruit/flower vegetables (including fruits, gourds, seeds, seed pods, and young flower buds), and (3) bulb/root vegetables (including bulbs and rhizomes). These three groups correspond to the first three chapters. These chapters focus on the scientific evidence related to the antioxidant, anticarcinogenic, antimutagenic, and immunoregulating properties of vegetables. In Chapter 1, the functions of eight common green vegetables in lowering cancer risk are discussed. *Allium* plants and *Brassica* plants are the two largest sources of green vegetables and provide remarkable contributions to human health. In addition to these commercialized vegetables, two wild vegetables—verdolaga (*Portulaca oleracea*) and the young leaves of cedar trees (*Cedrela sinensis*)—are mentioned for their significant activities in cancer prevention and tumor inhibition, but they are not available in most grocery stores. The functions and bioactivities of these two wild vegetables have been described in *Cancer Inhibitors from Chinese Medicines* published by CRC Press/Taylor & Francis group, at the end of 2016.

1. AMARANTH

Amarante   Amarant   Amaranto

莧菜　アマランス　아마란스

Amaranthus plants

Amaranthaceae

Amaranthus plants are distributed worldwide, growing under a wide range of climatic conditions. A variety of edible species of *Amaranthus* are consumed widely by all classes of people as leafy vegetable and grains around the world (especially in South Asian and some American regions) mainly for their high nutritional value, low cost, and taste. Thus, a number of *Amaranthus* species are being cultivated in South Asia and many tropical/subtropical areas for dietary consumption. By the color of leaves and stems, the amaranth vegetables can be classified into two kinds: (1) green plants (such as *A. spinosus* and *A. viridis*) and (2) red/reddish plants (such as *A. gangengitus* and *A. tricolor*). Generally, the leaves contain a high level of protein, fiber, vitamin C, unsaturated oil, and minerals such as potassium, calcium, magnesium, iron, and zinc, whereas the seeds are high in protein, lysine, vitamin B complex, fiber, antioxidant enzymes, and minerals such as magnesium, phosphorus, calcium, and potassium but lack leucine, threonine, and gluten. Aside from the great phytonutrients, amaranth has been reported to have biologically active phytoconstituents—that is, carotenoids, polyphenolics, glycolipids, and flavonoids in the leaves and stems and antimicrobial peptides, protease inhibitors, lectins, antioxidant compounds, and oily substances in the seeds. These natural substances from a diet of amaranth were found to play various biological roles, such as antioxidant, anti-inflammatory, anticancer, antiallergic, hematological parameters-improving, antihyperlipidemic, hepatoprotective, antidiabetic, immunostimulating, antiviral, and antiaging activities.[1-4] Because of their superior nutritional quality and nonallergenic and considerable functional potential, amaranth vegetables and seeds have gained much attention as a great food source for health promotion and cancer prevention.

SCIENTIFIC EVIDENCE OF CANCER-PREVENTIVE ACTIVITIES AND CONSTITUENTS

1. Anticancer properties of amaranth leaves and stems

Both grains and vegetables from the plants *A. hybridus* and *A. lividus* are popularly consumed in Southeast Asian countries such as Bangladesh. An extract (AL) was derived from the young leaves of *A. lividus*. In a mouse model, administration of 100 µg/mL/day of AL extract orally to mice for 6 days resulted in 45% suppression of the growth of Ehrlich ascites carcinoma (EAC) cells together with induction of mitochondria-mediated apoptosis of EAC cells via downregulation of Bcl-2 mRNA expression and upregulation of p53, Bax, and caspase-3 expressions. The AL extract also showed obvious antioxidant potential, with an IC_{50} value of 28 μg/mL.[5,6] Likewise, orally giving an ethanol extract of *A. spinosus* leaves to EAC-bearing mice at doses of 100 and 200 mg/kg for 16 days hampered the volume and viability of EAC tumors and extended survival, concomitant with the improvement of hematological and biochemical parameters to normal levels.[7]

A. viridis leaves have been used traditionally as an herb in the treatment of dysentery, hemorrhoids, enteritis, and kidney diseases in China and its young leaves are popularly consumed as a vegetable. Both ethyl ether extract (EEA) and ethyl acetate extract (EAA) of wild *A. viridis* (stems and leaves) showed not only strong anti-inflammatory activity on RAW 264.7 cells and DPPH-scavenging effect but also displayed suppressive activities against human HepG2 (liver) and HT-29 (colon) cancer cell lines. The antioxidant and anti-inflammatory activities of EAA were better than those of EEA, but the anticancer potency of EEA was much greater than that of EAA. At concentrations of 400 μg/mL, EEA treatment for 24 h deterred the growth of HepG2 and HT-29 cells by 85.9% and 96.9%, respectively, whereas EAA did not inhibit cancer cell growth.[6] An ethanolic extract of *A. gangeticus* was effective in suppressing the proliferation of human HepG2 (liver), MCF-7 (breast), and MDA-MB-231 (breast) cancer cell lines, with IC_{50}s of 27.75, 12.5, and 27.75 μg/mL, respectively, whereas an aqueous extract of *A. gangeticus* showed a lower inhibitory effect on the HepG2 (liver) and MCF-7 (breast) cancer cells, with IC_{50}s of 93.8 and 98.8 μg/mL, respectively. Both also had weak inhibition on Caco-2 colon cancer cells but not on normal Chang liver cells.[8] Further, a diet mixed with 10% of *A. gangeticus* aqueous extract fed to rats markedly repressed the activities of all tumor marker enzymes (such as uridyl diphosphoglucuronyl transferase, γ-glutamyl transpeptidase, glutathione *S*-transferase, and alkaline phosphatase). These enzymes were significantly elicited in the *in vivo* assay by chemical carcinogens 2-acetylamino-fluorene (AAF) and diethylnitrosamine (DEN). Thus, the findings indicated the extract of *A. gangeticus* has preventive activities against liver carcinogenesis.[8]

A fatty acid described as (14E,18E,22E,26E)-methyl nonacosa-14,18,22,26 tetraenoate (**1**) was separated from *A. spinosus*. In an *in vitro* assay with tetraenoic fatty acid (**1**), antiproliferative and proapoptotic effects against HepG2 human hepatoma cells with IC_{50} of 25.52 μmol/L occurred, whose potency was better than that of linoleic acid (a well-known fatty acid, IC_{50} of 38.65 μmol/L) but comparable to that of the chemodrug doxorubicin (IC_{50} of 24.68 μmol/L).[9] The antihepatoma mechanism was associated with (1) apoptosis induction via downregulation of Bcl-2 and upregulation of Bax and (2) G2/M cell-cycle arrest via downregulation of cyclin-B1.[9] Bioassay-guided isolation of *A. tricolor* leaves and stems uncovered three galactosyl diacylglycerols, (1) GD-A (**2**), (2) GD-B (**3**), and (3) GD-C (**4**). Their anticancer activity was observed in an *in vitro* model against the proliferation of human AGS (stomach), HCT-116 (colon), and MCF-7 (breast) carcinoma cell lines. The IC_{50} values were 49.1, 42.8, and 39.2 μg/mL for GD-A; 74.3, 71.3, and 58.7 μg/mL for GD-B; and 83.4, 73.1, and 85.4 μg/mL for GD-C, respectively. GD-A (**2**) was also moderately active in deterring the human SF-268 (CNS) and NCI-H460 (lung) cancer cells (IC_{50}s of 71.8 and 62.5 μg/mL, respectively).[10] In addition, owing to their potent suppressive activities on cyclooxygenases (COX)-1 and -2, the three galactosyl diacylglycerols showed good anti-inflammatory activity.[10]

2. Anticancer properties of amaranth seeds

Amaranth grain/seed is a highly nutritional pseudocereal. It contains a superior amount of proteins when compared to most cereal grains. In a mouse model, daily oral administration of *A. hybridus* seed extracts (AH) to mice in a dose of 100 μg/mL for 6 days resulted in 43% inhibition against the growth of EAC cells.[5] MPI, a protein isolated from the seeds of *A. mantegazzianus*, exerted different antiproliferative potencies against four cancer cell lines—namely, murine osteosarcoma (MC3T3E1 and UMR106) and human colon cancer (Caco-2 and TC7) cells *in vitro*—where the UMR106 cells were most sensitive to MPI (IC_{50} of 1 mg/mL), concomitant with the inhibition of cell adhesion and apoptosis. Depending on its concentration, MPI exerted both cytostatic and cytotoxic effects on cancer cells. After protease hydrolysis of MPI, the antiproliferative effect could be enhanced by 30% (IC_{50} of 0.5 mg/mL).[11] From the hydrophobic fractionation, a lectin fraction was partially purified. The *A. caudatus* lectin and *A. mantegazzianus* lectin showed well-promoted suppressive effect against the UMR106 cells, with IC_{50} values of 0.1 and 0.08 mg/mL, respectively, indicating that the lectin should be the major inhibitor in the amaranth seeds responsive to the antiproliferative, antiadhesive, and proapototic activities.[12] In addition, the total contents of phenolic compounds range around 56.22 mg/100 g in *A. paniculatus* seeds and 39.17 mg/100 g in *A. caudatus* seeds, which are a potential source of natural antioxidants.[13] The ingestion of amaranth seeds (310 and 155 g/kg of diet) exerted a dose-dependent protective effect against oxidative stress in the plasma, heart, kidney, and pancreas of rats via increase of antioxidant enzymes and decrease in malondialdehyde and lipid peroxidation. The interactions may help to alleviate the generation of free radicals during several pathological states, including carcinogenesis.[14] In addition, the germination of amaranth seeds would significantly amplify the total contents of phenolics and anthocyanins, thereby enhancing antioxidant capacity.[15]

Lunasin (18.5 kDa) is an anticarcinogenic peptide in amaranth seeds, which is also found in albumin, prolamin, and globulin amaranth protein fractions and even in popped amaranth seeds. Among the amaranth protein fractions, the glutelin fraction presented the highest lunasin content (3.0 μg/g) and was similar to that found in barley. In bioactivity tests, the glutelin showed an proapoptotic effect in HeLa cervical cancer cells and an antihypertensive effect. The amaranth lunasin-like peptide was also able to internalize into NIH-3T3 fibroblast cell nucleus, leading to blockage of carcinogen-induced NIH-3T3 cell transformation to cancerous foci and repression of H3 and H4 histone acetylation. The findings revealed the potential of the amaranth peptide fraction in cancer prevention. Significantly, it is identified that this amaranth lunasin-like peptide harmonizes with more than 60% of soybean lunasin peptide,[16,17] soybean peptide with 44 amino acids of which showed anticancer and anti-inflammatory properties in the investigations but the lunasin was absent in true cereals.[18] AmI (8 kDa) isolated from amaranth seeds is a trypsin–chymotrypsin inhibitor and a serine protease inhibitor with a single protein chain. AmI is stable at neutral and alkaline conditions and is relatively thermostable. Its partial amino acid sequence of 45 amino acids in AmI's amino terminus varied considerably from those of known protease inhibitor families from legume seed and cereal grain. In an *in vitro* model, AmI deterred the growth of MCF-7 breast cancer cells, showing a potential in anticarcinogenesis.[19]

According to UniProt database records, 14 main proteins/enzymes are present in amaranth seeds, which are 11S-globulin, 7S-globulin, α-amylase inhibitor, trypsin inhibitor, nonspecific lipid-transfer-protein-1, superoxide dismutase, ring-zinc finger protein, prosystemin, amaranth albumin-1, glucose-1-phosphate polyamine oxidase, granule-bound starch synthase-1, adenyltransferase, glucosyltransferase, and acetolactate synthase. Besides, the amaranth proteins showed high frequencies of angiotensin-converting enzyme-inhibitor peptides and dipeptidyl peptidase IV inhibitor and some of the proteins showed anticancer and antithrombotic sequences and antioxidative and glucose uptake-stimulating activities. Thus, it is clear now that amaranth seeds are a rich source of functional proteins and enzymic hydrolysis, and food processing may augment bioactive peptide production from the amaranth proteins. Although more scientific evidence is needed for the biological application of amaranth proteins and peptides, amaranth seeds are definitely a food alternative with health-promoting benefits.[1-4]

3. Cancer prevention from amaranth seed oil

The commercial amaranth oil is generally extracted from the seeds of two species, (1) *Amaranthus cruentus* and (2) *A. hypochondriacus*. The influence of amaranth oil on the liver antioxidant system and blood of tumor-bearing mice had been investigated. Diets containing amaranth oil given to mice bearing NK/Ly lymphoma in a daily dose of 1 μL/g (10 days before tumor inoculation and during tumor growth for 14 days) resulted in a series of interactions on the lipid peroxidation and antioxidant activity in hepatocytes and blood, including a marked increase in superoxide dismutase (SOD), preservation of catalase, and decline of glutathione peroxidase activities together with a simultaneous increase in hydroperoxide levels and decrease in thiobarbituric acid–reactive

subspecies. The modification of antioxidant activity elicited by the oil was helpful in the maintenance of oxygen homeostasis, morphofunctional state, and antioxidant defense, thereby leading to
restrained proliferation of tumor cells.[20]

NANOFORMULATION

rGO/AE/AuNPs was a composite hydrogel prepared with reduced graphene oxide (rGO), amaranth
leaf extract (AE), and gold nanoparticles (AuNPs). Owing to its well-promoted biocompatibility and
hydrophilicity for loading chemotherapeutics, the rGO/AE/AuNPs showed a remarkably improved
and synergistic cytotoxic effect against HeLa cervical cancer under laser irradiation, compared with
free AE and a complex of rGO/AE.[21]

CONCLUSION AND SUGGESTION

The comprehensive reviews of amaranth vegetables and seeds focus on the potential of amaranth
in the practice of cancer prevention and its possible benefits to human health. On the basis of
bioactivity-related phytochemical research, it is known that the leaves of amaranth contain carotenoids, polyphenolics, flavonoids, and glycolipids (such as amaranthine, isoamaranthine, hydrox-
ylcinnamates, nicotiflorin, rutin, quercetin, and kaempferol glycosides). The seeds of amaranth
contain bioactive lectins, protease inhibitors, lunasin peptides, and polyphenolics (such as rutin,
isoquercetin, and nicotiflorin and some phenolic acids and amides). These phytochemicals in the
amaranth plants synergistically play multiple health-promoting roles responsible for the antioxidant,
cancer prevention and intervention, anti-inflammation, and other biological properties of amaranth.
Therefore, due to the desirable high nutritional and functional values, we should encourage the use
of amaranth in traditional diets as an alternative and beneficial source of food for lowering the incidence of cancers, especially in the liver, breast, colon, and bone.

REFERENCES

1. Montoya-Rodriguez, A. et al., 2015. Comprehensive reviews in food. *Sci. Food Safety* 14(2): 139–158.
2. Caselato-Sousa, V.M. et al., 2012. State of knowledge on amaranth grain: A comprehensive review. *J. Food Sci.* 77(4): R93–R104.
3. Asha, S. et al., 2016. *Amaranthus spinosus*- A review. *Bull. Env. Pharmacol. Life Sci.* 5(9): 102–107.
4. Bulbul, I.J. et al., 2011. Antibacterial, cytotoxic and antioxidant activity of chloroform, n-hexane and ethyl acetate extracts of plant *Amaranthus spinosus. Int. J. Pharm. Tech. Res.* 3: 1675–1680.
5. Al-Mamun, M.A. et al., 2016. Assessment of antioxidant, anticancer and antimicrobial activity of two vegetable species of *Amaranthus* in Bangladesh. *BMC Comp. Alter. Med.* 16:157.
6. Yin, Y.S. et al., 2013. Antioxidant, antiinflammatory and anticancer activities of *Amaranthus viridis* L. extracts. *Asian J. Chem.* 25(16): 8901–8904.
7. Samuel, J.L. et al., 2010. Antitumor activity of the ethanol extract of *Amaranthus spinosus* leaves against EAC bearing Swiss albino mice. *Der Pharm. Lett.* 2: 10–15.
8. Sani, H.A. et al., 2004. Potential anticancer effect of red spinach (*Amaranthus gangengitus*) extract. *Asia Pac. J. Clin. Nutr.* 13(4): 396–400.
9. Mondal, A. et al., 2016. A novel tetraenoic fatty acid isolated from *Amaranthus spinosus* inhibits prolif-eration and induces apoptosis of human liver cancer cells. *Int. J. Mol. Sci.* 17: 1604.
10. Jayaprakasm, B. et al., 2004. Tumor cell proliferation and cyclooxygenase enzymes inhibitory com-pounds in *Amaranthus tricolor. J. Agric. Food Chem.* 52(23): 6939–6943.
11. Barrio, D.A. et al., 2010. Potential antitumor properties of a protein isolate obtained from the seeds of *Amaranthus mantegazzianus. Eur. J. Nutr.* 49(2): 73–82.
12. Quiroga, A.V. et al., 2015. Amaranth lectin presents potential antitumor properties. *LWT - Food Sci. Technol.* 60: 478–485.
13. Klimczak, I. et al., 2002. Antioxidant activity of ethanolic extracts of amaranth seeds. *Nahrung Food* 46: 184–186.

14. Pasko, P. et al., 2011. Effect of amaranth seeds in diet on oxidative status in plasma and selected tissues of high fructose-fed rats. *Food Chem.* 126: 85–90.
15. Pasko, P. et al., 2009. Anthocyanins, total polyphenols and antioxidant activity in amaranth and quinoa seeds and sprouts during their growth. *Food Chem.* 115: 994–998.
16. Silva-Sanchez, C. et al., 2008. Bioactive peptides in amaranth (*Amaranthus hypochondriacus*) seed. *J. Agricul. Food Chem.* 56(4): 1233–1240.
17. Maldonado Cervantes, E. et al., 2011. Characterization of amaranth-like lunasin: A novel cancer-preventive peptide. Abstracts of Papers, *241st ACS National Meeting & Exposition*, Anaheim, CA, March 27–31, (2011): AGFD-71; 2010. Amaranth lunasin-like peptide internalizes into the cell nucleus and inhibits chemical carcinogen-induced transformation of NIH-3T3 cells. *Peptides* 31(9): 1635–1642.
18. Alaswad A.A. et al., 2016. Immunological investigation for the presence of lunasin, a chemopreventive soybean peptide, in the seeds of diverse plants. *J. Agricul. Food Chem.* 64(14): 2901–2909.
19. Tamir, S. et al., 1996. Isolation, characterization, and properties of a trypsin-chymotrypsin inhibitor from amaranth seeds. *J. Protein Chem.* 15(2): 219–229.
20. Yelisyeyeva, O.P. et al., 2006. Effects of amaranth oil on the liver antioxidant system and blood of mice with tumor growth. *Ukrains'kii Biokhimichnii Zhurnal* 78(1): 117–123.
21. Chang, G.R. et al., 2015. Reduced graphene oxide/amaranth extract/AuNPs composite hydrogel on tumor cells as integrated platform for localized and multiple synergistic therapy. *ACS Appl. Mater. Inter.* 7(21): 11246–11256.

2. ASPARAGUS

Asperge   Spargel   Espárrago
蘆笋 アスパラ 아스파라거스
Asparagus officinalis

Liliaceae

1. $R_1 = -glc, R_2 = R_3 = -H.$
2. $R_1 = -glc, R_2 = -xyl, R_3 = -H.$
3. $R_1 = -glc, R_2 = -H, R_3 = -COCH_3$
4. $R_1 = R_2 = -rha, R_3 = -H.$

glc: beta-D-glucose; xyl : beta-D-xylose; rha : alpha-L-rhamnose

Asparagus originated from an herbaceous Liliaceae plant *Asparagus officinalis*. Its fresh and green stem is commonly used in cuisines. According to nutritional fact, asparagus contains high levels of vitamin K and folate, higher antioxidant nutrients (vitamins C, E, B6, and β-carotene), and minerals (zinc, iron, copper, phosphorus, manganese, and selenium). It is a very good source of dietary fiber, protein, riboflavin, rutin, folic acid, thiamin, niacin, and amino acids, as well as chromium, a trace functional mineral. Pharmacological data revealed that asparagus has hypolipemic, hepatoprotective, anti-^{60}Co γ radiodamage, immunopotentiating, antilipooxidative, and antifungal properties besides being anticarcinogenic.

SCIENTIFIC EVIDENCE OF CANCER-INHIBITORY AND CANCER-PREVENTIVE ACTIVITIES

The concentrated decoction of asparagus demonstrated an inhibitory effect against the growth of human hepatoma, gastric cancer (MGC903), and histiocytic lymphoma (U937) cell lines but weakly active to nasopharyngeal carcinoma cells *in vitro*. The asparagus juice exhibited significant cytotoxicity against human HeLa and JTC26 (cervix), Eca109 (esophagus), CNE (nasopharynx) cancer cell lines, and mouse LA-795 lung adenocarcinoma and P388 leukemia cell lines *in vitro*.[1-3] In addition, the DNA and RNA synthesis in the cultured sarcoma 180 cells was obviously restrained by asparagus.[4]

Administration of a concentrated decoction either intraperitoneally (IP) or orally hindered the tumor growth, diminished the tumor sizes in mice-implanted sarcoma 180, and prolonged the life span of mice-bearing EAC cells *in vivo*.[4,5] The extract prepared from the cultured asparagus callus also demonstrated the inhibitory effect against the entity sarcoma 180 cell growth and showed the postponement of tested animal lifetime in mice bearing ascite sarcoma 180.[6] Daily feed of asparagus extract to mice notably reduced dimethyl hydrazine-induced crypt foci in the colon, directly blocked nitrite amine synthesis *in vivo*, and hindered nitrite amine caused tumorigenesis along with an increase and activation of SOD in erythrocytes and diminution of radical damages.[7,8] Four percent (wt./wt.) of asparagus in the diet was the most effective dose in the protection of mice against benzo[a]pyrene-induced forestomach papillomagenesis and 7,12-dimethylbenz[a]anthracene-induced skin papillomagenesis. Simultaneously, asparagus restrained phase-I and stimulated phase-II system and antioxidant enzymes, indicating that cancer prevention by asparagus may also be contributed to by drug-metabolizing phase-I and phase-II enzymes and free-radical scavenging antioxidant enzymes.[9]

Steroidal saponins and polysaccharides are the major antitumor components in the asparagus plant. The following summary provides scientific evidences to encourage the consumption of asparagus as a functional food for lessening the carcinogenic rate.

1. Steroidal saponins

The total steroidal saponins in high dose exerted significant dose-dependent suppressive effects against the growth of sarcoma 180 cells and hepatoma H22 cells in mice, with 39.53% and 34.81% inhibition rates, respectively.[4,10] IP injection of the saponins to tumor-bearing mice noticeably obstructed the proliferation of ascite hepatoma cells by 82.6%.[4] The saponins isolated from old stems of asparagus exerted potential inhibitory activity on the cell growth and metastasis of breast, pancreatic, and colon cancer cell lines in a concentration-dependent manner. Comparing to its anti-growth effect, the saponins were more functional in blocking cell migration and invasion via marked activation of Cdc42 and Rac1 and inactivation of RhoA in cancer cells.[11] These observations proved the advantages of asparagus saponins for cancer prevention and treatment.

From the total saponins, many spirosteriol saponin compounds have been obtained in the separation. In an *in vitro* assay, the moderate inhibitory effect was achieved by asparanin-A (**1**) against KB (nasopharynx), LTEP-a-2 (lung), Eca109 (esophagus), MGC-803 (gastric), and L1210 (leukemic) cancer cell lines with respective IC_{50}s of 1.38–4.03 μM.[12] Likewise, the IC_{50} values were 1.46–2.91 μM for (25S)-5β-spirostan-3β-ol 3-*O*-β-D-glucosyl-(1-2)[β-D-xylosyl-(1-4)]-β-D-glucoside (**2**) in L1210, KB, LTEP-a-2, and Eca-109 cells and 5.5–10.57 μM for sarsasapogenin-O (**3**) in CNE, MGC-803, and A2780 cells.[12] (25S)-5β-spirostan-3β-ol 3-*O*-α-L-rhamnosyl-(1-2)-[α-L-rhamnosyl-(1-4)]-β-D-glucoside (**4**) exerted the inhibition only on CNE and Eca-109 cells (IC_{50}s 10.15–12.88 μM). Asparagoside-A and two spirostans termed sarsasapogenin and (25S)-neospirost-4-en-3-one were effective in hindering the growth of human ovarian cancer cell lines (A2780 and/HO8910).[12]

Moreover, in human HepG2 hepatoma cells, asparanin-A (**1**) downregulated cell-cycle–related proteins (cyclin-A, Cdk1, and Cdk4) to elicit G2/M cell arrest and upregulation of Bax and caspases to trigger cell apoptosis in a p53-independent manner.[13] The antitumor activity of asparanin-A (**1**) has been further verified in an *in vivo* model.[14] The anti-growth activity of asparagosides-C and -D was demonstrated against the mammary gland adenocarcinoma 755 cells and cancer cells of pancreas and cervix uteri in mice.[15] In addition, two oligofurostanosides elucidated as methyl protodioscin and protodioscin were separated from asparagus seeds, exhibiting a dose-dependent antiproliferative effect against human HL-60 leukemia cell lines together with blocking of macromolecular synthesis *in vitro*.[16] A steroidal saponin extract isolated from spears of wild triguero asparagus (which probably is a hybrid between *A. officinalis* and wild *A. maritimus*) was investigated *in vitro*, presenting the anticancer-related G0/G1 cell-cycle arrest and apoptosis-inducing effects in human HCT-116 colon cancer cells. The effects were mediated by hampering the signal transmissions of extracellular signal-regulated kinase (ERK), RAC-α serine/threonine–protein kinase (Akt) and S6 kinase (p70S6K), downregulating cyclins-D, -E, and -A expression, and promoting caspase-3 activation, poly(ADP-ribose) polymerase 1 (PARP-1) cleavage, and DNA fragmentation.[17]

2. Glutathione

Asparagus especially has a higher concentration of glutathione, a small micronutrient that is also made in the human body. As the body begins to age, its glutathione level needs to be maintained by dietary intake from other sources. A broad range of functions can be achieved with glutathione, including reduction of cancer risk by detoxifying oncogens, antioxidation, protection of damage from free radicals, boosting immunity by augmenting natural killer (NK) cells and lymphocytes (such as T and B cells), reducing inflammation and antiviruses, consequently helping to fight certain carcinomas such as bone, breast, colon, larynx, and lung.[9] However, both baking and frying processes notably diminished the content of asparagus glutathione, and only uncooked asparagus can afford rich glutathione. Accordingly, overcooking should be avoided.[18]

3. Polysaccharides

The cancer protecting function of asparagus was found to be contributed by its polysaccharides as well. The total asparagus polysaccharides (AOP) restrained the proliferation of ascite hepatoma cells and the growth of sarcoma 180 cells in mice.[19] AOP also reduced the migration of erythrocytes in the S180 mice and improved the erythrocyte function of S180 mice via significantly amplifying the numbers and activities of erythrocyte complement receptor-1, interactions of which might be related to its antitumor mechanisms.[19,20] Deproteinized AOPs exerted greater antioxidant and antitumor activities compared to the AOP. In human Hep3B and HepG2 hepatoma cells, the deproteinized AOPs selectively elicited the cell apoptosis and G2/M cell-cycle arrest, thereby exerted the anticancer effect and potentiated the cytotoxic effects of mitomycin both *in vitro* and *in vivo*.[21] Three main fractions labeled as AOP-4, AOP-6, and AOP-8 were separated from the AOP, which markedly suppressed the cell growth of HeLa cervical carcinoma and BEL-7404 hepatoma in a dose-dependent manner. AOP-4 (5.75×10^4 Da) demonstrated an 83.96% inhibitory rate against the growth of HeLa cells at a concentration of 10 mg/mL and showed marked function of scavenging hydroxyl radicals, whose activities were greater than those of other AOPs.[22]

CONCLUSION AND SUGGESTION

The bioactivity-guided chemical investigations of asparagus showed that the spirosteriol saponins and polysaccharides that were discovered may be potential preventive agents and therapeutic adjuvants against cancer and carcinogenesis. These bioactive constituents showed only moderate-to-weak degrees of cancer suppressive effects but they integrate with glutathione and some abundant nutrients in this vegetable make the dietary consumption of asparagus more attractive for cancer prevention. In addition, old stems, roots, leaves, and other wastes of the asparagus plant still have great value for further utilization owing to rich flavonoids that possess anti-inflammatory, antioxidant, and other biological activities.[23]

REFERENCES

1. Chen, L.M. et al., 1989. The antitumor activity of *Asparagus. Zhongchengyao* 11: 45.
2. Li, D.H. et al., 1988. The experimental and clinic studies of *Asparagus*-I. *J. Chinese Clin. Pharmacol.* 4: 32.
3. An, Y.H. et al., 1989. The observation of *Asparagus* oral solution and beverage on the inhibition of esophageal ECa109 cells. *Aizheng* 8: 306.
4. Guan, J. et al., 1991. The antitumor activity of *Asparagus* extracts. *Bangbu Yixueyuan Xuebao* 16: 116–118; 128.
5. Lin, X.S. et al., 1994. The antitumor effect of *Asparagus* juice. *Xiamen Daxue Xuebao* 33: 133–135.
6. Wang, Z.J. et al., 1990. Studies on the inhibitor effect and mechanism of *Asparagus* callus against the growth of mouse S180 cells. *Xiandai Shiyong Yaoxue* 7: 45.
7. Sun, H.X. et al., 1991. The significant reduction of *Asparagus* on the foci of crypt in colon epithelial cells induced by dimethyl hydrazine. *J. Henan Med. College* 16: 17.
8. Guo, B. et al., 1994. The protection of *Asparagus* against the toxic from endogenous nitrosamine in rats. *J. Guiyang Med. College* 19: 101–103.
9. Singh, M. et al., 2011. Chemomodulatory potential of *Asparagus adscendens* against murine skin and forestomach papillomagenesis. *Eur. J. Cancer Prevent.* 20: 240–247.
10. Song, Q. et al., 2010. In vivo antitumor activity of total saponins from *Asparagus officinalis. Shipin Kexue* 31: 273–275.
11. Wang, J.Q. et al., 2013. Saponins extracted from by product of *Asparagus officinalis* L. suppress tumour cell migration and invasion through targeting Rho GTPase signalling pathway. *J. Sci. Food Agricul.* 93: 1492–1498.

12. Huang, X.F. et al., 2008. Steroids from the roots of *Asparagus officinalis* and their cytotoxic activity. *J. Integr. Plant Biol.* 50: 717–722.

13. Liu, W. et al., 2009. Asparanin A induces G2/M cell cycle arrest and apoptosis in human hepatocellular carcinoma HepG2 cells. *Biochem. Biophys. Res. Commun.* 381: 700–705.

14. Li, X.M. et al., 2017. Two new phenolic compounds and antitumor activities of asparinin A from *Asparagus officinalis*. *J. Asian Nat. Prod. Res.* 19(2): 164–771.

15. Goryanu, G.M. et al., 1984. Steroid glycosides from *Asparagus officinalis* and their biological activity. *Nauka-Farm Prakt* 38–39. [C.A. 1986, 104: 373q.]

16. Shao, Y. et al., 1997. Steroidal saponins from *Asparagus officinalis* and their cytotoxic activity. *Planta Med.* 63: 258–262.

17. Jaramillo, S. et al., 2016. Saponins from edible spears of wild *Asparagus* inhibit AKT, p70S6K, and ERK signalling, and induce apoptosis through G0/G1 cell cycle arrest in human colon cancer HCT-116 cells. *J. Funct. Foods* 26: 1–10.

18. Drinkwater, J.M. 2015. Effects of cooking on rutin and glutathione concentrations and antioxidant activity of green *Asparagus* (*Asparagus officinalis*) spears. *J. Funct. Foods* 12: 342–353.

19. Ji, Y.B. et al., 2006. Effect analysis of *Asparagus* polysaccharide on erythrocytes of S180 mice by high performance capillary electrophoresis. *Harbin Shangye Daxue Xuebao, Science Edition* 22: 1–3.

20. Ji, Y.B. et al., 2009. Effects of *Asparagus* polysaccharide on number and activity of erythrocyte complement receptor 1 (CD35) of S180 mice. *Zhongguo Yaoxue Zazhi* 44: 1066–1069.

21. Xiang, J.F. et al., 2014. Anticancer effects of deproteinized *Asparagus* polysaccharide on hepatocellular carcinoma in vitro and in vivo. *Tumor Biol.* 35: 3517–3524.

22. Zhao, Q.S. et al., 2012. In vitro antioxidant and antitumor activities of polysaccharides extracted from *Asparagus officinalis*. *Carbohydr. Polym.* 87: 392–396.

23. Jiang, D. et al., 2014. Development of flavonoids in *Asparagus officinalis* L. *Shipin Gongye Keji* 35: 357–362.

3. BRASSICACEAE VEGETABLES

十字花科蔬菜

Brassica oleracea and its cultivars

Cruciferae

A Brassicaceae plant *Brassica oleracea* L. has been bred into a wide range of cultivars, which have been popular vegetables in human diets for a long time. Today the cultivars are divided into 11 major groups, including (1) broccoli (var. *italica*), (2) cabbage (var. *capitata*), (3) cauliflower (var. *botrytis*), (4) collard greens (var. *acephala*), (5) kale (var. *acephala*), (6) kohlrabi (var. *gongylodes*), (7) Brussels sprouts (var. *gemmifera*), (8) Chinese kale (var. *alboglabra*), (9) broccoflower (var. *botrytis*), (10) broccolini (var. *italica* × *alboglabra*), and (11) turnip (*B. rapa*). These cultivars of *B. oleracea* and some other Brassicaceae plants are the extensively consumed vegetables that provide great sources of vitamins, soluble fiber, and multiple components with interesting anticancer, anticarcinogenic, and antioxidant properties and other health functions.[1]

SCIENTIFIC EVIDENCE OF CANCER-INHIBITORY AND CANCER-PREVENTIVE ACTIVITIES

With the consumption of the Brassicaceae vegetables in our diet, the cancer-preventing, radical-scavenging, and health-enhancing functions can be promoted. *In vitro* assays showed that Brussels sprout extracts strongly inhibited the proliferation of MCF-7 (breast), AGS (stomach), PC3 (prostate), A549 (lung), Caki-2 (kidney), and Panc-1 (pancreas) cancer cell lines and U-87 glioblastoma and Daoy medulloblastoma cell lines by 30%–100% at 1/1000–1/100 dilution (3.32–33.2 mg raw vegetable/mL). Similarly, a broccoli extract exerted 30%–100% inhibitory effect against the same eight cancer cell lines but at 1/100–1/20 dilution (33.2–166 mg raw vegetable/mL).[2] Cabbage juice deterred the viability of human AGS (stomach), MCF7 (breast), Panc1 (pancreas), PC3 (prostate), A549 (lung), Daoy and U87 (brain), and Caki-2 (kidney) cancer cell lines and normal human dermal fibroblast cells. A 100% methanol extract of cabbage was effective in inhibiting the proliferation of Calu6 pulmonary carcinoma and SNU-601 gastric carcinoma cell lines, whereas an 80% acetone extract of cabbage was active to HepG2 hepatoma cells.[3] The cabbage extract not only exerted cytotoxic effects on rat AH109A ascite hepatoma cells but also stimulated rat spleen cells to produce TNF, revealing that the *in vivo* antitumor effect of cabbage could be partially implemented by enhancing the cytotoxicity of tumor-infiltrating macrophages besides its direct antitumor effect.[3] The anti-growth rates of kale juice and cabbage juice were 21% and 42%, respectively, on AGS gastric cancer cells *in vitro*. Combining of the two vegetable juices at a 3:7 ratio showed synergistic effects in hampering AGS cells by 65% and in scavenging DPPH radicals, the anti-AGS effect of which was accompanied by significant downregulation of inflammatory genes (TNF-α, IL-1β, iNOS, and COX-2).[2]

Meanwhile, the Brassicaceae vegetables in *in vivo* animal studies were protective against various classes of DNA-reactive carcinogens. A diet of Brussels sprouts fed to rats showed an inhibitory effect on breast carcinogenesis by 7,12-dimethylbenz[a]anthracene (DMBA).[4] A diet containing cauliflower (>70 g/kg) for 2 weeks could reduce the risk of carcinogenesis in lung and colon in a mouse model.[5] In an *in vivo* two-stage test in mice, a methanol extract of watercress (*Nasturtium officinale*) markedly obstructed skin carcinogenesis caused by DMBA as an initiator and TPA as a promoter.[6] Accordingly, this scientific evidence indicated that consumption of the Brassicaceae vegetables for a long period would be helpful for the prevention and treatment of various solid tumors.

SCIENTIFIC EVIDENCE OF CANCER-INHIBITORY AND CANCER-PREVENTIVE CONSTITUENTS

The increasing evidence showed that the chemopreventive properties of Brassicaceae vegetables are attributed to the additive/synergistic effects of several phytochemicals. The chemical biology-related approaches have revealed that the health benefits of Brassicaceae vegetables are mostly contributed by their bioactive components, such as sulforaphanes, carotenoids, polyphenolics, flavonoids, indol derivatives, and selenium, and the potential of cancer prevention primarily came from the decomposition products of glucosinolates, such as isothiocyanates, thiocyanates, nitriles, epithionitriles, and oxazolidines. Table 1.1 presents the most important cancer-preventive substances in 10 common Brassicaceae vegetables. Besides these bioactive components, triterpenoids (such as lupeol, α- and β-amyrins) are another kind of phytochemicals in the vegetables. They were also found in response to the inhibition of carcinogenesis.

1. Isothiocyanates and glucosinolates

The major components in Brassicaceae vegetables were isothiocyanates and glucosinolates, which are a family of sulfur-containing molecules that are converted to bioactive agents after chopping or chewing and then exerting the anticancer, anticarcinogenic, and antioxidant activities. However, cooking, particularly boiling and microwaving at high power, decreases their bioavailability.

TABLE 1.1
Cancer-Preventive Constituents Discovered from the Brassicaceae Vegetables

Vegetables	Cancer Inhibitors and Preventers
Broccoli and broccoli sprouts	Allyl isothiocyanate, β-carotene, choline, indole-3-carbinol and 3,3′-diindolyl-methane, kaempferol, sulforaphane, and soluble fiber
Brussels sprouts	Allyl isothiocyanate, indole-3-carbinol and 3,3′-diindolylmethane, phenethyl isothiocyanate, sulforaphane, β-carotene, choline, lutein, and soluble fiber
Cabbage	Allyl isothiocyanate, benzyl isothiocyanate, erucin, indole-3-carbinol, 3,3′-diindolylmethane, sulforaphane, β-carotene, choline, and lupeol
Cauliflower	Choline, indole-3-carbinol and 3,3′-diindolylmethane, and sulforaphane
Collard greens	β-carotene, lutein and other carotenoids, kaempferol, indole-3-carbinol, 3,3′-diindolylmethane, and several other isothiocyanates
Horseradish/Wasabi	Allyl isothiocyanate, phenethyl isothiocyanate, and sulforaphane
Kale	β-carotene, lutein, quercetin, kaempferol, indole-3-carbinol, 3,3′-diindolylmethane, and sulforaphane
Turnip radish	Benzyl isothiocyanate, indole-3-carbinol, and 3,3′-diindolylmethane
Turnip greens	β-carotene, kaempferol, allyl isothiocyanate, β-phenylethyl isothiocyanate, and various other isothiocyanates, including some sulforaphane
Watercress	Nasturtiin (a precursor of phenethylisothiocyanate), phenylethylisothiocyanate, benzyl isothiocyanate, indole-3-carbinol, 3,3′-diindolylmethane, and sulforaphane, lutein, β-carotene, and riboflavin

Isothiocyanates: *In vitro* assays revealed that sulforaphane (SFN, **1**) and 3-methylsulfinylpropyliso-thiocyanate (**2**) were inhibitors of leukemia cells but had very low toxicity to normal leukocytes.[7–10] SFN (**1**) exerted dose- and time-dependent growth inhibition and apoptosis-induction in ERMS and ARMS rhabdomyosarcoma cell lines.[11] SFN (**1**) also acted as a potent inhibitor against the viability of four different breast cancer cell lines (MDA-MB-231, MDA-MB-468, MCF-7, and SKBR-3), wherein upregulation of p53, Bax, Bad, Apaf-1, and AIF expressions and downregulation of Bcl-2, COX-2, HSPs, and HSF1 expressions occurred during the induced MCF-7 cell apoptosis and release of cytochrome c from mitochondria and activation of caspases-3, -9 happened in agreement with the apoptotic index values. Thus, the inhibitory effect was more prominent in MCF-7 (wild type) cells than in MDA-MB-231 (p53-mutant) cells, and the effect of SFN (**1**) could be synergistically enhanced when combined with gemcitabine (a chemotherapeutic drug).[12–14] SFN (**1**) and erucin (**3**) also deterred the viabilities of noninvasive (RT4) and invasive (J82, UMUC3) of human bladder neoplastic cell lines together with proapoptosis and G2/M cell-cycle arrest via downregulation of survivin, EGFR, and human epidermal growth factor receptor-2 (HER2/neu). The best IC_{50}s (in 48 h) were 5.66 μM for SFN (**1**) and 8.79 μM for erucin (**3**) in the UMUC3 cells.[15] The inhibitory rates on RT4 cells reached 64% for SFN (**1**) and 59% for erucin (**3**) after treatment for 48 h in 20 μM concentration, meanwhile, SFN (**1**) and erucin (**3**) had less inhibition on normal human urothelial cells. In a murine UMUC3 xenograft model, giving diets containing 4% broccoli sprout extract, 2% broccoli sprout isothiocyanate extract, 295 μmol/kg/day of SFN (**1**) or erucin (**3**) for 2 weeks reduced the tumor weight by 42%, 42%, 33%, and 58%, respectively.[15] When consumption of a diet with SFN (**1**) at an average daily dose of 7.5 μmol per animal for 21 days, SFN (**1**) hindered the growth of human PC3 prostate carcinoma cells by 40% in male nude mice, the effect of which was associated with the deactivation of histone deacetylases (HDACs).[16] Similarly, dietary isothiocyanates hampered HCT-116 colon cancer cells followed by lessening of HDACs and increasing in HDAC protein turnover, wherein SFN exceeds alkyl isothiocyanate.[17] By downregulation of prosurvival genes (cyclin-D2, integrin-β1, and Wnt-9A) and upregulation of proapoptotic genes (MBD4, TNFR-7, and TNF-11), the small intestinal polyps in ApcMin/+ mice were limited by SFN (**1**), leading to chemopreven-tion of colorectal carcinogenesis.[18] When combined with low doses of three common food phyto-chemicals (10 μM curcumin, 5 μM sulforaphane, and 1 mM aspirin), the treatment elicited ~70% viability reduction of human pancreatic cancer cell lines (MIA PaCa-2 and Panc-1) and promoted ~51% apoptotic death accompanied by activation of caspase-3 and poly(ADP-ribose) polymerase proteins, upregulation of P-ERK1/2, c-Jun, p38 MAPK, and p53 protein expressions, and blockage of NF-κB-DNA binding.[19]

Moreover, the anticarcinogenic potential of isothiocyanates has been further demonstrated by more *in vitro* and *in vivo* models. Oral administration of SFN (**1**) obstructed pulmonary carcinogenesis caused by benzo[a]pyrene in a daily dose of 9 μmol per mouse concomitant with elicited caspase-mediated apoptosis of the tumor cells.[20] The approaches showed that the chemopreventive activity of isothiocyanates was also mediated by modulation of Nrf2 (a redox-sensitive transcription factor). By augmenting Nrf2 levels and Nrf2 transcriptional activity, SFN (**1**) and resveratrol reduced benzo[a]pyrene-elicited ROS accumulation and benzo[a]pyrene-induced DNA damage, resulting in the anticarcinogenic effect against BRCA1-deficient breast epithelial cells.[21,22] Either in normal or Ehrlich ascites tumor-bearing BALB/c mice, administration of SFN notably enhanced the activity of NK cells and promoted the production of interleukin-2 and interferon-γ, leading to marked improvement of cell-mediated immune response and early antibody-dependent complement-mediated cytotoxicity.[23] In addition, SFN (**1**) was able to mitigate the genotoxicity induced by radiotherapies and chemotherapies in human lymphocytes.[24] SFN (**1**) was the most active substance in the *Brassica* vegetables for the increase in the anticarcinogenic phase-II enzymes in several different tissues of mice.[25] These provements showed that sulforaphane (**1**) is a highly promising dietary chemoprevention and therapeutic agent and has great ability for targeting several stages of cancer development.

Allyl isothiocyanate (AITC) is one of the most naturally occurring isothiocyanates, which are abundant in cabbage. When intake is oral, nearly 90% of AITC is absorbed. Its extremely high bio-availability is mostly effective in the protection from bladder cancer.[3] More experimental findings have proved that the isothiocyanates can reduce chemical-induced tumor formation, attenuate the negative effects of polycyclic aromatic hydrocarbons and nitrosoamines, and exert protective effects against heterocyclic amines.[25,26]

Glucosinolates: Glucoraphanin (**4**) accounts for 35%–50% of broccoli glucosinolates. It can be natu-rally converted to sulforaphane (**1**), a potent inducer of monofunctional phase-II enzymes.[25] Similar to isothiocyanates, glucoraphanin (**4**) and 3-methylsulphinypropyl glucosinolate (**5**) are potent induc-ers of two phase-II detoxication enzymes (quinone reductases and glutathione *S*-transferases). In an assay with murine Hepa 1c1c7 hepatoma cells, glucoraphanin (**4**) and glucosinolate (**5**) exerted potent protective effects against carcinogens and toxic electrophiles to diminish the risk of carcino-genesis.[24–28] A glucosinolate mixture was obtained from 70% methanolic extract of *B. oleracea* ripe seeds, and a major glucosinolate assigned as progoitrin (**6**) was separated from the mixture. Bioassay results showed that the inhibitory ratios on sarcoma 180 cells were 59.5% and 67.3%, respectively, after administering progoitrin (**6**) and the mixed glucosinolates in a dose of 60 mg/kg.[29,30]

2. Indoles

Indole-3-carbinol (**7**, I3C) was found at relatively high levels in broccoli, cauliflower, cabbage, Brussels sprouts, collard greens, and kale, which is a glucosinolate hydrolysis product of glucobras-sicin. I3C (**7**) was able to induce the growth arrest of human breast and prostate cancer cell lines and to boost DNA repair in the cells.[31,32] By stimulation of transcription of CDK2 inhibitor p21 and activation of p53 phosphorylation, I3C (**7**) elicited cell-cycle G1 arrest of human LNCaP pros-tate cancer cells.[33] I3C (**7**) and its condensation dimer 3,3′-diindolylmethane (**8**, DIM) at 1–5 μM could block androgen-mediated pathways and induce xenobiotic metabolic pathways in androgen-responsive LNCaP cells but not in androgen-nonresponsive PC3 prostate cancer cells. The inhibition of I3C (**7**) and DIM (**8**) on the cell growth was also related to downregulation of insulin-like growth factor-1 receptor expression. The effects thereby impacted the proliferation, cell cycle, and nuclear receptors–mediated pathways in the cancer cells.[34,35] Moreover, I3C (**7**) was able to efficiently induce apoptosis of Epstein–Barr virus (EBV)-positive Burkitt lymphomas (virus latency I/II) cells but not of EBV-negative Burkitt lymphoma cells.[36] In a mouse model, DIM (**8**) arrested the EBV-positive Burkitt lymphoma Daudi cells and prolonged the survival of tumor-bearing mice.[36] Ascorbigen is a chemical subtance found in cauliflower, broccoli, cabbage, and related vegetables and can be formed by I3C (**7**) spontaneously in the presence of vitamin C. Ascorbigen is a leading product from glu-cosinolate hydrolysis in fermented cabbage, and it significantly contributes to the anticarcinogenic properties as well.[3] The observations indicated the antitumor and antitumor-promoting activities of these indole derivatives. Besides, the chemotherapeutic effect of paclitaxel (an anticancer drug) could be additively augmented by two kale components: I3C (**7**) and quercetin.[37]

3. Flavonoids

Flavonoids were extracted from sun-dried broccoli flower buds with ultrasound-assisted 70% etha-nol and partially purified by AB-8 macroporous adsorptive resin. The flavonoid extract could dose-dependently inhibit the proliferation of SMMC7721 hepatoma cells *in vitro*.[38] The flavonoids extracted from broccolini leaves showed a dose-dependent antiproliferative effect in four human cancer cell lines (SW480, HepG2, HeLa, and A549) and apoptosis-inducing activity in the SW480 cell line.[39,40]

4. Polypeptide and protein

A polypeptide component-II derived from broccoli showed anti-growth effect against rat C6 glioma cells *in vitro* and *in vivo*. The polypeptide at a concentration of 10 μg/mL stimulated cell-cycle arrest and apoptotic death of C6 cells.[41,42] Similarly, through increasing Bax/Bcl-2 ratio and caspase-3 activation, the polypeptide at concentrations of 30 and 100 mg/L enhanced the apoptosis of human

SHG-44 glioma cells in the *in vitro* assay, indicating that the SHG-44 cells were less sensitive to the polypeptide compared to C6 cells.[43] A water-soluble fraction of kale (*B. oleracea* var. *acephala*) was able to promote the production of immunoglobulin (Ig) in human hybridoma HB4C5 cells and human peripheral blood lymphocytes, the bioactivity of which was found to attribute to a heat-stable protein with a molecular weight >50 kDa. This protein was identified as a ribulose-1,5-bisphosphate carboxylase/oxygenase (rubisco) by LC-ESI-MS/MS analysis. The discovery delivered additional beneficial aspects of kale as a health-promoting vegetable.[44]

5. Polysaccharides

A water-soluble polysaccharide (BPCa) was prepared from broccoli, which comprised arabinose, rhamnose, and galactose with a molar ratio of 5.3:1.0:0.8. α-L-1,5-Arabinofuranosyl and α-L-1,3,5-arabinofuranosyl unities were in the backbone of BPCa, and the α-L-arabinofuranosyl terminal was in its side chain. α-L-1,2-Rhamnopyranosyl was linked to α-L-1,5-arabinofuranosyl, and β-D-1,4-galactopyranosyl and α-D-1,4-galacturonic acid were also composed in the structure. In an *in vitro* assay, BPCa showed significant antiproliferation activities against human HepG2 (liver), Siha (cervix), and MDA-MB-231 (breast) carcinoma cell lines. The results indicated that BPCa had a good potential to be applied as a functional food supplement. After treatment with 2 mg/mL BPCa, the viabilities of HepG2, Siha, and MDA-MB-231 cell lines were diminished to 29.8%, 29.2%, and 22.4%, respectively.[45]

Nanoformulation

The phytochemicals (e.g., glucosinolates, isothiocyanates, and polyphenols) occurring in broccoli extract were proved to be a candidate class of cancer-preventive molecules. By interacting these broccoli phytochemicals with gold salt, the well-defined stable and biocompatible gold nanoparticles (B-AuNPs) were produced, the core sizes of which were 15 $\pm$ 2 nm and the hydrodynamic diameters were 100 $\pm$ 5 nm. The B-AuNPs showed moderate to weak cytotoxic effects against several human cancer cell lines. The IC_{50}s were 22, 80, and 160 μg/mL for T47D, SK-Br-3, and MDA-MB-231 breast cancer cells, respectively, 125 μg/mL for U266 myeloma cells, and 150 μg/mL for PC3 prostate cancer cells.[46] The B-AuNPs may have a potential for nanoparticulate-mediated molecular imaging and therapy.

A cauliflower water extract has been used in the green synthesis of magnesium oxide nanoparticles (particle sizes: 30–45 nm). After treatment with nanoparticles in a concentration of 31.2 μg/mL, the *in vitro* viability of HeLa cervical cancer cells was obstructed by 50% in association with stimulation of HeLa cell damage markedly. The magnesium oxide nanoparticles were also found to exert photocatalytic activity both under UV irradiation and sunlight, where the photocatalytic potency was dependent on their smaller size and higher surface area.[47] Similarly, an aqueous extract of fresh cauliflower floret was encapsulated by the silver nanoparticles, and the biosynthesized C-AgNPs demonstrated the promotion of antioxidant activity and the cytotoxicity on MCF-7 breast cancer cells.[48]

Conclusion and Suggestion

The summarized chemical biology studies have indeed revealed most of the health-promoting and cancer-preventive phytochemicals in the common Brassicaceae vegetables, such as glucosinolates/isothiocyanates, flavonoids, indol derivatives, polypeptide/protein, and polysaccharides. However, the major contributor should be isothiocyanates, although glucosinolates are exclusively present in Brassicaceae vegetables. The glucosinolates can be converted into isothiocyanates in our body to restrain the various solid tumor cell proliferation/growth, to lower the incidence of a variety of carcinogenesis, to induce cancer-destroying enzymes, and to counteract inflammatory pathways, exerting the cancer chemoprevention. Consequently, the scientific evidence recommends the consumption of

TABLE 1.2

The Spectrum of Cancer Prevention from Brassicaceae Vegetables

Vegetables	Spectrum of Cancer Prevention
Broccoli	Inhibit the carcinogenesis in urinary bladder and reduce the risk of multiple myeloma and cancers in lung, gallbladder, ovary, cervix, stomach, prostate, breast, small intestine, and colorectal/colon
Brussels sprouts	Reduce the risk of multiple myeloma and cancers in gallbladder, prostate, breast, lung, ovarian, cervix, and colorectal/colon, and suppress inflammation
Cabbage	Inhibit the carcinogenesis in urinary bladder and liver and reduce the risk of cancers in prostate, breast, lung, gallbladder, stomach, cervix, kidney, and colorectal/colon
Cauliflower	Inhibit the carcinogenesis in urinary bladder, small intestine, colorectal/colon, and liver; and reduce the risk of cancers in gallbladder, prostate, breast, lung, urothelial, and cervix
Horseradish and Wasabi	Inhibit the cancer-cell proliferation in colon, lung, pancreas, prostate, breast, and stomach
Kale	Reduce the risk of cancers in pancreas, lung, gallbladder, bladder, prostate, breast, ovarian, and colorectal/colon
Turnip	Reduce the risk of cancers in esophageal, lung, gastric, bladder, colorectal, prostate, and breast
Turnip green	Reduce the risk of cancers in stomach, bladder, prostate, and breast

Brassicaceae vegetables at least twice a week, a dietary habit that would be beneficial for lessening the risk for colon, kidney, esophagus, breast, prostate, pancreas, bladder, and/or oral cancers (Table 1.2) and providing protection at every stage of cancer progression. Moreover, food researchers disclosed that the methods of steaming, stir frying, and microwaving do not significantly decrease the levels of cancer-preventing constituents in Brassicaceae vegetables but that boiling losses are notable.[1,49]

OTHER BIOACTIVITIES OF THE CONSTITUENTS

3,3′-Diindolylmethane (**8**) is also a potent modulator of the innate immune response system with potent antiviral and antibacterial properties. However, the *Brassica* vegetables contain goitrogens, which in the absence of normal iodine intake can elicit hypothyroidism and goiter and restrain thyroid function.

REFERENCES

1. Song, L.J. et al., 2007. Effect of storage, processing and cooking on glucosinolate content of Brassica vegetables. *Food Chem. Toxicol.* 45: 216–224.
2. (a) Boivin, D. et al., 2009. Antiproliferative and antioxidant activities of common vegetables: A comparative study. *Food Chem.* 112: 374–380; (b) Hong, Y.J. et al., 2013. Inhibitory effects of cabbage juice and cabbage-mixed juice on the growth of AGS human gastric cancer cells and on HCl-ethanol induced gastritis in rats. *Han'guk Sikp'um Yongyang Kwahak Hoechi* 42(5): 682–689.
3. Šamec, D. et al., 2017. White cabbage (*Brassica oleracea* var. capitata f. alba): Botanical, phytochemical and pharmacological overview. *Phytochem. Rev.* 16: 117–135.
4. Steowsand, G.S. et al., 1988. Protective effect of dietary Brussels sprouts against mammary carcinogenesis in Sprague-Dawley rats. *Cancer Lett.* 39: 199–207.
5. van Breda, S.G. et al., 2005. Vegetables affect the expression of genes involved in carcinogenic and anticarcinogenic processes in the lungs of female C57BI/6 mice. *J. Nutr.* 135: 2546–2552; Vegetables affect the expression of genes involved in anticarcinogenic processes in the colonic mucosa of C57BI/6 female mice. *J. Nutr.* 135: 1879–1888.
6. Yasukawa, K. et al., 2016. Inhibitory effects of watercress on tumor promotion in a mouse model of two-stage skin carcinogenesis. *Jpn J. Complem. Alter. Med.* 13: 1–6.

7. Nakamura, O. et al., 2001. Methylsulfinylalkylisothiocyanates from *Brassica oleracea* italica and Eutrema wasabi Maxim. as new leukemia inhibitors. Jpn. Kokai Tokkyo Koho, JP 2001163775 A 20010619.

8. Mithen, R. et al., 1999. Breeding of Brassica hybrids for the elevated production of anticarcinogenic glucosinolates. Fr. Demande, FR 2778312 A1 19991112.

9. He, H.J. et al., 2003. Evaluation of glucosinolate composition and contents in Chinese Brassica vegetables. *Acta Horticult.* 620: 85–92.

10. Alan Crozier, A., Clifford, M.N. and Ashihara, H. 2007. Chapter 2. Sulphur-containing compounds. In: Mithen, R. (Ed.), *Plant Secondary Metabolites: Occurrence, Structure and Role in the Human Diet*, Blackwell Publishing, Oxford, UK, pp. 25–46. DOI:10.1002/9780470988558.ch2.

11. Bergantin, E. et al., 2014. Sulforaphane induces apoptosis in rhabdomyosarcoma and restores TRAIL-sensitivity in the aggressive alveolar subtype leading to tumor elimination in mice. *Cancer Biol. Ther.* 15: 1219–1225.

12. Hussain, A. et al., 2013. Sulforaphane inhibits growth of human breast cancer cells and augments the therapeutic index of the chemotherapeutic drug, gemcitabine. *Asian Pac. J. Cancer Prev.* 14: 5855–5860.

13. Sarkar, R. et al., 2012. Sulphoraphane, a naturally occurring isothiocyanate induces apoptosis in breast cancer cells by targeting heat shock proteins. *Biochem. Biophys. Res. Commun.* 427: 80–85.

14. Pawlik, A. et al., 2013. Sulforaphane inhibits growth of phenotypically different breast cancer cells. *Eur. J. Nutr.* 52: 1949–1958.

15. (a) Abbaoui, B. et al., 2012. Inhibition of bladder cancer by broccoli isothiocyanates sulforaphane and erucin: Characterization, metabolism, and interconversion. *Mol. Nutr. Food Res.* 56: 1675–1687; (b) Wood, D.P. 2013. Inhibition of bladder cancer by Broccoli isothiocyanates sulforaphane and erucin: Characterization, metabolism, and interconversion. *Reply J. Urol.* 190: 1956.

16. Myzak, M.C. et al., 2007. Sulforaphane retards the growth of human PC-3 xenografts and inhibits HDAC activity in human subjects. *Exp. Biol. Med.* (Maywood). 232: 227–234.

17. Rajendran, P. et al., 2013. HDAC turnover, CtIP acetylation and dysregulated DNA damage signaling in colon cancer cells treated with sulforaphane and related dietary isothiocyanates. *Epigenetics* 8: 612–623.

18. Khor, T.O. et al., 2006. Pharmacogenomics of cancer chemopreventive isothiocyanate compound sulforaphane in the intestinal polyps of ApcMin/+ mice. *Biopharm Drug Dispos.* 27: 407–420.

19. Thakkar, A. et al., 2013. The molecular mechanism of action of aspirin, curcumin and sulforaphane combinations in the chemoprevention of pancreatic cancer. *Oncol. Rep.* 29: 1671–1677.

20. Kalpana, D.P.D. et al., 2013. Apoptotic role of natural isothiocyanate from broccoli (*Brassica oleracea* italica) in experimental chemical lung carcinogenesis. *Pharm. Biol.* (London, UK) 51: 621–628.

21. Kang, H.J. et al., 2012. Bioactive food components prevent carcinogenic stress via Nrf2 activation in BRCA1 deficient breast epithelial cells. *Toxicol. Lett.* 209: 15–60.

22. Xu, T. et al., 2012. Dual roles of sulforaphane in cancer treatment. *Anticancer Agents Med. Chem.* 12: 1132–1142.

23. Thejass, P. et al., 2006. Augmentation of natural killer cell and antibody-dependent cellular cytotoxicity in BALB/c mice by sulforaphane, a naturally occurring isothiocyanate from broccoli through enhanced production of cytokines IL-2 and IFN-gamma. *Immunophar. Immunot.* 28: 443–457.

24. Katoch, O. et al., 2013. Sulforaphane mitigates genotoxicity induced by radiation and anticancer drugs in human lymphocytes. *Mut. Res. Genet. Toxicol. Environ. Mutagen.* 758: 29–34.

25. (a) Myzak, M.C. et al., 2006. Chemoprotection by sulforaphane: Keep one eye beyond Keap1. *Cancer Lett.* 233(2), 208–218; (b) Zhang, Y. et al., 1992. A major inducer of anticarcinogenic protective enzymes from broccoli: Isolation and elucidation of structure. *Proc. Natl. Acad. Sci. USA.* 89: 2399–2403.

26. Zareba, G. et al., 2004. Chemoprotective effects of broccoli and other *Brassica* vegetables. *Drugs Future* 29: 1097–1104.

27. Faulkner, K. et al., 1998. Selective increase of the potential anticarcinogen 4-methylsulphinylbutyl glucosinolate in broccoli. *Carcinogenesis* 19: 605–609.

28. Joseph M.-A. et al., 2004. Cruciferous vegetables, genetic polymorphisms in glutathione S-transferases M1 and T1, and prostate cancer risk. *Nutr. Cancer* 50: 206–213.

29. Zhou, J.L. et al., 2005. Purification and antitumor activity of major glucosinolates separated from *Brassica oleracea* rapeseed. *Yingyong Huaxue* 22:1075–1078.

30. Velasco, P. et al., 2011. Glucosinolates in *Brassica* and Cancer. In: Ronald, R.W. and Victor, R.P. (Eds.), *Bioactive Foods and Extracts, Cancer Treatment and Prevention*, CRC Press, Boca Raton, FL, pp. 3–30.

31. Fan, S. et al., 2006. BRCA1 and BRCA2 as molecular targets for phytochemicals indole-3-carbinol and genistein in breast and prostate cancer cells. *British J. Cancer* 94: 407–426.
32. Wu, Y.S. et al., 2010. A novel mechanism of indole-3-carbinol effects on breast carcinogenesis involves induction of Cdc25A degradation. *Cancer Prevent. Res.* 3: 818–828.
33. Hsu, J. et al., 2006. Indole-3-carbinol mediated cell cycle arrest of LNCaP human prostate cancer cells requires the induced production of activated p53 tumor suppressor protein. *Biochem. Pharmacol.* 72: 1714–1723.
34. Wang, T.T.Y. et al., 2012. Broccoli-derived phytochemicals indole-3-carbinol and 3,3'-diindolylmethane exerts concentration-dependent pleiotropic effects on prostate cancer cells: Comparison with other cancer preventive phytochemicals. *Mol. Carcinogenesis* 51: 244–256.
35. Vivar, O.-I. et al., 2009. 3,3'-Diindolylmethane induces a G1 arrest in human prostate cancer cells irrespective of androgen receptor and p53 status. *Biochem. Pharmacol.* 78: 469–476.
36. Perez-Chacon, G. et al., 2014. Indole-3-carbinol induces cMYC and IAP-family downmodulation and promotes apoptosis of Epstein-Barr virus (EBV)-positive but not of EBV-negative Burkitt's lymphoma cell lines. *Pharma. Res.* 89: 46–56.
37. Katrin, S. 2012. Chemotherapy and dietary phytochemical agents. *Chemother. Res. Practice* 2012: Article ID 282570.
38. Fang, X.B. et al., 2013. Preparation and antitumor activity of total flavonoids from Broccoli. *Jiangxi Yiyao* 48: 397–399.
39. Wang, X.Q. et al., 2010. Study of broccolini flavonoids on anticancer activity in vitro. *Anhui Nongye Kexue* 38: 20014–20015, 20024.
40. Wang, B.F. et al., 2012. Inhibitory effects of Broccolini leaf flavonoids on human cancer cells. *Scanning* 34: 1–5.
41. Xu, J.J. et al., 2012. Effect of broccoli polypeptide on C6 glioma cells of rat. *Zhongfeng Yu Shenjing Jibing Zazhi* 29: 1030–1031.
42. Qi, L. et al., 2014. Mechanism of broccoli polypeptide inhibited the growth of C6 glioma cells. *Zhongguo Yaoxue Zazhi* (Beijing, China) 49: 1027–1031.
43. Qi, L. et al., 2014. Effect of component II of broccoli polypeptide on glioma cell apoptosis. *Zhongguo Bingli Shengli Zazhi* 30: 1584–1589.
44. Nishi, K. et al. 2011. Immunostimulatory in vitro and in vivo effects of a water-soluble extract from kale. *Biosci. Biotechnol. Biochem.* 75: 40–46.
45. Xu, L.S. et al., 2015. Structural characterization of a broccoli polysaccharide and evaluation of anticancer cell proliferation effects. *Carbohydr. Polym.* 126: 179–184.
46. Khoobchandani, M. et al., 2013. Cellular uptake and cytotoxic effects of broccoli phytochemicals based gold nanoparticles (B-AuNPs): Enhanced cancer therapeutic efficacy. In: Laudon, M. and Romanowicz, B. (Eds.), *Nanotech Conference & Expo 2013: An Interdisciplinary Integrative Forum on Nanotechnology, Microtechnology, Biotechnology and Cleantechnology*, Washington, DC, May 12–16, 3, 422–425.
47. Sugirtha, P. et al., 2015. Green synthesis of magnesium oxide nanoparticles using *Brassica oleracea* and Punica granatum peels and their anticancer and photocatalytic activity. *Asian J. Chem.* 27(7): 2513–2517.
48. Ranjitham, A.M. et al., 2013. In vitro evaluation of antioxidant, antimicrobial, anticancer activities and characterisation of *Brassica oleracea*. var. bortrytis. L. synthesized silver nanoparticles. *Int. J. Pharm. Pharm. Sci.* 5(4): 239–251.
49. Matusheski, N.V. et al., 2006. Epithiospecifier protein from broccoli (*Brassica oleracea* L. Ssp. italica) inhibits formation of the anticancer agent sulforaphane. *J. Agricult. Food Chem.* 54: 2069–2076.

4. CELERY

Céleri   Sellerie   Apio

芹菜   セロリ   미나리

Apium graveolens

Apiaceae

4. R = –H
5. R = –OH

Celery (*Apium graveolens*, Apiaceae) is one of the most common vegetables in Western countries, and it has been cultivated as a vegetable since antiquity. Now it has been popularized more broadly in the world. Its crisp and thick stalk is often served as a plate vegetable and as an addition to salads and soups. Two other cultivars are also popular vegetables—that is, Chinese celery (*A. graveolens* var. *secalinum*) in Eastern Asia for its flavorful leaves and thinner stalks and celeriac (*A. graveolens* var. *rapaceum*) in Europe and the Mediterranean regions for its hypocotyl-formed large bulb. Celery is an excellent source of vitamin K and molybdenum and a good source of folate, potassium, dietary fiber, manganese, and pantothenic acid. For providing low-calorie dietary fiber bulk, celery is often used in weight-loss diets. It also helps to protect the digestive tract by decreasing gastric ulcers and lessens the risk of cardiovascular diseases—for example, high blood pressure and arteriosclerosis.[1] According to scientific investigation, celery and Chinese celery are known to provide similar levels of nutrition and health benefits. In addition, celery seed is employed as a spice and an herb.

Scientific Evidence of Cancer-Inhibitory and Cancer-Preventive Constituents

Celery is rich in phenolic phytochemicals such as flavonoids, dihydrostilbenoids, furanocoumarins, and vitamin C, so it has antioxidant, antitumor, and anti-inflammatory properties. The celery extract in a 1/20 dilution (corresponding to 166 mg raw vegetable per mL) showed moderate inhibitory effect against the proliferation of human cell lines such as PC3 (prostate cancer), U-87 (glioma), Panc-1 (pancreatic cancer), and Daoy (medulloblastoma) with the inhibitory rates of 50%–75% but weak effects on human MCF-7 (breast), Caki-2 (kidney), A549 (lung), and AGS (stomach) cancer cell lines *in vitro*.[2] The petroleum ether–acetone (7:3) extract of Chinese celery in an *in vitro* assay exerted obvious anti-growth effects against YTMLC-90 human lung squamous cell carcinoma cells. At a concentration of 5 mg/mL for 3 days, its suppressive rate reached 73.4%.[3] In addition, the juices of celery roots and leaves were demonstrated to be able to protect the side effects caused from doxorubicin, a chemotherapeutic drug.[4]

1. Monoterpenes

Volatile oils of celery have been demonstrated to have suppressive activity against a variety of cancer cell lines, the effect of which is largely attributed to monoterpene constituents. Three mono-terpenes assigned myrence (**1**), limonene (**2**), and 1,3,8-menthatriene (**3**) were isolated from the volatiles of *A. graveolens* var. *filicinum*. In an *in vitro* assay, the three moderately suppressed crown gall tumor, A549 lung carcinoma, MCF-7 breast cancer, and HT-29 colon adenocarcinoma cell lines

(ED_{50}: 2–<10 μg/mL).[5] Myrence (**1**) also showed the antiproliferative effect in HepG2 human hepatoma (IC_{50}: 9.23 μg/mL), B16-F10 mouse melanoma (IC_{50}: 12.27 μg/mL), and P388 mouse leukemia cell lines but no such effect in PBMC normal lymphocytes.[6,7] The essential oil (EO) extracted from celery seeds (*A. graveolens*) was active in the inhibition of benzo[a]pyrene-induced forestomach cancer in mice.[8] However, the major constituents isolated from the volatiles of leaves, stalks, and roots of Tunisian celery (*A. graveolens* var. *dulce*) have not been reported to have anticancer and anticarcinogenic activities, whose major molecules were identified as (Z)-3-buty-lidenephthalide, 3-butyl-4,5-dihydrophthalide, and α-thujene.[9]

2. Flavonoids

Celery is also an important food source of conventional antioxidant nutrients such as vitamin C, β-carotene, and manganese; the flavonoid component in celery exerts noticeable health benefit in cancer prevention and is an antioxidant as well. In an *in vitro* experiment, the hexanolic-extracted flavonoids from celery suppressed the proliferation of human HepG2 hepatoma and MCF-7 breast carcinoma cell lines in a dose-dependent manner.[10] Luteolin (**4**) and apigenin (**5**) are the two prominent flavonoids in celery, especially in celery leaves that have the contents of 187.2–250.4 mg/kg and 124.2–173.3 mg/kg, respectively.[11]

Luteolin: The anticancer property of luteolin (**4**) was revealed to be associated with the induction of apoptosis and inhibition of cell proliferation, metastasis, and angiogenesis. The *in vitro* experiments demonstrated that luteolin (**4**) was a marked inhibitor in mouse P388 leukemia and B16-4A5 melanoma cell lines (IC_{50}: 1–2.3 μM) and human lung carcinoma (A549), T-cell leukemia (CCRF-HSB-2), and gastric cancer (TGBC11TKB) cell lines (IC_{50}: 1.3–3.1 μM), and was a moderate inhibitor in human leukemia (HL-60), cervical cancer (HeLa), gastric cancer (AGS), head and neck cancer (Tu212), bladder cancer (J82), colon cancer (CoLo 320), hepatoma (HepG2, SK-Hep-1, PLC/PRF/5, Hep3B, and HA22T/VGH), lung cancer (GLC4, H661, and H292), squamous cell cancer (A431), and lung squamous carcinoma (CH27) cell lines (IC_{50}: 7–50 μM).[12,13] Luteolin (**4**) was also effective in hindering human leukemia (CEM-C7 and CEM-1), lung cancer (H520), bone cancer (U2OS), oral cancer (OSCC-1/KMC), melanoma (BCC-1/KMC), and kidney cancer (RTCC-1/KMC) cell lines.[12] The proliferation of both human LNCaP and PC3 prostate cancer cell lines was inhibited by luteolin (**4**) at 3 μM and was completely inhibited at 30 μM *in vitro*. Other studies reported that treatment with luteolin (**4**), kaempferol, or quercetin in 100-μM concentrations could completely obstruct the growth of human PC3 prostate cancer cells.[12]

The anticancer activity of luteolin (**4**) in most of the cases was closely related to its abilities in the induction of cell apoptosis and/or cell-cycle arrest. At concentrations from 20 to 60 μM, luteolin (**4**) efficiently elicited the apoptotic death of human HT-29 (colon) and NCI H460 (nonsmall cell lung) neoplastic cell lines with different mechanisms.[14,15] The apoptosis of HT-29 cells was promoted in a p53-independent manner by downregulation of p21CIP1/WAF1, survivin, Mcl-1, Bcl-xL, and Mdm-2 expression; activation of caspases-3, -7, and -9; and cleavage of poly(ADP-ribose) polymerase,[14] whereas the apoptosis of NCI H460 cells was induced by lessening of Bad expression and Bcl-2/Bax ratio and activation of caspase-3 via downregulation of Sirt1 expression.[15] During the luteolin (**4**) exposure, the cell-cycle arrest in HT-29 cells was also elicited, and the migration of NCI-H460 cells was blocked.[14,15] By blockage of Notch signaling via regulating miRNAs, luteolin (**4**) notably inhibited the cell survival, cell cycle, and tube formation in human MDA-MB-231 breast cancer cells *in vitro* and *in vivo*.[16] More investigations exposed that luteolin (**4**) acted as a potent HSP90 inhibitor as well in the HeLa, MCF-7, and Hep3B cancer cell lines to reduce STAT3 phosphorylation level and to suppress STAT3 transcriptional activity, in which STAT3 participates in the development of a wide variety of human cancers.[17]

The anticancer property of luteolin (**4**) was further confirmed in the *in vivo* models. Luteolin (**4**) in IP doses of 5–50 mg/kg/d inhibited tumor growth in nude mice with xenografted human SKOV3. ip1 ovarian carcinoma, in IP doses of 25–50 mg/kg/d repressed the volume of androgen-sensitive human prostate LNCaP adenocarcinoma in male nude mice with significantly reduced serum PSA levels, and in an IP dose of 10 mg/kg/d lessened the tumor weight of prostate cancer PC3 xenograft in nude mice. Likewise, luteolin (4) at an oral dose of 250 µg/mL/day (added to animals' water supply) restrained the growth of PC3 prostate cancer xenograft in nude mice. The in vivo effects of luteolin (4) were also demonstrated in murine models, leading to the suppression of Lewis lung carcinoma and HAK-1B hepatoma and the obstruction of benzo[a]pyrene-induced lung carcinogenesis.[12,18] In cMet-overexpressing patient-derived tumor xenograft models, luteolin (4) inhibited the proliferation and invasion of MKN45 and SGC7901 gastric cancer together with the promotion of cell apoptosis, activities that were achieved by blockage of cMet/Akt/ERK signaling, downregulation of cMet, MMP-9 and Ki-67 expression, and activation of caspase-3 and PARP-1.[19] Besides the antiproliferative effect, luteolin (4) concomitantly restrained the secretion and activities of MMP-2 and MMP-9 in human A431 epithelial cell cancer cells, implying the antimetastatic potential of luteolin.[12] Luteolin (4) and apigenin (5) also have a capacity to elicit morphological differentiation of the HL-60 cells into granulocytes in addition to the potent inhibitory effect against the growth of HL-60 human leukemia cells.[12]

Moreover, luteolin (4) is capable of amplifying the sensitivity of cancer cells to chemotherapeutic agent–induced cytotoxicity and enhancing the anticancer efficacy through stimulating p53-involved apoptosis pathways and blocking the cell-survival pathways such as PI3K/Akt, NF-κB, and XIAP.[20] The growth of two human hepatoma cell lines (Bel-7402 and HepG2) could be obstructed synergically by the combination of luteolin and 5-fluorouracil (5-FU) along with elicitation of the cell apoptosis and regulation of 5-FU metabolism.[21] The integration of gemcitabine (a drug for cancer therapy) with luteolin (4) promoted the apoptotic death of pancreatic cancer cells and the anticancer potency in vivo, the proapoptotic effect of which was mediated by blocking the K-ras/GSK3β/NF-κB signaling pathway, leading to reduction of the Bcl-2/Bax ratio, release of cytochrome c, and activation of caspase-3.[22]

Besides, luteolin (4) has been used for the formulation of water-soluble polymer-encapsulated nanoparticles and the formed Nano-Luteolin particles have an advantage in drug delivery. In an in vivo tumor xenograft mouse model, more significant anti-growth effect was exerted on Tu212 human head and neck squamous cell carcinoma in comparison to original luteolin.[13]

Apigenin: Similar to luteolin (4), apigenin (5) is a widely distributed flavonoid in many herbs and fruits as well, which has been shown to have antigenotoxic, antimutagenic, anticarcinogenic, and antioxidant activities. Its broad anticancer spectrum was demonstrated in many types of human neoplastic cells such as breast (MCF-7, MDA-MB-453, MDA-MB231, T47D, and SK-BR-3), prostate (PWR-1E, LNCaP, PC3, DU145, 22Rv1, and CA-HPV-10), lung (A549), liver (PLC/PRF/5, HepG2, and Hep3B), colon (HCT-116, SW480, HT-29, Caco-2, and MG63), ovary (HO-8910PM), cervix (HeLa and SiHa), leukemia (U937 and HL-60), adrenal cortical (H295R), thyroid (UCLA NPA-87-1, UCLA RO-82W-1, and UCLA RO-81A-1), stomach (SGC-7901), and brain (SH-SY5Y, SK-N-BE2, NUB-7, and LAN-5) cell lines in vitro.[23–28] Compared to PC3 and DU145 human androgen-refractory prostate cancer cells, LNCaP and PWR-1E human androgen-responsive prostate cancer cells were more susceptible to apigenin for the apoptotic induction.[25–26] Similarly, apigenin (5) was more sensitive to human MCF-7 (ER+), MDA-MB453 (AR+ and GR+), and HER2/neu overexpressing breast carcinoma cell lines than estrogen-insensitive breast carcinoma cell lines (MDA-MB231 and MDA-MB568).[27–31] Incubation of apigenin (5) enhanced the radiosensitivity and apoptosis in SQ-5 lung neoplastic cells significantly.[27] In murine models, apigenin (5) exerted an in vivo inhibitory effect against the prostate carcinogenesis, dimethyl benzanthracene-induced skin carcinogenesis, and N′-methyl-N′-nitro-N-nitroso-guanidine–triggered gastric carcinogenesis.[27,32] Other in vivo tests confirmed the protective effects of apigenin in a dose of 25 mg/kg/day for 2 weeks against N-nitrosodiethylamine—induced and phenobarbital-promoted hepatocarcinogenesis in rats together with diminishing oxidative stress and DNA damage caused by the carcinogens, and in doses of 5 and 20 µmol/day for 26 weeks against DMBA-initiated and TPA-promoted skin tumorigenesis along with repressing epidermal ornithine decarboxylase induced by TPA.[33,34] The efficacy of apigenin administration was also demonstrated against Lewis lung cancer C-6 glioma and DHDK-12 colonic cancer *in vivo*.[27,28] Administration of apigenin (**5**) was also effective in the prevention of UV-induced skin tumorigenesis by inducing ornithine decarboxylase activity, inhibiting cell-cycle and cyclin-dependent kinases, and prolonging tumor-free survival in mice.[27,28] A combination therapy with gemcitabine (a chemo-drug) and apigenin (**5**) enhanced the growth inhibition and proapoptosis efficacies were enhanced in pancreatic cancer cells (MiaPaca-2, AsPC-1) *in vitro* and *in vivo* in parallel to downregulation of NF-κB activity and suppression of Akt activation.[35] In a combination treatment, apigenin (**5**) could synergistically sensitize the cancer cells to paclitaxel-induced apoptosis through obstructing SOD activity, signifying that the combination of apigenin and paclitaxel was an effective way to reduce the dose of paclitaxel taken and to eliminate the side effects/toxicity of paclitaxel.[36] In addition, apigenin (**5**) is a radioprotector as well, which in doses of 2.5–10 μg/mL exerted the protective effect on δ-ray radiation-induced chromosomal damage in human lymphocytes.[37]

The antiproliferative effect of apigenin (**5**) in most of the cases is contributed by its ability to elicit apoptosis and/or cell-cycle arrest. The mechanisms in the diverse types of neoplastic cell lines were revealed to be mediated by characteristic pathways such as (1) p53-dependently caused G1-phase growth arrest and apoptosis by upregulation of p21/WAF1 and Fas/APO-1 and activation of caspase-3 in HeLa cells; (2) induced G2/M cell-cycle arrest and apoptosis through suppression of cdc2 kinase, reduction in cdc2 and cyclin-B1 proteins and increase of adenomatous polyposis coli (APC) expression, and p21/WAF1 expression in modifying p53 effects in various colon cancer cell lines, especially in p53-mutant HT-29 and MG63 cells and APC-mutated HT29-APC cells; (3) augmented ERK and p38 activities and modulated MAPK cascade in HCT-116 cells; (4) promoted HL-60 cells to apoptosis via increase in ROS production, loss of mitochondrial transmembrane potential, release of mitochondrial cytochrome c, induction of pro-caspase-9, and rapidly stimulated caspase-3 activity and proteolytic cleavage of poly(ADP-ribose) polymerase; (5) suppressed chymotrypsin-like activity of 20S and 26S proteasomes, increased putative ubiquitinated forms of two proteasome target proteins (Bax and IκBα), and activated caspase-3 and cleavage of poly(ADP-ribose) polymerase in Jurkat T cells; (6) initiated 22Rv1 cell apoptotic death by a ROS-dependent disruption of mitochondrial membrane potential through transcriptional-dependent and p53-independent pathways; (7) upregulated p53 and p21 activities, downregulated CDK4 expression, elevated intracellular ROS and hydrogen peroxide levels, transcriptionally lessened catalase activity and moderated sFas, Bcl-2, and Bax protein levels in HepG2 cells; (8) restrained HIF-1α and VEGF expression via HDM2/p53 and PI3K/Akt/p70S6K1 pathways in HO-8910PM cells; (9) obstructed aromatase activity and diminished cortisol production and 3β-HSD II P450c21 activities in H295R cells; (10) amplified wild-type p53 expression and p53-induced gene products p21WAF1/CIP1 and Bax, enlarged free Ca^{2+} and Bax/Bcl-2 ratio, and enhanced caspase-3 activity and PARP cleavage in brain cancer cell lines, and associated with an increase in intracellular, mitochondrial release of cytochrome c and activation of caspase-9, calpain, caspase-3, and caspase-12 as well in neuroblastoma SH-SY5Y cells; (11) augmented caspases-3 and, -7 activities and poly(ADP-ribose) polymerase cleavage in MDA-MB-231 cells; (12) blocked HER2/HER3-PI3K/Akt signalings in HER2/neu overexpressing breast cancer cells; (13) promoted cytochrome c level and dysfunction of mitochondria leading to release of cytochrome c, AIF and Endo G, and activation of caspases-9 and -3 in A549 cells; and (14) decreased levels of phosphorylated EGFR tyrosine kinase and MAPK and their nuclear substrate c-myc in anaplastic thyroid cancer cells.[27,28,38–45]

Furthermore, apigenin (**5**) has also shown promise in inhibiting tumor cell invasion and metastases along with regulating protease production and inhibiting angiogenesis. The treatments with apigenin (**5**) obstructed melanoma lung metastases by impairing interaction of tumor cells with endothelium and inhibiting hepatocyte growth factor-induced MDA-MB-231 breast carcinoma cell invasion and metastasis by blocking Akt, ERK, and JNK phosphorylation. Orally giving apigenin at doses of 20 and 50 μg/mouse/day, 6 days per week for 20 weeks, completely abolished distant-site metastases to lymph nodes, lungs, and liver besides significantly diminishing the volumes of prostate tumor.[46,47] By inhibiting a focal adhesion kinase (FAK), apigenin (5) restrained the motility and invasion of metastatic prostate carcinoma PC-3M cells and inhibited the migration, invasion, and metastasis of human ovarian cancer A2780 cells.[27,48] It has also been shown that oral administration of apigenin lessened the level of IGF-I in prostate tumor xenografts and raised the level of IGFBP-3, a binding protein that sequesters IGF-I in vascular circulation.[27] In the *in vivo* condition, apigenin (5) was effective in hindering TNFα-induced intracellular adhesion molecule-1 upregulation and suppressing vascular endothelial growth factor (VEGF) (an important factor in angiogenesis) expression via degradation of HIF-1α protein in human endothelial cells. Thus, exposure of nude mice with lung cancer to apigenin (5) inhibited the expressions of HIF-1α and VEGF in the tumor tissues, suggesting an antiangiogenic effect of apigenin.[27,49] The explorations showed that apigenin was capable of repressing Id1 protein in the A2780 cells via stimulating transcription factor 3 (ATF3).[49] In addition, in a B57BL/6N mouse model with B16–BL6 tumor cells, treatment with a single dose of an apigenin and quercetin combination significantly diminished the number of tumor cells adhering to lung vessels via impairment of endothelial interactions in malignant cells.[27,28]

CONCLUSION AND SUGGESTION

The summarized scientific evidence clearly established the advantages of dietary celery, especially luteolin (4) and apigenin (5) as the major flavonoids in celery. Their anticancer and anticarcinogenic activities and health-promoting and disease-preventing effects are intimately related to their antioxidant and free-radical scavenging abilities. On the basis of moderate to weak actions such as inhibiting tumor proliferation, diminishing oxidative stress, improving the efficacy of detoxification enzymes, inducing apoptosis and cell-cycle arrest, and stimulating the immune system, celery can be advocated as a functional vegetable and a food supplement for cancer prevention and the coordination of cancer therapy in clinics. For delivering the maximum health benefits of celery for our diet, blanching (3 min submersion in boiling water) and boiling (10 min) should be avoided because the two thermal processes result in substantial loss of the antioxidants in celery in a range of 38%–41%, whereas steaming keeps 83%–99% of the total phenolic antioxidants in celery even after 10 min of the process.[50] Of course, consumption of fresh celery without thermal processes (such as in salad) is best for 100% intake of the antioxidant nutrients from celery.

SIDE EFFECTS

Pharmacological experiments demonstrated the side effects of celery in reproductive system—that is, celery flavonoids could retard testosterone production and decrease the sperm count for males, and apigenin (5) could obstruct the secretion of female hormones and presentational hormones, the female, effects of which may be beneficial to birth control but disadvantageous for young couples who want a baby. Therefore, a frequent diet of celery should be avoided by some adults.[51] Because a stalk of celery contains nearly 35 mg of sodium, salt-sensitive individuals, especially the patients suffering from nephropathy, should keep track of their sodium when monitoring daily intake.

REFERENCES

1. Sowbhagya, H.B. et al., 2014. Chemistry, technology, and nutraceutical functions of celery (*Apium graveolens* L.): An overview. *Crit. Rev. Food Sci. Nutr.* 54: 389–398.
2. Boivin, D. et al., 2009. Antiproliferative and antioxidant activities of common vegetables: A comparative study. *Food Chem.* 112: 374–380.
3. He, T. et al., 1998. Influence on in vitro growth of human lung cancer cell line YTMLC-90 of vegetable fat-soluble crude extract. *Zhongguo Gonggong Weisheng Xuebao* 17: 88–89.

4. Kolarovic, J. et al., 2009. Protective effects of celery juice in treatments with doxorubicin. *Molecules* 14: 1627–1638.

5. Saleh, M.M. et al., 1998. Cytotoxicity and in vitro effects on human cancer cell lines of volatiles of *Apium graveolens* var. filicinum. *Pharm.Pharmacol. Lett.* 8: 97–99.

6. Ferraz, R.P.C. et al., 2013. Cytotoxic effect of leaf essential oil of Lippia gracilis Schauer (Verbenaceae). *Phytomedicine* 20: 615–621.

7. Okamura, K. et al., 1993. Biological activity of monoterpenes from trees. *Toyama-Ken Yakuji Kenkyusho Nenpo.* 20: 95–101.

8. Zheng, G. et al., 2012. Chemoprevention of benzo[a]pyrene-induced forestomach cancer in mice by natural phthalides from celery seed oil. *Nutr. Cancer* 19: 77–86.

9. Sellami, I.H. et al., 2012. Essential oil and aroma composition of leaves, stalks and roots of celery (*Apium graveolens* var. dulce) from Tunisia. *J. Essential Oil Res.* 24: 513–521.

10. Mahmood, A.S. et al., 2013. Extraction and purification flavonoid from celery plant and application on hepatic and breast cancer cells. *Int. J. Current Res.* 5: 2462–2465.

11. Silvia, T.-S. et al., 2013. Flavonols and flavones in some Bulgarian plant foods. *Pol. J. Food Nutr. Sci.* 63: 173–177

12. Günter, S. et al., 2008. Anti-carcinogenic effects of the flavonoid luteolin. *Molecules* 13: 2628–26251

13. Debatosh, M. et al., Luteolin nanoparticle in chemoprevention: In vitro and in vivo anticancer activity. *Cancer Prev. Res.* 7: 65–73.

14. Lim, D.Y. et al., 2007. Induction of cell cycle arrest and apoptosis in HT-29 human colon cancer cells by the dietary compound luteolin. *Am. J. Physiol.* 292(1, Pt. 1): G66–G75.

15. Ma, L.P. et al., 2015. Luteolin exerts an anticancer effect on NCI-H460 human non-small cell lung cancer cells through the induction of Sirt1-mediated apoptosis. *Mol. Med. Rep.* 12: 4196–4202.

16. Sun, D. W et al., 2015. Luteolin inhibits breast cancer development and progression in vitro and in vivo by suppressing notch signaling and regulating MiRNAs. *Cell Physiol. Biochem.* 37: 1693–1711.

17. Fu, J. et al., 2012. Luteolin induces carcinoma cell apoptosis through binding Hsp90 to suppress constitutive activation of STAT3. *PLoS ONE* 7: e49194.

18. Kasala, E.R. 2016. Antioxidant and antitumor efficacy of Luteolin, a dietary flavone on benzo(a)pyrene-induced experimental lung carcinogenesis. *Biomed. Pharm.* 82: 568–577.

19. Lu, J. et al., 2015. Luteolin exerts a marked antitumor effect in cMet-overexpressing patient-derived tumor xenograft models of gastric cancer. *J. Translat. Med.* 13: 42.

20. Lin, Y. et al., 2008. Luteolin, a flavonoid with potential for cancer prevention and therapy. *Curr. Cancer Drug Targets* 8: 634–646.

21. Xu, H. et al., 2016. Luteolin synergizes the antitumor effects of 5-fluorouracil against human hepatocellular carcinoma cells through apoptosis induction and metabolism. *Life Sci.* 144: 138–147.

22. Johnson, J.L. et al., 2015. Luteolin and gemcitabine protect against pancreatic cancer in an orthotopic mouse model. *Pancreas* 44: 144–151.

23. Chiang, L.C. et al., 2006. Anti-proliferative effect of apigenin and its apoptotic induction in human HepG2 cells. *Cancer Lett.* 237: 207–214.

24. Papachristou, F. et al., 2013. Time course changes of anti- and pro-apoptotic proteins in apigenin-induced genotoxicity. *Chinese Med.* (London, UK) 8: 9.

25. Shukla, S. et al., 2008. Apigenin-induced prostate cancer cell death is initiated by reactive oxygen species and p53 activation. *Free Radic. Biol. Med.* 44:1833–1845.

26. Shukla, S. et al., 2004. Molecular mechanisms for apigenin-induced cell-cycle arrest and apoptosis of hormone refractory human prostate carcinoma DU145 cells. *Mol. Carcinog.* 39: 114–126.

27. Patel, S.D. et al., 2007. Apigenin and cancer chemoprevention: Progress, potential and promise (Review). *Int. J. Oncol.* 30: 233–245.

28. Shukla, S. et al., 2010. Apigenin: A promising molecule for cancer prevention. *Pharm. Res.* 27: 962–978.

29. Nabavi, S. M. et al., 2015. Apigenin and breast cancers: From chemistry to medicine. *Anticancer Agents in Med. Chem.* 15: 728–735.

30. Choi, E.J. et al., 2009. Apigenin induces apoptosis through a mitochondria/caspase-pathway in human breast cancer MDA-MB-453 cells. *J. Clin. Biochem. Nutr.* 44: 260–265.

31. Choi, E.J. et al., 2009. Apigenin causes G2/M arrest associated with the modulation of p21 (Cip1) and Cdc2 and activates p53-dependent apoptosis pathway in human breast cancer SK-BR-3 cells. *J. Nutr. Biochem.* 20: 285–290.

32. Birt, D.F. et al., Inhibition of ultraviolet light induced skin carcinogenesis in SKH-1 mice by apigenin, a plant flavonoid. *Anticancer Res.* 1997, 17: 85–91.

33. Wei, H. et al., 1990. Inhibitory effect of apigenin, a plant flavonoid, on epidermal ornithine decarboxylase and skin tumor promotion in mice. *Cancer Res.* 50: 499–502.

34. Jeyabal, P.V.S. et al., 2005. Apigenin inhibits oxidative stress-induced macromolecular damage in N-nitrosodiethylamine (NDEA)-induced hepatocellular carcinogenesis in Wistar albino rats. *Mol. Carcinog.* 44: 11–20.

35. Lee, S.H. et al., 2008. Enhanced antitumor effect of combination therapy with gemcitabine and apigenin in pancreatic cancer. *Cancer Lett.* 259: 39–49.

36. Xu, Y. et al., 2011. Synergistic effects of apigenin and paclitaxel on apoptosis of cancer cells. *PLoS One.* 2011, 6: e29169.

37. Rithidech, K.N. et al., 2005. Protective effect of apigenin on radiation-induced chromosomal damage in human lymphocytes. *Mut. Res.* 585: 96–104.

38. Kuo, C.H. et al., 2014. Apigenin has anti-atrophic gastritis and anti-gastric cancer progression effects in Helicobacter pylori-infected Mongolian gerbils. *J. Ethnopharmacol.* 151: 1031–1039.

39. van Dross R. et al., The chemopreventive bioflavonoid apigenin modulates signal transduction pathways in keratinocyte and colon carcinoma cell lines. *J. Nutr.* 133 (Supp 1): 3800–3804.

40. Wang, W. et al., 2000. Cell-cycle arrest at G2/M and growth inhibition by apigenin in human colon carcinoma cell lines. *Mol. Carcinog.* 28: 102–110.

41. Miyoshi, N. et al., 2007. Dietary flavonoid apigenin is a potential inducer of intracellular oxidative stress: the role in the interruptive apoptotic signal. *Arch. Biochem Biophys.* 466: 274–282.

42. Valdameri, G. et al., 2011. Involvement of catalase in the apoptotic mechanism induced by apigenin in HepG2 human hepatoma cells. *Chem. Biol. Interact.* 193: 180–219.

43. Wang, I.K. et al., 1999. Induction of apoptosis by apigenin and related flavonoids through cytochrome c release and activation of caspase-9 and caspase-3 in leukaemia HL-60 cells. *Eur. J. Cancer.* 35: 1517–1525.

44. Lu, H.F. et al., 2010. Apigenin induces caspase-dependent apoptosis in human lung cancer A549 cells through Bax- and Bcl-2-triggered mitochondrial pathway. *Int. J. Oncol.* 36: 1477–1484.

45. Chung, C.S. et al., 2007. Impact of adenomatous polyposis coli (APC) tumor supressor gene in human colon cancer cell lines on cell cycle arrest by apigenin. *Mol. Carcinog.* 46: 773–782.

46. Lee, W.J. et al., 2008. Apigenin inhibits HGF-promoted invasive growth and metastasis involving blocking PI3K/Akt pathway and beta 4 integrin function in MDA-MB-231 breast cancer cells. *Toxicol. Appl. Pharmacol.* 226: 178–191.

47. Choi, E.J. et al., 2009. 5-Fluorouracil combined with apigenin enhances anticancer activity through induction of apoptosis in human breast cancer MDA-MB-453 cells. *Oncol. Rep.* 22: 1533–1537.

48. Hu, X.W. et al., 2008. Apigenin inhibited migration and invasion of human ovarian cancer A2780 cells through focal adhesion kinase. *Carcinogenesis* 29: 2369–2376.

49. Li, Z.D. et al., 2009. Apigenin inhibits proliferation of ovarian cancer A2780 cells through Id1. *FEBS Lett.* 583: 1999–2003.

50. Zhang, H.H. et al., 2013. Research progress in flavonoids from celery and the correlation with bioactivities. *Shipin Gongye Keji (Sci. Technol. Food Industry)* 34: 388–391.

51. (a) Yao, Y. et al., 2010. Effect of thermal treatment on phenolic composition and antioxidant activities of two celery cultivars. *LWT--Food Sci. Technol.* 44: 181–185; (b) Monmouth County's Ask The Doctor by Gunther Publications. Summer edition, May 27, 2014, p. 35.

5. CHIVE

Ciboulette   Schnittlauch   Cebollino

韭菜   ニラ   부추

Allium tuberosum

Amaryllidaceae

Chive is a useful vegetable around the world. Its leaves are widely used in Asian cuisine, whereas its seeds and roots are utilized as folk medicines in some countries. According to its nutritional analysis, it is a great source of vitamins K, A, E, and C and of dietary minerals such as molybdenum, magnesium, and phosphorus. Pharmacologically, chive leaves exhibited inhibitory effects on lipid, cholesterol, and platelet aggregation that help in the prevention of cardiovascular diseases. A dictionary of herbal medicines in East Asia indicated that chive leaves are traditionally employed for the treatment of abdominal pain, hematemesis, diarrhea, asthma, and snakebite, whereas the seeds are utilized as a tonic and aphrodisiac.

Scientific Evidence of Cancer-Inhibitory and Cancer-Preventive Constituents

1. Agents from leaves of Chinese chives

The extract of chive leaves demonstrated an *in vitro* suppressive effect against the growth of murine tumor cell lines (B16-F10 melanoma and M5076 sarcoma) and human cancer cell lines (Jurkat lymphoma, T24 bladder, and A549 lung epithelial) with IC_{50}s in a range of 2.5–13.0 mg (raw material)/mL. All the tested cancer cell lines underwent apoptotic death after being *in vitro* exposed to the extract for 4–6 h at 8–100 mg (raw material)/mL concentrations. Daily oral administration of the extract in doses equivalent to 2.5 or 12.5 mg/g (raw material/body weight) for 15 days reduced the lung metastatic colonies of B16–F10 melanoma in mice by 40%; however, IV injection of the extract showed inactive.[1] A fraction derived from the extract containing low-molecular-weight components significantly suppressed the tumor promotion induced by TPA in mouse epidermis.[2] An aqueous extract remarkably reduced the mutant incidents caused by oncogenic agents MNND and BAP *in vitro* together with activation of Rec-A expression and degradation of Lex-A protein.[3] In addition, chive leaf juice and phenolic components in the juice exerted a peroxyl radical (ROO*)-scavenging effect and showed an inductive effect on phenol sulfotransferases in human HepG2 hepatoma cells, showing the antioxidant and cancer-preventive potential of chives.[4,5]

Organosulfur components, such as ajoene, diallyl sulfides, *S*-allylcysteine, and thiosulfinate, have been isolated from the chives, being responsible for the preventive activity in chemical-induced animal carcinoma models and the inhibitory effects on the proliferation of cancer cells.[6,7] When assayed in several human neoplastic cell lines *in vitro*, the thiosulfinates obstructed the proliferation of HepG2 hepatoma cells and A549 lung cancer cells by >60% at a concentration of 20 µg/mL and promoted the apoptosis and cell-cycle arrest of HepG2 cells at a concentration of 30 µg/mL.[8] The thiosulfinates also prominently suppressed the viability of four other human carcinoma cell lines, HT-29 (colon), MCF-7 (breast), PC3, and RC-58T/h/#4 (prostate), together with the induction of cell apoptosis, the mechanism of which was substantiated to follow both caspase-dependent and caspase-independent proapoptotic pathways.[9–12] IP administration of the thiosulfinates to mice in a dose of 10–50 mg/kg for 7 days consecutively obviously prolonged the life span of mice-inoculated sarcoma 180.[12] *S*-Methyl-2-propene-1-thiosulfinate and *S*-methyl methanthiosulfinate were separated from the thiosulfinates and both exerted cytotoxic effects against MCF-7 breast cancer cells *in vitro*. The cytotoxicities were *S*-methyl-2-propene-1-thiosulfinate > thiosulfinates > *S*-methyl methanthiosulfinate.[12]

2. Agents from seeds of chives

Several steroidal saponins discovered from the seeds displayed significant antitumor and antimutant activities.[13] A spirostanol saponin assigned as tuberoside-M (**1**) exerted marked anti-growth effect on human HL-60 promyelocytic leukemia cells with an IC_{50} value of 6.8 µg/mL.[14] A furostanol saponin assigned as protodioscin (**2**) was found exerting the cytotoxic activity against most of the cell growth in a panel of NCI's human cancer cell lines, wherein it selectively suppressed the cell growth of Molt-C leukemia, A549 nonsmall cell lung carcinoma, HCT-116 and SW-620 colon carcinomas, SNB-75 CNS cancer, LOX IMVI melanoma, and renal cancer with GI_{50} values of ≤ 2.0–3.78 µM.[15–16] The growth inhibition on the HL-60 cells by protodioscin (**2**) was closely attributed to the induction of apoptosis, but it was weak to human KATO-III gastric carcinoma cells.[17] Other furostane-type steroidal oligoglycosides and pregnane-type oligoglycosides derived from the chive seeds exhibited lack of activity at their concentrations of 5 µM.[15,16] In addition, a polysaccharide isolated from the seeds at a dose of 40 µg/mL obviously hindered the proliferation of EC9706 human esophagus cancer cells *in vitro* in parallel with the induction of apoptotic death after 48 h of exposure.[18]

CONCLUSION AND SUGGESTION

The above-mentioned scientific investigations clearly substantiated the anticancer and anticarcinogenic properties of both leaves and seeds of chives. However, two different types of phytochemicals—that is, organosulfur components in the leaves and triterpene saponins in the seeds—were found to principally respond to the cancer-inhibitory activities. The chive leaves are the functional food, and it should be recommended for the human diet despite many people who do not like their flavor. Frequent intake of the vegetable would bring many health benefits, including free-radical scavenging and cancer prevention, especially protection of the liver, stomach, colon, lung, prostate, and breast, in addition to other positive health benefits.

OTHER BIOACTIVITIES OF THE CONSTITUENTS

Sulfur-containing compounds in the chives, especially allicin and ajoene, also possess antimicrobial activities, and *S*-allyl-cysteine displayed reductive effects on senescence-related symptoms, including cognition.

REFERENCES

1. Shao, J. et al., 2001. A pilot study on anticancer activities of Chinese leek. *J. Altern. Complem. Med.* 7: 517–522.
2. Shimpo, H. et al., 1998. Inhibitory effects of Kidachi aloe and Chinese chive extracts on TPA-induced tumor promotion in mouse epidermis. *Fujita Gakuen Igakkaishi* 22: 157–163.
3. Lu, D. et al., 1992. Identification of antimutagenic activity in Chinese Chives. *Acad. J. Second Military Med. Univ.* 13: 62–65.
4. Yeh, C.T et al., 2005. Effect of vegetables on human phenolsulfotransferases in relation to their antioxidant activity and total phenolics. *Free Radical Res.* 39: 893–904.
5. Jin, Z.Z. et al., 1994. Inhibitory effects of fifteen kinds of Chinese herbal drugs, vegetables, and chemicals on SOS response. *Zhonghua Yufang Yixue Zazhi* 28: 147–150.
6. Kim, H.J. et al., 1999. Biological functions of organosulfur compounds in Allium vegetables. *Han'guk Sikp'um Yongyang Kwahak Hoechi* 28: 1412–1423.
7. Block, E. et al., 1994. Flavorants from garlic, onion, and other alliums and their cancer-preventive properties. *ACS Symposium Series* 546 (Food Phyto-chemicals for Cancer Prevention I): 84–96.
8. Park, S.Y. et al., 2009. Effects of thiosulfinates isolated from *Allium tuberosum* L. on the growth of human cancer cells. *Han'guk Sikp'um Yongyang Kwahak Hoechi* 38: 1003–1007.
9. Lee, J.H. et al., 2009. Mechanisms of thiosulfinates from *Allium tuberosum* L.-induced apoptosis in HT-29 human colon cancer cells. *Toxicol. Lett.* 188: 142–147.
10. Kim, S.Y. et al., 2008. Induction of apoptosis by thiosulfinates in primary human prostate cancer cells. *Int. J. Oncol.* 32: 869–875.
11. Kim, S.Y. et al., 2008. Thiosulfinates from *Allium tuberosum* L. induce apoptosis via caspase-dependent and -independent pathways in PC-3 human prostate cancer cells. *Bioorg. Med. Chem. Lett.* 18: 199–204.
12. Park, K.W. et al., 2007. Cytotoxic and antitumor activities of thiosulfinates from *Allium tuberosum* L. *J. Agricul. Food Chem.* 55: 7957–7961.
13. Sang, S.M. et al., 2003. Chemistry and bioactivity of *Allium tuberosum* seeds. *ACS Symposium Series* 859 (*Oriental Foods and Herbs*), pp. 317–329.
14. Sang, S.M. et al., 2002. Tuberoside M, a new cytotoxic spirostanol saponin from the seeds of *Allium tuberosum*. *J. Asian Nat. Prods Res.* 4: 69–72.
15. Ikeda, T. et al., 2004. Pregnane- and furostane-type oligoglycosides from the seeds of *Allium tuberosum*. *Chem. Pharm. Bull.* 52: 142–145.
16. Hu, K. et al., 2002. Protodioscin (NSC-698796): Its spectrum of cytotoxicity against 60 human cancer cell lines in an anticancer drug screen panel. *Planta Med.* 68: 297–301.
17. Hibasami, H. et al., 2003. Protodioscin isolated from fenugreek (*Trigonella foenumgraecum* L.) induces cell death and morphological change indicative of apoptosis in leukemic cell line H-60, but not in gastric cancer cell line KATO III. *Int. J. Mol. Med.* 11: 23–26.
18. Zhang, H.B. et al., 2013. The effects of leek seed polysaccharide on the proliferation and apoptosis of human esophagus cancer cell EC9706. *Aibian, Jibian, Tubian* 25: 430–434.

6. CHINESE GARLIC AND SCALLION

薤白 らっきょう白 염교흰

Allium macrostemon and *A. chinense*

Amaryllidaceae

1. R$_1$ = –A, R$_2$ = –C.
3. R$_1$ = –B, R$_2$ = –C.
6. R$_1$ = –B, R$_2$ = –H.

2. R$_1$ = –A, R$_2$ = –C.

5. R$_1$ = –A, R$_2$ = –C.

4. R$_1$ = –B, R$_2$ = –C.

A : -Gal-(4-1)-Glc-(2-1)-Glc
(3-1)-Glc

B : -Gal-(2-1)-Glc　　　C : -Glc

Gal = beta-D-Galactose
Glc = beta-D-Glucose

7. R = –H.
8. R = –beta-D-glucose

The fresh bulbs and leaves of two Alliaceae plants, (1) Chinese garlic (*Allium macrostemon*) and (2) scallions (*A. chinense*), are broadly used as vegetables in East Asian dishes. Both dried bulbs are also used in folk medicine and as an herb. Pharmacological approaches have proved that Chinese garlic and scallion play a variety of biological roles in immunity enhancement, protective effects for myocardial damage, lipid decrease, antioxidants, vessel dilation, anti-inflammation, anticoagulation and antithrombosis, antiasthma, liver drug enzyme inhibition, antiobesity, and antibacterial effects, along with anticarcinogenic property.

SCIENTIFIC EVIDENCE OF CANCER-INHIBITORY AND CANCER-PREVENTIVE ACTIVITIES

These plants were reported to possess antimutation, anticarcinogenic, antitumor, and antioxidant properties. Both *in vitro* and *in vivo* experiments proved that the extracts of *A. macrostemon* could block the biosynthesis of nitrosamines, scavenge nitrites, and restrain mutagens (such as MMC and CP)-caused chromosomal mutation. Its bulb juice and its ether extract showed notable OH-scavenging and DNA-protecting functions in the assays. The extracts also have an ability to increase apoptotic death of sarcoma 180 cells and to inhibit the tumor growth in a mouse model. The TPA-stimulated phospholipid synthesis in HeLa cervical neoplastic cells could be obstructed by the alcoholic extract of Chinese garlic.[1,2] Antibacterial components extracted from *A. chinense* were found to suppress the proliferation of human HepG2 (liver) and HeLa (cervix) carcinoma cell lines along with arrested cell-cycle progression, wherein the components were more sensitive to HepG2 cells than to HeLa cells. When combined with 5-FU (a current anticancer drug), the bioactive components not only markedly enhanced the cytotoxicity of 5-FU against the proliferation of HeLa cervical cancer cells and BGC-823 gastric cancer cells but also diminished the toxicity and side effects of 5-FU on macrophages and lymphocytes. The major bioactive constituents in the components were analyzed to be allyl methyl disulfide, allyl methyl trisulfide, dimethyl tetrasulfide, and dimethyl trisulfide.[3,4]

SCIENTIFIC EVIDENCE OF CANCER-INHIBITORY AND CANCER-PREVENTIVE CONSTITUENTS

Investigations with modern phytochemical techniques found that the plants contained various con-stituents, such as organosulfur components, steroidal saponin, nitrogen compounds, volatile oil, acidic constituents, polysaccharides, proteins, and so on. Besides the organosulfur components were cancer inhibitors which are similar to those found in garlics and onions (see Sections 4 and 5 in Chapter 1) some of the other constituents were found to be also responsible for the cancer growth inhibition and cancer prevention. These findings of the diverse anticancer potentials clearly recom-mended that these vegetables may be beneficial for the prevention of malignant diseases.

1. Volatile oil

In vitro treatment with volatile oil prepared from *A. macrostemon* inhibited the growth of human SGC-7901 gastric carcinoma cells by 60.17% and 93.41%, respectively, in concentrations of 200 and 400 μg/mL.[5] Both *in vitro* and *in vivo* experiments showed that the volatile oil restrained the cell growth of sarcoma 180 and H22 hepatoma. The *in vitro* IC_{50} values were 145.97 and 153.16 μg/mL on S180 and H22 cells, respectively, and the *in vivo* inhibitory rates in high doses of the volatile oil were 60.86% and 52.99% on S180 and H22 cells, respectively.[6] During the treatments, the volatile oil ampli-fied the cell apoptosis in association with enhancing p53 expressions.[5,6] Simultaneously, the volatile oil also augmented the index of spleen and enhanced the proliferation of spleen cells and the phago-cytic function of macrophages in tumor-bearing mice.[7] Therefore, it is recognized that both apoptosis-stimulating and immunoregulating properties of the volatile oil contribute to the anti-growth effect against the neoplastic cells.

2. Steroidal saponins

Total saponins (100 and 200 μg/mL), which were prepared from *A. macrostemon*, could effectively suppress the proliferation and induce apoptosis in human HeLa cervical cancer cells, the mecha-nism of which might be mediated by downregulating Bcl-2 mRNA expression, upregulating Bax mRNA expression, decreasing mitochondrial membrane potential, and augmenting caspase-9 and -3 activities.[8] Many steroidal/furostanol saponins were isolated from the dried bulbs of Chinese garlic, and some of them exhibited selective cytotoxicity to human neoplastic cell lines *in vitro*. At a concentration of 25 μg/mL, macrostemonoside-C (1), XB-saponin-A (2), and XB-saponin-B (3) restrained the growth of SF-268 glioblastoma cells and NCI-H460 lung cancer cells.[9] The IC_{50} values of XB-saponin-C (4) were 25.7 and 35.4 μM, respectively, in NCI-H460 and SF-268 cell lines, and of XB-saponin-D (5) was 35.2 μM in SF-268 cells.[10] Macrostemonoside-O (6) and both 22-isomers of XB-saponin-B (3) were also effective to SF-268 cells (IC_{50}s 8.71, 8.15, and 11.74 μM, respectively), NCI-H460 cells (IC_{50}s 13.62, 10.87, and 26.09 μM, respectively), HepG2 hepatoma cells (IC_{50}s 16.34, 27.17, and 22.28 μM, respectively), and MCF-7 breast carcinoma cells (IC_{50}s 5.45, 12.17, and 24.46 μM, respectively). The saponins (6 and 3) exerted better suppressive effect against drug-resistant hepatoma R-HepG2 cells with IC_{50}s ranging between 8.15 and 11.41 μM.[11,12] Macrostemonoside-A also markedly inhibited the growth of Caco2 and SW480 human colorectal cancer cells together with the induction of cell-cycle arrest and apoptosis via increasing ROS gen-eration and annexin V positively stained cell population and activating caspases. In BALB/c nude mice with a colorectal carcinogenesis xenograft model, intraperitoneal injections of macroste-monoside-A remarkably inhibited tumor formation and reduced tumor volume and tumor weight when treated at daily dosages of 10–100 mg/kg for 35 days.[13]

Similarly, from the active fractions of the bulbs of *A. chinense*, a group of steroidal spirostane saponins were separated.[14] The *A. chinense* saponins (ACSs) in the *in vitro* models obviously elicited tumor cell death and inhibited the proliferation, cell migration, and colony formation of B16 melanoma and 4T1 breast carcinoma cell lines in a dose-dependent manner. IP injection of ACSs to tested mice earlier (on the following day after B16 tumor inoculation) in doses of 200 and 50 mg/mL for 18 days resulted in 62.74% and 54.94% suppressive rates against the growth of melanoma cells *in vivo*, respectively, and effectively protected the liver and spleen of mice from damage as well.[15] Xiebai-saponin-I and laxogenin 3-*O*-α-L-arabinopyranosyl-(1-6)-β-D-glucopyranoside displayed an *in vitro* inhibitory effect against TPA-stimulated[32] Pi-incorporation into phospholipids of human HeLa cervical cancer cells, indicating their cytotoxicity to HeLa cells. Notably, their aglycone named as laxogenin was demonstrated to have an antitumor-promoting activity by an *in vivo* experiment of two-stage lung carcinogenesis.[16]

3. Chalcones

Isoliquiritigenin (**7**) and isoliquiritigenin-4-*O*-glucoside (**8**) were isolated from scallion (*A. chinense*). The two bioactive chalcones showed the inhibitory effect against TPA-stimulated[32] Pi-incorporation into phospholipids in the HeLa cells *in vitro*, where isoliquiritigenin (**7**) exerted far more potent suppressive activity than its glucoside (**8**). In concentrations of 25–50 μg/mL, the inhibitory rates of isoliquiritigenin (**7**) on the viability of HeLa cells reached 95.3%–100%.[16]

4. Polysaccharides

Polysaccharides prepared from *A. chinense* were reported to possess antitumor property besides hypoglycemic, anti-inflammatory, antiviral, and anticoagulating activities.[17] From the dried bulbs of *A. macrostemon*, an active polysaccharide component PAM and three purified polysaccharides, (1) PAM-Ib, (2) PAM-IIa, and (3) PAM-III', were isolated. In *in vitro* antioxidant assays, PAM exhibited an anticarcinogenesis-related radical-scavenging effect, such as concentration-dependent scavenged •OH and $O^{2-•}$ free radicals. However, compared to PAM, PAM-Ib showed less ability in the scavenging of both •OH and $O^{2-•}$ free radicals, and PAM-IIa had no such function, whereas PAM-III' exerted great activity to scavenge •OH radicals only but not $O^{2-•}$ radicals.[18]

5. Proteins

By extraction with 100 mmol/L Tris-HCl buffer solution (pH 7.5) and salting out with ammonium sulfate at different degrees of saturation, several protein extracts were prepared from *A. chinense* bulbs. The protein extracts obtained with 20%–80% saturated ammonium sulfate exhibited potent cytotoxicity against both mouse B16 melanoma and Meth-A fibrosarcoma cell lines. The protein extract with the most potent cytotoxicity could be prepared by 80% saturated ammonium sulfate. Liquid Chromatography-Mass Spectrometry (LC-MS) analysis revealed that the most potent protein extract mainly consisted of alliinase, heat shock protein, lectin, cysteine synthase, and members of tumor necrosis factor receptor superfamily.[19]

CONCLUSION AND SUGGESTION

This scientific evidence highlighted the significance of two vegetables, (1) Chinese garlic and (2) scallion, in cancer prevention and cancer therapy as a supplemental and functional food. Similar to other *Allium* vegetables, the organosulfur components are the major contributors to the anticarcinogenic activities of Chinese garlic and scallion. In addition to those, steroidal saponins, some chalcones, and volatile oil from Chinese garlic and scallion were also found to play a role in the suppression of several types of carcinomas, whereas their macromolecules such as polysaccharides and proteins presented anticarcinogenesis-related radical-scavenging effect and cytotoxicity, respectively. Therefore, the consumption of Chinese garlic and scallion should be encouraged. Compared to the leaves, the bulbs of Chinese garlic and scallion possess more effective biological properties.

REFERENCES

1. Sheng, H.G. 2013. Research progress on chemical constituents and pharmacological actions of *Allium macrostemon* Bunge. *Yaowu Yanjiu (J. Pharm. Res.)* 12: 42–44.
2. Ding, F. et al., 2005. Experiment of Chinese garlic extracts in scavenging hydroxyl free radical and anti-DNA injury. *Zhongyaocai* 287: 592–593.

3. Sun, Y.J. et al., 2007. Roles of bioactive components of *Allium chinense* in increasing efficacy and decreasing toxicity of fluorouracil. *Shipin Kexue* (Beijing, China) 28: 462–465.
4. Sun, Y.J. et al., 2004. Anticancer effects and possible mechanism of antibacterial components from *Allium chinense*. *Shipin Kexue* (Beijing, China) 25: 295–299.
5. Wu, Z.M. et al., 2006. Apoptosis of human gastric cancer cells induced by bulbus of *Allium macrostemon* volatile oil. *Chin. J. Clin. Rehabilit.* 10: 115–117.
6. Zhang, Q. et al., 2003. Study of the volatile oil extracted from *Allium macrostemon* Bunge on antitumor effects. *Tumor* (3): 228–231.
7. Zhang, Q. et al., 2008. Influence of the volatile oil extracted from *Allium macrostemon* Bunge on immune function of mice bearing S18. *J. Med. College of Weifang* 24: 94–95.
8. Luo, T. et al., 2012. Effect of total saponins from *Allium macrostemon* Bunge on proliferation and apoptosis of cervix cancer HeLa cells. *Yinanbing Zazhi* 11: 762–765.
9. Chen, H.F. et al., 2005. Studies on bioactive steroidal saponins of *Allium macrostemon* Bunge. *Zhongguo Yaowu Huaxue Zazhi* 15: 142–147.
10. Chen, H.F. et al., 2009. Two new steroidal saponins from *Allium macrostemon* Bunge and their cytotoxity on different cancer cell lines. *Molecules* 14: 2246–2253.
11. Chen, H.F. et al., 2007. New furostanol saponins from the bulbs of *Allium macrostemon* Bunge and their cytotoxic activity. *Die Pharmazie* 62: 544–548.
12. XB-saponin-A (**2**): (25R)26- *O*-β-D-glucopyranosyl-22-hydroxy-furost-5(6)-en-3β,26-diol-3-*O*-β-D-gluco-pyranosyl(1-2) [β-D-glucopyranosyl(1-3)]-β-D-glucopyranosyl(1-4)-β-D-galactopyranoside; XB-saponin-B (**3**): (25R)26- *O*-β-D-glucopyranosyl-22-hydroxy-5β-furost-3β,26-diol-3-*O*-β-D-glucopyranosyl (1-2)-β-D-galactopyranoside; XB-saponin-C (**4**): 26-*O*-β-D-glucopyranosyl-5β-furost-20(22)-25(27)-dien-3β,12β,26-triol-3-*O*-β-D-gluco-pyranosyl (1-2)-β-D-galactopyranoside; XB-saponin-D (**5**): 26-*O*-β-D-glucopyranosyl-5α-furost-25(27)-ene-3β,12β,22,26-tetraol-3-*O*-β-D-gluco-pyranosyl(1-2) [β-D-glucopyranosyl(1-3)]-β-D-glucopyranosyl(1-4)-β-D-galactopyranoside.
13. Wang, Y.H. et al., 2013. Anti-colorectal cancer activity of macrostemonoside A mediated by reactive oxygen species. *Biochem. Biophys. Res. Commun.* 441: 825–830.
14. Jiang, Y. et al., 1998. Structural elucidation of the anticoagulation and anticancer constituents from *Allium chinense*. *Acta Pharm. Sinica* 33: 355–361.
15. Yu, Z.H. et al., 2015. Anticancer activity of saponins from *Allium chinense* against the B16 melanoma and 4T1 breast carcinoma cells. *Evid.-Based Complem. Alternat. Med.* Vol. 2015, Article ID 725023.
16. Baba, M. et al., 2000. Saponins isolated from *Allium chinense* G. Don and antitumor-promoting activities of isoliquiritigenin and laxogenin from the same drug. *Biol. Pharm. Bull.* 23: 660–662.
17. Xiao, X.N. et al., 2013. Method for preparing *Allium chinense* polysaccharides. *Faming Zhuanli Shenqing* CN 102850463 A 20130102.
18. Xia, X.K. et al., 2007. Studies on anti-oxidant activity of *Allium macrostemon* polysaccharides. *J. Xinyang agric. College* 17: 138–139.
19. Liu, W. et al., 2013. Isolation and antitumor activity of proteins from *Allium chinense* bulbs. *Shipin Kexue* (Beijing, China) 34: 300–302.

7. LEEK

Poireau Lauch Puerro

韭葱 リーキ 부추

Allium ampeloprasum var. *porrum, A. porrum*

Amaryllidaceae

1. R = − OH
3. R = −− OH

2. $R_1 = R_2 = H$
6. R1= =O, R2 = gal (4-1)-glc-(3-1)-xyl
    |
    (2-1)-glc

4

5

7. R = −rham
8. R = −rham-(4-1)-xyl

gal = beta-D-galactopyranose
glc = beta-D-glucopyranose
xyl = beta-D-xylopyranose
rham = alpha-L-rhamnopyranose

Leeks (*Allium ampeloprasum* var. *porrum* and *A. porrum*) are commonly employed as a vegetable in many parts of Europe, America, and Asia. Leeks have been cultivated in Central Asia and Europe for thousands of years and their wild original plant is native to Central Asia. Another two cultivars of *A. ampeloprasum* are kurrat (var. *kurrat*) and elephant garlic (var. *ampeloprasum*); kurrat is also called Egyptian leek. The three cultivars are all used as health-promoting vegetables. Nutritionally, leeks afford noteworthy vitamins such as vitamins K, C, and E and folate and small amounts of minerals such as potassium, iron, calcium, magnesium, and manganese. Their health benefits essentially present anti-oxidant, antibacterial, antiviral, antifungal, and anti-inflammatory activities. Due to having significant amounts of kaempferol, a diet of leeks helps to protect our blood vessels from damage in addition to its cytostatic and anti-inflammatory effects.[1] As an *Allium* vegetable, leeks have a mild onion-like taste and contain many health-supportive substances that are similar to those in onions and garlic.

SCIENTIFIC EVIDENCE OF CANCER-INHIBITORY AND CANCER-PREVENTIVE ACTIVITIES

In an *in vitro* assay, the juices of leek, green onion (shallot or scallion), yellow onion, and garlic (in 1/20 dilution of 166 mg raw vegetable per mL) showed antiproliferative effects against eight human cell lines such as MCF-7 mammary gland adenocarcinoma, AGS stomach adenocarcinoma, Panc-1 pancreatic carcinoma, A549 lung carcinoma, PC-3 prostatic adenocarcinoma, Daoy medulloblastoma, U-87 MG glioblastoma, and Caki-2 renal cancer, wherein AGS cells were mostly sensitive to these *Allium* samples and the following sensitivities were Daoy cells > U-87MG cells > MCF-7 cells > Panc-1 cells > PC3 cells > A549 cells > Caki-2 cells. Except garlic, leek and green onion exerted the second and third strongest inhibitory effect on the tested cell lines. However, in Caki-2 cells, the effect of leeks was more potent than that of garlic, whereas yellow onion had no inhibition. The experimental approaches noticeably evidenced the chemopreventive values of the five *Allium* vegetables, including leeks.[2]

SCIENTIFIC EVIDENCE OF CANCER-INHIBITORY AND CANCER-PREVENTIVE CONSTITUENTS

Bioactivity-combined phytochemical approaches revealed four types of bioactive components in leek—that is, (1) organosulfur components, (2) spirosteroid sapogenins and their saponins, (3) steroidal glycosides, and (4) flavonoids. Similar to other *Allium* vegetables (garlics and onions), organosulfur components in leeks served as the major inhibitors against cancer-cell proliferation, carcinogenesis, and oxidative damage (see Sections 4 and 5 in Chapter 1). Though leeks contain proportionately fewer thiosulfinites than garlic but the same as in onions, they still possess significant amounts of the organosulfur components such as diallyl disulfide, diallyl trisulfide, and allyl propyl disulfide. Moreover, some isolated spirosteroids and steroidal glycosides have also been reported to have anticancer properties, whereas the isolated flavonoids were significant antioxidants.

1. Spirosteroids

Several spirosteroid sapogenins were isolated from leeks and evaluated in an *in vitro* assay. Porrigenins-A (**1**), -B (**2**), agigenin (**3**), 12-keto-porrigenin (**4**), and 2,3-seco-porrigenin (**5**) showed moderate to weak suppressive effects on the proliferation of four types of tumor cell lines: (1) IGR-I human melanoma, (2) P388 murine lymphocytic leukemia, (3) WEHI164 murine fibrosarcoma, and (4) J774 murine monocyte/macrophage. Among them, the most potent activities were achieved by 2,3-seco-porrigenin (**5**) on P388 cells (IC_{50} of >30 μg/mL) and J774 cells (IC_{50} of >40 μg/mL) and next by porrigenin-B (**2**) on the four tumor cell lines (IC_{50}s 45–92 μg/mL, 72 h). The sensitivities of the tested cell lines to the spirosteroid sapogenins were P388 > J774 > IGR-I > WEHI 164.[3,4] Likewise, five spirostanol saponins separated from bulbs of *A. porrum* (collected in September) were effective to J-774 and WEHI-164 cell lines with IC_{50}s of 2.1–27.9 μg/mL and 1.9–21.1 μg/mL, respectively. The IC_{50}s of (25α)-3β,6β-dihydroxy-5α-spirostan-2,12-dione-3-*O*-*O*-β-D-glucosyl(1-2)-*O*-[β-D-xylosyl(1-3)]-*O*-β-D-glucosyl(1-4)-β-D-galactoside (**6**) were 5.8 μg/mL in J-774 cells and 4.3 μg/mL in WEHI-164 cells.[5] This evidence indicated that the saponins from leek bulbs were more potent than the sapogenins from leeks but that all of them can be used as cancer-preventing compounds.

2. Cholestane glycosides

From bulbs of *A. porrum* (collected in January), two cholestane glycosides elucidated as 22S-cholest-5-ene-1β,3β,16β, 22-tetrol 1-*O*-α-L-rhamnopyranosyl 16-*O*-β-D-galactopyranoside (**7**) and 22S-cholest-5-ene-1β,3β,16β,22-tetrol 1-*O*-[β-D-glucopyranosyl-(1-4)-α-L-rhamno-pyranoside] 16-*O*-β-D-galactopyranoside (**8**) were separated together with traces of the above-mentioned spirostanol saponins. These cholestane glycosides (**7** and **8**) exerted a similar level of inhibitory effect on the J-774 and WEHI-164 cell lines *in vitro* (IC_{50}s 4.0–5.8 μg/mL).[5]

CONCLUSION AND SUGGESTION

Similar to other *Allium* vegetables, organosulfur components in leeks served as the major inhibitors against cancer-cell proliferation and growth, carcinogenesis, and oxidative damage. When crushing and cutting leek stalk, the leek organosulfur compounds convert to allicin by enzymatic reaction, in which allicin plays remarkable biological functions in cancer prevention, suppression, and antioxidant (see Sections 4 and 5 in Chapter 1 and Sections 18 and 19 in Chapter 3). The discovered spirosteroids and cholestane glycosides from leek are also considered to be cancer preventers together with the leek organosulfur components. Therefore, leeks are obsolutely considered as a vegetable that can help us to prevent cancer initiation.

REFERENCES

1. Rajendran, P. et al., 2014. Kaempferol, a potential cytostatic and cure for inflammatory disorders. *Eur. J. Med. Chem.* 86: 103–112.
2. Dominique, B. et al., 2009. Antiproliferative and antioxidant activities of common vegetables: A comparative study. *Food Chem.* 112: 374–380.
3. Carotenuto, A. et al., 1997. Porrigenins A and B, novel cytotoxic and antiproliferative sapogenins isolated from *Allium porrum*. *J. Nat. Prod.* 60: 1003–1007.
4. Carotenuto, A. et al., 1997. 12-Keto-porrigenin and the unique 2,3-seco-porrigenin, new antiproliferative sapogenins from *Allium porrum*. *Tetrahedron* 53: 3401–3406.
5. Fattorusso, E. et al., 2000. Cytotoxic saponins from bulbs of *Allium porrum* L. *J. Agric. Food Chem.* 48: 3455–3462.

8. SPINACH

Épinard Spinat Espinaca

菠菜 ほうれん草 시금치

Spinacia oleracea

Amaranthaceae

1. R = –gal

2. R = –gal-(6-1)-gal

gal: beta-D-galactose

Spinach is one of the world's healthiest and favorite vegetables. It is an excellent source of vitamins K, A, and C and folic acid and a good source of manganese, magnesium, iron, and vitamin B2. Spinach embraces many health-promoting phytonutrients such as chlorophylls, carotenoids, polyphenols, and flavonoids; thus, it affords multiple functions such as powerful antioxidant protection, significant protection in the prostate and colon, bone health maintenance, anti-inflammatory, antihistaminic, CNS depressant, and γ-radiation protection.

SCIENTIFIC EVIDENCE OF CANCER-INHIBITORY AND CANCER-PREVENTIVE CONSTITUENTS

In an azoxymethane-induced rat model, a dietary supplement of spinach diminished the numbers of aberrant crypt foci in the colon and hampered the early initiation in colorectal carcinogenesis.[1] The consumption of spinach could retard the occurrence of aggressive prostate cancer. *In vitro* assay showed that the growth of human YTMLC-90 lung cancer cells was inhibited by a crude nonpolar extract of spinach.[2] Weak cytotoxic effects were observed against A549 lung cancer and K562 bone cancer cell lines after treatment with spinach ethanolic extract.[3] More experiments have been performed for exploring the correlation between spinach constituents and cancer prevention. The results revealed that chlorophylls, glycoglycerolipids, carotenoids, and polyphenols in spinach are responsible for spinach bioactivities, including anticarcinogenesis.

1. Chlorophyll-related compounds

Chlorophyll-a and chlorophyll-b are two lipid-soluble pigments that commonly exist in spinach and other green vegetables. In an *in vitro* assay, chlorophyll showed 60%–80% growth inhibitory effects against five human cancer cell lines such as HCT-116 (colon), AGS (stomach), NCI-H460 (lung), central nervous system (CNS), and MCF-7 (breast) cells, with IC_{50}s between 11 and 18 μg/mL.[4] Chlorophyll-a and chlorophyll-b at concentrations of >10 nM could suppress the proliferation of U87 glioblastoma cells. When the concentration was increased to 100 nM, the U87 cell proliferation was inhibited with decreased phosphorylation of phosphatase and tensin homolog deleted on chromosome 10 (PTEN), indicating the cytostatic activity of chlorophylls.[5] Likewise, the anti-carcinogenic, antimutagenic, and antigenotoxic properties of chlorophylls were demonstrated by both *in vitro* and *in vivo* investigations. *In vivo* approaches revealed that administration of chloro-phylls by gavage dose-dependently deterred the hepatic aflatoxin B1 (AFB1)-DNA adduction and dibenzo[a, l]pyrene (DBP)-DNA adduction to exert anticarcinogenic activity.[6,7] The genotoxicity of 4-nitroquinoline 1-oxide (4NQO) in *Drosophila* could be suppressed by simultaneous administra-tion of chlorophylls orally, and the mutagenicity of 3-hydroxyamino-1-methyl-5H-pyrido[4,3-b] indole in *Salmonella* could be inhibited by the chlorophylls.[8] Heme is produced after red meat consumption, and the heme enhances the cytotoxicity of colonic content and retards colonocyte proliferation in a rat model. However, the study revealed that spinach chlorophylls with heme were able to completely restrain the heme that caused detrimental, cytotoxic, and hyperproliferative effects, thereby lessening the risk of colon cancer.[9] Therefore, chlorophylls have been proven as an important contributor not only for nutrition but also for cancer prevention, and frequently intake of spinach as well as green vegetables should be highly encouraged.

2. Glycoglycerolipids

A glycoglycerolipid fraction extracted from spinach and some other green vegetables showed the inhibitory effects against DNA polymerases and cancer-cell proliferation *in vitro*. Its LD_{50}s were 58–70 µg/mL in human NUGC-3 gastric cancer and HL-60 promyelocytic leukemia cell lines.[10] In both *in vitro* and *in vivo* models, this fraction deterred the growth of human HeLa cervix carcinoma cells with LD_{50} of 57.2 µg/mL.[11] Oral administration of the fraction to mice in a dose of 20 mg/kg for 2 weeks hindered the growth of colon-26 tumor cells and lessened 56.1% solid tumor volume, associating with inhibition of proliferating cell nuclear antigen (PCNA) and cyclin-E and blockage of angiogenesis in tumor tissue.[10,12] Similarly, orally giving the glycolipid fraction (70 mg/kg) or a complex of the fraction and γ-cyclodextrin for 2 weeks reduced sarcoma formation with no adverse reactions in mice, and administration of the fraction resulted in the suppression on Greene melanoma in hamsters.[11,13] An acute toxicity test showed the oral dose for the glycoglycerolipid fraction safely reaching to 2000 mg/kg.[14] More studies further revealed that the glycoglycerolipid fraction also repressed the activity of DNA polymerases (α, δ, and ε) with IC_{50}s of 44.0–46.2 µg/mL, and the inhibitory effect on the polymerases may lead to the anti-growth and antiangiogenic effects.[10,14,15] Therefore, the glycoglycerolipid fraction of spinach is a safe and effective inhibitor for the anticarcinogenesis.

Three major glycoglycerolipids: (1) monogalactosyl diacylglycerol (MGDG, **1**), (2) digalactosyl diacylglycerol (DGDG, **2**), and (3) sulfoquinovosyl diacylglycerol (SQDG) were separated from the fraction, in which highest content of MGDG was found in spinach, kale, sugar peas, and green beans.[16–20] In TPA-induced Epstein–Barr virus (EBV) activation, both MGDG and DGDG showed antitumor-promoting activity.[17] MGDG and SQDG also inhibited microvessel growth in an *ex vivo* angiogenesis model and obstructed human umbilical vein endothelial cell (HVUEC) proliferation and tube formation in an *in vitro* HVUEC model.[18] The inhibitory potencies on DNA polymerases were MGDG (**1**) > SQDG > DGDG (**2**).[15] As a potent inhibitor of replicative DNA polymerases, MGDG (**1**) exerted an anti-growth effect on NUGC-3 gastric cancer cells, but DGDG (**2**) and SQDG had no such effect.[19] MGDG (**1**) also suppressed the proliferation of Colon-26 mouse colon cancer cells and human pancreatic cancer cell lines (BxPC-3, MIAPaCa2, and PANC-1). The LD_{50} was 24 µg/mL in Colon-26 cells *in vitro*. When a complex of MGDG and γ-cyclodextrin was admin-istered orally for 26 days in an equivalent dose of 20 mg/kg, the tumor volume of Colon-26 was reduced by ~60% and the mitosis of tumor cells was lessened via decrease of PCNA-positive cells, inhibition of CD31-positive tumor blood vessel growth, and increase of terminal deoxynucleotidyl transferase dUTP nick-end labeling (TUNEL)-positive apoptotic cells.[20] If MGDG is combined with gemcitabine (GEM, a chemotherapeutic drug often used for the treatment of pancreatic cancer), the effects could be synergistically enhanced in the inhibition of DNA replicative pols α and γ activities and of cancer-cell proliferation.[21] Moreover, liposomes (SLX-Lipo-MGDG) that were made of MGDG (1) and surface-bound sialyl Lewis X (SLX) demonstrated more potent inhibitory effect against human HT-29 colon adenocarcinoma in a nude model, indicating that the liposomes may be useful for actively targeting drug delivery systems.[22] On the basis of these results, MGDG (1) could be considered to have great potential for cancer prevention and chemotherapy as a food supplement.

3. Carotenoids

Neoxanthin (3), a 5,6-monoepoxy carotenoid isolated from spinach, was found to diminish the cell proliferation and viability via apoptosis induction in human prostate cancer cell lines. After 72 h treatment, neoxanthin (3) significantly reduced the prostate cancer-cell viability to 10.9% for PC3 cells, 15.0% for DU-145 cells, but nearly zero for LNCaP cells.[23] In an *in vivo* experiment, neoxanthin (3) by oral administration was partially converted into stereoisomers, 8'-R/S neochrome, by intragastric acidity before intestinal absorption. 8'-R/S-Neochromes and neoxanthin at ≥20 μmol/L concentration dose-dependently inhibited the proliferation of PC3 cells, but inhibition in the PC3 tumor cells was mediated by induction of cytostasis without obvious induction of apoptosis.[24] Spinach carotene and β-carotene could retrade 80%–85% viability of human leukemia cell lines: HL-60 (promyelocytic leukemia), ML-1 (acute myeloblastic leukemia), and ML-2 (acute myelo-monocytic leukemia). The spinach carotenoids also showed a weak differentiation-inducing activity on the three types of human leukemia cell lines, but purified neoxanthin and lutein showed no activity on the leukemia cells.[25]

4. Antioxidants

Dietary antioxidants present in vegetables contribute both the first and second defense lines against oxidative stress, leading to cancer prevention. The major antioxidants in vegetables are water-soluble polyphenols and vitamin C and lipid-soluble vitamin E and carotenoids. The phenolics, especially flavonoids, demonstrated remarkable biological activities, and the most important are antioxidant and ROS-scavenging activities, capillary protective effect, and inhibitory effect on various stages of tumor. Spinach has higher content of total phenolics than yellow onion, red pepper, carrot, cabbage, potato, lettuce, celery, and cucumber but less than broccoli.[26] The rich phenolics in spinach exerted marked inhibitory effects on human HepG2 hepatoma cells and on lipoxygenase and oxidation.[26] A water-soluble phenolic extract derived from spinach juice significantly scavenged hydroxyl radicals and retarded the viability of HL-60 leukemia cells to 47%.[27] In a mouse model, dietary spinach natural antioxidant (NAO) lessened oxidative/nitrosative injuries in the early stage of prostatic tumor lesions,[28] and in an *in vitro* model with PC3 prostate cancer cells, the spinach NAO arrested cell-cycle progression by downregulation of ppRb and E2F protein expression and reduction of cyclin-A and CDK-2 activities.[29] In addition, pretreatment with the spinach NAO in a cumulative dose of 130 mg/kg could reduce doxorubicin-induced heart injury via repressing catalase and enhancing superoxide dismutase activities.[30]

Two hydroxycinnamic acids termed E-ferulic acid and E-*p*-coumaric acid normally existed in the spinach cell wall by ester linkages with the cell wall polysaccharides. The hydroxycinnamic acids were capable of inhibiting xenobiotic-metabolizing enzyme activity, COX expression, and cytochrome P450 1A in HT-29 colon cancer cells, leading to protection against oxidative stress and genotoxicity.[31] Moreover, comparing the antioxidant potencies of common vegetables and foods disclosed the order of potencies to be garlic > asparagus > spinach > beet > bell pepper > mushroom > broccoli > cabbage > corn > onion > bean > carrot > cauliflower > sweet potato > tomato > potato > lettuce > squash > celery > cucumber. In addition, the antioxidative effect of spinach NAO was superior to that of green tea, *N*-acetylcysteine, butylated hydroxytoluene, and vitamin E.[32,33] Accordingly, the evidence implied that the function of these vegetables [spinach already included in list] may play an important role in the cancer prevention and the protection of cardio- and cerebrovascular systems, without any target-organ toxicity and side effects.[32,33]

5. Macromolecules

A nondialyzable extract from spinach showed the suppressive abilities against the mutagenicity of Trp-P-1, Trp-P-2, MNNG, BAP, and aflatoxin B1 on *Salmonella typhimurium* TA 100 and TA 98, and against the growth of neoplastic cell lines, such as MCF-7 breast cancer, HuH-7 differentiated hepatoma, QG-90 lung carcinoma, and other cancer cells. The extract can also activate macrophage-like cells to elicit the differentiation of human U937 and HL-60 leukemia cells into macrophage or monocyte cells and exert strong antioxidant effect against oxidation of linoleic acid.[34,35] By Sephadex G100 and G25 chromatographies, four fractions were derived from the nondialyzable extract. Among them, fractions SPW2-3 and SPW2-4 exhibited the anti-growth effect on MCF-7 cells, and SPW2-3 exerted antiviability on cancer cell lines such as HuH-7 hepatoma, PC-8 lung adenocarcinoma, QG-56 lung squamous carcinoma, and QG-90 lung anaplastic carcinoma as well, but less effect on normal cells. A heat-stable glycoprotein (m.w. 16,000) was detected as one of the bioactive principles in the SPW2-3 fraction.[35,36]

NANOFORMULATION

The aqueous extract of spinach has been utilized to synthesize bioinspired silver nanoparticles (AgNPs) and gold nanoparticles (AuNPs). The two types of nanoparticles were cytotoxic to mouse C2C12 myoblast cancer cells even at very low concentrations (5 μg/mL), associated with the induction of cell apoptosis via activation of caspases-3 and -7. However, in a zebrafish embryo toxicity model, the AgNPs at 3 μg/mL concentration caused 100% mortality potency of which was 100-fold higher than that of AuNPs.[37] When AuNPs combined with poly(ethylene glycol) double acrylates (PEGDA) to form a AuNRs/spinach extract/PEGDA composite hydrogel, it works as a photosensitizer to accelerate cytotoxic singlet oxygen (1O2) generation, resulting in the destruction of cancer cells and protection of normal tissues. Under NIP-light irritation, the photodynamic treatment with this nanocomposite hydrogel could synergistically and efficiently achieve its curative effect against the carcinomas.[38]

CONCLUSION AND SUGGESTION

The scientific evidence disclosed that the anticancer and anticarcinogenic properties of spinach should be attributed to the combinational effect of its bioactive components such as chlorophylls, glycoglycerolipids, carotenoids, antioxidants (phenolics and flavonoids), and some macromolecules. Most of these components are antioxidative agents, indicating that the cancer-suppressive activity of spinach is largely associated with their antioxidant and radical-scavenging potencies. The rich nutrients and biovaluable phytochemicals in spinach resulted in high benefits in cancer prevention and healing naturally. Hence, it is strongly recommended that frequent consumption of spinach either cooked or raw as in salad is a smart and safe means to help stave off this malignant disease.

REFERENCES

1. Rijken, P.J. 1999. Effect of vegetable and carotenoid consumption on aberrant crypt multiplicity, a surrogate end-point marker for colorectal cancer in azoxymethane-induced rats. *Carcinogenesis* 20: 2267–2272.
2. He, T. et al., 1998. Influence on in vitro growth of human lung cancer cell line YTMLC-90 of vegetable fat-soluble crude extract. *Zhongguo Gonggong Weisheng Xuebao* 17: 88–89.
3. Asija, R. et al., 2015. Evaluation of anticancer activity of ethanolic extract of *Spinacia oleracea* by high throughput screening. *Intl. J. Pharm. Sci. Rev. Res.* 33: 225–227.
4. Reddy, M.K. et al., 2005. Relative inhibition of lipid peroxidation, cyclooxygenase enzymes, and human tumor cell proliferation by natural food colors. *J.Agricult. Food Chem.* 53: 9268–9273.
5. Kim, S.A. et al., 2011. Growth inhibitory effect of chlorophylls in cultured U87 glioblastoma cells. *Curr. Top. Nutraceut. Res.* 9: 123–130.

6. Breinholt, V. et al., 1995. Mechanisms of chlorophyllin anticarcinogenesis against aflatoxin B1: Complex formation with the carcinogen. *Chem. Res. Toxicol.* 8: 506–514.

7. Harttig, U. et al., 1998. Chemoprotection by natural chlorophylls in vivo: Inhibition of dibenzo[a, l] pyrene-DNA adducts in rainbow trout liver. *Carcinogenesis* 19: 1323–1326.

8. Negishi, T. et al., 1997. Antigenotoxic activity of natural chlorophylls. *Mut. Res.* 376: 97–100.

9. de Vogel, J. et al., 2005. Green vegetables, red meat and colon cancer: Chlorophyll prevents the cytotoxic and hyperproliferative effects of haem in rat colon. *Carcinogenesis* 26: 387–393.

10. Maeda, N. et al., 2008. Inhibitory effects of preventive and curative orally administered spinach glycoglycerolipid fraction on the tumor growth of sarcoma and colon in mouse graft models. *Food Chem.* Volume Date 2009, 112: 205–210.

11. Maeda, N. et al., 2007. Antitumor effects of the glycolipids fraction from spinach which inhibited DNA polymerase activity. *Nutr. Cancer* 57: 216–223.

12. Maeda, N. et al., 2008. Antitumor effect of orally administered spinach glycolipid fraction on implanted cancer cells, Colon-26, in mice. *Lipids* 43: 741–748.

13. Maeda, N. et al., 2005. Effects of DNA polymerase inhibitory and antitumor activities of lipase-hydrolyzed glycolipid fractions from spinach. *J. Nutr. Biochem.* 16: 121–128.

14. Kuriyama, I. et al., 2005. Inhibitory effects of glycolipids fraction from spinach on mammalian DNA polymerase activity and human cancer cell proliferation. *J. Nutr. Biochem.* 16: 594–601.

15. Maeda, N. et al., 2011. Anticancer effect of spinach glycoglycerolipids as angiogenesis inhibitors based on the selective inhibition of DNA polymerase activity. *Mini-Rev. Med. Chem.* 11: 32–38.

16. Larsen, E. et al., 2007. Common vegetables and fruits as a source of 1,2-di-*O*-α-linolenoyl-3-*O*-β-D-galactopyranosyl-sn-glycerol, a potential anti-inflammatory and antitumor agent. *J. Food Lipids* 14: 272–279.

17. Shirahashi, H. et al., 1993. Isolation and identification of antitumor-promoting principles from freshwater cyanobacterium Phormidium tenue. *Chem. Pharm. Bull.* 41: 1664–1666.

18. Matsubara, K. et al., 2005. Inhibitory effect of glycolipids from spinach on in vitro and ex vivo angiogenesis. *Oncol. Rep.* 14: 157–160.

19. Murakami, C. et al., 2003. Effects of glycolipids from spinach on mammalian DNA polymerases. *Biochem. Pharmacol.* 65: 259–267.

20. Maeda, N. et al., 2013. Oral administration of monogalactosyl diacylglycerol from spinach inhibits colon tumor growth in mice. *Exper. Therap. Med.* 5: 17–22.

21. Akasaka, H. et al., 2013. Monogalactosyl diacylglycerol, a replicative DNA polymerase inhibitor, from spinach enhances the anti-cell proliferation effect of gemcitabine in human pancreatic cancer cells. *Biochimica et Biophysica Acta*, 1830: 2517–2525.

22. Mizushina, Y. et al., 2012. In vivo antitumor effect of liposomes with sialyl Lewis X including monogalactosyl diacylglycerol, a replicative DNA polymerase inhibitor, from spinach. *Oncol. Rep.* 28: 821–828.

23. Kotake-Nara, E. et al., 2001. Carotenoids affect proliferation of human prostate cancer cells. *J. Nutr.* 131: 3303–3306.

24. Asai, A. et al., 2004. An epoxide-furanoid rearrangement of spinach neoxanthin occurs in the gastrointestinal tract of mice and in vitro: Formation and cytostatic activity of neochrome stereoisomers. *J. Nutr.* 134: 2237–2243.

25. Takagi, S. et al., 1992. Effect of spinach carotenoids on differentiation of some human leukemia cell lines. *Okayama Daigaku Nogakubu Gakujutsu Hokoku* 80: 7–15.

26. Chu, Y.F. et al., 2002. Antioxidant and antiproliferative activities of common vegetables. *J. Agricul. Food Chem.* 50: 6910–6916.

27. Roy, M.K. et al., 2007. Antioxidant potential, anti-proliferative activities, and phenolic content in water-soluble fractions of some commonly consumed vegetables: Effects of thermal treatment. *Food Chem.* 103: 106–114.

28. Tam, N.N.C. et al., 2005. Differential attenuation of oxidative/nitrosative injuries in early prostatic neoplastic lesions in TRAMP mice by dietary antioxidants. *Prostate* (Hoboken, NJ, US) (2005), Volume Date 2006, 66: 57–69.

29. Bakshi, S. et al., 2004. Unique natural antioxidants (NAOs) and derived purified components inhibit cell cycle progression by downregulation of ppRb and E2F in human PC3 prostate cancer cells. *FEBS Lett.* 573: 31–37.

30. Breitbart, E. et al., 2001. Effects of water-soluble antioxidant from spinach, NAO, on doxorubicin-induced heart injury. *Human Exper. Toxicol.* 20: 337–345.

31. Ferguson, L.R. et al., 2005. Antioxidant and antigenotoxic effects of plant cell wall hydroxycinnamic acids in cultured HT-29 cells. *Mol. Nutr. Food Res.* 49: 585–593.

32. Sun, T. et al., 2007. Antioxidants and antioxidant activities of vegetables. *ACS Symposium Series*, 956 (*Antioxidant Measurement and Applications*), pp. 160–183.

33. Lomnitski, L. et al., 2003. Composition, efficacy, and safety of spinach extracts. *Nutr. Cancer* 46: 222–231.

34. Shinohara, K. et al., 1997. Anticancer functions of nondialyzable extracts of vegetables and fruits. In: Ohigashi, H. (Ed.), *Food Factors for Cancer Prevention*, (*International Conference on Food Factors: Chemistry and Cancer Prevention*), Hamamatsu, Japan, December 1995, pp. 170–173.

35. Kobori, M. et al., 1993. Effects of spinach extract on the differentiation of the human promyelocytic cell line HL-60. *Biosci. Biotech. Biochem.* 57: 1951–1952.

36. Shinohara, K. et al., 1993. Desmutagenic effect of vegetables on mutagens and carcinogens and growth-inhibiting effect of spinach components on cultured human cancer cells. In: Waldron, K.W., Johnson, I.T., and Fenwick, G.R. (Eds.), *Food and Cancer Prevention: Chemical and Biological Aspects*, Woodhead Publishing, Cambridge, UK, pp. 238–242.

37. Ramachandran, R. et al., 2017. Anticancer activity of biologically synthesized silver and gold nanoparticles on mouse myoblast cancer cells and their toxicity against embryonic zebrafish. *Mater. Sci. Eng. C.* 73: 674–683.

38. Wang, Y.L. et al., 2014. Preparation and multiple antitumor properties of AuNRs/Spinach Extract/PEGDA composite hydrogel. *ACS Appl. Mater. Inter.* 6(17): 15000–15006.

2 Cancer-Preventive Substances in Fruit and Flower Vegetables

9. Artichoke/*Cynara cardunculus* var. *scolymus*

10. Bitter Gourd or Bitter Melon/*Momordica charantia*

11. Cochinchin Gourd or Gac Fruit/*Momordica cochinchinensis*

12. Eggplant/*Solanum melongena*

13. Myoga Ginger/*Zingiber mioga*

14. Okra/*Abelmoschus esculentus*

15. Pumpkin/*Cucurbita moschata, C. pepo, C. maxima*

16. Tomato/*Lycopersicon esculentum* (= *Solanum lycopersicum*)

Probably 40 fruit vegetables and 6 flower vegetables are classified in the list of widespread vegetables. In the fruit vegetable category, almost 50% originate from the plants of Cucurbitaceae, commonly known as cucumbers, gourds, melons, squashes, zucchinis, pumpkins, and luffa; 25% are from the plants of Solanaceae, which include tomatoes, eggplants, and peppers, and several are from the plants of Fabaceae, which include peas and green beans. The fruit vegetables are tightly connected with human dietary life and nutritional intake. These fruits are higher in calories than green vegetables and are rich in vitamin C. Most fruit vegetables are also functional foods, as consumption is linked to their physiological activities such as antioxidant, anticarcinogenesis, antimutagenesis, anti-inflammation, antidiabetes, and several other health-improving benefits. This chapter selects five fruit vegetables as examples to extensively discuss their potential in cancer prevention and body safeguard action. Flower vegetables are a small group, with only six or seven types, so three of them that have body-protective functions are covered in this chapter. Broccoli and cauliflower may count as the most common flower vegetables, yet discussions regarding these two are combined into the section on Brassicaceae vegetables in Chapter 1.

9. ARTICHOKE

Artichaut   Artischocke   Alcachofa

洋薊 アーティチョーク 아티초크

Cynara cardunculus var. *scolymus*

Asteraceae

Artichoke (*Cynara cardunculus* var. *scolymus*) is an Asteraceae plant cultivated as a vegetable. Its edible portions are the flower buds, collected before the flowers bloom. The flower bud is broadly consumed in the Western diet, especially the Mediterranean diet. The United States Department of Agriculture (USDA) nutrition data showed that fresh artichoke (100 g) provides good sources of vitamins C (20%) and K (12%), folates (17%), dietary fiber (14%), vitamin B complex, and minerals (copper, iron, magnesium, manganese, and phosphorus). Pharmacological experiments have established that the flower buds of artichoke possess hepatoprotective, choleretic, cholesterol-lowering, bile-expelling, diuretic, antioxidative, anti-inflammatory, immunomodulating, antiatherosclerotic, antithrombotic, anti-HIV, and antibacterial properties.[1,2]

SCIENTIFIC EVIDENCE OF CANCER-PREVENTIVE ACTIVITIES AND CONSTITUENTS

The antitumor activity of artichoke flowers was shown in an *in vivo* mouse model, where its methanol extract exerted a remarkable inhibitory effect against two-stage carcinogenesis induced by 7,12-dimethylbenz[a]anthracene as an initiator and 12-*O*-tetradecanoylphorbol-13-acetate (TPA) as a promoter.[3] An ethyl acetate–soluble fraction derived from involucral bracts *C. cardunculus* at concentrations of 500–2500 μg/μL dose-dependently inhibited the growth of L1210 and HL-60 leukemia cells, together with induction of G0/G1 cell-cycle arrest after 24-h treatment. The antiproliferative activity of the fraction in HL-60 cells was associated with elicitation of apoptotic death apoptosis via a mitochondrial/caspase-dependent pathway, including an release of cytochrome-c, caspase-9/-3 activations, and specific proteolytic cleavage of poly(ADP-ribose) polymerase.[4] The hexane extracts of artichoke (collected in Turkey) in 0.1–1 mg/mL concentrations elicited apoptotic death of human DLD-1 colorectal cancer cells via an intrinsic apoptotic pathway, including an increase of the Bax/Bcl-2 ratio and upregulation of p21 (a cyclin-dependent kinase inhibitor).[5] In addition, a leaf extract of *C. scolymus* was highly effective in the suppression of cell proliferation and colony formation of mesothelioma cell lines (MSTO-211H, MPP-89, and NCI-H28) *in vitro* and *in vivo*, implying a therapeutic potential for treatment of mesothelioma.[6]

The edible parts in the flowers and leaves of artichokes represent a potent source of phenol fractions, which are potential chemopreventive and anticancer dietary components. As compared with the heart part of artichoke, the bracts of artichoke showed a higher content of total free phenolic compounds and higher free-radical scavenging and antioxidant activities, and both inner and outer parts of artichoke showed lower levels of bound phenolic compounds. After treatment with the free phenolic extract of bracts, the suppressive and apoptosis-triggering effects of the free phenolic extract were observed in HepG2 hepatoma cells.[7] Treatment with the phenolic-rich extract (100–400 μM) for 6 days resulted in an antiproliferative effect on estrogen receptor–negative MDA-MB-231 and BT549 and estrogen receptor–positive T47D and MCF-7 human breast cancer cell lines. The proliferation of MDA-MB-231 cells was completely obstructed at a 400-μM concentration and 60%, and more than 80% MDA-MB-231 cells died after treatment with the extract at 600 μM and 800 μM, respectively; however, it did not have any cytotoxic effect on MCF10A normal breast epithelial cells.[8] The high doses of phenolic extracts could induce apoptosis and decrease the invasive potential of the MDA-MB-231 cells via a p53-independent apoptotic pathway, a reactive oxygen species (ROS)-mediated mechanism, increase of p21(Waf1), increase of Bax:Bcl-2 ratio, loss of mitochondrial transmembrane potential, activation of caspase-9, and inhibition of MMP-2 activity.[8–10] The phenolic artichoke extracts also showed a marked antioxidative potential and protection of hepatocytes from oxidative stress.[10] These findings revealed that the artichoke phenolics may be a promising dietary tool, either in cancer chemoprevention or in cancer treatment as a non-conventional adjuvant therapy, especially for breast cancer and hepatoma.

Now, the major biologically active components in *C. scolymus* were revealed to be caffeoylquinic acid derivatives (such as cynarin, chlorogenic acid, caffeic acid, and ferulic acid), flavonoids (such as silymarin, luteolin, and apigenin), and terpenes (cynaropicrin). All the components are marked antioxidants, and artichoke also contains small amounts of other antioxidants such as carotene-β, lutein, and zeaxanthin. These artichoke antioxidants are capable of protecting the human body from harmful free radicals and carcinogenic agents. After exposure to 75–500 μM cynarin (**1**) for 3 days, the survival and growth of HeLa cervical cancer cells were diminished in a dose-dependent manner, and the longevity of normal cell lines (human FSF-1 skin fibroblasts and hTERT-MSC telomerase-immortalized mesenchymal stem cells) was also influenced. These effects were probably mediated by inducing the antioxidative heme oxygenase (HO)-1-dependent pathway (HO-1 is a mark of stress response). Cynarin (**1**) inhibited the growth of human MT-2 T-cell leukemia cells at 250-μM concentration as well, but there was no cytotoxic effects on Jurkat T-cells until 1000 μM.[11] Besides having significant activity against hepatotoxicity, silymarin (**2**), an antioxidant flavonoid derived from both artichoke and milk thistle, at a dose of 2 mg per mouse suppressed the tumor promotion induced by 12-*O*-tetradecanoylphorbol-13-acetate (TPA) and inhibited TPA-induced epidermal ornithine decarboxylase activity and mRNA level, exerting the cancer chemopreventive activity.[12] Cynaropicrin (**3**) deterred the proliferation of human HL-60 leukemia cells *in vitro*, with 50% inhibitory concentration (IC_{50}) value of 1.16 μM. Nevertheless, cynaropicrin and grosheimin only showed weak cytotoxicity against the MCF-7 cancer cells, and other compounds from artichoke had no activity against the MCF-7 cells.[13–15] Chlorogenic acid, the most representative agent in the phenol extract of artichoke, had no obvious inhibitory effects on MDA-MB-231 breast cancer cells.[8,9]

CONCLUSION AND SUGGESTION

Based on the above-summarized scientific evidence, artichoke was confirmed to be not only a nutritional food but also a cancer-preventive vegetable. By regular consumption of artichoke, the presence of bioactive components (such as polyphenolics and sesquiterpene lactone) and antioxidants (such as polyphenolics) in the artichoke flower buds may provide a earlier protective effect against the growth and survival of potentially cancerous cells in the human body.

REFERENCES

1. Lattanzio, V. et al., 2009. Globe artichoke: A functional food and source of nutraceutical ingredients. *J. Funct. Foods* 1: 131–144.
2. Sekara, A. et al., 2015. Globe artichoke—A vegetable, herb and ornamental of value in central Europe: A review. *J. Horti. Sci. Biotechnol.* 90: 365–374.

3. Yasukawa, K. et al., 2010. Inhibitory effect of the flowers of artichoke (*Cynara cardunculus*) on TPA-induced inflammation and tumor promotion in two-stage carcinogenesis in mouse skin. *J. Nat. Med.* 64: 388–391.

4. Nadova, S. et al., 2008. Growth inhibitory effect of ethyl acetate-soluble fraction of *Cynara cardunculus* L. in leukemia cells involves cell cycle arrest, cytochrome c release and activation of caspases. *Phytother. Res.* 22: 165–168.

5. Simsek, E.N. et al., 2013. *In vitro* investigation of cytotoxic and apoptotic effects of *Cynara* L. species in colorectal cancer cells. *Asian Pacific J. Cancer Prev.* 14: 6791–6795.

6. Claudio, P. et al., 2015. Cynara scolymus affects malignant pleural mesothelioma by promoting apoptosis and restraining invasion. *Oncotarget* 6: 18134–18150.

7. Zeinab, A.S. et al., 2013. Antioxidant and antiproliferative effects on human liver HepG2 epithelial cells from artichoke (*Cynara scolymus* L.) by-products. *J. Nat. Sci. Res.* 3: 17–24.

8. Mileo, A.M. et al., 2012. Artichoke polyphenols induce apoptosis and decrease the invasive potential of the human breast cancer cell line MDA-MB231. *J Cell Physiol.* 227: 3301–3309.

9. Mileo, A.M. et al., 2015. Long term exposure to polyphenols of artichoke (*Cynara scolymus* L.) exerts induction of senescence driven growth arrest in the MDA-MB231 human breast cancer cell line. *Oxid. Med. Cell. Longev.* 363827.

10. Miccadei, S. et al., 2008. Antioxidative and apoptotic properties of polyphenolic extracts from edible part of artichoke (*Cynara scolymus* L.) on cultured rat hepatocytes and on human hepatoma cells. *Nutr. Cancer.* 60: 276–283.

11. Gezer, C. et al., 2015. Artichoke compound cynarin differentially affects the survival, growth, and stress response of normal, immortalized, and cancerous human cells. *Turkish J. Biol.* 39: 299–305.

12. Agarwal, R. et al., 1994. Inhibitory effect of silymarin, an anti-hepatotoxic flavonoid, on 12-O-tetradecanoylphorbol-13-acetate-induced epidermal ornithine decarboxylase activity and mRNA in SENCAR mice. *Carcinogenesis* 15: 1099–1103.

13. Yoshizawa, Y. et al., 2013. Leukemia cell proliferation inhibiting composition containing artichoke or Senecio graveolens extract, their uses as pharmaceuticals, antitumor agents, and food, and treatment of nonhuman animals with the compositions. Jpn. Kokai Tokkyo Koho JP 2013180993 A 20130912.

14. Li, X.L. et al., 2005. Sesquiterpenoids from *Cynara scolymus. Heterocycles* 65: 287–291.

15. Yasukawa, Y. et al., 1996. Inhibitory effect of taraxastane-type triterpenes on tumor promotion by 12-O-tetradecanoylphorbol-13-acetate in two-stage carcinogenesis in mouse skin. *Oncology* 53: 341–344.

10. BITTER GOURD/BITTER MELON

Le melon amer   Bitterer Kürbis   El melón amargo

苦瓜　ニガウリ

Momordica charantia

Cucurbitaceae

1. $R_1 = -H$, $R_2 = -D$-beta-Glucosyl, $R_3 = D$
3. $R_1 = -H$, $R_2 = -D$-beta-Glucosyl, $R_3 = B$
5. $R_1 = -H$, $R_2 = -D$-beta-Glucosyl, $R_3 = A$
6. $R_1 = -H$, $R_2 = -D$-beta-Glucosyl, $R_3 = E$
7. $R_1 = -D$-beta-Glucosyl, $R_2 = -H$, $R_3 = -E$
8. $R_1 = -H$, $R_2 = -D$-beta-Glucosyl, $R_3 = F$
12. $R_1 = -H$, $R_2 = -OCH_3$, $R_3 = A$
13. $R_1 = -H$, $R_2 = -OCH_3$, $R_3 = B$

A
B. $R' = -H$
C. $R' = -CH_3$
E. $R' = -CH_2CH_3$

D. $R' = -CH_3$
F. $R' = -CH_2CH_3$

2. $R_1 = -D$-beta-allosyl, $R_2 = B$
4. $R_1 = -D$-beta-allosyl, $R_2 = -B$
9. $R_1 = -H$, $R_2 = -A$
10. $R_1 = -H$, $R_2 = -B$
11. $R_1 = -H$, $R_2 = -C$

11

12

13

14

Bitter gourd is the fruit of *Momordica charantia* L. (Cucurbitaceae). The plant is widely distributed in the tropical and subtropical regions of the world, and its edible fruits are one of the most common vegetables in South and East Asian countries, despite having some bitter taste. Bitter gourd is traditionally known as a useful herb and vegetable for human health, as it shows a number of potential biological activities, including antidiabetic, anti-obesity, anti-inflammation, anti-oviposition, anti-virus, anti–human immunodeficiency virus (HIV), antifeedant, and cholesterol-lowering activities, besides anticancer activity. Several recent preclinical efficacy studies recommended the use of bitter gourd in diabetic and cancer patients as a functional food supplement. Nutritionally, bitter gourd is an excellent source of vitamins (especially vitamins A, C, and B complex), carotenes, folates, and dietary minerals (such as iron, zinc, manganese, magnesium, and potassium).

SCIENTIFIC EVIDENCE OF CANCER-INHIBITORY AND CANCER-PREVENTIVE ACTIVITIES

Biological phytochemistry studies have revealed the suppressive efficacy of bitter gourd on various carcinoma cells, especially lymphoid leukemia, lymphoma, choriocarcinoma, melanoma, prostatic cancer, breast cancer, bladder cancer, squamous cancer of tongue and larynx, and Hodgkin's disease. The cancer-suppressive components were found primarily to be present in the fruits and seeds of the bitter gourd plant.

In vivo antitumor activity of a protein-rich aqueous extract from bitter gourd fruits was determined in animal models implanted with CBA/Dl or YAC-1 lymphomas, P388 or L1210 leukemias, or Molt-4 T-lymphocytic leukemia. By intraperitoneal (IP) injections for 42 or 30 days, the extract prominently inhibited tumor formation in mice without toxicity, wherein the optimum dose for biweekly IP administration was 8 μg. The cytotoxic effect on the leukemia lymphocytes was because the extract had the priority to inhibit soluble guanylate cyclase in the lymphocytes and to block thymidine incorporation into DNA.[1-3] Bitter gourd juice/extract (BMJ/BME) was effective in suppressing two human breast cancer cells (MCF-7 and MDA-MB-231) and human pancreatic cancer cells (BxPC-3, MiaPaCa-2, AsPC-1, and Capan-2) *in vitro*. The BMJ/BME treatment resulted in marked proapoptosis of the breast and the pancreatic cancer cell lines, together with downregulation of survivin and claspin expressions, cleavage of poly(ADP-ribose) polymerase, and activation of caspases. A G2/M cell-cycle arrest in MCF-7 cells was caused by the treatments through suppression of cyclins B1 and D1 expressions as well as enhancement of p53, p21, and pChk1/2 functions.[7,8] In an *in vivo* model, oral administration of lyophilized BMJ in a daily dose of 5 mg in 100 μL water per mouse for 6 weeks inhibited the growth of MiaPaCa-2 tumor xenograft by 60% in nude mice, without obvious toxicity observed. At the same time, BMJ also elicited proliferation of inhibition, apoptosis, and adenosine monophosphate-activated protein kinase (AMPK) activation.[8] In co-treatment with the aqueous extract and a guanylate cyclase inhibitor, the cell cycle was disturbed at the G2/M stage in rat implanted prostatic adenocarcinoma and the level of cycle GMP was reduced in the treated leukemia cells.[1-3] Moreover, the spleen cells from the treated mice markedly exhibited an enhanced mixed lymphocyte reaction when exposed to irradiated P388 stimulator cells. This finding demonstrated that *in vivo* enhancement of immune functions such as activation of lymphocyte, peritoneal exudate cells, and natural killer cells may contribute to the antileukemia effect of the extract.[1-3]

Meanwhile, the fruit juice of bitter gourd was found to significantly diminish forestomach papillomagenesis induced by 3,4-benzo[a]pyrene in mice. In both short- and long-term treatments, the total tumorigenic incidence was reduced remarkably by standard feed with the 2.5% or 5% fruit extract given to mice.[4] The juices or extracts prepared from the whole fruits, peels, pulps, and seeds of bitter gourd were employed to deter the carcinogenesis caused by 7,12-dimethylbenz[a]anthracene (DMBA) in both tumor preinitiation and tumor promotion stages. By the modulation of enzymes in the biotransformation and detoxification systems, the extracts markedly restrained mouse skin papillomagenesis and also protected lymphocytes from DNA damage, and the maximum preventive effect was shown by the peel juice.[5] Also, the fruit aqueous extracts could significantly elevate sulfhydryl (-SH) levels in both liver and skin tissues and augment cytosolic glutathione *S*-transferase (GST) and microsomal cytochrome-b in the liver tissue, thereby improving the host's detoxification system to prevent the carcinogenesis.[6]

Based on this positive evidence, the fruit is strongly suggested to be used in the diet for the prevention of cancer and promotion of the immune system.

Scientific Evidence of Cancer-Inhibitory and Cancer-Preventive Constituents

The bioactivity of components in bitter gourd such as triterpenes, steroids, alkaloids, organic acids, proteins, and polysaccharides has been reported from the multiple pharmaceutical studies; these are some of the components responsible for various pharmacological properties of bitter gourd, significantly including antitumor, antidiabetic, antiviral, and antifertile effects.

1. Ribosome-inactivating proteins

RIP and MAP30: A ribosome-inactivating protein (RIP) with molecular weight (MW) about 30,000 Da or 30 kDa. was purified from bitter gourd. The RIP displayed a powerful inhibitory effect against the protein biosynthesis in reticulocyte lysate, with IC_{50} of 5.3×10^{-10} mol/L, indicating that the RIP may be used in the treatment of certain tumors and viral infections.[7,8] The fruits and seeds of bitter gourd also contain an antineoplastic protein termed MAP30.[9]

MCL: *Momordica charantia* lectin (MCL) is an α-type II RIP (MW 130 kDa) prepared from bitter gourd, which exerted marked cytotoxicity toward two human nasopharyngeal carcinoma (NPC) cell lines: CNE-1 (IC_{50} 6.9 μM) and CNE-2 (IC_{50} 7.4 μM), but it minimally affected normal NP 69 cells. In a model with nude mice, IP injection of MCL at a dose of 1.0 mg/kg per day resulted in 45% remission of NPC xenograft tumors *in vivo*. The apoptosis, G1-cell arrest, DNA fragmentation, and mitochondrial injury were concurrently elicited by MCL in the both types of NPC cells, associated with (1) diminished phosphoretinoblastoma (Rb) protein and cyclin-D1 expression, (2) regulated mitogen-activated protein kinases (MAPK, including p38 MAPK, JNK, and ERK) phosphorylation, (3) promoted downstream NO production, (4) released cytochrome-c into cytosol, and (5) enhanced cleaved poly(ADP-ribose) polymerase (PARP) and activating caspases-8, -9, and -3.[10,11] In hepatocellular carcinoma (HCC) cells, MCL treatment triggered G2/M phase arrest, autophagy, DNA fragmentation, and mitochondrial injury and subsequently elicited the cell apoptosis via the activation of caspase and MAPK pathway and upregulation of truncated Bid.[12]

Immunotoxins: Momordin, a type-1 RIP purified from bitter gourd, was linked to an anti-CD5 monoclonal antibody to afford an immunotoxin. *In vitro* cytotoxicity of the immunotoxin was shown on isolated peripheral blood mononuclear cells (PBMC) and human T-cell leukemia Jurkat cells through the inhibition of protein and DNA synthesis. Its potency on PBMC was very high (IC_{50} 1^{-10} μM), but the immunotoxin was also very efficient in the inhibition of proliferative response in a mixed lymphocyte reaction (IC_{50} of 10 μM). The *in vivo* antineoplastic effect of the immunotoxin was confirmed in a model of nude mice bearing Jurkat leukemia, showing 80% inhibition against tumor development. The results suggest that the anti-CD5–momordin conjugate has the potential for further development in the treatment of CD5-positive leukemia and lymphoma.[13] When the momordin was coupled to OX7, a monoclonal anti-Thy 1.1 antibody by a disulfide bond, the prepared immunotoxin displayed specific cytotoxicity to Thy 1.1-expressing mouse lymphoma AKR-A cells *in vitro*, with IC_{50} of 10^{-9} M.[14] Another immunotoxin was constructed by chemically attaching the momordin to monoclonal mouse IgG2a antibody Fib75 by means of a disulfide linkage. The produced immunotoxin was toxic in tissue culture to EJ human bladder cancer cells expressing antigen Fib75, and the immunotoxin at a concentration of 8×10^{-10} M could obstruct the incorporation of leucine into the cancer cells by 50%.[15] According to the results, it is established that the immunotoxin formulation may pointedly amplify the target-aimed special efficiency of momordin, the finding that is probably useful for the development of new anticancer drugs.

2. Momorcharins

Two glycoproteins, α-momorcharin and β-momorcharin, were isolated from bitter gourd, both of which suppressed mouse sarcoma 180, with inhibitory rates of 71.2% and 68.6%, respectively, but they showed toxic side effects on mice and their immune organs. *In vitro* assays revealed that both the momorcharins showed significant inhibitory effects on syntheses of DNA, RNA, and proteins in NKM gastric cancer cells.[16] α-Momorcharin was also able to inhibit the incorporation of leucine and uridine into P388D1 mouse monocyte-macrophage–like tumor, JAR (human placental choriocarcinoma, J774 Balb/c macrophage-like tumor, and sarcoma 180 cells *in vitro*. Besides, in an *in vivo* model, α-momorcharin enhanced the tumoricidal effect of mouse macrophages on mouse P815 mastocytomal tumor cells.[17] α-Momorcharin exerted the growth-inhibiting and apoptosis-inducing effects on human breast cancer cells *in vivo* and *in vitro*, and the IC_{50} was 15.07 μg/mL in MDA-MB-231 cells, 33.66 μg/mL in MCF-7 cells, and 42.94 μg/mL in MDA-MB-453 cells. However, the gap between its active dose and toxic dose was too narrow; this result showed the limitation of α-momorcharin in clinical application.[18] If α-momorcharin was modified with polyethylene glycol (PEG), the toxicity could be lessened and the antitumor effect enhanced in murine EMT-6 breast cancer and human MDA-MB-231 mammary carcinoma transplanted mouse models.[19]

Likewise, a mixture of α,β-momorcharins (800 μM) was more effective in killing Sk-Mel melanoma and Corl-23 large cell lung cancer cell lines compared with Gos-3, U87-MG, and 1321N1 glioma cell lines. The cell death of Weri Rb-1 retinoblastoma was also enhanced by α,β-momorcharins. During the treatments, the proapoptosis of these tested cancer cell lines was evoked through significant induction of caspase-3 and -9 activities and cytochrome-c release, and the levels of $[Ca^{2+}]i$ in the tested glioma cell lines markedly elevated in a time-dependent manner.[20] In addition, the hepatotoxicity of α-momorcharin was confirmed in the normal liver L02 cell line.[21]

3. Peptide

A novel peptide designated as BG-4 was isolated from the seeds of *M. charantia*, which is a potent trypsin inhibitor. In an *in vitro* assay, it caused weak suppressive effect on HCT-116 and HT-29 human colon cancer cells, with 50% effective doses (ED_{50}s) of 134.4 and 217.0 μg/mL, respectively, after 48 h of treatment. Simultaneously, BG-4 promoted the apoptosis of the colon cancer cells through downregulation of Bcl-1 and XIAP expressions, upregulation of Bax and caspase-3 expressions, and modulation of cell cycle proteins p21 and CDK2. By treatment with 250 μg/mL of BG-4 for 48 h, the proliferation of HCT-116 cells was markedly hampered by 72.8%, whereas the proliferation of HT-29 cells was deterred by 65.8%. Similarly, at 125 μg/mL of BG-4, the capabilities of colon cancer cells to form colonies were reduced by 85.9% in HCT-116 cells but only 9.4% in HT-29 cells,[22] implying that the HCT-116 cells were more sensitive to BG-4, even though both are colon cancer cells.

4. Polysaccharides

Bitter gourd polysaccharides (MCP), as one of the major active ingredients of *M. charantia*, have attracted a great deal of attention because they possess various biological properties, such as antitumor, antioxidant, immunomodulation, radioprotection, antidiabetes, and hepatoprotection. The MCP was found to exert the antiproliferative effect against K562 human leukemia cell lines *in vitro*.[23] In two *in vivo* mouse models, transplanted sarcoma 180 and H22 hepatoma, MCP treatment not only restrained tumor growth but also augmented the indexes of the thymus and spleen.[23] The antitumor mechanisms of MCP were revealed to be associated with disturbing the cell cycle by interaction of tumor cell proliferation-related signals, enhancement of tumor death via up- and downregulation of proapoptotic and apoptotic gene expression, and regulation of various immunity-related bioactive serum factors.[23] Additionally, MCP also showed a neuroprotective effect in response to intracerebral hemorrhage; this effect was mediated by inhibiting the JNK3 signaling pathway and scavenging ROS.[24]

Moreover, a synthesized Eu-MCP subnanocomplex exhibited additive inhibition against the proliferation of esophagus cancer cells *in vitro* at a concentration of 100 g/mL.[23] MCP2 is a native polysaccharide separated from *M. charantia*. Its sulfated derivatives that have different degrees of substitution ranging from 0.56 to 1.10 and different MWs ranging from 7.2 to 9.3 kDa restrained the growth of HepG2 and HeLa neoplastic cell lines *in vitro*, inferring that the sulfated modification could enhance the antitumor activity of MCP2.[25]

5. Triterpenoids and saponins

A group of cucurbitane-type monoglycosides were isolated from dried immature fruits of *M. charantia* and evaluated against A549 lung cancer, U87 glioblastoma, and Hep3B hepatoma cell lines *in vitro*. Charantagenin-D (1) and goyaglycoside-D (2) evinced obvious antiproliferative effect against the tested cancer cell lines. The respective IC_{50}s in A549, U87, and Hep3B cells were 1.07, 1.08, and 14.01 μmol/L for charantagenin-D (1) and 5.30, 0.19, and 19.30 μmol/L for goyaglycoside-D (2). The anticancer activities were also exerted by momordicoside-K (3) on the U87 and A549 cell lines (IC_{50}s 0.60 and 4.89 μmol/L, respectively) and by charantagenin-E (4) and kuguaglycoside-C (5) on the A549 cells (IC_{50}s 4.46–4.89 μmol/L).[26] Kuguasaponins-B (6), -C (7), and -E (8) and kuguaglycoside-C (5) exhibited moderate cytotoxicity (IC_{50}s 7.81–19.76 μM) against human HEp-2 (larynx [?]), MCF-7 (breast), WiDr (colon), and Doay (medulloblastoma) cancer cell lines, but no activity was found on M10 human breast epithelial cells.[27] Kuguaglycoside-C (**5**) treatment also triggered the cytotoxicity against human IMR-32 neuroblastoma cells (IC_{50} 12.6 μM, 48 h) and elicited caspase-independent apoptotic death.[28]

Five cucurbitane-type triterpenoids (**9–13**) and 13 of [?] their glycosides (including charantosides I-VIII) showed the inhibitory effects on the activation of Epstein–Barr virus early antigen promoted by TPA in Raji cells *in vitro*. The triterpenoids **9** and **10** were able to markedly repress the *in vivo* skin carcinogenesis induced by both agents DMBA and peroxynitrite. The triterpenoids (**9–13**) also showed free-radical scavenging activity against NO generation by NOR-1 in a cultured cell system.[29] Some of the triterpenoids and their glycosides obtained from the herb were also reported to have antioxidant property.[30]

Moreover, compared with these monoglycosylcucurbitanes (**1–8**), other cucurbitanes displayed less active or non-suppressive effects on the tested tumor cell lines. 5β,19-Epoxy-23(R)-methoxycucurbita-6,24-dien-3β-ol, 25-methoxy-cucurbita-5,23(E)-diene-3β,19-diol, 3β-hydroxy-25-methoxycucurbita-6,23(E)-diene-19,5β-olide, and 7β-ethoxy-3β-hydroxy-25-methoxycucurbita-5,23(E)-diene-19-al displayed moderate to weak inhibitory effect against the viability of human SK-Hep1 hepatoma cells.[31,32] (23E)-3β,7β,25-Trihydroxycucurbita-5,23-diene-19-al moderately retarded the proliferation of human cancer cell lines, such as Du-145 (prostate), MCF-7 (breast), HepG2 (liver), Colo205 (colon), and HL-60 (leukemic), whereas (23E)-5β,19-epoxycucurbita-6,23,25(26)-triene-3β-ol showed only selectively weak effect against the MCF-7 cells.[33] Additionally, one isolated sterol compound assigned as stigmasta-7,25(27)-dien-3β-ol was found to exert moderate antiproliferative activity on the U87 and A549 cell lines (IC_{50}s 8.65 and 15.10 μmol/L, respectively).[26]

6. Glycoglycerolipids

Several monogalactosyl diacylglycerols (MGDGs) containing two α-linolenic acids (C18:3) were isolated from the juice of bitter gourd, which is a group of selective inhibitors of mammalian DNA polymerases. These MGDGs were effective in the suppression of the growth of human A549 (lung), NUGC-3 (stomach), HeLa (cervix), HCT116 (colon), BALL-1 (acute lymphoblastoid leukemic), and HL-60 (promyelocytic leukemic) carcinoma cell lines *in vitro*. Among the MGDGs, MGDG-C18:3-C18:3 (**11**) exerted the strongest growth-inhibitory effect on the cancer cell lines, with 50% lethal dose (LD_{50}) values of 26.3–35.4 μM.[34] Bitter gourd seed oil contained 50% α-eleostearic acid (α-ESA, **12**), which displayed growth suppression of human SKBR3 and T47D breast carcinoma cell lines, along with induction of G0/G1 and G2/M cell arrest and apoptosis via activating Akt/BAD/Bcl-2 apoptotic pathway, inhibiting Akt/GSK3β survival pathway, and declining HER2/HER3 heterodimer protein level, wherein SKBR3 cells were more sensitive to α-ESA (**12**) than T47D cells.[35] The findings implied that MGDGs and α-ESA may be considered beneficial dietary factors for the prevention and chemotherapy of certain carcinomas, and α-ESA is specifically effective to HER2-overexpressed invasive breast cancer cells.

7. Acyclic bis[bibenzyls]

The acyclic bis[bibenzyls] were not ingredients in bitter gourd but a peroxidase prepared from the fruit of *M. charantia* that could biologically transform dihydro-resveratrol (a major metabolite of resveratrol in humans) into six acyclic bis[bibenzyls]. Among them, two acyclic bis[bibenzyls], 14,6′-diDR (**13**) and 1-*O*-6′-diDR (**14**), displayed moderate antigrowth activity agains the human PC3 prostate cancer cell line *in vitro*, with IC_{50}s of 14 and 17 μM, respectively, being more potent than the parent molecules.[36]

8. Ribonuclease

RNase-MC2 is a 14-kDa ribonuclease isolated from dietary bitter gourd, which manifested antitumor potential against breast and liver cancer cells, concomitant with the induction of cell apoptosis in both *in vitro* and *in vivo* models. Treatment of MCF-7 breast cancer cells with RNase-MC2 caused nuclear damage (such as karyorrhexis, DNA fragmentation, and chromatin condensation) via increase of Bak, Akt, and MAPKs [p38, JNK, and extracellular-signal-regulated kinase (ERK)] and activation of caspases-8, -7, and -9 and cleavage of PARP. These events in turn contributed to early/late apoptotic responses.[37] Similarly, the predominant S-cell arrest and cell apoptosis induced by RNaseMC2 in HepG2 hepatoma cells were associated with the activation of both caspase-8– and caspase-9–regulated caspase pathways in HepG2 cells.[38] Consequently, the RNase MC2 from bitter gourd can be considered as a potential agent desirable for further exploitation in the worldwide fight against breast and liver carcinomas.

OTHER BIOACTIVITIES OF THE CONSTITUENTS

Some cucurbitane-type glycosides such as kuguasaponins-B, -C, -G, and -H and momordicine IV exhibited strong antihyperglycemic effects at 10 μM.[27] Total phenolics and total flavonoids extracted from bitter gourd showed positive correlations with antioxygenic activities. Protocatechuic acid is a major phenolic constituent in bitter gourd, exhibiting protective activity against cisplatin-induced oxidative nephrotoxicity in an *in vivo* rat model.[39] The antiviral effect of bitter gourd is mostly largely served by its glycolprotein (lectin) and protein components.[40]

CONCLUSION AND SUGGESTION

According to the well-structured scientific evidence, the cancer inhibition and prevention activities of bitter gourd can be attributed to both macroconstituents (such as polysaccharides, RIPs, momorcharin, peptide, and ribonuclease) and the constituents with small molecular weight (such as cucurbitane types of triterpenoids and saponins, monogalactosyl diacylglycerols, and α-eleostearic acid) in the fruits and seeds of *M. charantia*. Besides, a broad biological spectrum of activities such as antioxidant, antidiabetic, neuroprotective, hepatoprotective, anti-inflammatory, anthelmintic, hypotensive, antiobesity, immunomodulatory, antihyperlipidemic, antiviral, anti-HIV, antifungal, and antibacterial activities has also been demonstrated for bitter gourd. With such solid scientific support of so many health benefits, it is true that the consumption of bitter gourd is one of the best choices for the protection of the human body from the risk of malignant diseases, including tumors, as well as for health improvement. Nevertheless, bitter gourd is not a panacea.

REFERENCES

1. Jilka, C. et al., 1983. In vivo antitumor activity of the bitter melon (*Momordica charantia*). *Cancer Res.* 43: 5151–5155.
2. Cunnick, J.E. et al., 1990. Induction of tumor cytotoxic immune cells using a protein from the bitter melon (*Momordica charantia*). *Cell Immunol.* 126: 278–289.
3. Clafin, A.J. et al., 1978. Inhibition of growth and guanylate cyclase activity of an undifferentiated prostate adenocarcinoma by an extract of the balsam pear (*Momordica charantia* abbreviata). *Proc. Natl. Acad. Sci. USA.* 75: 989–993.
4. Deep, G. et al., 2004. Cancer preventive potential *Momordica charantia* L. against benzo(a)pyrene induced fore-stomach tumourigenesis in murine model system. *Ind. J. Exp. Biol.* 42: 319–322.
5. Singh, A. et al., 1998. *Momordica charantia* (Bitter Gourd) peel, pulp, seed and whole fruit extract inhibits mouse skin papillomagenesis. *Toxicol. Lett.* 94: 37–46.
6. Ganguly, C. et al., 2000. Prevention of carcinogen-induced mouse skin papilloma by whole fruit aqueous extract of *Momordica charantia*. *Eur. J. Cancer Prev.* 9: 283–288.
7. Ray, R.B. et al., 2010. Bitter melon (*Momordica charantia*) extract inhibits breast cancer cell proliferation by modulating cell cycle regulatory genes and promotes apoptosis. *Cancer Res.* 70: 1925–1931.
8. Kaur, M. et al., 2013. Bitter melon juice activates cellular energy sensor AMP-activated protein kinase causing apoptotic death of human pancreatic carcinoma cells. *Carcinogenesis* 34: 1585–1592.
9. Rothan, H.A. et al., 2015. Scalable production of recombinant membrane active peptides and its potential as a complementary adjunct to conventional chemotherapeutics. *PLoS One* 10: e0139248.

10. Meng, Y.F. et al., 2000. Study on characteristics and biological activity of ribosome inactivating protein (RIP) from *Momordica charantia*. *J.Lanzhou Univ. Sci. Edi.* 36: 80–87.
11. Fang, E.F. et al., 2012. *Momordica charantia* lectin, a type II ribosome inactivating protein, exhibits antitumor activity toward human nasopharyngeal carcinoma cells in vitro and in vivo. *Cancer Prev. Res.* 5: 109–121.
12. Zhang, C.Z.Y. et al., 2015. *Momordica charantia* lectin exhibits antitumor activity towards hepatocellular carcinoma. *Invest. New Drugs* 33: 1–11.
13. Porro, G. et al., 1993. In vitro and in vivo properties of an anti-CD5-momordin immunotoxin on normal and neoplastic T lymphocytes. *Cancer Immunol. Immunother.* 36: 346–350.
14. Stripe, F. et al., 1988. Selective cytotoxic activity of immunotoxins composed of a monoclonal anti-Thy 1.1 antibody and the ribosome-inactivating proteins bryodin and momordin. *British J. Cancer* 58: 558–561.
15. Wawrzynczak, E.J. et al., 1990. Pharmacokinetics in the rat of a panel of immunotoxins made with abrin A chain, ricin A chain, gelonin, and momordin. *Cancer Res.* 50: 7519–7526.
16. Qi, W.B. et al., 1999. Study on isolation, purification and antitumor activity of momorcharin. *Lizi Jiaohuan Yu Xifu* 15: 59–63.
17. Ng, T.B. et al., 1994. Action of α-momorcharin, a ribosome inactivating protein, on cultured tumor cell lines. *General Pharmacol.* 25: 75–77.
18. Cao, D.L. et al., 2015. α-Momorcharin (α-MMC) exerts effective anti-human breast tumor activities but has a narrow therapeutic window in vivo. *Fitoterapia* 100: 139–149.
19. Deng, N.H. et al., 2016. PEGylation alleviates the non-specific toxicities of alpha-momorcharin and preserves its antitumor efficacy in vivo. *Drug Deliv.* 23: 95–100.
20. Gunasekar, M. et al., 2014. Effect of α, β momorcharin on glioma cell viability, caspase activity, cytochrome c release and on cytosolic calcium levels. *Mol. Cell. Biochem.* 388: 233–240.
21. Wang, L. et al., 2016. Cytotoxicity mechanism of α-MMC in normal liver cells through LRP1 mediated endocytosis and JNK activation. *Toxicology* 357–358: 33–43.
22. Dia, V.P. et al., 2016. BG-4, a novel anticancer peptide from bitter gourd (*Momordica charantia*), promotes apoptosis in human colon cancer cells. *Sci. Rep.* 6: 33532.
23. Zhang, F. et al., 2016. A mini-review of chemical and biological properties of polysaccharides from *Momordica charantia*. *Int. J. Biol. Macromol.* 92: 246–253.
24. Duan, Z.Z. et al., 2015. Protection of *Momordica charantia* polysaccharide against intracerebral hemorrhage-induced brain injury through JNK3 signaling pathway. *J. Recept. Sig. Transd.* 35: 523–529.
25. Guan, L.X. 2012. Synthesis and antitumour activities of sulphated polysaccharide obtained from *Momordica charantia* Guan, Lingxiao. *Nat. Prod. Res.* 26: 1303–1309.
26. Wang, X.J. et al., 2012. Structures of new triterpenoids and cytotoxicity activities of the isolated major compounds from the fruit of *Momordica charantia* L. *J. Agricul. Food Chem.* 60: 3927–3933.
27. Zhang, L.J. et al., 2014. Cucurbitane-type glycosides from the fruits of *Momordica charantia* and their hypoglycaemic and cytotoxic activities. *J. Funct. Foods* 6: 564–574.
28. Tabata, K. et al., 2012. Kuguaglycoside C, a constituent of *Momordica charantia*, induces caspase-independent cell death of neuroblastoma cells. *Cancer Sci.* 103: 2153–2158.
29. Akihisa, T. et al., 2007. Cucurbitane-type triterpenoids from the fruits of *Momordica charantica* and their cancer chemopreventive effects. *J. Nat. Prods.* 70: 1233–1239.
30. Lin, K.W. et al., 2011. Antioxidant constituents from the stems and fruits of *Momordica charantia*. *Food Chem.* 127: 609–614.
31. Liao, Y.W. et al., 2012. Cucurbitane-type triterpenoids from the fruit pulp of *Momordica charantia*. *Nat. Prod. Commun.* 7: 1575–1578.
32. Liao, Y.W. et al., 2013. Cucurbitane triterpenoids from the fruit pulp of *Momordica charantia* and their cytotoxic activity. *J. Chin. Chem. Soc.* 60: 526–530.
33. Cao, J.Q. et al., 2011. Two new cucurbitane triterpenoids from *Momordica charantia* L. *Chin. Chem. Lett.* 22: 583–586.
34. Matsui, Y.K. et al., 2009. Structure and activity relationship of monogalactosyl diacylglycerols, which selectively inhibited in vitro mammalian replicative DNA polymerase activity and human cancer cell growth. *Cancer Lett.* 283: 101–107.
35. Zhuo, R.J. et al., 2014. α-eleostearic acid inhibits growth and induces apoptosis in breast cancer cells via HER2/HER3 signaling. *Mol. Med. Rep.* 9: 993–998.
36. Xie, C.F. et al., 2009. Biocatalytic production of acyclic bis[bibenzyls] from dihydroresveratrol by crude *Momordica charantia* peroxidase. *Chem. Biodivers.* 6: 1193–1201.

37. Fang, E.F. et al., 2012. RNase MC2: A new *Momordica charantia* ribonuclease that induces apoptosis in breast cancer cells associated with activation of MAPKs and induction of caspase pathways. *Apoptosis* 17: 377–387.

38. Fang, E.F. et al., 2012. In vitro and in vivo anticarcinogenic effects of RNase MC2, a ribonuclease isolated from dietary bitter gourd, toward human liver cancer cells. *Int. J. Biochem. Cell Biol.* 44: 1351–1360.

39. Yamabe, N. et al., 2015. Protective effects of protocatechuic acid against cisplatin-induced renal damage in rats. *J. Funct. Foods* 19(Part-A), 20–27.

40. Anilakumar, K.R. et al., 2015. Nutritional, pharmacological and medicinal properties of *Momordica charantia*. *Int. J. Nutr. Food Sci.* 4: 75–83.

11. COCHINCHIN GOURD/GAC FRUIT

Cochinchin gourde   Cochinchin Kürbis   Calabaza cochinchin

木鱉　木スッポン　박

Momordica cochinchinensis

Cucurbitaceae

The fruits of *Momordica cochinchinensis* have been traditionally used as both food and local medicine in the growing regions of gac fruit. Gac fruit is well known to contain high levels of carotenoids and vitamin E and also to contain nutrients such as vitamins C and F and minerals such as iron and zinc. The edible part of gac fruit is only red aril, which is oily pulp surrounding the seeds. The aril is rich in long-chain fatty acids, which can help the body absorb fat-soluble nutrients and drugs. The fruit is also enriched with valuable antioxidants. Because of the important phytonutrients, gac fruit is currently attracting more attention in the West. The fruit juice as a healthy beverage is beneficial for immunity, eyes, reproduction, skin, heart health, and the prostate. In addition, gac fruit seeds are used as an herb to treat a variety of internal and external medicinal problems in China.

SCIENTIFIC EVIDENCE OF CANCER-INHIBITORY AND CANCER-PREVENTIVE ACTIVITIES

The aqueous extract of gac fruits exhibited a clear suppressive effect *in vitro* toward the proliferation of 26-20 colon adenocarcinoma cells and HepG2 hepatoma cells, together with the induction of cell-cycle arrest at S phase. The extract elicited necrosis rather than apoptosis in the 26-20 cells. Administration of 250 mg/kg or 750 mg/kg doses of the extract to mice implanted the 26-20 tumor diminished 23.6% of tumor weight and blocked the vessels in the cancer tissue, where the active substance in the fruit extract was confirmed to be a protein (35 KDa).[1] Cochinchina momordica seed ethanolic extract (CMSEE) and cochinchina momordica seed water extract (CMSWE) are ethanolic extract and water extract, respectively, prepared from gac seeds. CMSEE significantly suppressed the proliferation of human A549 (lung), MDA-MB-231 (liver), and TE-13 (esophagus) carcinoma cell lines and mouse B16 melanoma cells *in vitro* by arresting the cell cycle and inducing apoptosis of tumor cells, while CMSWE had no such effects.[2] CMSEE was also able to elicit the differentiation of B16 F1 melanoma cells via modulating the activity of MAPKs.[3] Both CMSEE and CMSWE had no obvious influence on the growth of human normal peripheral blood mononuclear cells.[2]

The ethanol-soluble extract of gac seeds (ECMS) in an *in vitro* assay significantly obstructed the survival of human MKN-28 and SGC7901 gastric cancer cell lines in a dose- and time-dependent manner, concomitant with the induction of S-cell cycle arrest and apoptosis.[4] Moreover, ECMS dose-dependently decreased the survival rates of human A549 and H1299 lung cancer cell lines and hindered the migration and invasion of A549 cells. The proapoptotic and anti-invasive activities of ECMS in A549 cells were mediated by modulation of multiple molecular targets such as (1) upregulation of p53 and Bax and downregulation of Bcl-2 and PI3K/Akt signaling, (2) dissipation of mitochondrial membrane potential and sequential activation of caspase-3 cascade, and (3) increase of E-cadherin level, decrease of STAT3 and MMP-2 levels, and downregulation of vascular endothelial growth factor (VEGF) expression.[5] The MDA-MB-231 breast cancer cells treated with ECMS caused G2/M cell-cycle arrest and apoptotic death similarly via downregulation of cyclins-B1, PI3K, Akt, NF-κB, Bcl-2, and Cdk1 expressions and upregulation of p53, Bax, and caspase-3 functions.[6]

Scientific Evidence of Cancer-Inhibitory and Cancer-Preventive Constituents

For searching the cancer inhibitors, the gac fruits and seeds have been well investigated to show two types of components, (i) with macromolecules such as peptides/proteins and glycoproteins and (ii) with small molecules such as polyphenols and carotenoids being primarily responsible for the antitumor activity.

1. Peptides

From the seeds, two peptides were isolated and characterized: MCoCC-1 and MCoCC-2. The two peptides were composed of 33 and 32 amino acids, respectively, with similar sequences. Both showed cytotoxicity on human A549 (lung), HT29 (colorectal), and MM96L (skin) cancer cell lines *in vitro*. The highest levels of cytotoxicity found for MCoCC-1 and MCoCC-2 were against MM96L cells. The survival of MM96L melanoma cells was lessened by 57% in the presence of 2 μM MCoCC-1 and by 51% in the presence of 1.3 μM MCoCC-2. However, cytotoxicities of the two peptides were less than those of the aqueous extract of gac seeds on the tested cancer cell lines, implying that there are more effective substances in the extract.[7]

2. Glycoproteins

Two RIP-type glycoproteins, momorcochin-S and cochinin-B, were purified from gac seeds. Both could limit the protein biosynthesis in the cell-free rabbit reticulocyte lysate system and retard phenylalanine polymerization in the isolated ribosomes.[8,9] Cochinin-B (28 kDa), an isolated glycoprotein from gac seeds, demonstrated marked anti-growth activities on human HeLa (cervical epithelial), HEK293 (embryonic kidney), and NCI-H187 (small cell lung) neoplastic cell lines *in vitro*, with IC_{50}s of 16.9, 114, and 574 nM, respectively. An immunotoxin was synthesized by chemical attachment of momorcochin-S to a kind of monoclonal antibody (8A) of human plasmacytes. The constructed immunotoxin showed selective cytotoxicity toward the targeted tumor cells.[8,9]

3. Bioactive constituents with small molecules

The gac fruit is an exceptional source of lycopene (**1**) and β-carotene (**2**); these two carotenoids were claimed to be the major constituents in tomato and carrot, respectively. Both the carotenoids have been shown to have noticeable antioxidant and anticarcinogenic properties. (See section 16 in Chapter 2 and section 17 in Chapter 3.) A lycopene-enriched gac aril extract exerted cyto-toxic and antiestrogenic effects on human MCF-7 breast cancer cells, concomitant with the induc-tion of cell apoptosis via both intrinsic and extrinsic signaling pathways such as upregulation of Bax and activation of caspases-6, -8, and -9.[10] Eight constituents with small molecules were isolated from the ethanolic extract of gac seeds (CMSEE). p-Hydroxycinnamaldehyde (**3**) at con-centrations of 20 and 40 μmol/L inhibited the proliferation of B16 melanoma cells by 37.70% and 42.17%, respectively, and it also effectively attenuated metastasis and remarkably reduced colony-forming capacity in the B16 cells. The anticancer mechanism was possibly mediated by the activation of p38 and JNK signaling pathways.[11] Six Five isolated compounds, p-hydrox-ylcinnamaldehyde (**3**), ligballinol (**4**), erythro-guaiacylglycerol-β-coniferylaldehyde ether (**5**), threo-guaiacyl-glycerol-β-coniferylaldehyde ether, 3-[2-(4-hydroxyphenyl)-3-hydroxy-methyl-2,3-dihydro-1-benzofuran-5-yl]propan-1-ol (**6**), and chushizisin-E (**7**), could prompt the differ-entiation of B16 F1 melanoma cells, wherein p-hydroxylcinnamaldehyde (**3**) was more powerful compound than others.[3]

OTHER BIOACTIVITIES OF THE CONSTITUENTS

Lycopene and/or β-carotene possess multiple biological functions such as promoting heart health by specifically combating atherosclerosis, protecting against the risk of heart attack, helping to develop white blood cells (including lymphocytes) for enhancement of the body defense, and mitigating oxidative damage in skin tissue to promote skin health. The bioactive constituents also support healthy reproductive function by up-production of sperm and lowering prostatic hyperplasia. Another carotenoid, zeaxanthin, in gac fruit is beneficial to enhance overall eye health.[12]

CONCLUSION AND SUGGESTION

Based on the biology-based phytochemical investigations, the antioxidant, anticancer, and anticar-cinogenic activities of gac (cochinchin gourd) are attributed mostly to the four types of bioactive components—that is, carotenoids, polyphenols, peptides/proteins, and glycoproteins, especially two prominent carotenoids, lycopene (**1**) and β-carotene (**2**), both of which are enriched in the fruit aril (an edible portion). The beneficial bioactivities of gac fruit may surely help decrease the risk of some types of carcinomas. More recently, owing to the higher phytonutrient contents, the gac fruit juice and its soft capsules have begun to be marketed outside of Asia as dietary supplements.

REFERENCES

1. Tien, P. et al., 2005. Inhibition of tumor growth and angiogenesis by water extract of gac fruit (*Momordica cochinchinensis* Spreng). *Int. J. Oncol.* 26: 881–889.
2. Zhao, L.M. et al., 2010. Antitumor activity of cochinchina momordica seed extract. *Aibian, Jibian, Tubian* 22: 19–23.
3. Zhao, L.M. et al., 2012. An ester extract of Cochinchina momordica seeds induces differentiation of melanoma B16 F1 cells via MAPKs signaling. *Asian Pacific J. Cancer Prevent.* 13: 3795–3802.
4. Liu, H.R. et al., 2012. Cochinchina momordica seed extract induces apoptosis and cell cycle arrest in human gastric cancer cells via PARP and p53 signal pathways. *Nutr. Cancer* 64: 1070–1077.
5. Shen, Y. et al., 2015. Cochinchina momordica seed suppresses proliferation and metastasis in human lung cancer cells by regulating multiple molecular targets. *Am. J. Chinese Med.* 43: 149–166.
6. Meng, L.Y. et al., 2011. Cochinchina momordica seed extract induces G2/M arrest and apoptosis in human breast cancer MDA-MB-231 cells by modulating the PI3K/Akt pathway. *Asian Pacific J. Cancer Prevent.* 12: 3483–3488.
7. Chan, L.Y. et al., 2009. Isolation and characterization of peptides from *Momordica cochinchinensis* seeds. *J. Nat. Prod.* 72: 1453–1458.

8. Bolognesi, A. et al., 1989. Purification and properties of a new ribosome-inactivating protein with RNA N-glycosidase activity suitable for immunotoxin preparation from the seeds of *Momordica cochinchinensis*. *Biochim. et Biophys. Acta* 993: 287–292.

9. Chuethong, J. et al., 2007. Cochinin B, a novel ribosome-inactivating protein from the seeds of *Momordica cochinchinensis*. *Biol. Pharm. Bull.* 30: 428–432.

10. Petchsak, P. et al., 2015. *Momordica cochinchinensis* Aril extract induced apoptosis in human MCF-7 breast cancer cells. *Asian Pac. J. Cancer Prev.* 16: 5507–5513.

11. Zhao, L.M. et al., 2014. Effect and mechanisms of p-hydroxylcinnamaldehyde from *Cochinchina momordica* seed on differentiation of mouse melanoma B16 cells in vitro. *Zhongguo Zhongliu Shengwu Zhiliao Zazhi* 21: 282–287.

12. Chuyen, H.V. et al., 2015. Gac fruit (*Momordica cochinchinensis* Spreng.): A rich source of bioactive compounds and its potential health benefits. *Int. J. Food Sci. Technol.* 50: 567–577.

12. EGGPLANT

Aubergine   Auberginen   Berenjena

茄子 ナス 가지

Solanum melongena

Solanales

1. R = –glc-(2-1)-rham
   └(4-1)-rham
2. R = –H
3. R = –gal-(2-1)-rham
   └(3-1)-glc

4. R_1 = –glc R_2 =
5. R_1 = –glc R_2 =

6. R_1 = R_2 = –H
7. R_1 = –glc R_2 = –A

The fruits of eggplant are one of the most broadly consumed vegetables in the world. The eggplant fruits have a typical dark purple and glossy skin, which can be eaten raw, cooked, or pickled. The fruits with different size, shape, and color are produced by different varieties of the *Solanum melongena* plant, but the most widely cultivated varieties of eggplant today are like a pear-shaped egg in Europe and North America and like a narrower shaped cucumber in East Asia. Eggplant is a very good source of dietary fiber, vitamin B1, and copper and a good source of manganese, vitamin B6, niacin, potassium, folate, and vitamin K.

Scientific Evidence of Cancer-Inhibitory and Cancer-Preventive Constituents

Several classes of bioactive phytochemicals are concentrated in eggplant fruits, including glycoalkaloids, saponins, flavonoids, anthocyanidins, and phenolic compounds, which are responsible for the activities of eggplants, such as analgesic, anti-anaphylactic, anti-inflammatory, antipyretic, antioxidant, intraocular pressure-reducing, central nervous system–depressing, hypolipodemic, and hypotensive effects.[1] In Japan, the calyx of eggplants has been used as a folk remedy for human papilloma virus (HPV)-caused common warts. In an anticancer exploration, the incubation with a 1/20 dilution (corresponding to 166 mg raw eggplants per milliliter) of an eggplant extract for 48 h resulted in the antiproliferative effect against human cancer cell lines such as Panc-1 (pancreas), A549 (lung), Caki-2 (renal), PC3 (prostate), AGS (stomach), and DAOY medulloblastoma, but no such effect was found on MCF-7 breast cancer and U87 MG glioblastoma cell lines. Eggplant fruit juice also exhibited the inhibitory effect in a mutagenic experiment.[2–4]

1. Glycoalkaloids

The major bioactive constituents in eggplant fruits are glycoalkaloids, whose content generally increased during fruit development and ripening. A class of glycoalkaloids—namely, solasodine rhamnosyl glycosides, was isolated from the fruits and elucidated as solamargine, solasonine, solanine, and di- and monoglycosides of solasodine. The components were revealed to be responsible for biological effects, including cytotoxic, antiproliferative, proapoptotic, and lasting immunological effects, toward a variety of cancer cells.[3] Due to the presence of rich glycoalkaloids, a methanol extract of eggplant peels (MEP), which were cultivated in Egypt, showed a clear antiproliferative effect against all tested human carcinoma cell lines such as HepG2 (liver), HCT116 (colon), HeLa (cervix), HEp2 (larynx), and MCF-7 (breast) cell lines, with IC_{50}S of 2.14–6.56. The isolated solamargine (1) and its aglycon solasodine (2) exerted a slightly better or similar degree of inhibition (IC_{50}s 2.51–3.43), whereas solasonine (3) had a lower inhibitory effect (IC_{50}s of 4.34–9.07) in the same *in vitro* assay. Among these cell lines, the most sensitive cell line was HepG2 hepatoma cells.[3–7] The antiproliferative effects of solamargine (1) and solasonine (3) were also observed in other *in vitro* tests with human HT-29 (colon); MCF-7 (breast); HeLa (cervix) HepG2 (liver); MO59J, U343, and U251 (brain); and H441, H520, H661, and H69 (lung) cancer cell lines; and murine melanoma B16F10 cells (IC_{50}s of 4.58–18.23 µg/mL). The lowest IC_{50}s were 3.0, 6.7, 7.2, 5.8 µM and 4.58 µg/mL for solamargine (1) in H441, H520, H661, and H69 cells and HepG2 cells, respectively, and 6.01 µg/mL for solasonine (3) in HepG2 cells. Solasonine (3) was also effective in the inhibition of Ehrlich carcinoma and K562 leukemia cell lines in a dose-dependent manner, whereas solanine was moderately effective to HepG2 cells (IC_{50} of 14.5 µg/mL) but weak to human SGC-7901 (gastric) and LS-174 (colon) cancer cell lines. As compared with chemodrugs (cisplatin, methotrexate, epirubicin, 5-fluorouracil, cyclophosphamide, paclitaxel, vinblastine, camptothecin, vincristine (VCR), gemcitabine, and doxorubicin), solamargine (1) displayed a more pronounced cytotoxic effect against breast cancer cells.[3–7] Moreover, the methanol extract of eggplants (MEP) in two doses of 100 and 200 mg/kg obstructed CCl_4-induced rat hepatocellular carcinoma (HCC) in an *in vivo* experiment, via lessening α-fitorotein to stabilize the hepatocytes and restoring the levels of aspartate transaminase (AST), alanine aminotransferase (ALT), and albumin in a dose-dependent manner.[3–5] A mixture of solasodine rhamnosyl glycosides (SRG), which contains 33% solamargine, 33% solasonine, and 34% di- and monoglycosides of solasodine, was effective in the suppression of murine sarcoma 180 *in vivo*. Interestingly, the mice cured by the treatment were resistant to the re-inoculated terminal doses of cancer, indicating that the SRG stimulated lasting immunity against cancer. Several SRG formulations have been successfully used in mouse models to treat human basal cell carcinomas and squamous cell carcinoma of skin and in clinics to treat basal cell carcinoma in patients, with cure rates of 66% at 8-week and 78% at 1-year follow-up.[3–11]

Furthermore, the *in vitro* examinations revealed the broad spectrum of solamargine (1) and solasonine (3) in proapoptosis of human cancer cell lines such as K562 (leukemic); HT-29 and HCT-15 (colon); A549 and H441 (lung); PLC/PRF/5, SMMC-7721, HepG2, and HepB3 (liver); AGS (stomach); MIA and PaCa-2 (pancreas); 786-0 (kidney); HeLa 229 (uterine); JAM (ovarian); DV-145, LNCap, and PC3 (prostate); T47D and MDA-MB-231 (breast); and U87-MG (brain) carcinomas; A431, SCC4, SCC9, SCC25 (squamous cell) carcinomas and A2058 melanoma, NO36 mesothelioma, and U20S osteosarcoma, as well as murine Ehrlich tumor.[7] However, in the similar concentrations, solamargine (1) and solasonine (3) did not cause apoptosis in normal cells such as bone marrow cells, fibroblasts, normal hepatocyte cells HL7702, and H9C2.[7] An exploration of the mechanisms further discovered that proapoptosis in the malignant cells was primarily mediated by (1) triggering extrinsic and intrinsic apoptotic pathways in cancer cells by upregulating the expressions of external death receptors, such as tumor necrosis factor receptor 1 (TNFR-1), Fas receptor, TNFR-1–associated death domain, and Fas-associated death domain, (2) enhancing intrinsic ratio of Bax/Bcl-2 by upregulating Bax and downregulating Bcl-2 and Bcl-xL expressions, (3) leading to loss of mitochondrial potential and releasing cytochrome-c, (4) activating caspase-8, -9, and -3 in cancer cells,

(5) increasing p53 and Bax mRNA and protein expression and inducing mitochondrial translocation of p53 (such as in U20S osteosarcoma cells), (6) downregulating hILP/XIAP, Apaf-1, and Bax (such as in WM115 and WM239 melanoma cells),[12] (7) enlarging the binding activities of tumor necrosis factor (TNF)-α and TNF-β to lung cancer cells (such as H441, H520, H661, and H69 cells),[13] (8) eliciting the phosphorylation of p38 MAPK, repressing Stat3 expression, and upregulating p21 (such as in nonsmall cell lung cancer [NSCLC] cells), and (9) increasing intracellular calcium level and inducing an early lysosomal rupture to initiate plasma membrane perturbation and disruption (such as in K562 cells).[3–15] The investigations of the mechanism also discovered that solamargine (**1**) at low concentrations kills cancer cells by proapoptosis and at high doses kills cancer cells by oncosis, and both types of cell death are induced by intermediate concentrations of solamargine (**1**). Also, solamargine (**1**) caused cell-cycle arrest at the G2/M phase in human SMMC-7721 and HepG2 hepatoma cells. After the treatment, Hep3B hepatoma cells in the G2/M stage were susceptible to solamargine (**1**)-elicited apoptotic death.[3–5]

In addition to inducing apoptosis and cell-cycle arrest, solamargine (**1**) was capable of sensitizing some cancer cells to chemotherapies, reversing multidrug resistance (MDR), and killing a range of MDR tumor cell lines; its cytotoxicity against MDR-tumor cells was nearly equal to or even more potent than that against the corresponding parental non–MDR tumor cells. The anti-MDR tumor effect (such as in K562/AO2) was largely attributed to the ability of solamargine (**1**) in the suppression of P-glycoprotein activity. By combining cisplatin with solamargine (**1**), the inhibitory effect on cisplatin-resistant cancer cells, particularly lung carcinoma and breast cancer, was effectively boosted. In association with inhibition of topoisomerase-IIα and promotion of chemotherapy-induced apoptosis through increase of Fas expression and decrease of HER2 expression, the co-treatment with solamargine (**1**) and epirubicin resulted in synergistic cytotoxic effects in NSCLC cells and breast cancer cells. Similarly, solamargine (**1**) could synergistically augment the effect of trastuzumab in eliciting apoptotic death and inhibiting the proliferation of breast cancer cells. Also, solamargine (**1**) has antimutagenic properties but does not exert any mutagenic effects. Thus, in both V79 cells and micronuclei in Swiss mice, solamargine (**1**) markedly lessened the frequency of chromosomal aberrations induced by the chemotherapeutic agent doxorubicin.[3–5]

The investigations on the structure–activity relationship demonstrated that the presence of the terminal rhamnosyl moiety of solasodine glycosides (such as solamargine, solasonine, and solanine) was required to exert the greater cytotoxicity and anticancer activities, wherein the rhamnosyl residue played a crucial role in eliciting the cell death by apoptosis and oncosis.[3–5,12] Taken together, the glycoalkaloids, especially solamargine (**1**), are the biologically active and eggplant-related natural components that can play important roles in cancer chemotherapy as an adjuvant and in cancer prevention as a supplement.

2. Steroidal glycosides

Two steroidal glycosides identified as β-sitosterol-3-O-β-D-glucoside (**4**) and poriferasterol-3-O-β-D-glucoside (**5**) were isolated from the methanol extract of eggplant fruit peels. Both the agents in an *in vitro* assay exerted antiproliferative effects against human cancer cell lines such as HepG2 (liver), MCF-7 (breast), and HCT116 (colon) cells (respective IC_{50}s of 2.12–2.36 and 3.52–5.20) but fewer effects on HEp2 (larynx) and HeLa (cervix) cancer cell lines (IC_{50}s of 10–13.4). Their anticancer activity was comparable to that of solamargine (**1**) and solasonine (**3**) in the hepatoma, breast cancer, and colon cancer cell lines.[5]

3. Antioxidants

Significantly, eggplant fruits contain various types of antioxidant components such as anthocyanin, polyphenolics, and flavonoids, having advantages for limitation of oxidative stress that is correlated with promotion of many diseases. The aqueous extract of eggplant peel presented a strong suppressive effect on the infiltration of HT-1080 human fibrosarcoma cells to block the invasion and metastasis of HT-1080 cells, wherein the effective component in the peel was identified as delphinidin (**6**), a flavonoid pigment. However, the extract and delphinidin (**6**) did not affect tumor cell adhesion to Matrigel or haptotactic migration to Matrigel. Delphinidin (**6**) slightly inhibited the activity of matrix metalloproteinases (MMPs)-2 and -9; this inhibition might be partially responsible for the anti-invasive effect.[16,17] Nasunin (**7**) is a remarkable anthocyanin that was separated from purple eggplant peels. It characterizes 70%–90% of the total anthocyanins in the eggplant skin. Due to nasunin (**7**), eggplant is not only a potent free-radical scavenger but also an iron chelator. It is capable of lessening free-radical formation, restraining blood cholesterol from peroxidation, and protecting free-radical–caused cellular damage by chelating iron. Thus, the carcinogenesis and lipid peroxidation of brain homogenates can be effectively retarded, and the cardiovascular system can be kept healthy. Nasunin (**7**) has also been shown to have antiangiogenic properties—that is, blocking the development of new blood vessels in the tumor tissue to starve the cancer cells.[18]

Likewise, eggplant fruits are rich sources of other types of phenolic compounds. Besides 13 phenolic acids isolated from eggplant, chlorogenic acid (**8**) is a predominant phenolic compound found in the commercial cultivars of eggplant, which was revealed to have anticarcinogenesis-related health benefits, including free-radical scavenging and antimutagenic activities, as well as antiviral, bad cholesterol–reducing, and antimicrobial activities. In addition, flavonoids (i.e., myricetin and kaempferol) and carotenoids (i.e., lycopene, lutein, and α-carotene) in the eggplants have been reported to possess the antioxidative function.[19]

4. Long-chain compounds

Two long-chain fatty acid ketodienes identified as 9-oxo-(10E,12E)-octadecadienoic acid (9-EE-KODE, **9**) and 9-oxo-(10E,12Z)-octadecadienoic acid (9-EZ-KODE, **10**) were isolated from eggplants as active ingredients, exhibiting the suppressive effect on human ovary cancer (HRA) cells *in vitro*, where the approximate anti-growth effect of 9-EE-KODE (**9**) was 10-fold higher than that of 9-EZ-KODE (**10**). Human HRA ovarian cancer cells were relatively sensitive to 9-EE-KODE (**9**) (IC_{50} of 6.48 μM), but human MCF-7 breast cancer cells were resistant (IC_{50} of 74.0 μM). The 9-EE-KODE (**9**) also exerted 5–8.5-fold lower cytotoxicity on other tested human tumor cell lines such as Mia-PaCa-2 pancreatic cancer, HT-1080 fibrosarcoma, KB cervical cancer, and ACC-MESO-1 malignant mesothelioma, as well as on P388 mouse leukemia cells, compared with that on HRA cells. After treatment with 9-EE-KODE (**9**), the apoptosis of HRA cells was enhanced via a mitochondrial regulation pathway—that is, downregulation of Bcl-2 expression and upregulation of Bax expression level, dissipation of mitochondrial membrane potential, release of cytochrome-c to cytosol, and increase of caspase-3/7 activities. The content of 9-EE-KODE (**9**) in the edible part of eggplant was less than that in its calyx part,[20,21] showing that the calyx part of eggplant still has a value.

In addition, solanesol (**11**), a long-chain polyisoprenoid alcohol with nine isoprene units, was separated from eggplants. It also mainly accumulates in other solanaceous crops, including tobacco, tomato, potato, and pepper plants. Solanesol (**11**) possesses multiple bioactivities, including antibacterial, antifungal, antiviral, anticancer, anti-inflammatory, and antiulcer activities. In the pharmaceutical industry, it is broadly employed as an intermediate for the synthesis of ubiquinone drugs, such as coenzyme Q10 and vitamin K2. Some synthesized derivatives from solanesol (**11**) showed *in vitro* antitumor activities to synergistically enhance the curative effect of VCR.[22]

5. Pheophytin

From Japanese eggplant fruits, pheophytin, an Mg-free derivative of chlorophyll, was identified. In an Ames test, pheophytin deterred mutagenesis of *Salmonella typhimurium* TA98 against several mutagens such as 2-amino-anthracene, 2-amino-3-methyl-9H-pyrido 2,3-b indole, 3-amino-1-methyl-5H-pyrido 4,3-b indole, 2-aminofluorene, and 2-nitrofluorene. The desmutagenic effect was found to be contributed by the phorbin skeleton of pheophytin.[23]

6. Macromolecules

A non-dialyzable extract derived from eggplants exhibited the suppressive effects against the mutagenicity of 3-amino-1,4-dimethyl-5H-pyridol[4,3-b]-indole (Trp-P-1), benzo[a]pyrene (BAP), 3-amino-1-methyl-5H-pyridol[4,3-b]indole (Trp-P-2), aflatoxin B1, and/or N-methyl-N′-nitro-N-nitroso-guanidine (MNNG) on *S. typhimurium* TA100 or TA 98. In an *in vitro* assay, the non-dialyzable extract was able to induce the differentiation of human U937 and HL-60 leukemia cell lines into macrophage or monocyte cells and to trigger antioxidant effects against the oxidation of linoleic acid.[24]

CONCLUSION AND SUGGESTION

The extensive studies on chemical biology of eggplant fruit clearly showed that the vegetable contains various types of constituents, such as glycoalkaloids, steroidal glycosides, pheophytin, antioxidants (polyphenolics, flavonoids, and anthocyanin), and long-chain fatty acid ketodienes. Many of the constituents in eggplant fruit have been proven to play multiple roles in the suppression of tumor cell growth, proliferation, and/or invasion; in the induction of tumor cell death by apoptosis and/or oncosis; in the reversal of drug resistance in cancer cells; in the inhibition of angiogenesis in tumor tissues; as antioxidant; and/or in antimutagenesis. Among these bioactive components, the prominent cancer inhibitors in eggplants should be glycoalkaloids, especially solamargine (**1**), solasodine (**2**), and solasonine (**3**), not only showing a broad anticancer spectrum but also having higher contents in eggplant fruit. By the integrative effects from these bioactive components, eggplant can provide medical and health advantages for cancer prevention and treatment. Therefore, frequent consumption of eggplant fruits in our diet is recommended to help lower the risk of cancer.

REFERENCES

1. Sun, J. et al., 2013. Research advances on chemical constituents of *Solanum melongena* and their pharmacological activities. *Zhongcaoyao* 44: 2615–2622.
2. Dominique, B. et al., 2009. Antiproliferative and antioxidant activities of common vegetables: A comparative study. *Food Chem.* 112: 374–380.
3. Friedman, M. 2015. Chemistry and anticarcinogenic mechanisms of glycoalkaloids produced by eggplants, potatoes, and tomatoes. *J. Agric. Food Chem.* 63: 3323–3337.
4. Cham, B.E. 2013. Drug therapy: Solamargine and other solasodine rhamnosyl glycosides as anticancer agents. *Mod. Chemother.* 2: 33–49.
5. Shabana, M.M. et al., 2013. In vitro and in vivo anticancer activity of the fruit peels of solanum melongena against hepatocellular carcinoma. *J. Carcinogen. Mut.* 4: 1000149.
6. Kuo, K.W. et al., 2000. Anticancer activity evaluation of the Solanum glycoalkaloid solamargine: Triggering apoptosis in human hepatoma cells. *Biochem. Pharmacol.* 60: 1865–1873.
7. Cham, B.E. 2007. Solasodine rhamnosyl glycosides in a cream formulation is effective for treating large and troublesome skin cancers. *Res. J. Biol. Sci.* 2: 749–761.
8. Punjabi, S. et al., 2008. Solasodine glycoalkaloids: A novel topical therapy for basal cell carcinoma. A double-blind, randomized, placebo-controlled, parallel group, multicentre study. *Int. J. Dermatol.* 47: 78–82.
9. Cham, B.E. 2011. Topical solasodine rhamnosyl glycosides derived from the eggplant treats large skin cancers: Two case reports. *Int. J. Clin. Med.* 2: 473–477.
10. Cham, B.E. 2012. Intralesion and CuradermBEC5 topical combination therapies of solasodine rhamnosyl glycosides derived from the eggplant or devil's apple result in rapid removal of large skin cancers. Methods of treatment compared. *Int. J. Clin. Med.* 3: 115–124.
11. Sana, S. et al., 2016. Solamargine triggers cellular necrosis selectively in different types of human melanoma cancer cells through extrinsic lysosomal mitochondrial death pathway. *Cancer Cell Int.* 16:11.
12. Liu, L.F. et al., 2004 Action of solamargine on human lung cancer cells-enhancement of the susceptibility of cancer cells to TNFs. *FEBS Lett.* 577: 67–74.
13. Li, X. et al., 2011. Solamargine induces apoptosis associated with p53 transcription-dependent and transcription-independent pathways in human osteosarcoma U2OS cells. *Life Sci.* 88: 314–321.
14. Lee, K.R. et al., 2004. Glycoalkaloids and metabolites inhibit the growth of human colon (HT29) and liver (HepG2) cancer cells. *J. Agric. Food Chem.* 52: 2832–2839.

15. Sato, T. et al., 1995. Development of cancer-metastasis inhibitory medicines based on crude drug principles. *Ikagaku Oyo Kenkyu Zaidan Kenkyu Hokoku* Vol. Date 1994, 13: 198–207.
16. Nagase, H. et al., 1998. Inhibitory effect of delphinidin from *Solanum melongena* on human fibrosarcoma HT-1080 invasiveness in vitro. *Planta Med.* 64: 216–219.
17. Noda, Y. et al., 1998. Antioxidant activity of nasunin, an anthocyanin in eggplant. *Res. Commun. Mol. Pathol. Pharmacol.* 102: 175–187.
18. Igarashi, K. et al., 2000. Physiological functions of food component anthocyanins. *Foods Food Ingredients J. Jpn* 187: 17–29.
19. Zhao, B.Y. et al., 2015. 9-Oxo-(10E,12E)-octadecadienoic acid, a cytotoxic fatty acid ketodiene isolated from eggplant calyx, induces apoptosis in human ovarian cancer (HRA) cells. *J. Nat. Med.* 69: 296–302.
20. Zhao, B.Y. et al., 2014. Cytotoxic fatty acid ketodienes from eggplants. *Nippon Shokuhin Kagaku Gakkaishi* 21: 42–47.
21. Yan, N. et al., 2015. Solanesol: A review of its resources, derivatives, bioactivities, medicinal applications, and biosynthesis. *Phytochem. Rev.* 14: 403–417.
22. Yoshikawa, K. et al., 1996. Desmutagenic effect of pheophytin from Japanese eggplant against several mutagens. *Shokuhin Eiseigaku Zasshi* 37: 295–300.
23. Shinohara, K. et al., 1995. Anticancer functions of nondialyzable extracts of vegetables and fruits. In: Ohigashi, H. (Ed.), *Food Factors for Cancer Prevention*, (*International Conference on Food Factors: Chemistry and Cancer Prevention*), Springer, Hamamatsu, Japan, December 1995 (1997), pp. 170–173.

13. MYOGA GINGER

蘘荷　みょうが　양하

Zingiber mioga

Zingiberaceae

Myoga ginger, or *Zingiber mioga*, is a perennial plant distributed in warm regions of East Asia. Its flower buds can be used as a fresh vegetable in East Asian cuisines, especially in Japanese cooking. Nutritionally, the flower bud is an excellent source of vitamin K, manganese, and molybdenum and a good source of vitamins B1, B2, and B6; folate; niacin; pantothenic acid; magnesium; potassium; copper; iron; zinc; and calcium. The young flesh stems of the myoga plant are also edible vegetables in the growing areas. The rhizome, flower, and fruit of myoga ginger are individually utilized as Chinese folk medicines.

SCIENTIFIC EVIDENCE OF CANCER-INHIBITORY AND CANCER-PREVENTIVE CONSTITUENTS

1. Diterpenoids

Galanals-A (**1**) and -B (**2**) separated from the flower buds of myoga demonstrated moderate inhibitory activity against KB nasopharynx carcinoma cells, with IC_{50}s of 3.25 and 15 µg/mL, respectively, and also exerted potent cytotoxicity on human Jurkat T-lymphoma cells *in vitro*. The treatment with the diterpenoids could promote cell apoptosis characterized by DNA fragmentation, mitochondrial transmembrane potential alteration, cytochrome-c release, and caspase-3 activation.[1,2] From the flower buds and rootstalks of myoga, labda-12-ene-15,16-dial and its salt were isolated, showing *in vitro* activity to deter the proliferation of skin cutaneous melanoma, leukemia, breast cancer, lung cancer, and hepatoma cell lines.[3,4]

The chloroform extract of myoga rhizomes displayed potent suppressive effects on the generation of nitric oxide (NO) and superoxide (O^{2-}) by both NAD(P)H oxidase and xanthine oxidase, implying that the rhizome possesses antitumorigenic activity.[5,6] Aframodial (**3**), a labdane diterpene isolated from myoga, markedly obstructed mouse L1210 leukemia cells (ED_{50} of 2.5 µg/mL) and strongly restrained the mutagenicity of AS52 cells by 95.9%; the AS52 tumor was caused by the stimulated human HL-60 leukemia cells.[5] Moreover, aframodial (**3**) at a 20-µM concentration exerted distinct inhibitory effects on the generation of 12-*O*-tetradecanoylphorbol-13-acetate (TPA)-induced O^{2-} in human HL-60 leukemia cells and on the generation of lipopolysaccharide/interferon-γ–induced nitric oxide in mouse macrophage RAW264.7 cells, with 84.6% and 95.9% inhibitory rates, respectively, wherein the NF-κB expression was also completely repressed by aframodial (**3**). These results implied that aframodial (**3**) may be a promising drug candidate in the prevention of carcinogenesis, owing to its potent antioxidative, antimutant, and anti-inflammatory potentials.[5]

2. Polysaccharide

A polysaccharide component prepared from myoga exerted significant scavenging effects in free-radical 2,2-diphenyl-1-picrylhydrazyl (DPPH) and nitrate (NO^{2-}) experiments. At a concentration of 5 mg/mL, the NO^{2-} scavenging rate of myoga polysaccharide reached 72.6%. The results implied that the myoga polysaccharide is able to inhibit the formation of nitrite amine (a strong carcinogenic substance) by scavenging free radicals, displaying a potential to diminish the probability of some types of carcinogenesis.[7]

CONCLUSION AND SUGGESTION

The flower buds and flesh stems of myoga are a kind of high-nutritional vegetables. Based on the results of current scientific research, the discovered diterpenoids (galanal-A, galanal-B, and aframodial) are important cancer inhibitors with a moderate grade of cancer-suppressive activity in myoga, and myoga polysaccharide is a remarkable free-radical scavenger and a potential cancer-preventing constituent. Considering the higher quality of nutrition provided from myoga, the dietary intake of myoga vegetables is definitely beneficial for cancer prevention.

REFERENCES

1. Morita, H. et al., 1988. Cytotoxic and antifungal diterpenes from the seeds of *Alpinia galangal*. *Planta Med.* 54: 117–120.
2. Miyoshi, N. et al., 2003. Dietary ginger constituents, galanals A and B, are potent apoptosis inducers in human T-lymphoma Jurkat cells. *Cancer Lett.* 199: 113–119.
3. Lee, Y.J. et al., 2006. Composition comprising compound isolated from *Zingiber mioga* for inhibiting proliferation of cancer by inducing apoptosis of cancer cells. *Repub. Korean Kongkae Taeho Kongbo* KR 2004-82269 20041014.
4. Jang, K.C. et al., 2005. Labda-12-ene-15,16-dial compound or pharmaceutically acceptable salt thereof and purified from *Zingiber mioga* Roscoe. *Repub. Korean Kongkae Taeho Kongbo* KR 2003-61429 20030903.
5. Kim, H.W. et al., 2005. Suppressive effects of mioga ginger and ginger constituents on reactive oxygen and nitrogen species generation, and the expression of inducible pro-inflammatory genes in macrophages. *Antioxid. Redox Signal.* 7: 1621–1629.
6. Kim, O.K. et al., 1998. Screening of edible Japanese plants for nitric oxide generation inhibitory activities in RAW 264.7 cells. *Cancer Lett.* 25: 199–207.
7. Tan, Z.W. et al., 2008. Study on the antioxidant prosperity in vitro of water soluble polysaccharide in *Zingiber mioga*. *Anhui Nongye Kexue* 36: 433–434.

14. OKRA

Gombos   Okra   Okra

秋葵　オクラ　오크라

Abelmoschus esculentus

Malvaceae

Okra is the edible immature green seed pod of a Malvaceae plant (*Abelmoschus esculentus* = *Hibiscus esculentus*), which is native to West Africa, and it is cultivated in tropical, subtropical, and warm temperate regions around the world. The raw okra offers high to moderate amounts of vitamins C, K, B6, and A; dietary fibers; and necessary minerals such as magnesium, phosphorus, calcium, and iron. Okra also has been found to have the health-promotive advantages of being antioxidant, antistress, and antifatigue and lowering cholesterol. Accordingly, it is often recommended by nutritionists in cholesterol-controlling and weight-reduction programs and in diabetes-treating diets. Also, the flowers of okra plant are similar to those of hibiscus and have ornamental value.

SCIENTIFIC EVIDENCE FOR CANCER-INHIBITORY AND CANCER-PREVENTIVE CONSTITUENTS

The cancer research on okra is just beginning, but four types of macromolecules (protein/peptides, polysaccharides, lectin, and pectin) that displayed *in vitro* cancer-suppressive properties have been discovered from okra. However, small molecules with cancer inhibitory activity have not been reported yet from the okra research.

1. Protein/peptides

By extraction with 0.05 N H_2SO_4 solutions, the total protein component was prepared from defatted okra seeds. In a cytotoxic test for 3H-thymidine incorporation into cellular DNA, the protein component exerted growth inhibition against murine KML melanoma cells at a concentration of 100 µg/mL. Three peptide fractions I–III were derived from separation of the okra proteins in a column of Sephadex G-50. The inhibitory activity of peptide fraction-1 reached 39% in the KML cells, but others reached only 8%.[1]

2. Lectin

Abelmoschus esculentus Lectin (AEL), a lectin isolated from okra in the *in vitro* model, significantly elicited 63% growth inhibition against MCF-7 human breast cancer cells, concomitant with the promotion of apoptotic death of MCF-7 cells by 72% via increase of Bax/Bcl-2 ratio and upregulation of proapoptotic caspase-3, caspase-9, and p21 gene expression. However, it showed no such suppression on the tested skin fibroblast (CCD-1059 sk) cell line.[2] In addition, the AEL also showed anti-inflammatory and antinociceptive properties.[2]

3. Pectin

A highly branched pectin rhamnogalacturonan, labeled as okra RG-I, was isolated from the skin of okra pods by hot buffer extraction, which is carrying very short galactan side chains to 2D (on tissue culture polystyrene, tPS) and 3D (on poly[2-hydroxyethyl-methacrylate], polyHEMA) cultures of highly metastatic B16F10 mouse melanoma cells. Thus, incubation with okra RG-I altered the morphology of B16F10 cells and significantly reduced the proliferation and survival of B16F10 cells by 75% after 48 h of treatment. At the same time, okra RG-I induced the apoptosis and G2/M cell arrest in B16F10 cells by interacting with galectin-3 protein.[3]

4. Polysaccharides

A raw polysaccharide (RPS) was extracted by water and ethanol from fresh okra fruit and then was purified by diethyl-aminoethyl group (DEAE) anion exchange chromatography to give three fractions, E1–E3. After 72-h treatment, RPS and E1 at a concentration of 800 μg/mL lessened the survival rates of OVCAR-3 human ovarian cancer cells from 100% to 72.30% and 52.31%, respectively, but E2 and E3 were inactive to OVCAR-3 cells. E3 at a concentration of 800 μg/mL retarded human HeLa (cervix) and MCG803 (stomach) cancer cell lines and at a concentration of 200 μg/mL hindered the growth of human HeLA, MCG803, and MCF-7 carcinoma cells, with the lowest survival rates of 63.51%, 67.71%, and 63.90%, respectively.[4,5] OFPS11, a water-soluble polysaccharide prepared from okra flowers, is mainly composed of galactose and rhamnose in a molar ratio of 2.23:1, with molecular mass of 1700 kDa. OFPS11-pretreated mouse RAW264.7 macrophage cells could notably inhibit the proliferation of human HepG2 hepatoma cells; the antitumor activity of OFPS11 was revealed to be mediated by stimulation of macrophage activities through a nuclear NF-κB pathway, including elevation of NO production, TNF-α and IL-1β secretion, and upregulation of iNOS protein and inducible nitric oxide synthase (iNOS) and TNF-β mRNA expression in RAW264.7 cells.[6]

NANOFORMULATION

The green syntheses of gold nanoparticles (AuNPs) and silver nanoparticles (AgNPs) were prepared with okra pulp extract, with average nanoparticle sizes ~14 nm. In *in vitro* assays, Jurkat human acute myeloid leukemia was mostly sensitive to AuNPs and AgNPs, and their IC_{50} values were 8.17 μg/mL and 16.15 μg/mL, respectively. At 25 μg/mL and 50 μg/mL concentrations, the antiviability rates of the Jurkat cells were 81.3% and 87.2%, respectively, for AuNPs and 85.4% and 91.6%, for the AgNPs, respectively,[7,8] while AuNPs arrested the viability of K562 chronic myeloid leukemia cells by 38.4% and 50.2% and of Dalton's lymphoma cells by 28.5% and 48.2%, respectively.[7] On the other hand, no significant antiviability effect was observed in peripheral blood lymphocytes (PBLs) at doses of AuNPs up to 25 μg/mL, and 38.27% inhibition in PBLs was noted when the dose of AuNPs increased to 50 μg/mL[8]. These approaches displayed that the formulated okra-green nanoparticles (especially AuNPs) may have excellent potential for the treatment of leukemias as adjuvants.

CONCLUSION AND SUGGESTION

As a healthy vegetable, okra has been widely consumed around the world. According to the limited scientific evidence, it is clear that okra may provide protection against carcinogenesis in the skin, breast, liver, and ovary, besides other advantages in health improvement and nutrition. The anti-cancer activity of macromolecules from okra has gained more attention in recent years, but the exploration of bioactive components with small molecules has not been reported yet. Nonetheless, the consumption of okra is one of the choices encouraged for lowering the risk of cancer.

REFERENCES

1. Pshenichnov, E.A. et al., 2005. Bioactive protein components from *Hibiscus esculentus* seeds. *Chem. Nat. Compds.* 41: 82–84.
2. Monte, L.G. et al., 2014. Lectin of *Abelmoschus esculentus* (Okra) promotes selective antitumor effects in human breast cancer cells. *Biotechnol. Lett.* 36: 461–469.
3. Ren, D.D. et al., 2010. Inhibition effect of okra polysaccharides on proliferation of human cancer cell lines. *Shipin Kexue* (Beijing, China) 31: 353–356.
4. Zheng, W. et al., 2014. Purification, characterization and immunomodulating activity of a polysaccharide from flowers of *Abelmoschus esculentus*. *Carbohydr. Polym.* 106: 335–342.

5. Vayssade, M. et al., 2010. Antiproliferative and proapoptotic actions of okra pectin on B16F10 mela-noma cells. *Phytother. Res.* 24: 982–989.
6. Mollick, R.M. et al., 2014. Anticancer (*in vitro*) and antimicrobial effect of gold nanoparticles synthe-sized using *Abelmoschus esculentus* (L.) pulp extract via a green route. *RSC Advan.* 4(71): 37838–37848.
7. Mollick, R.M. et al., 2015. Studies on green synthesized silver nanoparticles using *Abelmoschus escu-lentus* (L.) pulp extract having anticancer (in vitro) and antimicrobial applications. *Arabian J. Chem.* Available online 2015, May 5. (http://dx.doi.org/10.1016/j.arabjc.2015.04.033).

15. PUMPKIN

Citrouille   Kürbis   Calabaza

南瓜　パンプキン　호박

Cucurbita moschata, C. pepo, C. maxima

Cucurbitaceae

1. R = −galactosyl (1-6)-galactosy (1-6)-galactose
3. R = −galactosyl (1-6)-galactosy (1-6)-galactosyl (1-6)-galactose

2. R = −galactosyl (1-6)-galactosy (1-6)-galactose
4. R = −galactosyl (1-6)-galactosy (1-6)-galactosyl (1-6)-galactose

5. R = −ribose (f)
6. R = −H.

7

Pumpkin is one of the common cultivars of Cucurbitaceae plants, which are native to Central and northern South America. Today, it is grown worldwide for uses as a vegetable and for decoration at Halloween. Three most widespread pumpkin varieties, *C. moschata*, *C. maxima*, and *C. pepo*, have great commercial value, with high production. Pumpkin fruits are covered with a thick shell but contain edible pulp and seeds with very few calories. The pulp is a great source of dietary fibers, antioxidants, vitamins (such as vitamins A, C, E, and B complex), β-carotene (provitamin A), antioxidants, carbohydrates, and minerals (such as phosphorus, copper, calcium, and potassium), while the seeds are rich in protein, antioxidants, vitamins, and omega-3 fatty acids. The variety of *C. moschata* is most often used for commercial production of pumpkin pie mix. The large red-orange squash (*C. maxima*) is seen at Halloween in the United States, and the orange-type summer squash (*C. pepo*) is used to make jack-o-lanterns; however, the nutritional and functional values of the two types of pumpkins are ignored in some areas.

Scientific Evidence of Cancer-Inhibitory and Cancer-Preventive Constituents

According to ethnopharmacological studies, pumpkin can provide an excellent source of many natural polyphenolic flavonoids, β-carotenes (such as cryptoxanthin, lutein, and zeaxanthin), polysaccharides, and proteins. During the past decade, pumpkin has been reported to possess antitumor, cancer-preventive, antidiabetic, antihypercholesterolemic, intestinal antiparasitic, antihypertensive, antibacterial, anti-inflammatory, immunomodulatory, and analgesic properties. Some of the phytochemicals from both pulp and seeds of pumpkin have been found to have anticancer potentials and to play a preventive role in certain cancers. Besides the antioxidant activity, zeaxanthin and lutein may offer a protective effect against age-related macular lutea in eyes.

1. Glycoglycerolipids

Six glycoglycerolipid monomers termed GCL-I–VI were discovered from *n*-butanol extract of pumpkin, but GCL-I and -II were isomer mixtures. The structures of other GCLs were determined as 1-O-(9Z,12Z,15Z-octadecatrienoyl)-3-O-[β-D-galactosyl-(1-6)-β-D-galactosyl-(1-6)-β-D-galacosyl]-glycerol for GCL-III (**1**) and 1-O-(9Z,12Z-octadecadienoyl)-3-O-[β-D-galactosyl-(1-6)-β-D-galactosyl-(1-6)-β-D-galacosyl]-glycerol for GCL-IV (**2**), as well as for GCL-V (**3**) and -VI (**4**). In addition to their blood sugar–lowering, anti-inflammatory, and antioxidant activities, the antiproliferative effect of GCLs was observed in human Colo205 (colon), and A549 (lung) carcinoma cell lines and murine B16-F10 melanoma cells *in vitro*. As compared with A549 cells, Colo205 and B16-F10 cells were more sensitive to the GCLs. The preliminary analysis of the structure–activity relationship pointed out that the cancer-inhibitory potencies of GCLs were in dependent on glycerol–sugar backbone and the saturated degree of fatty acid moieties. The efficacy of GCLs in tumor suppression would be attenuated with lessening of galactosyl groups and amplified with increase of double bonds. Accordingly, the GCL-I, -II, and -III presented relatively higher activities on these cell lines.[1]

2. Triterpenes

Cucurbitacins are well-known triterpenes isolated from *Cucurbita* plants for the marked cytotoxic behavior and broad range of anticancer, anti-inflammatory, anthelmintic, cardiovascular, and antimicrobial activities. Cucurbita glycosides-A (**5**) and -B (**6**), two cucurbitane triterpenoids with a purine unit, were discovered from the fruits of *C. pepo* cv. *dayangua* (collected in Jilin, China), showing moderate cytotoxic activity against human HeLa cervical cancer cells, with IC_{50}s of 17.2 μg/mL and 28.4 μg/mL, respectively, in an *in vitro* model.[2] Several multiflorane-type triterpenes were separated from seeds of *C. maxima* (collected in Japan) as cancer inhibitors. Among them, 7-oxomultiflor-8-ene-3α,29-diol 3-acetate-29-benzoate (**7**), multiflora-7,9(11)-diene-3α,29-diol 3-p-hydroxybenzoate-29-benzoate, multiflora-5,7,9(11)-triene-3α,29-diol 3,29-dibenzoate, 7α-hydroxymultiflor-8-ene-3α,29-diol 3-acetate-29-benzoate, and 7β-methoxymultiflor-8-ene-3α,29-diol 3,29-dibenzoate exerted moderate to weak inhibitory activities against the proliferation of two tested leukemia cell lines, human HL-60 and mouse P388 cell lines, *in vitro*, and the most potent inhibitor was 7-oxomultiflor-8-ene-3α,29-diol 3-acetate-29-benzoate (**7**), which exhibited single-digit micromolar cytotoxicity against HL-60 and P388 cells (respective IC_{50}s of 7.0 and 9.5 μM), and the IC_{50}s of other active triterpenes were in the range of 34.5–93.7 μM.[3] Likewise, cucurbitacin-B presents in pumpkins, gourds, and squashes as a bioactive constituent. It showed the inhibitory effects against the proliferation and viability of human non small cell lung cancer cell lines such as epidermal growth factor receptor (EGFR)-wild type (A549 and H1792) and EGFR-mutant type (H1650 and H1975) at nanomolar concentrations (0.2–0.6 μM, 24 h). It also was able to elicit these lung cancer cells to apoptosis, where sestrin-3 was found to play an important role in proapoptosis of both EGFR wild-type and EGFR mutant-type lung cancer cells in the cucurbitacin-B treatment.[4]

3. Proteins

Cucurmosin is a novel type 1 RIP isolated from sarcocarp of pumpkin (*C. moschata*). In *in vitro* models, cucurmosin demonstrated the suppressive effect against the proliferation of human pancreatic cancer (SW-1990, BxPC-3, and PANC-1), cystic fibrosis pancreatic adenocarcinoma (CFPAC-1), and hepatoma (HepG2) cell lines, concomitantly with elicitation of the cell apoptotic death. Proapoptosis in the pancreatic cancer cell lines was mediated by blocking the PI3K/Akt/mechanistic target of rapamycin (mTOR) signaling pathway, downregulation of EGFR, and/or platelet-derived growth factor receptor (PDGFR)-B expression and activation of caspases-3 and -9 and in the hepatoma cell line was associated with an increase of the Bax/Bcl-2 ratio and activation of caspase-3.[5–9] When combined with gefitinib (an EGFR inhibitor), the antiproliferative effect of cucurmosin on PANC-1 cells could be enhanced.[7] The suppressive effects against SW-1990, PANC-1, and HepG2 tumors were further proved in the *in vivo* mouse models.[7–9] *In vivo* treatment with cucurmosin in a dose of 0.5 mg/kg showed 53.45% growth inhibition against human K562 chronic myeloid leukemia in mice and 36% survival extension of the tested mice.[10] In association with downregulation of P210bcr/abl, disruption of Hsp90 molecular chaperone functions, decline of Bcl-2/Bax ratio, and activation of caspase-3, cucurmosin triggered the K562 cells to apoptosis.[11]

In addition, another novel RIP designated Moschatin was purified from mature seeds of pumpkin (*C. moschata*), whose molecular weight was approximately 29 kDa. Moschatin in an *in vitro* assay displayed potent antiproliferative effects against human M21 melanoma cells, with IC_{50} of 59.0 nM. When an immunotoxin termed Moschatin-Ng76 was prepared by using antihuman melanoma McAb Ng76 and Moschatin, the suppression on the M21 cells could be augmented remarkably by 1500 times (IC_{50} of 0.04 nM).[12]

All these scientific results have demonstrated that the protein components such as cucurmosin and Moschatin are the major contributors to the cancer-preventive potential of pumpkin and pumpkin seeds. The preparation of immunotoxin from the pumpkin proteins may be a promising clue to the discovery and development of a new therapeutic agent for cancer treatment.

4. Enzyme

An ascorbic oxidase was isolated from Japanese pumpkin (*C. moschata*), which could hinder the growth of sarcoma 180 after being injected into tested mice subcutaneously SC. Because of its affinity for thymus DNA, the pumpkin ascorbate oxidase is able to induce the cleavage of DNA molecules by the formation of DNA–oxidase complexes. Its biological character was possible to relate to the antitumor effect of pumpkin.[13]

5. Seed extract

A hydroalcoholic extract derived from seeds of the Styrian pumpkin (*C. pepo* var. *styriaca*) showed a weak inhibitory effect on human neoplastic cell lines such as LNCaP (androgen-sensitive prostate), DU145 (androgen-insensitive prostate), MCF-7 (estrogen receptor alpha (ERα)-positive breast), and Caco-2 (colorectal), as well as on human benign prostate hyperplasia (BPH-1) cells *in vitro*. By treatment with the extract in a 100-μg/mL concentration, cell growth inhibition of about 40%–50% was observed in these cancer cell lines and BPH-1 cells, but only inhibition of ~20% was observed in human HDF-5 fibroblast cells.[14] Moreover, a phytoestrogen-rich extract (PSE) was isolated from pumpkin seeds, which was found to contain polyphenolics such as lignans and flavones. After PSE treatment, the levels of estradiol production were elevated in human Jeg3 and BeWo choriocarcinoma and human MCF-7 breast cancer cells in a dose-dependent manner. At the same time, a significant upregulation of progesterone receptor and a prominent downregulation of estrogen receptor-α were elicited in MCF-7 cells.[15] These findings therefore disclosed that pumpkin seed consumption may be safe to protect prostate, colon, breast, and hormone-related female organs from cancer.

CONCLUSION AND SUGGESTION

The cancer prevention-related phytochemicals in pumpkin pulp and seeds have been summarized earlier, wherein glycoglycerolipids, cucurbita glycosides, major proteins (cucurmosin and Moschatin), and ascorbic oxidase are weak cancer inhibitors, but they are believed to have applications in lowering the risk of certain cancers by dietary intake of pumpkin fruits and seeds. Meanwhile, β-carotenes (such as cryptoxanthin, lutein, and zeaxanthin) present in the pumpkin pulp also have potential for cancer prevention in some cases, especially lessening the risk of cancer in lung, stomach, and lymphocytes (see section 17 in Chapter 3), besides antioxidant and free-radical scavenging activities.[16] In addition, pumpkin flower is used as a vegetable and a folk medicine in some areas. Its contents are rich in β-carotene, vitamins C and A, and folic acid, and thus, it may also be helpful as an anticarcinogen. Consequently, this evidence provided the rationale to consume pumpkin frequently as both a nutritional and functional food to benefit our health.

REFERENCES

1. Jiang, Z.G. et al., 2013. Preparation separation and antioxidant activities of glycoglycerolipids from pumpkin and antitumor activity. *Zhongguo Liangyou Xuebao* 28(7): 88–92, 98.
2. Wang, D.C. et al., 2008. Purine-containing cucurbitane triterpenoids from *Cucurbita pepo* cv dayangua. *Phytochemistry* 69: 1434–1438.
3. (a) Kikuchi, T. et al., 2013. Three new multiflorane-type triterpenes from pumpkin (*Cucurbita maxima*) seeds. *Molecules* 18: 5568–5579; (b) Kikuchi, T. et al., 2014. Three new triterpene esters from pumpkin (*Cucurbita maxima*) seeds. *Molecules* 19: 4802–4813.
4. Khan, N. et al., 2017. Sestrin-3 modulation is essential for therapeutic efficacy of cucurbitacin B in lung cancer cells. *Carcinogenesis* 38(2): 184–195.
5. Zhang, B.M. et al., 2012. Cucurmosin induces apoptosis of BxPC-3 human pancreatic cancer cells via inactivation of the (EGFR) signaling pathway. *Oncol. Rep.* 27: 891–897.
6. Xie, J.M. et al., 2013. Cucurmosin induces the apoptosis of human pancreatic cancer CFPAC-1 cells by inactivating the (PDGFR-B) signaling pathway. *Pharmacol. Rep.* 65: 682–688.
7. Wang, C.F. et al., 2014. PANC-1 pancreatic cancer cell growth inhibited by cucurmosin alone and in combination with an epidermal growth factor receptor-targeted drug. *Pancreas* 43: 291–297.
8. Xie, J.M. et al., 2013. Cucurmosin kills human pancreatic cancer SW-1990 cells in vitro and in vivo. *Anticancer Agent Med. Chem.* 13: 952–956.
9. Xie, J.M. et al., 2012. Antiproliferative effects of cucurmosin on human hepatoma HepG2 cells. *Mol. Med. Rep.* 5: 196–201.
10. Liu, T.B. et al., 2013. Effect of cucurmosin on chronic myeloid leukemia K562 cell line. *Zhongguo Shiyan Xueyexue Zazhi* 21: 891–894.
11. Xie, J.M. et al., 2011. Antitumor effects of cucurmosin in human chronic myeloid leukemia occur through cell cycle arrest and decrease the Bcl-2/Bax ratio to induce apoptosis. *Afr. Pharm. Pharmacol.* 5: 985–992.
12. Xia, H.C. et al., 2003. Purification and characterization of Moschatin, a novel type I ribosome-inactivating protein from the mature seeds of pumpkin (*Cucurbita moschata*), and preparation of its immunotoxin against human melanoma cells. *Cell Res.* 13: 369–374.
13. (a) Omura, H. et al., 1974. Antitumor potentiality of the enzyme preparations, pumpkin ascorbate oxidase and shiitake mushroom polyphenol oxidase. *J. Fac. Agricul. Kyushu Univ.* 18: 191–200; (b) Omura, H. et al., 1973. Antitumor action of an ascorbate oxidase preparation and its interaction with deoxyribonucleic acid. *J. Fac. Agricul. Kyushu Univ.* 17: 187–194.
14. Svjetlana, M. et al., 2016. Pumpkin seed extract: Cell growth inhibition of hyperplastic and cancer cells, independent of steroid hormone receptors. *Fitoterapia* 110: 150–156.
15. Richter, D. et al., 2013. Effects of phytoestrogen extracts isolated from pumpkin seeds on estradiol production and ER/PR expression in breast cancer and trophoblast tumor cells. *Nutr. Cancer* 65: 739–745.
16. Colagar, A.H. et al., 2012. Review of pumpkin anticancer effects. *Quran Med.* 1: 77–88.

16. TOMATO

Tomates   Tomaten   Tomate

番茄 トマト 토마토

Lycopersicon esculentum (= Solanum lycopersicum)

Solanaceae

2. R = –OH
3. R = –H

4. R = –beta-D-glucosyl(2-1)-alpha-L-rhamnosyl,
7. R = –H

5. R$_1$ = –A, R$_2$ = –H, R$_3$ = –CH$_3$
6. R$_1$ = –A, R$_2$ = –CH$_2$O-beta-D-glucosyl, R$_3$ = –H

The tomato is native to western South America and Central America, but its fruit is now found all over the world as an important healthy vegetable. Originally called the cherry tomato (var. *cerasiforme*), many cultivars have been developed as an edible vegetable. The Roma tomato is one of the cultivars available, developed in the 1950s by the USDA as a fusarium wilt-resistant cultivar. Tomatoes and their products (sauce, paste, and juice) are now often employed in cuisines or drinks. Being rich in vitamins C and A, carotene, and lycopene, tomatoes are considered to be one of the most powerful natural antioxidants, which may improve the skin's ability to protect against harmful ultraviolet (UV) rays and sunburn, may relieve the oxidative stress of people who already have diabetes or other related diseases, and may help delay free-radical–induced aging and diminish the risk of angiocardiopathy, besides resisting cancer initiation.

SCIENTIFIC EVIDENCE OF CANCER-INHIBITORY AND CANCER-PREVENTIVE ACTIVITIES

Tomatoes have been subjected to various investigations in cancer prevention and carcinogenesis inhibition for a long time. Giving drinking water–diluted tomato juice to male rats for 12 weeks resulted in a suppressive effect against *N*-butyl-*N*-(4-hydroxybutyl)nitrosamine (BBN)-caused urinary bladder carcinogenesis.[1] An *in vivo* approach exhibited that drinking tomato juice daily enhanced the anticancer properties of saliva to protect against carcinogenesis.[2] Tomato juices that were made of either tomato (CK) or two mutant tomatoes (M1 and M2, by space mutation breeding) exerted anticancer activity against human colon cancer cell lines (SW480 and HT-29). The juices of M1 and M2 were able to arrest cell cycle at G0/G1 and/or G2/M phases and to inhibit the growth of cancer cells by maximum 30%, showing more effectiveness than the CK juice, wherein SW480 cells were more sensitive to the M1 and M2 juices as compared with HT-29 cells.[3] Feeding 5% tomato powder to rats decreased the rate of aberrant crypt foci (ACF) and impeded the development of azoxymethane (AOM)-induced colorectal adenocarcinoma; the preventive effect was mediated by inhibition of COX-2 expression via the NF-κB pathway and promotion of apoptosis, as well as regulation of Nrf2/HO-1 signaling pathway.[4] In a mouse model with transgenic prostate adenocarcinoma, a diet of tomato delayed the progression from prostatic intraepithelial neoplasia to adenocarcinoma and lessened the incidence of poorly differentiated carcinoma, leading to prolonging the overall survival of the tested mice.[5] An n-hexane extract of tomato paste (TP) at a 5-μM concentration induced the G0/G1 and G2/M cell-cycle arrests and late-stage apoptosis, thereby restraining the proliferation of human LNCaP prostate cancer cells by 67% after 48-h incubation, whereas whole TP and its water extract only showed modest growth inhibition in the same *in vitro* assay.[6] A tomato extract PLX (which included 2% lycopene) and tomato chitooligosaccharides showed *in vitro* cytotoxic effects in the LNCaP cells, together with downregulation of prostate-specific antigen (PSA) and 5α-reductase expression.[7] Likewise, a diet of tomato powder diminished the incidence of prostate carcinogenesis caused by *N*-methyl-*N*-nitrosourea and testosterone in male rats and reduced the tumor weights in rats implanted with R3327-H prostate adenocarcinoma.[8] During the treatment, tomato-elicited events such as augmenting serum antioxidative activity and lessening serum inflammatory/angiogenic biomarkers were particularly involved in the inhibition of prostate carcinogenesis.[5]

In addition, a fraction derived from 82% methanol extract of tomato plant leaves exhibited a cytotoxic effect toward the human MCF-7 breast cancer cell line, with an IC_{50} value of 5.85 µg/mL, but it was harmless to Vero normal kidney epithelial cells (IC_{50} of 765.6 µg/mL).[9]

SCIENTIFIC EVIDENCE OF CANCER-INHIBITORY AND CANCER-PREVENTIVE CONSTITUENTS

1. Lycopene

A carotenoid termed lycopene (**1**) is the predominant constituent in tomatoes and tomato-based foods, as well as in other fruits or plants such as gac, pink grapefruit, watermelon, pink guava, red carrot, and papaya.[10] The average content of lycopene in tomatoes is 11.6–14 mg/kg of tomato weight.[11] Lycopene, in chemistry, is a symmetrical tetraterpene assembled from eight isoprene units. Naturally, lycopene is present in the all *trans*-isomer form in plants, but a total of 72 geometric isomers of the molecule are sterically possible. On exposure to light and heat, lycopene can undergo isomerization to produce various forms of mono- and poly-*cis* isomers. The studies revealed that *cis*-lycopene predominated in some benign and malignant tissues after tomato consumption, and the poly-*cis* isomers can establish more than 60% of total lycopene in human bloodstream concentration. The findings indicated that tomato tissue isomerases are involved in isomerization of lycopene from all-*trans* form to various *cis* forms, and the *cis*-isomers of lycopene are possibly more bioavailable than the *trans*-lycopene *in vivo*.[12] Likewise, the food cooking can increase *cis* forms of lycopene (**1**) far more than it is destroyed during the processing, leading to improvement of the bioavailability of lycopene.

In first, Lycopene (**1**) as a potent antioxidant may play an important role in reducing the risk of some types of cancers through scavenging of free radicals, induction of apoptosis, and inhibition of cellular proliferative processes. *In vitro* assay revealed that lycopene (**1**) was effective in inhibiting the proliferation of multiple human cancer cell lines, such as prostate (PC3, LNCaP, and DU145), breast (ER/PR-positive MCF-7, MDA-MB-231, MDA-MB-235, HER2-positive SK-BR-3, and triple-negative MDA-MB-468), liver (Hep3B and SK-Hep1), lung (NCI-H226 and BEN), colon (T-84 and HT-29), leukemic (K562, Raji, B-CLL), and endometrial (Ishikawa), as well as rat R3327-H prostate adenocarcinomas. The antiproliferative effect was associated with the induction of cell-cycle arrest and/or apoptosis, and the IC_{50} values were 1–2 µM in Ishikawa, MCF-7, and NCI-H226 cell lines,[8–30] whose inhibitory potencies were 4-fold higher than α-carotene or 10-fold higher than β-carotene,[16] and the IC_{50} values were 9, 22, and 30 µg/mL in HCT-116 (colon), MCF-7 (breast), and AGS (stomach) cancer cell lines, respectively. Similarly, lycopene (**1**) impeded the growth of SF-268 central nervous system (CNS) cancer cells by 35% and NCT-H460 lung cancer cells by 25% at 60 µg/mL concentration.[17] After 96 h of treatment, lycopene (**1**) reduced the viabilities of MCF-7, MDA-MB-231, and MDA-MB-235 cells by 30%, 75%, and 20%, respectively.[17] The *in vivo* capacities of lycopene (**1**) were further proved in inhibiting *N*-nitrosodiethylamine-induced hepatocarcinogenesis, inducing apoptosis in female Balb/c mice,[11,18] and activating antioxidant enzymes and immunity function in *N*-methyl-*N'*-nitro-*N*-nitrosoguanidine-induced gastric carcinoma in rats.[19] Daily consumption of spaghetti sauce (containing 30 mg of lycopene in 200 g of sauce) in pasta dishes for 3 weeks prior to radical prostatectomy resulted in clearly lower oxidative DNA damage in prostate tissue and higher apoptotic rate in prostate cancer epithelial cells.[8]

Moreover, combining lycopene with vitamin E hindered cancer progression and extended the median survival of nude mice burdened with prostate cancer.[8] Lycopene beadlet (LB) formation contains lycopene plus 5% ascorbyl palmitate and 1.5% D,L-α-tocopherol as antioxidants. In a mouse model transplanted with prostate adenocarcinoma, intake of lycopene from TP or LB for 20 days provided the same 28 mg lycopene in per-kg diet, leading to marked lessening of prostate cancer incidence by 20% in the TP group and by 40% in the LB group. The results exhibited that an LB-enriched diet (which combined lycopene with antioxidants) achieved better chemopreventive activity against prostate cancer.[20] Also, when co-treated with 1,25-dihydroxy-vitamin D3, lycopene (1) in low concentrations synergistically elicited the cell-cycle arrest and differentiation of human HL-60 promyelocytic leukemia cells.[21]

More broad explorations provided a mechanistic insight into the anticarcinogenic effects of lycopene, revealing that it was associated with (1) induction of retinoic acid receptors/retinoid-X receptor activation pathways (particularly mediated by lycopene metabolites),[22] (2) modulation of growth factors and growth factor receptors, including insulin-like growth factor-1 and platelet-derived growth factor-BB,[16,22] (3) blockage of COX pathways, control of ROS-mediated cell growth, and prevention of cell oxidative damage and its influence on cell growth,[23] (4) alteration of the mevalonate pathway and Ras signaling and lessening of Ras-dependent activation of NF-κB,[24] (5) upregulation of connexin-43 and enhancement of gap junction communication,[24,25] (6) inhibition of high-mobility group box-1 (HMGB1)-induced proinflammatory responses,[26] (7) block of PI3K/Akt signaling pathway and upregulation of IGFBP-3, c-fos, and uPAR (especially in prostate cancer),[10,27] and (8) multi-immuno-modulatory activity—that is, restoration of the decreased viability and cytotoxicity of NK cells and limitation of NK cell apoptosis, enhancement of IFN-γ expression, lymphocyte proliferation, and IL-2 secretion, and inactivation of intrathymic T-cell differentiation in tumorous body,[28] besides induction of cell apoptosis and cell-cycle arrest. In triple-negative MDA-MB-468 breast cancer cells, the inhibition of lycopene was mediated by the stop of Akt phosphorylation and its downstream molecule mTOR and subsequent upregulation of proapoptotic Bax and p21 expressions.[29]

Furthermore, the suppressive effect of lycopene on the cell adhesion, invasion, and migration was observed in SK-Hep1 human hepatoma cells. Incubation of SK-Hep1 cells with lycopene (1) for 1 h markedly deterred cell adhesion to Matrigel-coated substrate in a concentration-dependent manner and sequentially for 24 h arrested cell invasion and migration, concomitant with lessening of gelatinolytic activities of MMP-2 and MMP-9, demonstrating the antimetastatic potential of lycopene. During the treatment in the SK-Hep1 cells, the cell growth was inhibited by 40% at 50 mM lycopene for 24 h and the cell invasion was significantly reduced to 61.9% of the control level at 10 mM lycopene.[30]

2. Flavonoids

Tomato contains several flavonoids such as quercetin, kaempferol, naringin, naringenin, rutin, and luteolin. Quercetin (2) and kaempferol (3) exhibited dose-dependent inhibition of growth and induced G2/M cell-cycle arrest in AT6.3 rat prostate cancer cells (IC_{50}s of 25–40 μmol/L), while rutin was less potent (IC_{50} of >60 μmol/L). The inhibitory effect was associated with repression of insulin-like growth factor-I (IGF-I)–induced proliferation and induction of apoptosis in AT6.3 cells via inhibition of multiple intracellular signaling pathways.[31] Both cellular and xenograft breast cancer models proved that treatment with kaempferol restrained estrogen-caused growth of human MCF-7 breast cancer cells.[32] Likewise, naringin (4) demonstrated the chemopreventive and anticancer activities in various models of oral, breast, colon, liver, lung, and ovarian cancers.[34] Pretreatment of naringin (4) shortened the survival of human cervical SiHa carcinoma cells (IC_{50} of 750 μM), along with the stimulation of death receptor and mitochondria-mediated apoptosis. By activating the Ras/Raf-dependent ERK signaling pathway, naringin (~150 μM) dose-dependently hindered the growth and proliferation of human 5637 bladder cancer cells. Naringin (4) was also effective in the *in vitro* inhibition of human MDA-MB-435 (breast) and A549 (lung) cancer cell lines and in the *in vivo* suppression of carcinogenesis in colorectal (induced by 1,2-dimethylhydrazine), colon (induced by azoxymethane), liver (induced by N-nitrosodiethylamine), oral (induced by DMBA), and skin (caused by UV-A radiation) cancers [?].[33] The *in vivo* antigrowth effect of naringin also occurred in mice bearing sarcoma 180 and in rats bearing Walker 256 carcinosarcoma. Impressively, administration of naringin orally in a dose of 25 mg/kg impeded the growth of W256 tumor by 75%, along with a decrease in interleukin (IL)-6 and TNF-α levels.[33] The cytotoxicity of irinotecan (50 mg/kg, a chemotherapeutic agent) could be augmented by naringin (100 mg/kg) in co-treatment of Ehrlich ascites tumor in mice.[33] Consequently, these research results revealed that the flavonoids of tomato are able to neutralize the risk of some solid carcinogeneses, and their weak inhibitory potencies are propitious in cancer prevention.

3. Glycoalkaloids

Tomato glycoalkaloid tomatine is a steroid-alkaloid glycoside that was especially isolated from green tomatoes. A mixture of α-tomatine (**5**) and dehydrotomatine (~10:1) demonstrated marked growth inhibition against both human colon and liver cancer cell lines *in vitro*. The mixture in the *in vivo* experiment diminished the incidence of liver and stomach tumors caused by a multiorgan carcinogen dibenzo[a,l]pyrene.[34] The inhibitory effect of purified α-tomatine (**5**) was much stronger than that of dehydrotomatine, which differs from α-tomatine by only a double bond presented in ring B. Their aglycons tomatidine and tomatidenol exerted a moderate effect against some of tested cancer cell lines. Cytotoxicity experiments showed that α-tomatine was capable of inducing about 50% lysis of CT-26 colon cancer cells at 3.5 μM after 24 h of treatment and eliciting apoptosis of CT-26 cells via caspase-independent signaling pathways, including increase of nuclear translocation of Apoptosis-inducing factor (AIF) and downregulation of survivin expression. The cancer inhibition of α-tomatine (**5**) was further proved in a mouse model implanted with CT-26 cancer, without causing changes of body and organ weight. The antigrowth rate was 38% after intraperitoneal (IP) administration of α-tomatine (5 mg/kg body weight) for 2 weeks.[35] In concentrations between 0.1 μg/mL and 100 μg/mL, α-tomatine (**5**) achieved 38.0%–81.5% inhibition against HT-29 colon cancer cells and 46.3%–89.2% suppression against HepG2 hepatoma cells. However, it also showed a similar degree of inhibition on normal human Chang liver cells.[37] The antiproliferative effect of α-tomatine (**5**) was also observed in human prostate (PC3), breast (MCF-7 and MDA-MB-231), gastric (KATO-III), and leukemic (Molt-4) cancer cell lines and normal human lung (Hel299) cells *in vitro*. Of these cell lines, PC3 prostatic adenocarcinoma cells were highly susceptible to α-tomatine, with IC_{50} of 1.67 μM; the higher inhibition was probably attributed to proapoptosis through both intrinsic and extrinsic pathways and the reduction in TNF-α levels by α-tomatine (**5**). An *in vivo* approach further confirmed the anti-growth effect of α-tomatine (in doses of 5–10 mg/kg IP) on the PC3 prostate cancer, without inducing overt toxicity.[36] Another glycoalkaloid assigned as esculeoside-A (**6**) was separated from ripe tomatoes. Its antiproliferative effect presented in mouse B16F2F melanoma and human MCF-7 breast carcinoma cell lines, with 50% reduction in growth of cancer cells (GI_{50}s) of 7.9–13.3 μM.[38]

Moreover, α-tomatine (**5**) was capable of restraining the invasion and migration of A549 and NCI-H460 nonsmall cell lung cancer cell lines; its antimetastatic potential was associated with the inactivation of PI3K/Akt or ERK1/2 signaling pathways, inhibition of NF-κB or AP-1 binding activities, and/or inactivation of MMPs-2 and -9 and urokinase-type plasminogen activator (u-PA).[36] α-Tomatine has a tetrasaccharide chain in its structure. When the side saccharide chain was shortened by partial hydrolysis, the anticancer potency would be attenuated.[37,38] According to these findings, it is clear that α-tomatine (**5**), esculeoside-A (**6**), and tomatine-rich green tomatoes may be helpful in the prevention and chemotherapy of colon cancer and hepatoma. However, overdoses of tomato glycoalkaloids may have safety problem. Immature tomato generally contains higher content of glycoalkaloids.

NANOFORMULATION

Lycopene (**1**) is an important functional constituent of tomatoes. A lycopene-nanogold nano-emulsion was created, which was composed of gold nanoparticles (AN) 0.16 ppm and lycopene (LP) 0.4 μM. This nanoformulation could synergistically amplify the abilities to induce the early apoptotic death of HT-29 colon cancer cells by 15-fold and to deter the migration and invasion of HT-29 cells significantly, indicating a promising potential for further development in colon cancer chemotherapy.[39]

CONCLUSION AND SUGGESTION

This research indicates that tomatoes, tomato juices, and tomato products (which presumably contain lycopene and other antioxidants) exert the inhibitory and preventive effects against the development of carcinogenesis. The anticancer-related components have been disclosed to be lycopene (1), flavonoids, and glycoalkaloids such as α-tomatine (5) and esculeoside-A (6). When the tomatoes ripen, the content of lycopene (1) is amplified to high levels, along with a great decrease of the glycoalkaloid contents in tomatoes. The green tomatoes contain the highest level of glycoalkaloids, which would gradually decline during fruit ripening and in preservation. The flavonoid and lycopene components are primarily responsible to the antioxidant activities of tomatoes. There is no doubt that tomato and its products deserve to be used as dietary supplements for chemoprevention, especially for protecting colon, liver, prostate, and urinary bladder from oncogenesis. Hence, frequent consumption of tomato, tomato juice, and other products is highly encouraged. Cooking tomatoes for a longer time promotes the conversion of natural all-*trans* forms of lycopene to *cis* forms, since the *cis* forms of lycopene are more bioavailable in cancer prevention and are more delicious.

OTHER BIOACTIVITIES OF THE CONSTITUENTS

Besides having antioxidant, anticarcinogenic, and anti-inflammatory properties, lycopene (1) possesses multiple capabilities such as repressing neuroinflammation and hepatic steatosis, protecting cardiovascular from oxidative stress and heart lysosomal damage, recovering liver and kidney tissue injuries, reducing DNA damage, and defending skin against sunburn.[36] Moreover, naringenin (7) displayed a potential for the treatment of neurodegenerative disorders such as Parkinson's and Alzheimer's,[40] and esculeoside-A (6) showed an ability to lessen the levels of cholesterol, triglycerides, and low-density lipoprotein (LDL)-cholesterol in serum.[41]

REFERENCES

1. Okajima, E. et al., 1998. Inhibitory effect of tomato juice on rat urinary bladder carcinogenesis after N-butyl-N-(4-hydroxybutyl) nitrosamine initiation. *Jpn J. Cancer Res.* 89: 22–26.
2. Toda, M. et al., 2008. Tomato and anticancer properties of saliva. In: Preedy, V.R. and Watson, R.R. (Eds.), *Tomatoes & Tomato Products*, Science Publishers, Enfield, NH, pp. 377–384.
3. Shi, J.H. et al., 2010. Induction of apoptosis by tomato using space mutation breeding in human colon cancer SW480 and HT-29 cells. *J. Sci. Food Agric.* 90: 615–621.
4. Tuzcu, M. et al., 2012. Tomato powder impedes the development of azoxymethane-induced colorectal cancer in rats through suppression of COX-2 expression via NF-κB and regulating Nrf2/HO-1 pathway. *Mol. Nutri. Food Res.* 56: 1477–1481.
5. Pannellini, T. et al., 2010. A dietary tomato supplement prevents prostate cancer in TRAMP mice. *Cancer Prev. Res.* 3: 1284–1291.
6. Hwang, E.-S. et al., 2005. Effects of tomato paste extracts on cell proliferation, cell-cycle arrest and apoptosis in LNCaP human prostate cancer cells. *BioFactors* 23: 75–84.
7. Kang, H.S. et al., 2007. The effect of the compound of tomato extract to the prostatic cancer cell and the prostate of the rat model of benign prostatic hyperplasia. *Saengyak Hakhoechi* 38: 197–203.
8. Wang, Y. et al., 2016. Lycopene, tomato products and prostate cancer-specific mortality among men diagnosed with nonmetastatic prostate cancer in the Cancer Prevention Study II Nutrition Cohort. *Intl. J. Cancer* 138: 2846–2855.
9. Chik, W.D.W. et al., 2010. Purification and cytotoxicity assay of tomato (*Lycopersicon esculen tum*) leaves methanol extract as potential anticancer agent. *J. Appl. Sci.* 10: 3283–3288.
10. Chen, J.Z. et al., 2014. The effect of lycopene on the PI3K/Akt signalling pathway in prostate cancer. *Anti-Cancer Agent. Med. Chem.* 14: 800–805.

11. Gupta, P. et al., 2013. Spectroscopic characterization of lycopene extract from *Lycopersicum esculentum* (Tomato) and its evaluation as a chemopreventive agent against experimental hepatocarcinogenesis in mice. *Phytother. Res.* 27: 448–456.

12. Avci, A. et al., 2008. Tomato juice, prostate cancer and adenosine deaminase enzyme. In: Preedy, V.R. and Watson, R.R. (Eds.), *Tomatoes & Tomato Products*, Enfield, NH, pp. 457–474.

13. Nda, S. et al., 2013. Influence of lycopene on cell viability, cell cycle, and apoptosis of human prostate cancer and benign hyperplastic cells. *Nutr. Cancer* 65: 1076–1085.

14. Tang, F.Y. et al., 2008. Lycopene inhibits growth of human colon cancer cells via suppression of the Akt signaling pathway. *Mol. Nutr. Food Res.* 52: 646–654.

15. Salman, H. et al., 2007. Lycopene affects proliferation and apoptosis of four malignant cell lines. *Biomed. Pharmacother.* 61: 366–369.

16. Levy, J. et al., 1995. Lycopene is a more potent inhibitor of human cancer cell proliferation than either α-carotene or β-carotene. *Nutr. Cancer* 24: 257–266.

17. Gloria, N.F. et al., 2014. Lycopene and beta-carotene induce cell-cycle arrest and apoptosis in human breast cancer cell lines. *Anticancer Res.* 34: 1377–1386.

18. Gupta, P. et al., 2013. Evaluating the effect of lycopene from *Lycopersicum esculentum* on apoptosis during NDEA induced hepatocarcinogenesis. *Biochem. Biophys. Res. Commun.* 434: 479–485.

19. (a) Luo, C. et al., 2011. Lycopene enhances antioxidant enzyme activities and immunity function in N-methyl-N′-nitro-N-nitrosoguanidine-induced gastric cancer rats. *Int. J. Mol. Sci.* 12: 3340–3351; (b) Yang, T.S. et al., 2013. The role of tomato products and lycopene in the prevention of gastric cancer: A meta-analysis of epidemiologic studies. *Med. Hypoth.* 80: 383–388.

20. Konijeti, R. et al., 2010. Chemoprevention of prostate cancer with lycopene in the TRAMP model. *Prostate* (Hoboken, NJ) 70: 1547–1554.

21. Amir, H. et al., 1999. Lycopene and 1,25-dihydroxyvitamin D3 cooperate in the inhibition of cell cycle progression and induction of differentiation in HL-60 leukemic cells. *Nutr. Cancer.* 33: 105–112.

22. (a) Aydemir, G. et al., 2013. Lycopene-derived bioactive retinoic acid receptors/retinoid-X receptors-activating metabolites may be relevant for lycopene's anticancer potential. *Mol. Nutr. Food Res.* 57: 739–747; (b) Sharoni, Y. et al., 2012. The role of lycopene and its derivatives in the regulation of transcription systems: Implications for cancer prevention. *Am. J. Clin. Nutr.* 96: 1173S–1178S.

23. Palozza, P. et al., 2011. Role of lycopene in the control of ROS-mediated cell growth: Implications in cancer prevention. *Current Med. Chem.* 18: 1846–1860.

24. Paola, P. 2010. Lycopene induces cell growth inhibition by altering mevalonate pathway and Ras signalling in cancer cell lines. *Carcinogenesis* 31: 1813–1821.

25. Palozza, P. et al., 2011. Tomato lycopene and lung cancer prevention: From experimental to human studies. *Cancers* 3: 2333–2357.

26. Lee, W.W. et al., 2012. Inhibitory effects of lycopene on HMGB1-mediated pro-inflammatory responses in both cellular and animal models. *Food Chem. Toxicol.* 50: 1826–1833.

27. Talvas, J. et al., 2010. Differential effects of lycopene consumed in tomato paste and lycopene in the form of a purified extract on target genes of cancer prostatic cells. *Am. J. Clini. Nutr.* 91: 1716–1724.

28. (a) Qi, L. et al., 2014. Lycopene prolongs the lifespan and enhances the cytotoxicity of NK cells after ex vivo expansion. *Bioeng. Biosci.* 2: 23–30: (b) Kobayashi, T. et al, 1996, Effects of lycopene, a carotenoid, on intrathymic T cell differentiation and peripheral CD4/CD8 ratio in a high mammary tumor strain of SHN retired mice. *Anticancer Drugs* 7(2): 195–8.

29. Takeshima, M. et al., 2014. Anti-proliferative and apoptosis-inducing activity of lycopene against three subtypes of human breast cancer cell lines. *Cancer Sci.* 105: 252–227.

30. Hwang, E.S. et al., 2006. Inhibitory effects of lycopene on the adhesion, invasion, and migration of SK-Hep1 human hepatoma cells. *Exp. Biol. Med.* (Maywood). 231: 322–327.

31. Wang, S.H. et al., 2003. Tomato and soy polyphenols reduce insulin-like growth factor-I-stimulated rat prostate cancer cell proliferation and apoptotic resistance in vitro via inhibition of intracellular signaling pathways involving tyrosine kinase. *J. Nutri.* 133: 2367–2376.

32. Kim, S.H. et al., 2016. Treatment with kaempferol suppressed breast cancer cell growth caused by estrogen and triclosan in cellular and xenograft breast cancer models. *J. Nutri. Biochem.* 28: 70–82.

33. Bharti, S. et al., 2014. Preclinical evidence for the pharmacological actions of naringin: A review. *Planta Med.* 80: 437–451.

34. Friedman, M. et al., 2010. Review of anticarcinogenic and anticholesterol effects of the tomato glycoalkaloid tomatine. *Abstracts of Papers, 239th ACS National Meeting*, San Francisco, CA, March 21–25, (2010), AGRO-41.

35. Kim, S.P. et al., 2015. The tomato glycoalkaloid α-tomatine induces caspase-independent cell death in mouse colon cancer CT-26 cells and transplanted tumors in mice. *J. Agricul. Food Chem.* 63: 1142–1150.
36. Friedman, M. et al., 2013. Anticarcinogenic, cardioprotective, and other health benefits of tomato compounds lycopene, α-tomatine, and tomatidine in pure form and in fresh and processed tomatoes. *J. Agricul. Food Chem.* 61: 9534–9550.
37. Lee, K.R. et al., 2004. Glycoalkaloids and metabolites inhibit the growth of human colon (HT29) and liver (HepG2) cancer cells. *J. Agric. Food Chem.* 52: 2832–2839.
38. Murakami, Y. et al., 2010. Edible dry tomato powders containing tomato steroid glycosides, their manufacture, and their uses. Jpn. Kokai Tokkyo Koho JP 2010273593 A 20101209.
39. Huang, R.F.S. et al., 2015. Inhibition of colon cancer cell growth by nanoemulsion carrying gold nanoparticles and lycopene. *Int. J. Nanomed.* 10: 2823–2846.
40. Wu, L.H. et al., 2016. Naringenin suppresses neuroinflammatory responses through inducing suppressor of cytokine signaling 3 expression. *Mol. Neurobiol.* 53: 1080–1091.
41. Nohara, T. et al., 2010. The tomato saponin, esculeoside A. *J. Nat. Prod.* 74: 1734–1741.

3 Cancer-Preventive Substances in Root Vegetables

17. Carrot/*Daucus carota* subsp. *sativus*

18. Garlic/*Allium sativum*

19. Onion/*Allium cepa*

20. Konjac or Moyu/*Amorphophallus rivieri*

21. Potato/*Solanum tuberosum*

22. Red Beet or Chard/*Beta vulgaris* and its varieties

23. Sweet Potato/*Ipomoea batatas*

The root vegetables are a large and important group in the vegetable category. Many kinds of plant tubers, rhizomes, true roots, and bulbs are commercialized as nutritional foods for human daily life, including carrots, potatoes, yams, beets, parsnips, turnips, rutabagas, daikon, radishes, yucas, taros, celeriacs, onions, and garlics. Growing underground, the root vegetables absorb a large amount of nutrients from the soil and store high concentrations of biologically active chemicals such as antioxidants, polyphenolics, fibers, vitamins, iron, and several types of carbohydrates. Root vegetables not only contribute their nutritional values to human living but also exert functional characteristics for human health promotion through dietary intake. This chapter highlights seven common and popular root vegetables in day-to-day life and discusses their remarkable potentials for anticarcinogenesis, antioxidant, immunoregulation, and other functions regarding health improvement. Daily consumption of these seven roots/bulb-representative root vegetables is highly recommended to lessen the incidence of malignant tumors and chronic diseases. Furthermore, intake of both steamed and baked potatoes and sweet potatoes/yams as a staple food is a good idea.

In addition to these common root vegetables, the true roots of an herbal plant named fishwort (*Houttuynia cordata*) have been popularized as a wild vegetable in some local cities of China. The roots of three herbal plants—Chinese yam (*Dioscorea polystachya*), kudzu (*Pueraria lobata*), and great burdock (*Arctium lappa*)—are often used as natural medicines and consumed for cooking in common medicinal recipes in East Asian regions. These four roots are characterized as having moderate health-helping bioactivities. The latter three roots are often sold in the Asian food markets, whereas the first is only available in some local markets of China. The cancer-inhibiting and cancer-preventing functions of these roots have been summarized in *Cancer Inhibitors from Chinese Medicines*, an excellent reference book published by CRC Press at the end of 2016.

17. CARROT

Carottes   Karotten   La zanahoria

胡蘿卜 にんじん 당근

Daucus carota subsp. *sativus*

Apiaceae

Carrot is one of the 10 most economically important vegetable crops in the world today. Actually, it used to be a folklore herb and then gradually became a nutritional food. Carrot has five cultivated varieties with different colors: yellow, orange, red, black, and purple. The most popular carrot is orange cultivar but black or purple carrots have been increasingly consumed in Western Europe. The orange carrot has significant sources of vitamins A, B, and C and trace elements (K, Na, Ca, Mg, P, Mn, Fe, Cu, and Zn). Orange carrots are enriched in lipid-soluble carotenoids, which are the important antioxidants and micronutrients, and contain bioactive polyphenols such as anthocyanins, flavonoids, and polyacetylenes. But water-soluble anthocyanins are predominantly present in black and purple carrots, with high lycopene content in red carrots and high lutein in yellow carrots. All the phytochemicals exert numerous nutritional and health benefits such as antioxidant, immunoenhancing, digestion-improving, hepatoprotective, renoprotective, cholesterol and cardiovascular disease lowering, and antidiabetic properties.[1] Because of these marked health advantages, worldwide carrot consumption has been growing in recent years.

Scientific Evidence of Cancer-Inhibitory and Cancer-Preventive Constituents

Carrots and carrot juices are a major source of provitamin A in the diet. The anticarcinogenic effect of carrot juice extract was demonstrated in an *in vitro* assay against myeloid and lymphoid leukemia cell lines. The ability of carrot juice to induce apoptosis and cell-cycle arrest was observed in leukemia cell lines but was seen less in myeloid cells and hematopoietic stem cells.[2] Impressively, smokers who eat carrots ≥1 time per week have a lower risk of lung cancer compared to smokers without carrot intake.[3] However, the antioxidant features of black carrot extract were significantly higher than those of orange carrots.[4] Similar to other colored vegetables, carrots are seen as the gold mine of antioxidants today. The major bioactive constituents such as carotenoids, polyacetylenes, polyphenols, anthocyanins, and vitamins present in carrots were demonstrated to synergistically contribute to the cancer chemopreventive activities—that is, antioxidant, anticarcinogenesis, anti-mutagenesis, and immunopotentiation.

Anticarcinogenic Agents from *D. carota* Rhizomes

1. Carotenoids

Carotenoids that are widely distributed in orange carrots and the major unoxygenated carotenoids are lycopene, α-carotene, and β-carotene (1). Carrot is rich in β-carotene (0.01%), which is a potent antioxidant to scavenge free radicals, to neutralize the effects of free radicals, and to obstruct lipid peroxidation and COX-1 and -2 activities;[7] thus, carotenoids play an important role in protecting the cells and organisms. Both α-carotene and β-carotene can be converted to vitamin A. The studies showed that a deficiency in vitamin A not only causes vision problems but also relates to higher incidence of carcinogenesis. Vitamin A especially showed suppressive effects against the proliferation of stomach, colon, bladder, and breast cancer cell lines. Diets rich in β-carotene could protect against prostate carcinogenesis, and high intake of carotenoids is linked with a significant decrease in postmenopausal breast cancer. Therefore, daily intake of carrots is able to effectively reduce the risk of several types of cancers.[3,5] A case-control analysis was conducted by Memorial Sloan-Kettering Cancer Center in the United States from 1993 to 1997. The results revealed that an increase in plasma carotenoids (such as lutein, α-carotene, zeaxanthin, β-cryptoxanthin, and lycopene) was accompanied with a lowered risk of bladder cancer with dose-response gradients.[6] In the *in vitro* assays, β-carotene (1) in a concentration of 45 µg/mL hampered the proliferation of AGS (stomach), SF-268 (CNS), and HCT-116 (colon) human cancer cell lines by 26%, 43%, and 43%, respectively, and in a concentration of 60 µg/mL it retarded the proliferation of NCI-H460 (lung) and MCF-7 (breast) cancer cells by 30% and 45%, respectively.[7] β-Carotene (1) in higher concentrations was able to promote the apoptosis of HL-60 and Molt-4 leukemia, HT-29 colon cancer, SK-MEL-2 melanoma, and MCF-7 breast cancer cell lines, mechanisms of which were mediated by multiple interactions—that is, (1) increase of ROS production and induction of O_2 formation, leading to decreasing mitochondrial membrane potential and release of cytochrome c from mitochondrion; (2) upregulation of p21 protein and downregulation of COX-2 and Bcl-2 expression; (3) activation of caspase-8, cleavage of Bid, and shift of tBid to mitochondrion to release cytochrome c and activation of caspases-9 and -2 (in HL-60, HT-29, and SK-MEL-2 cells); (4) upregulation of caspase-2 activity and cleavage of Bcl-xL (in Molt-4 cells); and (5) upregulation of PPAR-γ or elicitation of PGE2 (in MCF-7 and HT-29 cells).[8–12]

Besides the anticancer properties, an *in vivo* experiment demonstrated that administration of carrot-extracted carotenoids markedly augmented monocytes, lymphocytes, eosinophils, and platelet concentration in rats, specifying the immunostimulating functions of carrots, which is definitely good for indirect cancer prevention.[13]

2. Polyacetylenes

Falcarinol types of aliphatic C17-polyacetylenes are present in many Umbelliferae food plants such as carrot, celeriac, parsnip, and parsley, which are responsible for a variety of bioactivities. From carrot extracts, three polyacetylenes (falcarinol, falcarindiol, and falcarindiol-3-acetate) were separated along with two carotenoids (β-carotene and lutein). In an *in vitro* assay, the separated polyacetylenes dose- and time-responsively repressed the proliferation of three human lymphoid leukemia cell lines associated with the elicitation of apoptosis and cell-cycle arrest, but the individual carotenoids showed less effect as compared to the mixture of carotenoids. In addition, falcarinol (2) and falcarindiol-3-acetate were more cytotoxic than falcarindiol (3) to the tested lymphoid leukemia cells.[14,15]

The polyacetylenes exerted obvious inhibitory effects against the proliferation of both normal (FHs 74 Int.) and cancer (Caco-2) human intestinal epithelial cell lines, wherein the inhibitory potency was falcarinol (2) > falcarindiol (3). At a 20-μg/mL concentration, the maximal inhibitory effect reached to 95% and 80% in FHs 74 Int and Caco-2 cells, respectively.[15,16] Combination of falcarinol and falcarindiol could synergistically restrain the proliferation of the normal and cancer cells.[16] Falcarinol (2) was also reported to be effective in the suppression of human gastric adenocarcinoma (MK-1) and murine leukemia (L1210), melanoma (B16), and fibroblast-derived cells (L929), the effective dose$_{50}$ (ED$_{50}$) of which were 0.027, 1.23, and 2.50 μg/mL in MK-1, B16, and L929 cell lines, respectively. The ED$_{50}$ data in MK-1 cells were almost 20 times lower than those in normal human fibroblast cells (MRC-5), indicating that falcarinol (2) may be helpful in cancer prevention and chemotherapy.[17,18] Moreover, in an *in vivo* rat model, dietary intake of falcarinol (35 μg/g, per feed) for 18 weeks retarded the development of large aberrant crypt foci (ACF) and colon preneoplastic lesions caused by azoxymethane (AOM).[19] Falcarinol types of polyacetylenes were also inhibitors of BCRP/ABCG2, a breast cancer resistance protein.[17] This evidence inferred that the treatment with falcarinol or carrot may have a potential to prevent some types of carcinogeneses. Moreover, the combination of falcarinol (2) and falcarindiol (3) has shown a synergistic inhibitory effect against AOM-prompted neoplastic lesions in rat colorectal cancer *in vivo*.[20] Nevertheless, absolute configuration of falcarinol (2) in carrots has not been clearly determined, but the falcarinol (2) used in the assay with colon cells was assigned a 3R-configuration.[19]

3. Phenylpropanoids

From ether extract of carrots, four phenylpropanoids were isolated. Laserine (4) showed only weak cytotoxicity, but 2-epilaserine (5) exerted significant cytotoxicity against human HL-60 leukemia cells, with an IC$_{50}$ value of 0.52 μM. Both phenylpropanoids had no cytotoxic activity against human A549 lung cancer and rat PC12 pheochromocytoma cell lines.[21]

4. Anthocyanins

The anthocyanins present in black carrots (*D. carota* ssp. *sativus* var. *atrorubens*) were markedly acylated, and their levels were found to correspond to 25%–50% of the total phenolic content. Exposure of a black carrot anthocyanin-rich extract (~2 mg/mL) to cancer cells resulted in a dose-dependent antiproliferative effect toward the two tested human cancer cell lines (HT-29 colorectal adenocarcinoma and HL-60 promyelocytic leukemia).[22] The black carrot anthocyanins have been encapsulated into silica-PAMAM dendrimer hybrid nanoparticles, and the synthesized hybrid nanoparticles exerted the antiproliferative effects against Neuro 2A neuroblastoma cells. During treatment, release of the anthocyanin content totally ended at day six, and the inhibitory rate reached 87.9% in 134 h.[23]

5. Polysaccharides

Carrots contain 0.01% β-carotene and 0.8% pectins. Binding of β-carotene to carrot pectic polysaccharide (CRPP) formed a natural carbohydrate polymer. The β-carotene–CRPP complex could reduce the prooxidant effect of β-carotene, enhance the proapoptotic effect of β-carotene, and strengthen the anticancer potential of CRPP via galectin-3 inhibition.[24]

Anticarcinogenic Agents from *D. carota* Fruits or Umbels
6. Sesquiterpenoids

One eudesmane-type sesquiterpenoid and two glucopyranosides were isolated from *D. carota* fruits. Daucucarotol weakly inhibited human BGC-823 gastric cancer cells by 13.3% and showed almost no effect on AGS gastric cancer cells *in vitro*. Daucucarotol-10-*O*-β-D-glucopyranoside (6) and decahydro-7-[(2-*O*-β-D-glucopyranosyl)-isopropyl]-1β, 4aα-dimethyl-(1α,4α,8aβ)-naphthalenetriol (7) exerted moderate suppression against human ECA-109 esophageal squamous carcinoma cells *in vitro* (IC$_{50}$s of 23.22 and 26.76 μM, respectively).[25,26]

Oil Extract from Umbels of Wild *D. carota*

The chemopreventive effects of oil extract of *D. carota* umbels were demonstrated in a mouse model against 7,12-dimethyl benz(a)anthracene (DMBA)-initiated and 12-*O*-tetradecanoyl Phorbol-13-acetate (TPA)-promoted skin carcinogenesis. Topical treatment with 0.2 mL of 50% oil for 20 weeks restrained tumor incidence and yield by 30% and 83%, respectively, and the tumor volume was lessened by 91%. Intraperitoneal (IP) treatment with 0.3 mL of 2% oil for 20 weeks inhibited the tumor yield by 43% and diminished the tumor volume by 85%; however, gavage treatment with 0.02 mL of 100% oil showed only minimal effects. The intraperitoneal (IP) and topical treatment also reduced infiltration and hyperplasia with an increase in hyperkeratosis.[27] In an *in vitro* assay, the carrot oil exhibited a dose-dependent inhibitory effect against several human neoplastic cell lines *in vitro*, which was particularly observed in Caco-2 and HT-29 (colon), MCF-7, and MDA-MB-231 (breast) cancer cells. After treatment with oil in a 50-μg/mL concentration for 48 h, the percentages of dead HT-29, MCF-7, and MDA-MB-231 cells were between 70% and 80%, whereas the percentage of dead Caco-2 cells was 44%.[28] The IC_{50}s were 46.20 mg/L in HuH7 hepatoma cells and 61.76 mg/L in NCI-H446 lung cancer cells after exposure to the oil extract for 24 h.[29]

A pentane fraction and a pentane-diethyl ether (1:1) fraction from the oil extract showed better cytotoxic effect against both MCF-7 and MDA-MB-231 breast cancer cell lines together with the induction of apoptotic death and cell-cycle arrest via obvious blockage of the Erk pathway.[30] Similarly, through inhibition of MAPK/Erk and PI3K/Akt pathways, the pentane-based fractions elicited cell-cycle arrest and apoptosis in HT-29 colon cancer cells, leading to an antiproliferative effect.[31] The pentane-diethyl ether (1:1) fraction also showed a pronounced lessening of the cell motility in four cancer cell lines such as MDA-MB231 breast carcinoma, A549 lung adenocarcinoma, SF-268 glioblastoma, and B16F-10 melanoma.[32] GC-MS analysis identified 31 compounds in the oil extract, and the major constituent was assigned as β-bisabolene accounting for 63.06% of the total oil.[29] In addition, the antioxidant activity of the oil extract was proved by the assays of DPPH free-radical scavenging, ferrous ion chelating, and ferric-reducing antioxidant power.[26] A sesquiterpene assigned as β-2-himachalen-6-ol (**8**) was isolated from the wild carrot oil, and it showed moderate anticancer activity against B16F-10 (skin), Caco-2 (colon), MB-MDA-231 (breast), A549 (lung), and SF-268 (brain) cancer cell lines, with IC_{50}s of 18–58 μM or 4–13 μg/mL, wherein SF-268 cells were the most sensitive. In the SF268 astrocytoma brain cells, β-2-himachalen-6-ol not only induced cell apoptosis but also markedly reduced the cell motility and invasion and amplified the cell adhesion.[33] These studies established that wild carrot umbel oil also has both antioxidant and promising anticancer activities.

CONCLUSION AND SUGGESTION

As an important nutritional vegetable, carrots have rich β-carotene and pectins, as well as flavonoids, polyacetylenes, phenylpropanoids, and vitamins, all of which display numerous health benefits. β-carotene and some polyacetylenes, phenylpropanoids, anthocyanins, and polysaccharides in carrot have also been demonstrated to have biological activities related to cancer inhibition, cancer prevention, and antioxidant. Therefore, it is noteworthy that the intake of carrots that contain a variety of bioactive components can provide not only nutrition supplements but also health improvement and cancer prevention. The extended investigations further proved that carrot by-products (such as its fruits and umbels) may be still useful in food manufacturing owing to their positive anticarcinogenic and anticancer potentials.

REFERENCES

1. Dias, J.C.D.S. et al., 2014. Nutritional and health benefits of carrots and their seed extracts. *Food Nutr. Sci.* 5: 2147–2156.
2. Zaini, R. et al., 2011. Bioactive chemicals from carrot (*Daucus carota*) juice extracts for the treatment of leukemia. *J. Med. Food* 14: 1303–1312.

3. Oszmianski, J. et al., 2002. Improvement of carotenoid content and color in carrot juice concentrate. *Fruit Proc.* 12: 70–73.

4. Algarra, M. et al., 2014. Anthocyanin profile and antioxidant capacity of black carrots (*Daucus carota* L. ssp. sativus var. *atrorubens Alef.*) from Cuevas Bajas, Spain. *J. Food Compos. Anal.* 33: 71–76.

5. Wu, K. et al., 2004. Plasma and dietary carotenoids, and the risk of prostate cancer: A nested case-control study. *Cancer Epidemiol. Biomarkers Prev.* 13: 260–269.

6. Hung, R.J. et al., 2006. Protective effects of plasma carotenoids on the risk of bladder cancer. *J. Urol.* 176: 1192–1197.

7. Reddy, M.K. et al., 2005. Relative inhibition of lipid peroxidation, cyclooxygenase enzymes, and human tumor cell proliferation by natural food colors. *J. Agricult. Food Chem.* 53: 9268–9273.

8. Palozza, P. et al., 2003. Mechanism of activation of caspase cascade during β-carotene-induced apoptosis in human tumor cells. *Nutr. Cancer.* 47: 76–87.

9. Prasad, V. et al., 2006. ROS-triggered caspase-2 activation and feedback amplification loop in β-carotene induced apoptosis. *Free Radic. Biol. Med.* 41: 431–442.

10. Cui, Y.H. et al., 2007. β-Carotene induces apoptosis and upregulates peroxisome proliferator-activated receptor expression and reactive oxygen species production in MCF-7 cancer cells. *Eur. J. Cancer.* 43: 2590–2601.

11. Wang, J.C. et al., 2008. Advance in antitumor activity and molecular mechanism of β-Carotene. *Food Sci.* (Chinese) 29: 665–669.

12. Palozza, P. et al., 2002. Regulation of cell cycle progression and apoptosis by β-carotene in undifferentiaed and different and differentiated HL-60 leukemia cells: Possible involvement of a redox mechanism. *Int. J. Cancer* 97: 593–600.

13. Ekam, V.S. et al., 2006. Comparative effect of carotenoid complex from golden neo-life dynamite and carrot extracted carotenoids on immune parameters in Albino Wistar rats. *Nigerian J. Physiol. Sci.* 21: 1–4.

14. Zaini, R.G. et al., 2012. Effects of bioactive compounds from carrots (*Daucus carota* L.), polyacetylenes, β-carotene and lutein on human lymphoid leukaemia cells. *Anticancer Agents Med. Chem.* 12: 640–652.

15. Christensen, L.P. et al., 2011. Aliphatic C17-polyacetylenes of the falcarinol type as potential health promoting compounds in food plants of the Apiaceae family. *Recent Pat. Food Nutr. Agri.* 3: 64–77.

16. Purup, S. et al., 2009. Differential effects of falcarinol and related aliphatic C17-polyacetylenes on intestinal cell proliferation. *J. Agri. Food Chem.* 57: 8290–8296.

17. Corinna, D. et al., 2015. Bioactive C17-polyacetylenes in carrots (*Daucus carota* L.): Current knowledge and future perspectives. *J. Agri. Food Chem.* 63: 9211–9222.

18. Matsunaga, H. et al., 1990. Cytotoxic activity of polyacetylene compouds in Panax ginseng C.A. Meyer. *Chem. Pharm. Bull.* 38: 3480–3482.

19. Yang, R.L. et al., 2008. Cytotoxic phenylpropanoids from carrot. *J. Agric. Food Chem.* 56: 3024–3027.

20. Kobaek-Larsen, M. et al., 2017. Dietary polyacetylenes, falcarinol and falcarindiol, isolated from carrots prevents the formation of neoplastic lesions in the colon of azoxymethane-induced rats. *Food Func.* 8: 964–974.

21. Kobk-Larsen, M. et al., 2005. Inhibitory effects of feeding with carrots or (-)-falcarinol on development of azoxymethane-induced preneoplastic lesions in the rat colon. *J. Agri. Food Chem.* 53: 1823–1827.

22. Netzel, M. et al., 2007. Cancer cell antiproliferation activity and metabolism of black carrot anthocyanins. *Innov. Food Sci. Emer. Technol.* 8: 365–372.

23. Yesil-Celiktas, O. et al., 2017. Synthesis of silica-PAMAM dendrimer nanoparticles as promising carriers in Neuro blastoma cells. *Analyt. Biochem.* 519: 1–7.

24. Natarajmurthy, S.H. et al., 2016. A novel β-carotene-associated carrot (*Daucus carota* L.) pectic polysaccharide. *Nutrition* (NY, US) 32(7–8): 818–826.

25. Xu, J.K. et al., 2015. Two new eudesmane-type glucopyranosides from the fruits of *Daucus carota* L. *Nat. Prod. Res.* 29: 1903–1908.

26. Fu, H.W. et al., 2009. A new sesquiterpene from the fruits of *Daucus carota* L. *Mol.* 14: 2862–2867.

27. Abu, Z. et al., 2011. Chemopreventive effects of wild carrot oil against 7,12-dimethyl benz(a)anthracene-induced squamous cell carcinoma in mice. *Pharm. Biol.* (London, UK) 49: 955–961.

28. Shebaby, W.N. et al., 2013. The antioxidant and anticancer effects of wild carrot oil extract. *Phytother Res.* 27: 737–744.

29. Li, M. et al., 2012. Constituents and biological activity of volatile oil from umbels of *Daucus carota* Linn. *Zhongguo Liangyou Xuebao* 27: 112–115.
30. Shebaby, W.N. et al., 2014. *Daucus carota* pentane-based fractions arrest the cell cycle and increase apoptosis in MDA-MB-231 breast cancer cells. *BMC Complem. Alternat. Med.* 14: 1–21.
31. Shebaby, W.N. et al., 2015. *Daucus carota* pentane-based fractions suppress proliferation and induce apoptosis in human colon adenocarcinoma HT-29 cells by inhibiting the MAPK and PI3K pathways. *J. Med. Food* 18: 745–752.
32. Zgheib, P. et al., 2015. *Daucus carota* pentane/diethyl ether fraction inhibits motility and reduces invasion of cancer cells. *Chemother.* (Basel, Switzerland) 60: 302–309.
33. Taleb, R. I. et al., 2016. β-2-himachalen-6-ol: A novel anticancer sesquiterpene unique to the Lebanese wild carrot. *J. Ethnopharmacol.* 190: 59–67.

18. GARLIC

Ail   Knoblauch   Ajo

大蒜   ニンニク   마늘

Allium sativum

Amaryllidaceae

Garlic is the bulbous roots of one of the most recognized Liliaceae plant *Allium sativum* L. Garlic has a long history for more than 2000 years being utilized for both culinary and medicinal purposes in many areas. Besides, garlic cloves provide high levels of vitamins (B6 and C) and minerals (magnesium and manganese); modern scientific approaches have revealed that garlic possesses multiple beneficial effects such as antimicrobial, antithrombotic, hypolipidemic, hypoglycemic, antiarthritic, and antitumorigenic activities. More results suggested the health-improving properties of garlic in the treatment of drug toxicity, diabetes, and osteoporosis and prevention of cancer.

SCIENTIFIC EVIDENCE OF CANCER-INHIBITORY AND CANCER-PREVENTIVE ACTIVITIES

Anticarcinogenic and detoxic effects: The roles of garlic in the prevention and treatment of cancer have received increasing attention. Epidemiological and experimental studies showed that high intake of garlic exerted protective effects against carcinogenesis in prostate, colorectal, and stomach cancers and showed obvious antitumor efficacy against bladder carcinoma.[1-3] Oral administration of garlic effectively diminished the incidence of 4-nitroquinoline 1-oxide (4NQO)-induced tongue carcinogenesis, diethylnitrosoamine (DEN)-induced hepatomagenesis, and 7,12-dimethylbenz[a]anthracene

(DMBA)-caused oral tumorigenesis.[4–6] The chemopreventive effects were contributed by modulating lipid peroxidation and enhancing antioxidant status such as augmenting the levels of GSH, GPx, and GST and the activities of SOD and catalase.[5,6] Garlic was also capable of exerting the detoxification of aflatoxin B1 to lower the incidence of carcinogenesis and diminishing chrysotile asbestos-induced genotoxicity in human peripheral blood lymphocytes associated with amplifying the levels of GST-A5 and aldehyde reductase and hampering the activities of glutathione S-transferase (GST), UDP glucuronosyl transferase, and hepatic ethoxyresorufin ethylase.[7,8] In more tests, an n-butanolic extract of garlic showed high nitrite scavenging and inhibitory effects against the tumor formation by dimethylnitrosamine (DMN), which is highly carcinogenic.[9] The aged garlic was more effective than the fresh garlic in the protection of intestinal damage from 5-fluorouracil and methotrexate and in the reduction of cardiotoxicity of doxorubicin, a chemodrug.[10,11] Moreover, in an *in vitro* assay, garlic extract potently suppressed the proliferation of neoplastic cell lines such as AGS (stomach), PC3 (prostate), MCF-7 (breast), Pac-1 (pancreas), Caki-2 (kidney), and A549 (lung) cancer cell lines, U-87 glioblastoma, and Daoy medulloblastoma cell lines at a 1/1000 (corresponding to 3.32 mg raw vegetable/mL) dilution of the extract.[12]

Se-enriched garlic: The trace element nutrient selenium has been shown to possess cancer-preventive activity in both animal models and humans. Se-enriched garlic displayed an anticancer effect in murine renal cell cancer *in vivo*, an effect that was partly attributed to the increase of selenium in the tumor tissue.[13] Intake of Se-enriched garlic to nude mice in over 1.67% of diet led to growth suppression of human MGC803 gastric carcinoma cells by 29.92%, the potency of which was greater than that of normal garlic.[14] In addition, the Se-enriched garlic could markedly lessen the intratumoral microvessel density in mice bearing breast carcinoma—that is, antiangiogenic activity.[15]

Synergistic antitumor effects: The anticancer and anticarcinogenic properties of garlicin can be potentiated in combination with certain treatments. Simple administration of garlic together with tomato was effective in repressing the development of hamster buccal pouch carcinoma and promoting cell apoptosis *in vivo*.[16,17] Fed with aqueous suspensions of garlic and tomato to rats also synergistically obstructed AOM-elicited colon carcinogenesis and reduced preneoplastic lesions and the incidence of ACF by 71.62%,[18] and markedly retarded the frequencies of DMBA-induced bone marrow micronuclei together with diminishment of DMBA-induced oxidative stress and genotoxicity.[19] When garlic was mixed with vitamin C in *in vitro* treatments, the synergistic growth inhibition was observed in human HT-29 (colon), HRT-18 (rectal), and HepG2 (liver) carcinoma cell lines. By feeding the mixture of garlic and vitamin C, the survival was prolonged in mice burdened with sarcoma 180.[20] Though garlic showed a definite inhibition against the growth of bladder cancer in a murine model, the combination of garlic and suicide gene therapy achieved a more effective and additive treatment modality for the suppression of bladder cancer.[21]

Immunoenhancing effects: Garlic was also reported to have the ability to stimulate host immunity, including activation of NK cells, LAK cells, and macrophage and to increase IL-2, TNF, and interferon-γ. These cytokines are closely associated with the beneficial Th1 antitumor response, which is a characteristic of effective cancer immunotherapies. Due to augmentation and proliferation of macrophages and lymphocytes, garlic could effectively protect the host immunity from the toxicities caused by both or either chemotherapy and/or ultraviolet radiation.[22]

SCIENTIFIC EVIDENCE OF CANCER-INHIBITORY AND CANCER-PREVENTIVE CONSTITUENTS

Organosulfur compounds (OSCs) in garlic are recognized as the major and most important constituents with obvious health benefits in chemoprevention and chemotherapies. Meanwhile, lectin, oligosaccharide, and superoxide dismutase derived from garlic bulbs were also reported to have an inhibitory effect on cancer and carcinogenesis.

1. Organosulfur compounds

The major functional characteristics of the OSCs include (1) inactivation of carcinogen; (2) arrest of cell cycle and induction of apoptosis in tumor cells; (3) repression of tumor metastasis and angiogenesis; (4) blockage of DNA adduct formation and chromosomal damage; (5) scavenging of radicals; and (6) activation of various phase II detoxifying enzymes. Garlic OSCs are shown to be metabolized into two groups, oil-soluble OSCs and water-soluble OSCs. The oil-soluble OSCs (such as diallyl sulfide, diallyl disulfide, and diallyl trisulfide) are usually more effective in obstructing cancer cells than the water-soluble OSCs (such as S-allylcysteine and S-allylmercaptocysteine).[23] More than 20 kinds of anticarcinogenic OSCs have been separated from garlic; however, their functions were not found to be the same, showing their own characteristics. The selenium-enriched garlic OSCs might provide more potent protection against various types of carcinogeneses and better cancer inhibition than normal garlic OSCs.[24]

a. *Allyl sulfides*: The major naturally occurring organosulfides in garlic are diallyl sulfide (DAS), diallyl disulfide (DADS), and diallyltri-sulfide (DATS), as well as less content of ally sulfide (AS) and diallylpentasulfide (DPS). All these organic sulfides were reported of having anticarcinogenesis and antimutagenesis properties, but the oil-soluble DADS (**1**) was the most significant one, and DAS (**2**) was the second most potent based on the extensive evidence from *in vitro* and *in vivo* studies.

DADS: DADS (**1**) exerted a marked antiproliferative effect on human leukemia (HL-60 and WEHI-3),[25] colorectal cancer (HCT-116 and HCT-15), lung tumor (A549, H460, and H1299), prostate cancer (PC3 and LNCaP), bladder cancer (T24), esophagus cancer (CE 81T/VGH), and melanoma cell lines, *in vitro* and/or *in vivo*, concomitant with the induction of apoptotic death and cell-cycle arrest.[26] The key mechanisms were found to extensively correlate with (1) triggering mitochondria-mediated signaling pathways; (2) binding directly to tubulin, disrupting microtubule assembly, and arresting cells in mitosis (such as in colon cancer cells); (3) notably increasing the intracellular ROS and oxidative stress (such as in A549 and HL-60 cells);[27–29] (4) blocking thymidine incorporation and causing DNA damage (such as in PC3 cells);[30] (5) reducing N-acetyltransferase (NAT) activity and 2-aminofluorene (AF)-DNA adduct formation (such as in HL-60 and CE 81T/VGH cells);[31,32] (6) elevating p53 and cyclin levels and reducing CDK2 gene expression (such as in T24 cells);[33,34] and (7) modulating phase I and II enzyme activities.[35] Compared to the inhibition in wild-type p53 cell lines (such as HCT-116 colorectal cancer and H460 NSCLC) and p53 null-type cells (such as H1299 NSCLC), DADS (**1**) was less effective in p53 mutant cell lines (such as PC3 prostate cancer and HCT-15 colon cancer).[36,37] In addition, treatment with DADS arrested human MDA-MB-435 breast cancer cells in mitosis and elicited the cells to apoptosis.[37]

Moreover, DADS (**1**) at a concentration of 25 M exerted synergistic effect to greatly potentiate the cytotoxicity of daunorubicin (100 nM) on human HL-60 leukemia cells and prevented severe side effects of the therapeutic drug.[38] DADS (**1**) could also hinder the invasion of human LNCaP prostate cancer cells via blocking MMP-2 and -9 activities and augmenting the tightness of tight junctions (TJ).[39] During DADS (**1**), the antitumor effect of cisplatin was amplified, and multidrug resistance protein-2 (Mrp2) was expressed by 30-fold in renal brush-border membranes.[40]

DAS: Diallyl sulfide (DAS, **2**) is second important sulfur-containing volatile compound present in garlic. The *in vivo* experiments revealed that DAS was effective in the suppression of oncogen-induced carcinogenesis. For instance, DAS (**2**) played protective roles against rat hepatocarcinogenesis by repressing DEN-initiated and 2-acetylaminofluorene-promoted hepatic foci of preneoplasm,[41] against rat breast carcinogenesis by reducing diethylstilbestrol (DES)-caused lipid hydroperoxides in the breast tissue[42] against apoptosis in hypodiploid region and oxidative damage in mouse liver induced by DMBA,[43] and against mouse melanomagenesis caused by benzo[a]pyrene (BAP) or DMBA.[44] The anticancer effect of DAS (2) in mouse Hepa-1c1c7 hepatoma cells was found to partially correlate with the activation of GST[45] and in human promyelocytic leukemia cells (HL-60) and human colon cancer cell lines (colo 205, colo 320 DM, and colo 320 HSR) was also found closely in association with the reduction of N-acetyltransferase (NAT) activity and/or 2-AF-DNA adduct formation.[32,46] Similarly, the antiproliferation DAS (2) on p53 wild-type H460 nonsmall cell lung cancer (NSCLC) cells was mediated by a rise in the expression levels of Bax and p53 and a fall in the expression level of Bcl-2.[34]

Moreover, a multidrug-resistant (MDR) reversing property of DAS (2) was confirmed in K562/R10 cells (VBL-resistant human leukemia cells) in vitro and in vivo. At a nontoxic concentration (8.75×10^{-3} M), DAS (2) was able to enhance the cytotoxic effects of vinblastine (VBL) and vincristine (VCR) time-dependently against the K562/R10 cells, although it had no effect on the parent (K562/S) cells. The anti-MDR activity of DAS (2) resulted by lessening the expression and level of P-glycoprotein (P-gp).[47]

DATS: Diallyltrisulfide (DATS, 3), the third major allyl sulfides derived from garlic, also showed inhibitory and proapoptotic effects on cancer cells. Similar to DADS (1), DATS (3) is capable of disturbing microtubule network formation and microtubule fragments in the tumor cells.[48] The growth of human colon cancer cells (HCT-15 and DLD-1) was significantly obstructed by DATS in vitro, and 70% inhibition was achieved by DATS in nude mice xenografted HCT-15 cells.[49] Fifty- or 100-μM DATS (3) considerably attenuated the viability of human J5 hepatoma cells and elicited the cell-cycle G2/M arrest.[50] The DATS (10 μM) effectively promoted the apoptosis of A549 lung cancer cells as well, where a progressive increase of intracellular Ca^{2+} by DATS might importantly participate in the initiation of apoptosis.[51]

In addition, a sample-A, which consisted of DATS (3), diallyltetrasulfide, and diallylpentasulfide (5.3:3:1), exerted a selective inhibition against the activities of mammalian family X-DNA polymerases in vitro. The inhibition of X-DNA polymerases was found to reflect the growth suppression of certain human tumor cell lines and the potency order on the family X-DNA polymerases was sample-A >DATS (3) >DADS (1) >DAS (2).[52] Structure–activity relationship analysis integrated with the above-described evidence disclosed that the numbers of both allyl and sulfide moieties in the OSCs are important features for antiproliferative and chemopreventive potencies.[27]

b. *Allicin*: Allicin (4) is a major component present in freshly crushed garlic that has marked antitumor and immunostimulatory activities. By activation of caspases, cleavage of poly(ADP-ribose) polymerase, and increase in apoptotic body formation, allicin (4) exerted great growth inhibitory and chemopreventive effects against cancer cells in murine and human origins.[53] In vitro approaches confirmed that allicin (4) was effective in deterring the proliferation and inducing apoptosis of murine EL-4 T-lymphoma cells through a mitochondrial pathway.[54] Multiple IP administrations of allicin (4) resulted in marked antitumor effect in mice inoculated with B16 melanoma or MCA-105 fibrosarcoma. Concurrently, allicin (4) stimulated thymidine incorporation in splenocytes and enhanced the cytotoxicity of human peripheral mononuclear cells.[55] More evidence displayed that the anticancer activity of allicin (4) was also closely correlated with its synergistic effect of immunostimulatory and antioxidant properties.[53-55]

c. *Ajoene*: Ajoene that showed to be a mixture of E- and Z-isomers is one of the main sulfur compounds formed from heating crushed garlic. Ajoene (5) displayed a broad spectrum of biological activities that include anticancer activity with no obvious side effects. Its cytotoxicity occurred in various cancer cells in parallel with caspase-activated and mitochondrial-dependent apoptosis. Ajoene (5) repressed the viability of murine B16F10 melanoma cells (IC$_{50}$ 62 μM) and promoted cell apoptosis. At a 25-μM concentration, ajoene also significantly diminished the adhesion of B16F10 cells to endothelial cell monolayer.[56] Treatment with ajoene (5) elicited apoptosis promotion and growth inhibition in human CD34$^-$ leukemia cells (such as U937, HL-60, HEL, and OCIM-1 lines). The apoptosis of myeloblasts from chronic myeloid leukemia patienst could be partially increased by ajoene (5) but not affect the peripheral mononuclear blood cells of healthy donors. The proapoptotic effect of anticancer agents (cytarabine and fludarabine) could be profoundly augmented by ajoene (5) in human CD34$^+$ drug-resistant myeloid leukemia cells.[57,58] The findings suggested a promising treatment for refractory and relapsed acute myeloid leukemia patients (CD34$^+$) and elderly AML patients.[57] Furthermore, ajoene (5) had been used to topically treat 21 patients with either nodular or superficial basal cell carcinoma (BCC). The tumor sizes of 17 patients were notably reduced concomitant with inducing the mitochondria-dependent route of apoptosis.[59]

Structure–activity relationship studies have revealed that the Z-isomer of ajoene is moderately more active than its E-isomer in inhibiting tumor cell growth. Z-ajoene displayed an inhibitory effect against the growth of two leukemia cell lines (U937 and HL-60), with similar IC$_{50}$s of 10 μmol/L. By treatment with Z-ajoene (20 μmol/L) for 24 h, the apoptosis and G2/M cell arrest of U937 cells were enhanced, but mitotic blocking and interruption of tubulin assembly could be provoked by Z-ajoene (5) earlier than the proapoptosis.[60] In addition, several derivatives were synthesized by substitution of the terminal-end allyl groups in ajoene (5) for the groups of alkyl, aromatic, or heteroaromatic, showing superior anticancer potencies to ajoene (5) *in vitro*.[61]

d. *Thiacremonone*: Thiacremonone (6) is a main sulfur component isolated from heated garlic bulbs, which acts as an inhibitor of NF-κB. By decreasing DNA binding activity of NF-κB and suppressing NF-κB target antiapoptotic genes (cIAP1/2, Bcl-2, and XIAP), thiacremonone (6) dose-dependently retarded the growth of human SW620 and HCT-116 colon carcinoma cells followed by the induction of apoptosis but showed no cytotoxicity on Caco-2 colon cells. The IC$_{50}$s (48 h) were 105 and 130 μg/mL in the SW620 cells and HCT-116 cells, respectively. The growth inhibition was also accompanied to activate apoptotic genes (Bax, caspase-3, and cleaved PARP) and to inhibit inflammatory genes (iNOS and COX-2).[62] A combination of thiacremonone (50 μg/mL) with lower doses of a chemotherapeutic agent docetaxel (5 nM) was more effective in the growth inhibition of colon carcinoma cells and prostate cancer cells. Thiacremonone (6) could also increase susceptibility of PC3 and DU145 prostate cancer cells and SW620 and HCT-116 colon neoplastic cells to docetaxel via significant inhibition of NF-κB activity. Therefore, thiacremonone (6) may be useful as an adjuvant agent for cancer chemotherapy and chemoprevention.[63,64]

e. *Cysteine S-conjugates*: Cysteine S-conjugates, including S-allyl-L-cysteine (SAC, 7), S-methyl-L-cysteine (SMC, 8), and S-allyl mercapto-L-cysteine (SAMC, 9), are a group of water-soluble organosulfur garlic derivatives, which have been demonstrated as suppressive agents against tumors and oxidation. Oral administration of SAC (7) markedly inhibited DMBA-induced hamster buccal pouch tumorigenesis and lipid peroxidation in the oral tissue together with the elevation of GSH, GPx, and GST levels.[65] SMC (8) chemopreventively obstructed diethyl nitrosamine-induced hepatocarcinogenesis in F344 male rats.[66] The antineoplastic effect of SAMC (9) was related to the decrease of proliferation and the increase of apoptosis and necrosis of cancer cells. Treatment with SAMC (9) was effective in the growth inhibition of a panel of human colorectal/colon carcinoma cell lines (SW480, SW620, Caco-2, and HT-29). The cell-cycle progression in HT-29 and SW480 cells was blocked at the G2/M phase, and the mitosis was specifically arrested by SAMC (**9**), leading the cells to apoptosis.[66–68] The antiproliferative effects exerted by SAMC (150 μM) in SW480 cells and NIH3T3 fibroblast cells were found to be mediated by directly binding to tubulin and disrupting microtubule assembly, thereby triggering JNK1 and caspase-3 signaling pathways to arrest the cells in mitosis and to promote apoptosis.[69] *In vivo* tests further corroborated the antiproliferative and antimetastatic effects of SAMC (**9**) in luciferase-expressing SW620 colon cancer xenografts in mice.[68] Coadministration of SAMC (**9**) with sulindac sulfide (one of the well-established preventive agents for colon cancer) could enhance the anti-growth effects on the colon cancer cells.[66] The growth of human gastric cancer cells implanted in nude mice was inhibited by 31.36%–37.78%, and the apoptosis was promoted at doses of 100–300 mg/kg of SAMC (**9**), where oral administration of SAMC (**9**) in a relatively large dose showed no apparent toxic side effect on the vital organs of mice.[67–71] Moreover, both SAC (**7**) and SAMC (**9**) were capable of repressing the proliferation and invasion of androgen-independent prostate cancer (PCa) cells via induction of mesenchymal-to-epithelial transition. In the treatments with SAC (**7**) or SAMC (**9**), the restoration of E-cadherin expression at transcription and protein levels played an important role for the inhibition of invasive growth as well in the treatment of prostate, ovarian, nasopharyngeal, and esophageal carcinoma cells.[72]

In addition, alliin (**10**) is a natural cysteine sulfoxide in fresh garlic, which is able to repress both FGF2 and VEGF secretion from human fibrosarcoma cells in a concentration-dependent manner, implying that alliin (**10**) may have an ability to obstruct angiogenesis. Combinational use of vitamins C and E with alliin (**10**) could markedly enhance the efficacy of alliin (**10**) in the growth suppression of colon cancer and fibrosarcoma cells.[73] However, when fresh garlic is chopped or crushed, the enzyme alliinase converts the alliin (**10**) into allicin (**4**). On the basis of the evidence, the cysteine *S*-conjugates and garlic are known to be useful for cancer prevention.

2. Lectin

A cytotoxic lectin (≈23 kDa) was prepared from a hot water extract of garlic bulbs, which might be a dimer. The garlic lectin could inhibit the growth of human U937 lymphoma and HL-60 leukemia cell lines *in vitro*, accompanied with strong reduction of DNA synthesis and blockage of thymidine incorporation in these cells. At a low concentration, the garlic lectin induced the U937 cell apoptosis. Other reports showed that the garlic lectin was able to bind to the cellular membrane of tumor cells and then exert the cytotoxic effect. When garlic lectin was incubated with a protease at a concentration ratio of lectin and protease (5:1), the garlic lectin was highly resistant to *in vitro* digestion by the proteases, implying that the garlic lectin can withstand proteolysis in the intestinal tract. The results showed a rational basis for its effectiveness, but the value of garlic lectin in clinical application for antitumor needs further investigation.[74]

3. Oligosaccharide

From fractionation of garlic hot water extract, an oligosaccharide (MW [molecular weight] >1800) was purified by ammonium sulfate partition, gel filtration, and ion exchange chromatography, the structure of which was 10 fructose units connected by a β-(1-2) linkage to a terminal glucose. *In vitro* assay showed that the oligosaccharide had cytotoxicity against human U937 malignant lymphoma cells and WiDr colon adenocarcinoma cells, and it also exerted immunoenhancing activities such as stimulation of human peripheral blood lymphocyte to produce interferon-γ. The anticancer effect was further demonstrated in an animal model-implanted colon-26 murine colon adenocarcinoma, indicating that the tumor growth inhibition is partially mediated by the activation of immunological pathways *in vivo* in addition to its direct cancer inhibition.[75]

4. Superoxide dismutase

A manganese superoxide dismutase (MnSOD) was isolated from garlic bulbs, the enzymes of which have a specific activity equal to 55 U/mg. The treatment of two cell lines (mouse melanoma cells and porcine endothelial cells) with MnSOD showed an inhibitory effect on the proliferative capacity and the multiplication of the cells. The effect of MnSOD was found to correlate with the upregulation of phosphoextracellular signal-regulated kinases, leading to several biological processes, including anticancer and anticarcinogenic effects.[76]

CONCLUSION AND SUGGESTION

These scientific observations disclosed that garlic contains the richest organosulfur compounds (OSCs) in the *Allium* plants, consequently providing the strongest fighting power against cancer, particularly against cancers and carcinogenesis in the stomach, esophagus, and colon. The most prominent OSCs should be diallyltri sulfide (DATS) in garlic. The naturally enriched allyl sulfides in garlic can usually be transferred to other types of OSCs (such as allicin, ajoene, thiacremonone, and systeine *S*-conjugates) when in contact with oxygen in air during the cooking process, exerting a broader spectrum of inhibitory effects against a variety of cancer cell growth, proliferation, and invasion. Thus, fresh, chopped, or squeezed garlic is essential for cancer inhibition and prevention. Besides, the lectin, oligosaccharide, and superoxide dismutase found in garlic bulbs were also cytotoxic to some neoplastic cells, and garlic was also capable of potentiating the host immune system and protecting the human body against the side effects from radiotherapy and chemotherapy, particularly DNA and chromosome damage. It is no doubt that garlic serves as a naturally occurring powerful and safe weapon against cancer. More common use of garlic in our daily menu may be a smart choice for lowering cancer risk despite its pungent taste and smell.

REFERENCES

1. Fleischauer, A.T. et al., 2000. Garlic consumption and cancer prevention: Meta-analyses of colorectal and stomach cancers. *Am. J. Clin. Nutr.* 72: 1047–1052.
2. Riggs, D.R. et al., 1997. *Allium sativum* (garlic) treatment for murine transitional cell carcinoma. *Cancer* 79: 1987–1994.
3. Howard, E.W. et al., 2008. The use of garlic and its derivatives in the prevention and treatment of prostate cancer. *Nat. Prod. Future Med. Agents* 141–163.
4. Samaranayake, M.D. et al., 2000. Inhibition of chemically induced liver carcinogenesis in Wistar rats by garlic (*Allium sativum*). *Phytother. Res.* 14: 564–567.
5. Balasenthil, S. et al., 2001. Prevention of 4-nitroquinoline 1-oxide-induced rat tongue carcinogenesis by garlic. *Fitoterapia* 72: 524–531.
6. Balasenthil, S. et al., 2001. Garlic inhibits experimentally induced hamster buccal pouch carcinomas. *J. Biochem. Mol. Biol. Biophy.* 5: 261–266.
7. Berges, R. et al., 2004. Comparison of the chemopreventive efficacies of garlic powders with different alliin contents against aflatoxin B1 carcinogenicity in rats. *Carcinogenesis* 25: 1953–1959.
8. Bhattacharya, K. et al., 2004. Reduction of chrysotile asbestos-induced genotoxicity in human peripheral blood lymphocytes by garlic extract. *Toxicol. Lett.* 153: 327–332.
9. Choi, S.Y. et al., 2006. Effect of garlic (*Allium sativum* L.) extracts on formation of N-nitrosodimethylamine. *Han'guk Sikp'um Yongyang Kwahak Hoechi* 35: 677–682.
10. Horie, T. et al., 2001. Alleviation by garlic of antitumor drug-induced damage to the intestine. *J. Nutr.* 131(3S): 1071S–1074S.
11. Borek, C. 2001. Antioxidant health effects of aged garlic extract. *J. Nutr.* 131(3S): 1010S–1015S.
12. Boivin, D. et al., 2009. Antiproliferative and antioxidant activities of common vegetables: A comparative study. *Food Chem.* 112: 374–380.
13. Kashiwabara, Y. 2005. Inhibition of tumor-growth and changes of selenium concentration in tissues by the garlic in murine renal carcinoma. *Iwate Igaku Zasshi* 57: 41–46.

14. Tang, F. et al., 2001. In vivo and in vitro effects of selenium-enriched garlic on growth of human gastric carcinoma cells. *Zhonghua Zhongliu Zazhi* 23: 461–464.

15. Jiang, C. et al., 1999. Selenium-induced inhibition of angiogenesis in mammary cancer at chemo-preventive levels of intake. *Mol. Carcinogenesis* 26: 213–225.

16. Bhuvaneswari, V. et al., 2004. Combination chemoprevention by tomato and garlic in the hamster buc-cal pouch carcinogenesis model. *Nutr. Res.* (NY, U.S.) 24: 133–146.

17. Bhuvaneswari, V. et al., 2004. Altered expression of anti and proapoptotic proteins during chemo-prevention of hamster buccal pouch carcinogenesis by tomato and garlic combination. *Clin. Chimica Acta* 350: 65–72.

18. Sengupta, A. et al., 2004. Modulatory influence of garlic and tomato on cyclooxygenase-2 activity, cell proliferation and apoptosis during azoxymethane induced colon carcinogenesis in rat. *Cancer Lett.* 208: 127–136.

19. Mohan, K.V.P. et al., 2004. Protective effects of a mixture of dietary agents against 7,12-dimethyl-benz[a]anthracene-induced genotoxicity and oxidative stress in mice. *J. Med. Food* 7: 55–60.

20. Sohn, H.-E. et al., 2001. Enhancement of anticancer activity by combination of garlic (*Allium sativum*) extract and vitamin C. *Han'guk Sikp'um Yongyang Kwahak Hoechi* 30: 372–376.

21. Moon, D.G. et al., 2000. *Allium sativum* potentiates suicide gene therapy for murine transitional cell carcinoma. *Nutr. Cancer* 38: 98–105.

22. Lamm, D.L. et al., 2000. The potential application of *Allium sativum* (garlic) for the treatment of bladder cancer. *Urol Clin North Am* 27: 157–162.

23. Thomsom, M. et al., 2003. Garlic (*Allium sativum*): A review of its potential use as an anticancer agent. *Curr. Cancer Drug Targets* 3: 67–81.

24. Seki, T. et al., 2012. Anticancer property of allyl sulfides derived from garlic (*Allium sativum* L.) *J. Food Drug Analysis* 20(Suppl. 1): 309–312.

25. Yang, J.S. et al., 2006. Diallyl disulfide inhibits WEHI-3 leukemia cells in vivo. *Anticancer Res.* 26: 219–225.

26. Karmakar, S. et al., 2011. Molecular mechanisms of anticancer action of garlic compounds in neuroblas-toma. *Anti-Cancer Agent Med. Chem.* 11: 398–407.

27. Xiao, D.H. et al., 2005. Effects of a series of organosulfur compounds on mitotic arrest and induction of apoptosis in colon cancer cells. *Mol. Cancer Therap.* 4: 1388–1398.

28. Wu, X.J. et al., 2005. The role of reactive oxygen species (ROS) production on diallyl disulfide (DADS) induced apoptosis and cell cycle arrest in human A549 lung carcinoma cells. *Mutat. Res. Fund. Mole. Mech. Mut.* 579: 115–124.

29. Kwon, K.B. et al., 2002. Induction of apoptosis by diallyl disulfide through activation of caspase-3 in human leukemia HL-60 cells. *Biochem. Pharmacol.* 63: 41–47.

30. Arunkumar, A. et al., 2005. Growth suppressing effect of garlic compound diallyl disulfide on prostate cancer cell line (PC-3) in vitro. *Biol. Pharm. Bull.* 28: 740–743.

31. Yu, F.S. et al., 2005. Diallyl disulfide inhibits N-acetyltransferase activity and gene expression in human esophagus epidermoid carcinoma CE 81T/VGH cells. *Food Chem. Toxicol.* 43: 1029–1036.

32. Lin, J.G. et al., 2002. Effects of garlic components diallyl sulfide and diallyl disulfide on arylamine N-acetyltransferase activity and 2-amino-fluorene-DNA adducts in human promyelocytic leukemia cells. *Am. J. Chin. Med.* 30: 315–325.

33. Lu, H.F. et al., 2004. Diallyl disulfide (DADS) induced apoptosis undergo caspase-3 activity in human bladder cancer T24 cells. *Food Chem. Toxicol.* 42: 1543–1552.

34. Hong, Y.S. et al., 2000. Effects of allyl sulfur compounds and garlic extract on the expressions of Bcl-2, bax, and p53 in non-small cell lung cancer cell lines. *Exp. Mol. Med.* 32: 127–134.

35. Morris, C.R. et al., 2004. Inhibition by allyl sulfides and phenethylisothiocyanate of methyl-n-pentylnitrosaminedepentylation by rat esophageal microsomes, human and rat CYP2E1, and rat CYP2A3. *Nutr. Cancer* 48: 54–63.

36. Bottone, F.G. et al., 2002. Diallyl disulfide (DADS) induces the antitumorigenic NSAID-activated gene (NAG-1) by a p53-dependent mechanism in human colorectal HCT 116 cells. *J. Nutr.* 132: 773–778.

37. Lund, T. et al., 2005. Garlic arrests MDA-MB-435 cancer cells in mitosis, phosphorylates the proapop-totic BH3-only protein BimEL and induces apoptosis. *British J. Cancer* 92: 1773–1781.

38. Koo, B.S. et al., 2003. Diallyl disulfide enhances daunorubicin-induced apoptosis of HL-60 cells. *Hanguk Yongyang Hakhoechi* 36: 828–833.

39. Shin, D.Y. et al., 2010. Anti-invasive activity of diallyl disulfide through tightening of tight junctions and inhibition of matrix metallo-proteinase activities in LNCaP prostate cancer cells. *Toxicol. Vitro* 24: 1569–1576.

40. Demeule, M. et al., 2004. Diallyl disulfide, a chemopreventive agent in garlic, induces multidrug resistance-associated protein 2 expression. *Biochem. Biophy. Res. Commun.* 324: 937–945.
41. Singh, A. 2004. Modulation of altered hepatic foci induction by diallylsulphide in Wistar rats. *Eur. J. Cancer Prev.*13: 263–269.
42. Gued, L.R. et al., 2003. Diallyl sulfide inhibits diethylstilbestrol-induced lipid peroxidation in breast tissue of female ACI rats: Implications in breast cancer prevention. *Oncol. Rep.* 10: 739–743.
43. Prasad, S. et al., 2007. Regulation of oxidative stress-mediated apoptosis by diallyl sulfide in DMBA-exposed Swiss mice. *Human Experim. Toxicol.* 27: 55–63.
44. Singh, A. et al., 1998. Antitumor activity of diallyl sulfide on polycyclic aromatic hydrocarbon-induced mouse skin carcinogenesis. *Cancer Lett.* 131: 209–214.
45. Chen, Y.H. et al., 2000. Enhancement of glutathione S-transferase using diallyl sulfide from garlic in Hepa-1c1c7 cells. *Zhonghua Minguo Yingyang Xuehui Zazhi* 25: 1–8.
46. Chung, J.G. et al., 2004. Inhibition of N-acetyltransferase activity and gene expression in human colon cancer cell lines by diallyl sulfide. *Food Chem. Toxicol.* 42: 195–202.
47. Arora, A. et al., 2004. Reversal of P-glycoprotein-mediated multidrug resistance by diallyl sulfide in K562 leukemic cells and in mouse liver. *Carcinogenesis* 25: 941–949.
48. Seki, T. et al., 2008. Anticancer effects of diallyltrisulfide derived from garlic. *Asia Pac. Clin. Nutr.* 17(Suppl.1): 249–252.
49. Ariga, T. 2008. Anticancer effects of garlic-derived scents "organosulfur compounds." *Aroma Res.* 9: 176–180.
50. Wu, C.C. et al., 2004. Differential effects of allyl sulfides from garlic essential oil on cell cycle regulation in human liver tumor cells. *Food Chem. Toxicol.* 42: 1937–1947.
51. Sakamoto, K. et al., 1997. Allyl sulfides from garlic suppress the in vitro proliferation of human A549 lung tumor cells. *Nutr. Cancer* 29: 152–156.
52. Nishida, M. et al., 2008. Diallyl sulfides: Selective inhibitors of family X DNA polymerases from garlic (*Allium sativum* L.). *Food Chem.*108: 551–560.
53. Oommen, S. et al., 2004. Allicin (from garlic) induces caspase-mediated apoptosis in cancer cells. *Eur. J. Pharmacol.* 485: 97–103.
54. Wang, Z. 2012. Allicin induces apoptosis in EL-4 cells in vitro by activation of expression of caspase-3 and -12 and up-regulation of the ratio of Bax/Bcl-2. *Nat. Prod. Res.* 26: 1033–1037.
55. Patya, M. et al., 2004. Allicin stimulates lymphocytes and elicits an antitumor effect: A possible role of p21ras. *Int. Immunol.* 16: 275–281.
56. Ledezma, E. et al., 2004. Apoptotic and anti-adhesion effect of ajoene, a garlic derived compound, on the murine melanoma B16F10 cells: Possible role of caspase-3 and the $\alpha4\beta1$ integrin. *Cancer Lett.* (Amsterdam, Netherlands) 206: 35–41.
57. Hassan, H.T. et al., 2004. Ajoene (natural garlic compound): A new anti-leukaemia agent for AML therapy. *Leukemia Res.* 28: 667–671.
58. Dirsch, V.M. et al., 1998. Ajoene, a compound of garlic, induces apoptosis in human promyelo-leukemic cells, accompanied by generation of reactive oxygen species and activation of nuclear factor-κB. *Mol. Pharmacol.* 53: 402–407.
59. Tilli, C. et al., 2003. The garlic-derived organosulfur component ajoene decreases basal cell carcinoma tumor size by inducing apoptosis. *Archiv. Dermatol. Res.* 295: 117–123.
60. Li, M. et al., 2004. Mechanism of growth inhibition of Z-ajoene on U937 cells. *Zhongguo Yaolixue Tongbao* 20: 688–693.
61. Kaschula, C.H. et al., 2010. Garlic-derived anticancer agents: Structure and biological activity of ajoene. *BioFactors* 36: 78–85.
62. Ban, J. et al. 2007. Inhibition of cell growth and induction of apoptosis via inactivation of NF-κB by a sulfur compound isolated from garlic inhuman colon cancer cells. *J. Pharmacol. Sci.* 104: 374–383.
63. Ban, J. et al., 2009. Thiacremonone augments chemotherapeutic agent–induced growth inhibition in human colon cancer cells through inactivation of nuclear factor-κB. *Mol. Cancer Res.* 7: 870–879.
64. Ban, J. et al., 2009. Anticancer effect of the combination of thiacremonone and docetaxel by inactivation of NF-κB in human cancer cells. *Biomol. Therap.* 17: 403–411.
65. Balasenthil, S. et al., 2000. Inhibition of 7,12-dimethylbenz[a]anthracene-induced hamster buccal pouch carcinogenesis by S-allylcysteine. *Oral Oncol.* 36: 382–386.
66. Takada, N. et al., 1997. S-methylcysteine and cysteine are inhibitors of induction of glutathione S-trans-ferase placental form-positive foci during initiation and promotion phases of rat hepatocarcinogenesis. *Jpn J. Cancer Res.* 88: 435–442.

67. Shirin, H. et al., 2001. Antiproliferative effects of S-allylmercaptocysteine on colon cancer cells when tested alone or in combination with sulindac sulfide. *Cancer Res.* 61: 725–731.
68. Liang, D. et al., 2011. S-allylmercaptocysteine effectively inhibits the proliferation of colorectal cancer cells under in vitro and in vivo conditions. *Cancer Lett.* 310: 69–76.
69. Xiao, D.H. et al., 2003. Induction of apoptosis by the garlic-derived compound S-allylmercapto-cysteine (SAMC) is associated with microtubule depolymerization and c-Jun NH2-terminal kinase 1 activation. *Cancer Res.* 63: 6825–6837.
70. Lee, Y. et al., 2011. Anticancer activity of S-allylmercapto-L-cysteine on implanted tumor of human gastric cancer cells. *Biol. Pharm. Bull.* 34: 677–681.
71. Lee, Y. et al., 2008. Induction of apoptosis by S-allylmercapto-L-cysteine, a biotransformed garlic derivative, on a human gastric cancer cell line. *Int. J. Mol. Med.* 21: 765–770.
72. Chu, Q.J. et al., 2006. A novel anticancer effect of garlic derivatives: Inhibition of cancer cell invasion through restoration of E-cadherin expression. *Carcinogenesis* 27: 2180–2189.
73. Mousa, A.S. et al., 2005. Anti-angiogenesis efficacy of the garlic ingredient alliin and antioxidants: Role of nitric oxide and p53. *Nutr. Cancer* 53: 104–110.
74. Karasaki, Y.J. et al., 2001. A garlic lectin exerted an antitumor activity and induced apoptosis in human tumor cells. *Food Res. Int.* 34: 7–13.
75. Tsukamoto, S. et al., 2008. Purification, characterization and biological activities of a garlic oligosac-charide. *J. UOEH* 30: 147–157.
76. Sfaxi, I.H. et al., 2009. Inhibitory effects of a manganese superoxide dismutase isolated from garlic (*Allium sativum* L.) on in vitro tumoral cell growth. *Biotechnol. Prog.* 25: 257–264.

19. ONION

Oignon   Zwiebel   Cebolla

洋蔥 たまねぎ 양파

Allium cepa

Amaryllidaceae

1. $R_1 = -OH, R_2 = -H$
2. $R_1 = R_2 = -H$
3. $R_1 = R_2 = -OH$

Onion, the bulbs of *Allium cepa*, has been one of the most common vegetables in diets for 1000 years. The onions are normally available in three color varieties: yellow, purple, and white. Similar to other *Allium* vegetables, onion has beneficial effects on the cardiovascular and immune systems and has antidiabetic and anticarcinogenic effects. Pharmacological approaches have proved that onions also possess antimicrobial, antithrombotic, hypolipidemic, antiasthmatic, antiplatelet, and hypoglycemic activities. Onions are good sources of vitamin C, folate, and fiber, without cholesterol and fat. In freshly cut onions, a pungent volatile gas (*syn*-propanethial-*S*-oxide) is released that irritates the eyes.

Scientific Evidence of Anticarcinogenic Activities

In addition to their well-known medicinal value, onions also showed preventive benefits against chemical-induced carcinogenesis and a suppressive effect against cancer-cell proliferation. In the investigations, oral administration of 20% onion extract in water significantly hindered the buccal pouch carcinoma formation induced by DMBA *in vivo*, and exposure to 25% onion extract inhibited the growth of hamster buccal pouch carcinoma HCPC-1 cells by 54%–89% *in vitro*.[1,2] With the onion treatment, proliferation of Caco-2 colon cancer and HepG2 hepatoma cell lines was arrested dose-dependently.[3] Dietary supplementation of onion deterred DEN-elicited preneoplastic foci formation in rat liver, accompanied by a significant decrease in GST activity and oxidative stress.[4] Feeding 1% or 5% onion in the diet to rats dose-dependently restrained the mutagenicity induced by either BAP or 3-methylcholanthrene and recovered the mutagen-caused damages in kidney and liver tissues through protection of the peripheral blood lymphocytes.[5] Both water and ethanol extracts of onion were able to dose- and time-dependently suppress the proliferation of human colorectal cancer cell lines (Lovo, SW480, HCT-8, and HT-29) and the water extract exerted more significant inhibitory effect than the ethanol extract. The apoptosis elicited by the water extract was greater than by the ethanol extract in SW480 and HCT-8 cell lines but lower than the ethanol extract in HT-29 cells. Phytochemical analysis showed the content of flavonoids extracted by water was higher than by ethanol.[6]

Moreover, in association with activation of the ROS-dependent pathway and downregulation of phospho-cdc2 and phosphocyclin-B1 expression, onion oil at a 12.5-μg/mL concentration mark-edly enlarged the apoptotic rate of human A549 lung cancer cells and caused cell-cycle arrest at the G2/M stage. When treated with 25 μg/mL of onion oil, the percentage of G2/M cells could be amplified almost six fold, and the collapse of mitochondrial membrane potential was elicited, infer-ring that mitochondrial dysfunction may be related to oxidative burst and proapoptosis.[7] Similarly, onion extract has capacities to promote apoptosis and/or necrosis in Lucena MDR–human K562 erythroleukemic and its parental cell lines through provoking oxidative stress and DNA damage.[8] Twenty μg/mL of onion oil exerted marked growth inhibition on HL-60 promyelocytic leukemia cells and elicited differentiation of HL-60 cells. In combination with the oil with all-*trans* retinoic acid or DMSO, more effective synergistic differentiation of HL-60 cells would result.[9,10] *In vivo* mouse models with papillomas induced by two-stage promotion with DMBA and mezerein/TPA were further used to evaluate the bioactivity of onion oil. The number of papillomas per mouse and the percentage of mice with papillomas were noticeably reduced after onion oil treatment.[11] The scientifically established proofs proposed that onion is a functional vegetable that can be consumed in human diets to prevent carcinogenesis and to avert toxic effects of environmental carcinogens/genotoxicants.

SCIENTIFIC EVIDENCE OF CANCER-INHIBITORY AND CANCER-PREVENTIVE CONSTITUENTS

Biology-related phytochemical research revealed that onion is a rich source of three chemical groups: (1) polyphenols, (2) flavonoids, and (3) organosulfurs. Their valuable health benefits have been perceived, particularly cancer chemoprevention through the diet.

1. Polyphenols

A mixture of polyphenols was extracted from lyophilized *A. cepa*, which demonstrated an inhibitory effect against the proliferation of human leukemia cell lines (THP-1, K562, and U937) and AGS gastric cancer cells together with induction of caspase-dependent apoptosis.[12,13] The apoptosis of leukemia cells was triggered by both extrinsic and intrinsic pathways. However, the apoptosis of these cancer cell lines elicited by onion polyphenols was found to be also partially associated with the blockage of a phosphatidylinositol 3-kinase (PI3K)/Akt signaling pathway.[12,13] These findings showed that the onion polyphenols are promising contributors to cancer prevention.

2. Flavonoids

Two flavonoid subgroups, anthocyanins and flavanols, were found in onion. Anthocyanins impart a red/purple color to certain onion varieties, whereas flavanols are responsible for yellow/brown skins of other varieties.[14,15] The flavonoids prepared from yellow onion exerted significant anti-tumor activity against human Lovo, SW480, HT-29, and HCT-8 colorectal cancer cell lines and human HepG2 hepatoma cells, and the flavonoids extracted by 50% ethanol exhibited the most notable inhibitory effect.[16,17]

Quercetin (**1**) is the most important flavanol in onion, which exhibited moderate antiproliferative effects against various malignant tumor cells, such as human HT-29 (colon), HeLa (cervical), and A549 (lung) cancer cells *in vitro*.[18] By the upregulation of Bax expression and downregulation of Bcl-xL and Bcl-2 expressions in a p53-independent manner, the apoptosis of human PC3 prostate cancer cells is elicited by quercetin (**1**). It also concurrently increased the level of insulin-like growth factor–binding protein (IGFBP)-3 and significantly reduced the levels of insulin-like growth factors, IGFI, and IGFII, interactions of which were believed to contribute to the anti-growth effect against PC3 cells.[19] The quercetin-inhibited A549 cell proliferation was found to correlate with extracellular signal-regulated kinase (ERK) activation,[20] whereas the quercetin-promoted HeLa cell apoptosis was associated with an ERα-dependent mechanism involving the activation of caspase and p38 kinase.[21] The suppression of COX and PGE-2 was revealed to contribute to the preventive efficacy of quercetin (**1**) in the treatment of human HCA-7 colon cancer cells and other human colon epithelial cells.[22] An *in vivo* experiment in rats confirmed that quercetin (**1**) was able to selectively inhibit the growth of transformed tumorigenic cells and restrained the neoplastic transformation of mouse embryonic fibroblast NIH/3T3 cells with oncogene H-ras.[15] Quercetin (**1**), quercetin-4'-*O*-glucoside, and two isomeric quercetin dimers (10 μM for each) isolated from the brownish scale components of onion showed an ability to reduce the fluidity of tumor cell membranes. The membrane-targeted flavonoids at concentrations of 10–100 μM could exert the anti-growth activity against mouse myeloma cells and their potencies that were in order as quercetin-4'-O-glucoside < quercetin (**1**) < isomeric quercetin dimers.[23]

More data showed that quercetin (**1**) is capable of reducing the cell growth and metastasis and highly protecting the carcinogenesis in breast, prostate, lung, and other types of cancers. The inhibition of migration and invasion of human SAS oral cancer cells by quercetin was associated with the inhibition of MMP-2 and -9 and NF-κB expression via downregulating PKC and RhoA activities and blocking MAPK and PI3K/Akt signaling pathways.[24] When the quercetin (**1**) was used in the cotreatment with D,L-sulforaphane (a cruciferous vegetable-derived isomer isolated from broccoli), the migration of B16F10 melanoma cells was more effectively deterred than either of the compounds used alone, because the cotreatment predominantly diminished MMP-9 expression in the tumors.[25] In addition, the effects of quercetin (**1**) on murine WEHI-3 leukemia cells were investigated *in vivo*, suppressive activity of which on the WEHI-3 leukemia was attributed to the promotion of immune responses such as stimulation of natural killer cell activity and macrophage phagocytosis of peritoneum.[26] Besides, treatment of the onion flavonol extracts together with human gut bacterial glucosidases could efficiently release quercetin (**1**) by deglycosylation of the quercetin glucosides, indicating that the glucosides can be biotransferred to quercetin (**1**) in the host.[14]

Two other flavonoids identified as luteolin (**2**) and myricetin (**3**) present in various vegetables (including onion and broccoli) also exerted antitumor-related activities. In particular, luteolin (**2**) reduced UVB-induced melanoma incidence, multiplicity, and overall size of tumor in SKH-1 hairless mice by attenuating the activities of PKC ε and Src kinase, inhibiting mitogen-activated protein kinases and the Akt signaling pathway, and markedly lessening the levels of COX-2, TNF-α, and proliferating cell nuclear antigen.[27] Myricetin (**3**) could obstruct UVB-induced VEGF and MMP expression, restrain PI-3 kinase activity and Akt/p70(S6K) phosphorylation, and subsequently repress UVB-elicited angiogenesis in the skin of SKH-1 hairless mice.[28] These findings showed that luteolin (**2**) and myricetin (**3**) are effective in the chemoprevention and/or antiangiogenesis of melanoma.

3. Organosulfur components

OSCs derived from onion and other *Allium* vegetables were extensively proved to have chemopreventive, anticarcinogenic, and antigenotoxic activities. The resultant evidence revealed that higher intake of onion included *Allium* plants that could lessen the risks of some carcinogenesis.[29,30] Oil-soluble OSCs such as diallyl sulfide, diallyl disulfide, and diallyl trisulfide were highly effective in their protection against carcinogenesis caused by a variety of chemical mutagens. Some naturally occurring OSC analogs were capable of retarding the proliferation and growth of transplanted cancer cell xenografts and homografts *in vivo* by inducing cell apoptosis and perturbing cell-cycle progression.[31] In association with the targeting of Cdc25 phosphatases, which are crucial enzymes of the cell cycle, the growth of both drug-sensitive and drug-resistant human breast cancer cell lines (MCF-7 and MCF-7 Vcr-R) was significantly inhibited by diallyl- and dipropyl-tetrasulfides, together with obvious elicitation of G2/M cell-cycle arrest.[32]

Diallyl disulfide was capable of reducing the mutagenicity of N-nitrosomorpholine (NDEA, a hepatocarcinogen) and depressing the formation of nitrosamine.[33] When orally administered 48–96 h prior to NDEA, the induced forestomach type of cancer would be separately obstructed by diallyl disulfide, allyl mercaptan, and allyl methyl disulfide. Of these, the most potent was diallyl disulfide, which diminished forestomach tumor formation by >90% and blocked pulmonary adenoma formation by 30%.[34] Treatment with diallyl sulfide or diallyl disulfide notably inhibited skin papilloma formation induced by DMBA plus TPA and expressively elongated the survival periods in a murine model.[35] Methylpropyl disulfide and propylene sulfide demonstrated significant inhibitory effects against the polyamine biosynthesis and the development of glutathione S-transferase placental (GST-P)–positive foci in the liver of rats, thereby achieving the antihepatocarcinogenic and antiproliferative effects.[36] Water-soluble OSCs such as S-methylcysteine and cysteine showed similar activity to lessen GST-P focus formation. The inhibitory potential on carcinogenesis in colon and renal cancers was also confirmed in rats treated with diallyl disulfide, S-methyl cysteine, or cysteine.[37] Similarly, the modulation of cytochrome P450–dependent monooxygenases and induction of phase II enzymes (quinone reductases, glutathione transferases, etc.) by OSCs were also responsible for lessening of carcinogen activation and toxification and to the protection of chemical-induced carcinogenesis in various cancer cells.[31,38,39]

S-alk(en)yl-l-cysteine sulfoxides (alliins) are another group of active OSCs in onion, such as thiosulfinates and thiosulfonates.[12] During onion tissue damage, S-alk(en)yl cysteine sulfoxides are converted to thiosulfinates or propanethial-S-oxide by the action of the enzyme alliinase.[40,41] Two alk(en)yl thiosulfates such as sodium propyl thiosulfate (NPTS) and sodium 2-propenyl thiosulfate (2PTS) dose-dependently inhibited the growth of three human tumorigenic cell lines (WiDr, 293, and HL-60) in vitro. NPTS and 2PTS were able to cause oxidative damage in HL-60 leukemia cells and then induce apoptosis, implying that the antitumor effect of the alk(en)yl thiosulfates should be mediated by the induction of oxidative stress-initiated apoptosis.[42]

4. Selenocompounds

Onion also has the ability to accumulate selenium (Se) from Se-rich soil. The Se-enriched onion presents a greater anticarcinogenic activity than the common onions. Three selenocompounds, selenomethionine, selenocysteine, and Se-methylselenocysteine, have been identified from onions.[43–46]

5. Other active compounds

2,3-Dihydro-3,5-dihydroxy-6-methyl-4H-pyranone (DDMP, **4**) isolated from the onions is an NF-κB inhibitor. Treatment with DDMP (**4**) in concentrations of 0.5–1.5 mg/mL could inhibit the growth of SW620 and HCT116 colon cancer cell lines followed by the induction of apoptotic death via inhibiting the expressions of NF-κB and Bcl-2 and promoting the expression of apoptotic genes (Bax, caspase-3, and cleaved PARP).[47] Onionin-A (**5**) is a sulfur-containing compound isolated from the acetone extract of onion bulbs. Its inhibitory activity on the proliferation of tumor cells was reported to be mediated by restraining CD163 expression and M2-macrophage polarization.[48]

OTHER BIOACTIVITIES OF THE CONSTITUENTS

Quercetin (**1**) as an important component in the onion also exerts many beneficial effects on human health such as cardiovascular protection, antiallergy, antiviral, antiulcer, cataract prevention, and anti-inflammatory activities besides anticarcinogenesis.

CONCLUSION AND SUGGESTION

Similar to the *Allium* vegetables such as garlic, chives, leeks, and scallions, the pungent, stinky, tear-inducing organosulfur components in onions have been proven to be major contributors to halting cancer-cell growth, cancer prevention, detoxifying carcinogens, antioxidants, and other bioactivities. The organosulfurs are usually released when onions are chopped, crushed, or chewed. However, in contrast to other *Allium* vegetables, onions are rich in flavonoids as well, and the predominant flavonoid in all onions is quercetin. The flavonoids are also responsible for the medicinal benefits of onions in antioxidant, anticarcinogenesis, DNA protection, and health promotion. The dark yellow and red varieties of onions contain more flavonoids and exhibit more antioxidant activity than pure white onions, and the outer layers of onions contain higher flavonoids. Overall, as with other *Allium* vegetables, dietary onion should be encouraged. It is without question that regular consumption of onions is one of the best choices for lowering the occurrences of carcinogenesis.

REFERENCES

1. Niukian, K. et al., 1987. Effects of onion extract on the development of hamster buccal pouch carcinomas as expressed in tumor burden. *Nutr. Cancer* 9: 171–176.
2. Niukian, K. et al., 1987. In vitro inhibitory effect of onion extract on hamster buccal pouch carcinogenesis. *Nutr. Cancer* 10: 137–144.
3. Yang, J. et al., 2004. Varietal differences in phenolic content and antioxidant and antiproliferative activities of onions. *J. Agri. Food Chem.* 52: 6787–6793.
4. Bang, M.-A. et al., 2010. Dietary supplementation of onion inhibits diethylnitrosamine-induced rat hepatocellular carcinogenesis. *Food Sci. Biotechnol.* 19: 77–82.
5. Polasa, K. et al., 2006. Inhibitory effect of unprocessed/processed alliums under in vitro/in vivo conditions on carcinogen induced mutagenesis using different assays. *Int. J. Cancer Res.* 2: 199–211.
6. Zhou, A.C. et al., 2012. Influence of *Allium cepa* extracts on apoptosis and cell cycle of colorectal cancer. *Shizhen Guoyi Guoyao* 23: 809–8011.
7. Wu, X.J. et al., 2006. The production of reactive oxygen species and the mitochondrial membrane potential are modulated during onion oil-induced cell cycle arrest and apoptosis in A549 cells. *J. Nutr.* 136: 608–613.
8. Votto, A.P.S. et al., 2010. Toxicity mechanisms of onion (*Allium cepa*) extracts and compounds in multidrug resistant erythroleukemic cell line. *Biol. Res.* 43: 429–437.
9. Ariga, T. et al., 2000. Antithrombotic and antineoplastic effects of phyto-organosulfur compounds. *BioFactor* 13: 251–255.
10. Seki, T. et al., 2000. Garlic and onion oils inhibit proliferation and induce differentiation of HL-60 cells. *Cancer Lett.* 160: 29–35.
11. Perchellet, J.P. et al., 1990. Inhibition of DMBA-induced mouse skin tumorigenesis by garlic oil and inhibition of two tumor-promotion stages by garlic and onion oils. *Nutr. Cancer* 14: 183–193.
12. Han, M.H. et al., 2013. Polyphenols isolated from *Allium cepa* L. induces apoptosis by suppressing IAP-1 through inhibiting PI3K/Akt signaling pathways in human leukemic cells. *Food Chem. Toxicol.* 62: 382–389.
13. Lee, W. et al., 2014. Polyphenols Isolated from *Allium cepa* L. induces apoptosis by induction of p53 and suppression of Bcl-2 through inhibiting PI3K/Akt signaling pathway in AGS human cancer cells. *J. Cancer Prev.* 19: 14–22.
14. Leighton, T. et al., 1992. Molecular characterization of quercetin and quercetin glycosides in Allium vegetables. Their effects on malignant cell transformation. In *Phenolic Compounds in Food and Effects on Health. II Antioxidants and Cancer Prevention*, Huang, M.-T., Ho, C.-T., and Lee, C. Y. Eds., ACS Symposium Series 507, American Chemical Society, Washington, DC, 220–238.
15. Griffiths, G. et al., 2002. Onions: A global benefit to health. *Phytotherapy Res.* 16: 603–615.
16. Wei, Y.X. et al., 2008. Effects of flavonoid extracts from onion by different methods on HepG2 cells. *Huaxi Yaoxue Zazhi* 23: 315–317.
17. Zhou, A.C. et al., 2011. *Allium cepa* extracts inhibit the proliferation of colorectal cancer in vitro. *Shijie Huaren Xiaohua Zazhi* 19: 2011–2015.
18. Wenzel, U. et al., 2004. Protein expression profiling identifies molecular targets of quercetin as a major dietary flavonoid in human colon cancer cells. *Proteomics* 4: 2160–2174.
19. Vijayababu, M.R. et al., 2006. Quercetin induces p53-independent apoptosis in human prostate cancer cells by modulating Bcl-2-related proteins: A possible mediation by IGFBP-3. *Oncol. Res.* 16: 67–74.
20. Hung, H. 2007. Dietary quercetin inhibits proliferation of lung carcinoma cells. *Forum Nutr.* 60 (Nutrigenomics), 146–157.
21. Galluzzo, P. et al., 2009. Quercetin-induced apoptotic cascade in cancer cells: Antioxidant versus estrogen receptor α-dependent mechanisms. *Mol. Nutr. Food Res.* 53: 699–708.
22. Al-Fayez, M. et al., 2006. Differential modulation of cyclooxygenase-mediated prostaglandin production by the putative cancer chemo-preventive flavonoids tricin, apigenin and quercetin. *Cancer Chemother. Pharmacol.* 58: 816–825.
23. Furusawa, M. et al., 2006. Cell growth inhibition by membrane-active components in brownish scale of onion. *J. Health Sci.* 52: 578–584.
24. Lai, W.W. et al., 2013. Quercetin inhibits migration and invasion of SAS human oral cancer cells through inhibition of NF-κB and matrix metalloproteinase-2/9 signaling pathways. *Anticancer Res.* 33: 1941–1950.
25. Pradhan, S.J. et al., 2010. Quercetin and sulforaphane in combination suppress the progression of melanoma through the down-regulation of matrix metalloproteinase-9. *Exp. Therap. Med.* 1: 915–920.

26. Yu, C.S. et al., 2004. Quercetin inhibited murine leukemia WEHI-3 cells in vivo and promoted immune response. *Phytotherapy Res.* 24: 163–168.
27. Byun, S. et al., 2010. Luteolin inhibits protein kinase C. vepsiln and c-Src activities and UVB-induced skin cancer. *Cancer Res.* 70: 2415–2423.
28. Jung, S.K. et al., 2010. Myricetin inhibits UVB-induced angiogenesis by regulating PI-3 kinase in vivo. *Carcinogenesis* 31: 911–917.
29. LeBon, A.M. et al., 2000. Organosulfur compounds from Allium and the chemoprevention of cancer. *Drug Metab. Drug Interact.* 17: 51–79.
30. Kris-Etherton, P.M. et al., 2002. Bioactive compounds in foods: Their role in the prevention of cardiovascular disease and cancer. *Am. J. Med.* 113: 71S–88S.
31. Herman-Antosiewicz, A. et al., 2004. Signal transduction pathways leading to cell cycle arrest and apoptosis induction in cancer cells by Allium vegetable-derived organosulfur compounds: A review. *Mutat. Res.* 555: 121–131.
32. Viry, E. et al., 2011. Antiproliferative effect of natural tetrasulfides in human breast cancer cells is mediated through the inhibition of the cell division cycle 25 phosphatases. *Int. J. Oncol.* 38: 1103–1111.
33. Dion, M.E. et al., 1997. S-allyl cysteine inhibits nitrosomorpholine formation and bioactivation. *Nutr. Cancer* 28: 1–6.
34. Wattenberg, L.W. et al., 1989. Inhibition of N-nitrosodiethylamine carcinogenesis in mice by naturally occurring organosulfur compounds and monoterpenes. *Cancer Res.* 49: 2689–2692.
35. Dwivedi, C. et al., 1992. Chemoprevention of chemically induced skin tumor development by diallyl sulfide and diallyl disulfide. *Pharm. Res.* 9: 1668–1670.
36. Matsuda, T. et al., 1994. Dose-dependent inhibition of glutathione S-transferase placental form-positive hepatocellular foci induction in the rat by methyl propyl disulfide and propylene sulfide from garlic and onions. *Cancer Lett.* 86: 229–234.
37. Fukushima, S. et al., 1998. The inhibitory effects of organosulfur compounds on chemical carcinogenesis of rats. In Prasad K.N. and Cole, W.H. (Eds.) *Cancer Nutrition*, Amsterdam, the Netherlands: IOS Press, pp. 157–165.
38. Herman-Antosiewicz, A. et al., 2004. Signal transduction pathways leading to cell cycle arrest and apoptosis induction in cancer cells by Allium vegetable-derived organosulfur compounds: A review. *Mutat. Res.* 555: 121–131.
39. Takada, N. et al., 1994. Enhancement by organosulfur compounds from garlic and onions of diethylnitrosamine-induced glutathione S-transferase positive foci in the rat liver. *Cancer Res.* 54: 2895–2899.
40. Munday, R. et al., 2001. Relative activities of organosulfur compounds derived from onions and garlic in increasing tissue activities of quinone reductase and glutathione transferase in rat tissues. *Nutr. Cancer* 40: 205–210.
41. Rose, P. et al., 2005. Bioactive S-alk(en)yl cysteine sulfoxide metabolites in the genus Allium: The chemistry of potential therapeutic agents. *Nat. Prod. Rep.* 22: 351–368.
42. Chang, H.S. et al., 2005. Growth inhibitory effect of alk(en)yl thiosulfates derived from onion and garlic in human immortalized and tumor cell lines. *Cancer Lett.* 223: 47–55.
43. Ip, C. et al., 1994. Characterization of tissue selenium profiles and anticarcinogenic responses in rats fed natural sources of selenium-rich products. *Carcinogenesis* 15: 573–576.
44. Ip, C. et al., 1994. Enrichment of selenium in allium vegetables for cancer prevention. Carcinogenesis 15: 1881–1885.
45. Auger, J. et al., 2004. High-performance liquid chromatographic-inductively coupled plasma mass spectrometric evidence for Se-"alliins" in garlic and onion grown in Se-rich soil. *J. Chromatog. A* 1032: 103–107.
46. Arnault, I. et al., 2006. Seleno-compounds in garlic and onion. *J. Chromatog. A* 1112: 23–30.
47. Ban, J.-O. et al., 2007. Anti-proliferate and pro-apoptotic effects of 2,3-dihydro-3,5-dihydroxy-6-methyl-4H-pyranone through inactivation of NF-κB in human colon cancer cells. *Archiv. Pharmacal Res.* 30: 1455–1463.
48. El-Aasr, M. et al., 2010. Onionin A from *Allium cepa* inhibits macrophage activation. *J. Nat. Prod.* 73: 1306–1308.

20. KONJAC/MOYU

魔芋 こんにゃく 구약나물

Amorphophallus rivieri

Araceae

Konjac/Moyu is an herbaceous Araceae plant, *Amorphophallus rivieri*, native to eastern Asia. Its large starchy corms are often utilized to create flour and jelly for cuisines of the area. The flours are ordinarily used to make noodles and foods and to make jelly Moyu-tofu/Konjac-tofu because it provides several nutrients, such as proteins, carbohydrates, lipids, vitamins A, E, D, B1, B2, B6, B12, and C, pantothenate, niacin, fatty acids, folic acid, dietary fiber, and minerals (magnesium, iron, phosphorus, copper, and zinc). Thus, it is also used as a vegan substitute for gelatin, and it is useful in the weight control as well. Scientific approaches have established that Konjac/Moyu possesses hypoglycemic, vasodilative, hypolipemic, antiatherosclerosis, anti-inflammatory, antibacterial, slimming, laxative, and hemostatic activities.

Scientific Evidence of Antitumor Activities and Constituents

In an *in vitro* assay, a petroleum-ether extract of konjac suppressed the proliferation of human SGC-7901 gastric cancer cells by activating the MAPK signaling pathway.[1] An ethyl acetate extract and the petroleum-ether extract from Moyu exerted inhibitory effects on human HepG2 hepatoma cells and rat C6 glioma cells in a dose-dependent manner.[2] The water extract of Moyu showed an anti-growth effect against sarcoma 180 by 49.8% in mice.[3] The *in vivo* inhibitory rates could be 40.86%–59.74% against murine Ehrlich tumor, HepS hepatoma, and U14 cervical cancer.[4] Konjac also enhanced the function of the immune system via increasing macrophage phagocytosis and T-lymphocyte conversion to impede the tumor cell growth *in vivo*.[4]

The major antitumor component in Moyu is a polysaccharide assigned as glucomannan (GM). The Moyu powder contains 84.8% glucomannan, which is composed of 1,4-linked β-D-glucose and β-D-mannose with minor 1,3-linked branches.[5] A diet that includes 10% Konjac powder significantly diminished the incidence of intestinal neoplasms and colon cancer induced by 1,2-dimethylhydrazine in mice.[6] A diet mixed with 8% Moyu powder was fed to mice injected with an oncogenic agent MNNG for long-term treatment, exerting a marked inhibitory effect on lung carcinogenesis and precancerous lesions. The cancer incidence rate declined from 70.87% to 19.38%, and the survival rate was enlarged in the tested animals.[7] The Moyu powder also could reduce the incidence of spontaneous hepatoma in mice.[8,9]

KF1 was a β-mannanase hydrolysis product from the konjac glucomannan (KGM), and KF2 was an enzymically hydrolyzed product after ^{60}Co γ-irradiation pretreatment. In an *in vivo* model, either KF1 or KF2 by intragastric administration significantly deterred the growth of mouse EAC tumor and resulted in different enhancement effects in the rates of life prolongation, spleen, and thymus indexes and the activity on macrophages of the celiac plexus. KF2 displayed greater anti-growth effect and more enhanced macrophage activity compared to KF1.[10]

Conclusion and Suggestion

The *in vitro* and *in vivo* investigations have demonstrated that both polar and nonpolar extracts of Konjac and both types of components with small molecules (organic solvent extracts) and macromolecules (such as polysaccharides) were able to suppress the proliferation and growth of certain carcinoma cells and to hinder chemical oncogen-induced carcinogenesis. In addition, the extract and the polysaccharide component are capable of stimulating the immune system and enhancing the antitumor activities of macrophages and T-lymphocytes. Consequently, dietary intake of

Konjac/Moyu and its products may help the human body to prevent and resist cancer initiation probably in the stomach, liver, lung, and/or pancreas. However, overdose of Konjac at one time may cause acute toxicity but the toxicity will not occur when the same dose is divided several times in administration. There was no obvious toxicity to be found when Konjac was orally administrated at a dose of 10.8 g/kg per day to rats for 3 months continuously.[11]

REFERENCES

1. Pan, L. et al., 2013. Impact of konjac extract on MAPK signal pathway of human gastric cancer cells SGC-7901. *Zhongguo Zhongyiyao Keji* 20: 254–256.
2. Chang, Z.F. et al., 2012. Screening of antitumor active components from extracts of Rhizoma Amorphophalli and primary analysis on chemical composition. *Shizhen Guoyi Guoyao* 23: 580–581.
3. Yang, C.L. et al., 1993. *Duyao Bencao*, 1st ed. Beijing, China: Chinese Medicine Publisher, p. 94.
4. Huang, M.F. et al., 2010. Healthy functions of konjac dietary fiber. *Food China* (5): 75–77.
5. Ohya, Y. et al., 1994. Preparation and biological properties of dicarboxy-glucomannan: Enzymic degradation and stimulating activity against cultured macrophages. *Carbohydr. Polym.* 25: 123–130.
6. Liang, Y.G. et al., 1995. Influence of Konjac flour on fecal neutral steroids discharged from dimethylhydrazine-induced rat colon cancer. *Jiefangjun Yufang Yixue Zazhi* 13: 27–32.
7. Luo, D.Y. et al., 1992. Inhibitory effect of refined Amorphophallus Konjac on MNNG-induced lung cancers in mice. *Zhonghua Zhongliu Zazhi* 14: 48–50.
8. Mizutani, T. et al., 1982. Effect of Konjac mannan on spontaneous liver tumorigenesis and fecal flora in C3H/He male mice. *Cancer Lett.* 17: 27–32.
9. Mizutani, T. et al., 1983. Effect of Konjac mannan on 1,2-dimethylhydrazine-induced intestinal carcinogenesis in Fischer 344 rats. *Cancer Lett.* 19: 1–6
10. Li, C.G. et al., 2012. Effect of γ-irradiation pretreatment on antitumor activity for enzymatic hydrolysis of konjac glucomannan. *Xinan Shifan Daxue Xuebao, Ziran Kexueban* 37: 46–50.
11. Cui, X. et al., 1995. Studies on the bioactivities of Kanjac. *Zhongyaocai* 18: 368.

21. POTATO

Pomme de terre   Kartoffel   Patata

土豆 ジャガイモ 감자

Solanum tuberosum

Solanaceae

1. R = –glc-(2-1)-rham
          └ (4-1)-rham

2. R = –gal-(2-1)-rham
          └ (3-1)-glc

glc: beta-D-glucose; gal: beta-D-galactose
rham: alpha-L-rhamnose

Potato is an edible tuberous crop from a perennial Solanaceae plant *Solanum tuberosum*. It was believed to be native to multiple locations in South America. The potato has become the fourth largest food crop in the world for human consumption because its nutrients have a clear impact on the dietary population. Nutritionally, potatoes provide high vitamin C, are a good source of vitamin B complex and potassium, and provide trace amounts of folate, niacin, iron, zinc, magnesium, and phosphorus. There are various potato cultivars with diverse color commercially in the markets today. Many phytochemicals in the potato cultivars contribute to antioxidant activity, but the cultivars with pigmented flesh seem more valuable. However, nutrient availability of the potato can be significantly affected by storage and cooking methods.

SCIENTIFIC EVIDENCE OF CANCER-INHIBITORY AND CANCER-PREVENTIVE CONSTITUENTS

Potato tuber is a carbohydrate-rich and energy-providing comestible with little fat and fairly low protein content. It contains a number of naturally occurring defense substances such as glycoalkaloids and polyphenolics that are largely concentrated in potato peels. A recent investigation revealed that basal glycoalkaloid levels in potatoes varied between potato cultivars. The stress treatments such as wounding and light exposure can augment the level of glycoalkaloids in potato tuber.[1] Almost 90% of natural polyphenols in potato peels are chlorogenic acid.[2] These constituents are believed to be responsible for the biological benefits of potato tubers, including antioxidant and anticarcinogenic activities.

1. Glycoalkaloids

Steroidal glycoalkaloids are nitrogen-containing secondary metabolites found in numerous solanaceous plants, which have been demonstrated of possessing anticarcinogenic, antiglycemic, antimalarial, antipyretic, and anti-inflammatory properties.[3] Up to 95% of total glycoalkaloids in potatoes, especially in potato skin, were identified as α-chaconine (**1**) and α-solanine (**2**). Structurally, both glycoalkaloids consist of the same steroidal aglycone called solanidine and a different oligosaccharide chain that is attached at the C-3 hydroxyl group of solanidine. In the *in vitro* experiments, α-chaconine (**1**) and α-solanine (**2**) demonstrated a suppressive effect against six tested human neoplastic cell lines such as MCF-7 breast cells, HepG2 liver cells, U937 leukemic monocyte lymphoma cells, HFFF2 fetal foreskin fibroblasts, Jurkat T-lymphocytes, and Caco-2 epithelial colorectal cells, where α-chaconine (**1**, IC_{50}s of 2–4 μg/mL) was more active than α-solanine (**2**, IC_{50}s of 6–15 μg/mL) and the inhibitory effects of α-chaconine (**1**) were similar to those of tamoxifen (a chemodrug for breast cancer therapy) on cell viability. Compared to the two glycoalkaloids, their aglycone solanidine showed lower inhibition on the six neoplastic cell lines (IC_{50}s of 14–40 μg/mL), suggesting the importance of rhamnose-terminated trisaccharide moiety in the α-chaconine (**1**) and α-solanine (**2**) for the anticancer activity.[4] Similarly, α-chaconine (**1**) and α-solanine (**2**) were also effective in inhibiting human cervical (HeLa), liver (HepG2), lymphoma (U937), and stomach (AGS and KATO III) cancer cell lines in a concentration range of 0.1–10 μg/mL (0.117–11.7 nmol/mL).[5] α-Chaconine (**1**) in a concentration of 5 μg/mL exerted antiproliferative properties and increased cyclin-dependent kinase inhibitor p27 levels in two human prostate cancer cell lines (LNCaP and PC3), whereas α-solanine (**2**) restrained the viability and proliferation of human SMMC-7721 (liver), NCI-H460, and A549 (lung) cancer cell lines (respective IC_{50}s of 14.4, 39.0, and 35.7 μm).[6,7] Normally, the effectiveness of α-chaconine (**1**) against HepG2 hepatoma cells was greater than against HT-29 colon cancer cells. The suppressive potential of α-chaconine (**1**) at a concentration of 1 μg/mL on hepatoma cells was superior to the anticancer drugs doxorubicin and camptothecin.[8] In both *in vitro* and *in vivo* models, α-solanine (**2**) significantly obstructed the growth of mouse mammary cancer cells and completely stopped the tumor growth rate at a concentration of 5 mg/kg.[9]

α-Chaconine (**1**) was also reported to have an ability to induce apoptosis of HT-29 human colon cancer cells via activation of caspase-3 and blockage of ERK 1/2 phosphorylation[4,10] of LNCaP prostate cancer cells via a caspase-dependent signaling pathway with the activation of c-Jun *N*-terminal protein kinase (JNK) and a caspase-independent pathway with the initiation of nuclear translocation of endonuclease-G, and of PC3 prostate cancer cells via caspase-independent pathway plus endo-G nuclear translocation.[6] Interestingly, α-chaconine (**1**) and α-solanine (**2**) were poor in the induction of apoptosis in the cancer cell lines (MCF-7, HFFF2, U937, Jurkat, and/or HepG2).[4] The antihepatoma effect by α-solanine (**2**) in HepG2 cells was primarily achieved by disruption of cell membranes via lessening of the cell membrane potential, opening ion channels, increasing calcium concentrations, and finally triggering the apoptotic pathway.[11] The inhibition of α-solanine (**2**) on PC3 androgen-independent prostate cancer cells was found to correlate with the induction of S-phase cell-cycle arrest and apoptosis as well as upregulation of IκBα expression and downregulation of Bcl-2 expression.[12]

Furthermore, by the repression of MMP-2 and NF-κB activities and blockage of JNK and PI3K/Akt signaling pathways, α-chaconine (**1**) in nontoxic doses dose-dependently obstructed the proliferation of bovine aortic endothelial cells (BAECs) and markedly obstructed migration, invasion, and tube formation of BAECs, indicating an antiangiogenetic potential for α-chaconine.[13] By the similar mechanism—that is, reducing MMP-2 and -9 and NF-κB activities and hindering JNK and PI3K/Akt signaling pathways—α-chaconine (**1**) and α-solanine (**2**) restrained the invasion and migration of human A549 lung adenocarcinoma cells[14] and human A2058 melanoma cells,[15] respectively, displaying the potential of α-chaconine and α-solanine in antimetastatic treatment. Besides the dose-dependent antiproliferative effects *in vitro* against three pancreatic cancer cell lines (Panc-1, sw1990, and Mia-PaCa-2), α-solanine (**2**) also suppressed migration and invasion of these pancreatic cancer cells in nontoxic doses and limited angiogenesis in the tumor tissues in addition to its antiproliferative activity, antipancreatic cancer mechanisms of which were found to be mediated by (1) downregulated MMP-2 and -9 and impeded CD44, extracellular inducer of MMP, eNOS, and E-cadherin expression in Panc-1 cells; (2) obviously hindering the VEGF expression and tube formation of endothelial cells; (3) blocked Akt, Stat3, and mTOR phosphorylation; and (4) amplified β-catenin phosphorylation and diminished nuclear translocation of NF-κB, β-catenin, and TCF-1.[14] The inhibition on the pancreatic cancer cells was further proved in an *in vivo* xenograft mouse model, where the tumor volume and tumor weight were decreased to 61% and 43%, respectively, after treatment with α-solanine (**2**) in a dose of 6 μg/kg for 2 weeks.[16] The anti-invasive effect by α-solanine (**2**) in PC3 prostate cancer cells at nontoxic doses was found to be mediated by (1) blockage of epithelial–mesenchymal transition (EMT); (2) reduction of MMP-2 and -9 mRNA levels and extracellular induction of MMP; (3) downregulation of miR-21 and upregulation of miR-138; and (4) limiting ERK and PI3K/Akt signaling pathways.[17] In addition, the antiangiogenetic effect of α-solanine (**2**) occurred in a breast cancer model.[9]

Taken together, the summarized scientific data clearly demonstrated the properties of two major glycoalkaloids in potatoes in the suppression of proliferation, metastasis, and angiogenesis, showing valuable chemoprotective and chemotherapeutic potential on some types of carcinomas, especially in liver, prostate, breast, and colon. However, the similar level of inhibition was observed in normal liver (Chang) cells and normal colon cells as well as after treatment with the two glycoalkaloids.[4,5] Thus, cancer chemotherapy with α-chaconine (**1**) and α-solanine (**2**) should be safely guided; however, the general amount of steroidal glycoalkaloids in the dietary intake of potato is acceptable for the cancer prevention.

2. Polyphenolic acids and anthocyanins

Potato is also an excellent source of dietary polyphenols, including phenolic acids and anthocyanins. However, the contents of polyphenolic acids and anthocyanins in diverse cultivations signify difference, which impacts the antioxidant and anticarcinogenic potencies of potatoes.

Polyphenolics: The antioxidant extracts were prepared from four potato cultivars (Northstar, Mountain Rose, Purple Majesty, and Bora Valley). The contents of total phenolics in the potato extracts were revealed to be Bora Valley (skin/flesh: purple/purple) > Purple Majesty (purple/ purple) > Mountain Rose (purple/red) >>> Northstar (white/white), the contents of anthocyanins were Purple Majesty > Bora Valley > Mountain Rose >>> Northstar, and the contents of chlorogenic acid were Bora Valley > Mountain Rose > Purple Majesty >>> Northstar. Thus, the DPPH-scavenging assay indicated that the antioxidant activities were Bora Valley > Purple Majesty > from Mountain Rose >> Northstar. In 400-μg/mL concentrations, the extract from Northstar exerted the lowest antiproliferative effect against human Caco-2 (colon) and HepG2 (liver) cancer cell lines. Despite the fact that all the extracts had weak inhibition on the cancer cell lines, the results revealed that Caco-2 cells were more sensitive to potato extracts than HepG2 cells, and the correlation between antioxidant activity and anticancer activity was significant.[18] Similarly, the ethanolic extract of Purple Majesty potatoes (purple-fleshed) demonstrated more potent inhibitory effects than the extracts of Atlantic (white-fleshed) and Yukon Gold (yellow-fleshed) potatoes in HT-29 (p53-mutated; ras wild-type) and HCT-116 (p53 wild-type; ras-mutated) colon cancer cell lines.[19]

The radical-scavenging and antiproliferative activities were also found in the ethanol extracts of white (Superior) and colored potatoes (Red, Rose, Haryoung, Blue, Jaseo, and Jasim), which were collected in Korea. The color-fleshed potato extracts of Rose, Blue, Jaseo, and Jasim displayed higher radical-scavenging activities than the general white potato extract, and Blue and Jasim potato extracts showed the highest cytotoxic activity on HepG2 hepatoma cells at a concentration of 100 μg/mL and on THP-1 leukemia monocytic cells at concentrations of 30–100 μg/mL.[20]

Anthocyanins: Vitelotte is a potato variety (dark blue-fleshed) enriched with anthocyanins. An anthocyanin-rich extract derived from the Vitelotte cultivar potatoes in an *in vitro* assay exerted antiproliferative activity on four human solid cancer cell lines such as HeLa (cervix), LnCaP (prostate), MCF-7, and MDA-MB-231 (breast) cells and on human hematological cancer cells such as U937 and NB4 myeloid leukemia cell lines. Simultaneously, the four solid cancer cell lines responded with proapoptosis in a dose-dependent manner. The anthocyanin extract blocked the Akt-mTOR signaling pathway in U937 acute myeloid leukemia (AML) cells and MDA-MB-231 breast cancer cells.[21] The anthocyanin extract was also able to disturb cell-cycle progression and induce differentiation of U937 cells, interactions of which might contribute to strengthen anti-AML activity.[22] Further, two active anthocyanins termed malvidin 3-*O*-*p*-coumaroyl-rutinoside-5-*O*-glucoside and petunidin 3-O-p-coumaroyl-rutinoside-5-O-glucoside were found to be in high content in Vitelotte cultivar potatoes.[21]

Similarly, the fractions of phenolic acids and anthocyanins were extracted from four specialty potato cultivars (CO112F2-2, PATX99P32-2, ATTX98462-3, and ATTX98491-3, which were grown in Texas in the United States). An extract and its anthocyanin fractions from CO112F2-2 cultivar at concentrations equivalent to 5 μg/mL chlorogenic acid inhibited the proliferation of both LNCaP and PC3 prostate cancer cell lines concomitantly with caspase-independent proapoptosis and increase in the p27 (a cyclin-dependent kinase inhibitor) level. The apoptosis induction was mediated by activation of mitogen-activated protein kinase (MAPK), c-Jun N-terminal kinase (JNK), nuclear translocation of endonuclease-G (Endo G), and apoptosis-inducing factor. However, proapoptosis was observed in LNCaP cells only in a caspase-dependent manner.[23]

3. Starch

Potatoes enriched with carbohydrate and the predominant form of carbohydrate are termed starch. Most of the potato starch can be digested, but a small and significant portion of the starch is resistant to digestion by enzymes in the digestive tract. The resistant starch called fiber exerts health benefits, including protection against colon carcinogenesis as well as improvement of glucose tolerance and insulin sensitivity and reduction of plasma cholesterol and triglyceride concentrations. Cooking and then cooling can markedly enlarge the amount of resistant starch in cooked potatoes. In addition, the potato skins afford substantial dietary fiber.[24]

4. Melanoidins

Melanoidins are commonly generated from foods such as potato, barley malts, bread crust, bakery products, and coffee. During the food process, sugars and amino acids combine through Maillard reaction at high temperatures and low water activity to form melanoidins, which are nitrogen-containing brown heterogeneous polymers with high molecular weight. *In vitro* experiments revealed that the melanoidin complexes containing water extract of heated potato fiber Potex (180°C for 2 h) exerted antiproliferative effects against human LS180 colon cancer and rat C6 glioma cells. HMW and LMW, two fractions with high- and low-molecular-weight melanoidins isolated from the extract, were found to contribute to the inhibitory activity against LS180 and C6 tumor cells.[25] Compared to LMW, HMW was responsible for stronger antiproliferative effect in C6 cells (IC_{50} of 115.8 μg/mL). Simultaneously, both fractions modulated MAPK and Akt signaling pathways and elevated p21 levels together with decreasing cyclin D1, leading to G0 cell-cycle arrest in LS180 colon cancer cells and G1/S cell-cycle arrest in C6 glioma cells. At a concentration of 1000 μg/mL, HMW and LMW deterred the growth of LS180 cells by 69% and 54%, respectively.[25] HMWF1–4 subfractions were derived from fractionation of HMW by size-exclusion chromatography. Of them, HMWF1 and HMWF4 showed significantly higher antiproliferative effects on C6 cells (IC_{50}s of 7.4 and 21.6 μg/mL, respectively).[26] Therefore, it is recommended to use heated potato fiber Potex as a functional food ingredient for chemoprevention.

5. Lectins

STL-S and STL-D were two 20 kDa chitin-binding lectins isolated from two potato cultivars, Sheelbilatee and Deshi, which were collected in Bangladesh. The lectins showed no specificity to animal and human erythrocytes, and their LC_{50} values were 75 and 90 μg/mL, respectively, having a dose-dependent intermediary toxic effect. In a mouse model, treatment with the lectins at a dose of 1.38 mg/kg/day for 5 consecutive days resulted in 79.84% and 83.04% of growth inhibition against Ehrlich ascites carcinoma (EAC) cells, respectively. At the same time, STL-S and STL-D augmented the levels of hemoglobin and white blood cells and reduced the level of red blood cells.[27]

6. Noclosan and Loxat

Noclosan and Loxat are two bioactive macromolecules separated from the potato tuber (*S. tuberosum*) by an ion-exchange chromatography eluted with increasing concentrations of NaCl. Two fractions obtained from 0.78 M and 1.02 M NaCl elusions were labeled as Noclosan and Loxat, respectively. Both the macromolecules were effective in growth suppression and apoptosis induction in seven human cell lines such as MR65 (nonsmall cell lung cancer) and NCI-H125 (lung adenocarcinoma), MCF-7 (breast cancer), Caco-2 (colon cancer), OVCAR3 (ovarian cancer), U937 (monocytic leukemia), and Jurkat (T-cell lymphoma). Both Noclosan and Loxat could dose-dependently disturb cell-cycle progression and elicit apoptosis in all the tested cancer cell lines. At high doses (10–20 mg/mL), the cell cycle was completely arrested and apoptosis was promoted via an SAPK/JNK pathway and by both mitochondrial and nonmitochondrial routes. Noclosan and Loxat also could act synergistically in the induction of apoptosis in the *in vitro* test. Moreover, Loxat dose-dependently triggered HUVEC cell apoptosis up to 80% at a 10-mg/mL concentration, implying the potential of angiogenesis supression.[28]

7. Proteins and proteinase inhibitors

Potato protein component mainly consists of 40-kDa glycoprotein and 5–25-kDa protease inhibitors as well as ~10% of other proteins with large molecular weights. In an *in vitro* experiment, the potato crude protein and protease inhibitor prepared from potato tuber and juice exerted an inhibitory effect against the proliferation of B16 melanoma cells, with inhibitory rates of 54% and 45%, respectively. The potato protein component showed good solubility, emulsifiability, foaming ability, and foam stability.[29] Inh-1 and Inh-2, which were isolated from potato tubers, were effective proteinase inhibitors of chymotrypsin and trypsin. Both Inh-I and Inh-II upregulated AP-1 constituent proteins (JunD and Fra-2) and suppressed c-Jun and c-Fos expression, leading to blockage of UVB irradiation-induced activator protein-1 (AP-1) activation effectively in mouse JB6 epidermal cells, indicating their preventive potential on skin carcinogenesis.[30,31]

8. Pectin

Pectin is one of the important dietary components in all fruits and vegetables. A rhamnogalacturonan-I domain-rich pectin was prepared from potato, which in an *in vitro* assay downregulated cyclin-B1 and cyclin-dependent kinase-1 expression, thereby significantly inducing G2/M cell-cycle arrest and proliferative suppression of human HT-29 colon cancer cells.[32]

9. Antitumor activity of transgenic potatoes

Human interleukin-12 (hIL-12) is expressed and extracted from transgenic potatoes, which in the *in vitro* assays actively obstructed the survival of human hepatocarcinoma HepG22.2.15 cells and promoted cell apoptosis.[33] The hIL-12 extracted from transgenic potato leaves or tubers at a 200-μg/mL concentration elicited 28.42% and 32.3% apoptotic death of human K562 leukemia cells, respectively, and at 25–400-μg/mL concentrations stimulated human peripheral blood monocyte (PBMC) to secrete IFN-γ.[34] The hIL-12–activated PBMC and IFN-γ was capable of killing the tested HepG22.2.15 and K562 cells. These apoptosis-inducing and PBMC-activating activities of hIL-12 from transgenic potatoes were greater than those of hIL-12 from natural potatoes.[34,35]

CONCLUSION AND SUGGESTION

Despite many types of components in potatoes have been reported to have antitumor potentials, such as polyphenolics, anthocyanins, pectins, lectins, proteins, melanoidins, and dietary fibers, the steroidal glycoalkaloids especially α-chaconine (**1**) and α-solanine (**2**) were the most potent inhibitors on cancer growth and proliferation. The polyphenolic and anthocyanin components in potatoes are primarily responsible for the prominent antioxidant and anticarcinogenic activities; however, their contents vary because of the different colors in the skin and flesh of the diverse potato cultivars. It is recognized that all the potato constituents can contribute to the antioxidant, cancer-suppressive, and cancer-preventive properties of potatoes. Consequently, the dietary potato should be a good choice for cancer prevention and nutritional supplementation.

However, the glycoalkaloids, including α-chaconine (1) and α-solanine (2), are also the major toxic compounds in various potato cultivars. The glycoalkaloid content is normally lowest in the tuber flesh but highest in sprouts and flowers of potatoes, though the cultivars contain different levels of glycoalkaloids. Cooking potatoes can partly destroy the glycoalkaloids but potatoes that are sprouted or green below the skin must be discarded for safe consumption. In addition, it is necessary to use fresh or well-preserved potatoes when cooking because light exposure, physical damage, and age amplifies the content of glycoalkaloids within the potato tuber. If doing so carefully, the poisoning from potatoes occurs very rarely. Poisoning from potatoes rarely occurs when they are cooked carefully.

REFERENCES

1. Petersson, E.V. et al., 2013. Glycoalkaloid and calystegine levels in table potato cultivars subjected to wounding, light, and heat treatments. *J Agric. Food Chem.* 61: 5893–902.
2. Schieber, A. et al., 2009. A source of nutritionally and pharmacologically interesting compounds—A review. *Food* 3: 23–29.
3. Friedman, M. et al., 2015. Chemistry and anticarcinogenic mechanisms of glycoalkaloids produced by eggplants, potatoes, and tomatoes. *J. Agricul. Food Chem.* 63: 3323–3337.
4. Kenny, O.M. et al., 2013. Cytotoxic and apoptotic potential of potato glycoalkaloids in a number of cancer cell lines. *J. Agricul. Sci. Applic.* 2: 184–192.
5. Friedman, M. et al., 2005. Anticarcinogenic effects of glycoalkaloids from potatoes against human cervical, liver, lymphoma, and stomach cancer cells. [Erratum to document cited in CA143:126101] *J. Agricul. Food Chem.* 53: 6162–6169.
6. Reddivari, L. et al., 2010. The bioactive compounds α-chaconine and gallic acid in potato extracts decrease survival and induce apoptosis in LNCaP and PC3 prostate cancer cells. *Nutr. Cancer* 62: 601–610.
7. Zhang, Z.Q. et al., 2013. Five new steroidal alkaloid glycosides from *Solanum tuberosum. Helv. Chim. Acta* 96: 931–940.
8. Lee, K.R. et al., 2004. Glycoalkaloids and metabolites inhibit the growth of human colon (HT29) and liver (HepG2) cancer cells. *J. Agric. Food Chem.* 52: 2832–2839.
9. Mohsenikia, M. et al., 2013. The protective and therapeutic effects of α-solanine on mice breast cancer. *Eur. J. Pharmacol.* 718: 1–9.
10. Yang, S.-A. 2006. α-Chaconine, a potato glycoalkaloid, induces apoptosis of HT-29 human colon cancer cells through caspase-3 activation and inhibition of ERK 1/2 phosphorylation. *Food Chem. Toxicol.* 44: 839–846.
11. Ji, Y.B. et al., 2008. Induction of apoptosis in HepG2 cells by solanine and Bcl-2 protein. *J. Ethnopharmacol.* 115: 194–202.
12. Zhang, J. et al., 2011. Inhibitory effect of solanine on prostate cancer cell line PC-3 in vitro. *Zhonghua Nankexue* 17: 284–287.
13. Lu, M.K. et al., 2010. α-Chaconine inhibits angiogenesis in vitro by reducing matrix metalloproteinase-2. *Biol. Pharm. Bull.* 33: 622–630.
14. Shih, Y.W. et al., 2007. α-Chaconine-reduced metastasis involves a PI3K/Akt signaling pathway with downregulation of NF-κB in human lung adenocarcinoma A549 cells. *J. Agric. Food Chem.* 55: 11035–11043.
15. Lu, M.K. et al., 2010. α-Solanine inhibits human melanoma cell migration and invasion by reducing matrix metalloproteinase-2/9 activities. *Biol. Pharm. Bull.* 33: 1685–1691.
16. Lv, C. et al., 2014. Antitumor efficacy of α-solanine against pancreatic cancer in vitro and in vivo. *PLoS One* 9: e87868.

17. Shen, K.H. et al., 2014. α-Solanine inhibits invasion of human prostate cancer cell by suppressing epithelial–mesenchymal transition and MMPs expression. *Molecules* 19: 11896–11914.
18. Wang, Q.Y. et al., 2011. Inhibitory effect of antioxidant extracts from various potatoes on the proliferation of human colon and liver cancer cells. *Nutr. Cancer* 63: 1044–1052.
19. Madiwale, G.P. et al., 2012. Combined effects of storage and processing on the bioactive compounds and pro-apoptotic properties of color-fleshed potatoes in human colon cancer cells. *J. Agri. Food Chem.* 60: 11088–11096.
20. Jang, H.L. et al., 2012. Biological activities and total phenolic content of ethanol extracts of white and flesh-colored Solanum tuberosum L. potatoes. *Han'guk Sikp'um Yongyang Kwahak Hoechi* 41: 1035–1040.
21. Bontempo, P. et al., 2013. Antioxidant, antimicrobial and anti-proliferative activities of *Solanum tuberosum* L. var. Vitelotte. *Food Chem. Toxicol.* 55: 304–312.
22. Bontempo, P. et al., 2015. Anticancer activities of anthocyanin extract from genotyped *Solanum tuberosum* L. "Vitelotte" *J. Func. Foods* 19(A): 584–593.
23. Reddivari, L. et al., 2007. Anthocyanin fraction from potato extracts is cytotoxic to prostate cancer cells through activation of caspase-dependent and caspase-independent pathways. *Carcinogenesis* 28: 2227–2235.
24. Camire, M.E. et al., 2009. Potatoes and human health. *Criti. Rev. Food Sci. Nutri.* 49: 823–840.
25. Langner, E. et al., 2013. Melanoidins isolated from heated potato fiber (Potex) affect human colon cancer cells growth via modulation of cell cycle and proliferation regulatory proteins. *Food Chem. Toxicol.* 57: 246–255.
26. Ewa, L. et al., 2011. Antiproliferative activity of Melanoidins isolated from heated potato fiber (Potex) in glioma cell culture model. *J. Agri. Food Chem.* 59: 2708–2716.
27. Hasan, I. et al., 2014. Antiproliferative activity of cytotoxic tuber lectins from *Solanum tuberosum* against experimentally induced Ehrlich ascites carcinoma in mice. *Afr. J. Biotech.* 13: 1679–1685.
28. Schutte, B. et al., 2004. Inhibition of the cell cycle and induction of apoptosis by Noclosan and Loxat in cell lines irrespective of their origin. *Int. J. Oncol.* 24: 1357–1367.
29. Li, G.M. et al., 2013. Preliminary study on the properties of crude protein and protease inhibitor from potato fruit juice. *China Food Addi.* 1: 58–61.
30. Huang, C.S. et al., 1997. Proteinase inhibitors I and II from potatoes specifically block UV-induced activator protein-1 activation through a pathway that is independent of extracellular signal-regulated kinases, c-Jun N-terminal kinases, and P38 kinase. *Proc. Nat. Aca. Sci. USA* 94: 11957–11962.
31. Liu, G.M. et al., 2001. Proteinase inhibitors I and II from potatoes block UVB-induced AP-1 activity by regulating the AP-1 protein compositional patterns in JB6 cells. *Proc. Nat. Acad. Sci. USA* 98: 5786–5791.
32. Cheng, H.R. et al., 2013. The inhibitory effects and mechanisms of rhamnogalacturonan I pectin from potato on HT-29 colon cancer cell proliferation and cell cycle progression. *Int. Food Sci. Nutr.* 64: 36–43.
33. Chen, J.Y. et al., 2010. The in vitro anti-hepatocarcinoma effects of human interleukin-12 from transgenic potato. *Anhui Nongye Kexue* 38: 11069–11070, 11074.
34. Chen, J.Y. et al., 2010. Bioactivity of human interleukin-12 from transgenic potatoes. *Di-San Junyi Daxue Xuebao* 32: 1632–1634.
35. Luo, G. et al., 2010. Analysis on bioactivity of human interleukin 12 purified from transgenic potato. *J. Anhui Agric. Sci.*, 38(3): 1173–1176.

22. RED BEET OR CHARD

Betterave rouge   Rote rüben   Remolacha roja

紅甜菜   レッドビート   붉은사탕무우

Beta vulgaris and its varieties

Chenopodiaceae

3. R = −beta-D-glucose-(2-1)-beta-D-xylose(p)

Red beet/chard is a nutritional vegetable, which originated from varieties of *Beta vulgaris* var. *cicla* and var. *conditiva*. The original plant is believed to be native to the Mediterranean coast, dating to the second millennium B.C. The vegetable has many cultivated varieties, which are grown for their taproots, leaves, or swollen midribs, which are favorable in diets for healthful nutrition and delicious taste. Nutritionally, red beet/chard is a great source of vitamins K, A, and C and minerals (magnesium, manganese, iron, and potassium). Biological approaches have confirmed that beetroot can provide multiple health benefits such as antioxidant, anti-inflammatory, antiradiation, antifatigue, immunoregulating, and hepatoprotective detoxification besides lowering oncogenesis. The chard vegetable is also employed as an alternative hypoglycemic agent by diabetics.

SCIENTIFIC EVIDENCE OF CANCER-INHIBITORY AND CANCER-PREVENTIVE CONSTITUENTS

1. Anticancer activities and agents from red beet leaves

The investigation found that beet leaves contained 1195 mg of polyphenolics in 100 g fresh weight.[1] The ethanolic extract of beet leaves (*B. vulgaris*) exerted marked antioxidative effect in both DPPH- and ABTS-radical scavenging assays and inhibitory activity against cancer-cell proliferation in *in vitro* assays. The extract restrained the proliferation of all tested human MKN-45 (stomach), HCT-116 (colon), NCI-H460 (lung), and MCF-7 (breast) cancer cell lines, and the inhibitory rates ranged from 57.6% to 66.4%.[1] A diet of beet leaf fiber to rats prominently diminished the number of 1,2-dimethylhydrazine-caused colon carcinogenesis.[2] The beet leaves collected in Egypt exhibited marked antioxidative and antileukemia activities. Their ethanolic and methanol/dichloromethane (1:1) extracts at a 20-μg/mL concentration showed 85% and 60% suppressive rates against acute lymphocyte leukemia cells and obstructed the viability of acute myeloid leukemia cells by 81% and 83%, respectively, at a 200-μg/mL concentration, after 24 h of incubation. At the same concentrations, the two extracts showed very low cytotoxicity on normal bone marrow cells (6% and 14%, respectively), and the aqueous extracts had weak activity against other two types of leukemia cells.[3] Oral administration with the ethanolic extract to nude mice in a daily dose of 20 mg for 8 weeks resulted in 40% inhibition against the growth of HeLa cells and prompted the tumor cells to necrosis.[4] However, the ethanolic extract showed no activity in a mouse model implanted with Ehrlich ascites tumor cells.[3]

Modern phytochemical studies further revealed that the chard (*B. vulgaris* var. *cicla*) contains apigenin flavonoids: vitexin, vitexin-2-*O*-rhamnoside, and vitexin-2-*O*-xyloside. The antiproliferative effect of these flavonoids was shown in the tested cancer cell lines.[5] P2, a phenolic fraction derived from chard leaves (*B. vulgaris* subsp. *cycla*) showed the antiproliferative effect against human MCF-7 cancer cells (IC_{50} of 9 μg/mL) without inducing apoptosis but also no toxicity to human lymphocytes and slight toxicity to macrophages. The primary components of P2 were identified as vitexin-2″-O-rhamnoside, its demethylated form 2″-xylosylvitexin, rutin, and isorhamnetin 3-gentiobioside. These components in combination exerted the inhibitory effect against the DNA synthesis in MCF-7 cells.[6] In addition, beet greens are a valuable source of lutein/zeaxanthin, which is usually known to play an important role in eye health. The anticarcinogenic potential of lutein/zeaxanthin has been observed in several tumor tissues, though high doses of β-carotene failed to exhibit chemotherapeutic activity in clinical trials.[7]

2. Anticancer activities and agents from red beetroot

Beetroots have been used for centuries as a natural coloring agent in many traditional cuisines and as a nutritional vegetable with unexpected health benefits. In recent investigations, beetroot pigments have been shown to reduce carcinogenesis via a number of mechanisms: antioxidant activity, inhibition of proinflammatory enzymes (specifically, cyclooxygenase) and cytochrome P450 activity (such as CYP1A1 and 1A2), and an increase in phase II enzymes (such as quinone reductase).[8,9] Oral consumption of red beetroot-derived food color resulted in an inhibitory effect against N-nitroso-methylbenzylamine (NMBA)-induced esophageal tumors in rats. Concurrently, the apoptosis was enhanced, and the levels of angiogenesis and inflammation were impeded in beetroot color-consuming animals.[10,11] *In vivo* models also revealed a significant antitumor-promoting activity of beetroot extract on the carcinogenesis in mice skin and lung.[12] Feeding with beetroot juice could lessen the activities of CYP1A1 and 1A2 and augment phase II enzymes, leading to reduction of DMBA-induced damage in the liver and mammary gland of female rats, and the root juice could also induce GST levels in the mammary gland.[7] Moreover, the researchers found that beetroot extract was dose-dependently cytotoxic to androgen-independent human PC3 prostate cancer cells and estrogen receptor–positive human MCF-7 breast cancer cells but significantly had low cytotoxicity to normal human FC skin and HC liver cell lines.[13] With treatment using the beetroot, the cytotoxicity of doxorubicin (an anticancer drug) was synergistically potentiated against human pancreatic (PaCa), breast (MCF-7), and prostate (PC3) tumor cell lines.[14]

Furthermore, red beetroots contain a specific class of antioxidants collectively named betalains, which have been shown to possess multiple biological benefits. Four predominant betalains—that is, two betacyanins (betanin and isobetanin) and two betaxanthins (vulgaxanthin-I and miraxanthin-V)—were isolated from the beetroots. Betanin (**1**) and vulgaxanthin-I (**2**) were the major compounds in the extracts of red and yellow beetroots, respectively, and they comprised >90% of the betalain content in many cultivars of *B. vulgaris*.[15] The anticarcinogenic and antitumor-promoting effects of betanin (**1**) were shown in mouse models with two-stage carcinogenesis induced by DMBA and 12-O-tetra-decanoylphorbol-13-acetate (TPA). The marked inhibitory effects of betanin (**1**) also were observed in two-stage carcinogenesis of mouse lung tumor (induced by 4-nitroquinoline-N-oxide as an initiator and glycerol as a promoter) and of murine hepatoma (induced by N-nitrosodiethylamine as an initiator and phenobarbital as a promoter).[16,17] Oral consumption of betanin (**1**) in drinking water diminished tumor multiplicity and tumor load by 20% and 39% in a vinyl carbamate–elicited lung cancer model and by 46% and 65% in a benzo[a]pyrene-induced lung cancer model, respectively.[18] During lung tumor suppression, betanin (**1**) lessened the number of CD31+ endothelial microvessels and amplified the expression of caspase-3, implying that betanin (**1**) stimulated the cell apoptosis and retarded the angiogenesis. An *in vitro* model correspondingly proved that betanin (**1**) enhanced apoptosis via activation of caspases and PARP in human lung cancer cell lines.[18] Similarly, betanin (**1**) at a 200-μg/mL concentration restrained the proliferation of the human HepG2 hepatoma cell line by 49%, whereas betaine (trimethyl-glycine), another type of component in beetroot, only yielded a 25% inhibitory effect on the HepG2 cells at a 800-μg/mL concentration.[15] Betanin (**1**), however, showed weak growth inhibition on human HCT-116 (colon), NCI-H460 (lung), AGS (stomach), MCF-7 (breast), and central nervous system (CNS) cancer cell lines, with IC_{50}s between 147 and 164 μg/mL.[19] Furthermore, by deterring basic fibroblast growth factor (bFGF), MMP-2 and -9 and inhibiting NF-κB and Akt activation, betaine (1) obstructed the angiogenic cascade, tube formation, migration, and invasion of human umbilical vein endothelial cells (HUVECs) *in vitro*. The antiangiogenic effect of betaine was further observed in an *in vivo* mouse model.[20]

Accordingly, these positive data evidenced that betanin (1) may be beneficial to the cancer chemoprevention and treatment of certain types of cancers, strongly suggesting that long-term consumption of beetroot should be an efficient cancer prevention and cancer therapy supplement for humans.

3. Anticancer activities and agents from red beet seeds

From ethyl-acetate extract of beet seeds, a fraction labeled as P4 was fractionated. Isolation of the P4 gave a group of apigenin-glycosides that were identified as 2,4,5-trihydroxybenzaldehyde, 2,5-dihydroxybenzaldehyde, vanillic acid, xylosylvitexin, glucopyranosylglucopyrasylrhamnetin, and glucopyranosylxylosylrhamnetin. Of them, xylosylvitexin (3) is a main constituent that showed an efficient chemopreventive effect. *In vitro* experiments revealed that xylosylvitexin (3) was remarkably active in the antiproliferation of human RKO colon cancer cells and the induction of cell-cycle arrest and apoptosis. The treatment could also obviously stimulate the proliferation of normal human fibroblast HF cells.[21]

4. Anticancer activities and agents from sugar beet pectin

Sugar beet is a different cultivar of *Beta vulgaris*, which is grown commercially for sugar production. In the past years, sugar beet pectin has been subjected to several investigations, including antitumor assays. The pectic extract at a concentration range of 12.5–25 mg/mL killed 80.6% of the tested human MCF-7 breast cancer cells *in vitro*. Its antiproliferative activity was greater than that of 4-hydroxytamoxifen (a classic anticancer drug), which killed 56.5% of the MCF-7 cells in the experiment.[22] A pectin prepared from sugar beet has been used to formulate an injectable and biodegradable sugar beet pectin/gelatin hydrogel. Using the pectin-produced gel combined with doxorubicin (an anticancer drug) could notably suppress the growth of mouse B16F1 melanoma cells in nude mice, showing more usefulness in cancer chemotherapy.[23]

NANOFORMULATION

A conjugation of *Beta vulgaris* extract with hydroxyapatite nanoparticles and functionalized multi-walled carbon nanotubes was prepared by using a grafting technique. The created nanocomposites showed marked improvement of long-term stability in aqueous solution and dispersibility of the nanotube and exhibited greater enhancement of the free-radical scavenging activity and cytotoxicity on EAC cells.[24]

CONCLUSION AND SUGGESTION

According to the scientific research results shown earlier, the red beet and chard have been confirmed to have significant antioxidant and moderate to weak levels of anticancer properties, the activities of which should be attributed to a significant amount of phenolics, flavonoids, and betalain-type alkaloids. The studies showed that red beet and chard may be good for protecting against carcinogenesis in the liver, stomach, colon, lung, breast, and prostate and for additively enhancing certain chemotherapies. Significantly, both roots and leaves of red beet/chard are recommended as dietary food supplements for health promotion and cancer prevention.

OTHER HEALTH BENEFITS

The aqueous extract of chard leaves showed benefit to hinder valproic acid (VPA)-induced cardiac damage.[25]

REFERENCES

1. Kim, H.K. et al., 2007. Antioxidant and antiproliferative activities of methanol extracts from leafy vegetables consumed in Korea. *Food Sci. Biotechnol.* 16: 802–806.
2. Aritsuka, T. et al., 1989. Protective effect of beet dietary fiber on 1,2-dimethylhydrazine-induced carcinogenesis in rats. *Nippon Nogei Kagaku Kaishi* 63: 1221–1229.
3. Nassr-Allah, A.A. et al., 2009. Anticancer and anti-oxidant activity of some Egyptian medicinal plants. *J. Med. Plants Res.* 3: 799–808.
4. Luo, Q.J. et al., 2012. Effect of red beet extract on HeLa cell proliferation in vitro and tumor growth in tumor-bearing mice. *Drug Eva. Res.* 35: 10–13.
5. Tanaka, T. et al., 2012. Cancer chemoprevention by carotenoids. *Molecules* 17: 3202–3242.
6. Ninfali, P. et al., 2007. Characterization and biological activity of the main flavonoids from Swiss chard (*Beta vulgaris* subspecies cycla). *Phytomedicine* 14: 216–221.
7. Ninfali, P. et al., 2013. Nutritional and functional potential of *Beta vulgaris* cicla and rubra. *Fitoterapia* 89: 188–199.
8. Szaefer, H. et al., 2014. Evaluation of the effect of beetroot juice on DMBA-induced damage in liver and mammary gland of female Sprague-Dawley rats. *Phytother. Res.* 28: 55–61.
9. Georgiev, V.G. et al., 2010. Antioxidant activity and phenolic content of Betalain extracts from intact plants and hairy root cultures of the red beetroot beta vulgaris cv. Detroit Dark Red. *Plant Food Human Nutri.* (New York) 65: 105–111.
10. Kapadia, G.J. et al., 1996. Chemoprevention of lung and skin cancer by *Beta vulgaris* (beet) root extract. *Cancer Lett.* 100: 211–214.
11. Lechner, J. et al., 2010. Drinking water with red beetroot food color antagonizes esophageal carcinogenesis in N-nitrosomethylbenzylamine-treated rats. *J. Med. Food.* 13: 733–739.
12. Parkin, K.L. et al., 2003. Betalain-based cancer chemopreventive agents from beet. *U.S. Pat. Appl. Publ.* US 20030036565 A1 20030220.
13. Kapadia, G.J. et al., 2011. Cytotoxic effect of the red beetroot (*Beta vulgaris* L.) extract compared to doxorubicin (adriamycin) in the human prostate (PC3) and breast (MCF-7) cancer cell lines. *Anti-Cancer Agent Med. Chem.* 11: 280–284.
14. Kapadia, G.J. et al., 2013. Synergistic cytotoxicity of red beetroot (*Beta vulgaris* L.) extract with doxorubicin in human pancreatic, breast and prostate cancer cell lines. *J. Complementary Integr. Med.* 10: 113–122.
15. Lee, E. et al., 2014. Betalain and betaine composition of greenhouse- or field-produced beetroot (*Beta vulgaris* L.) and inhibition of HepG2 cell proliferation. *J. Agri. Food Chem.* 62: 1324–1331.
16. Konoshima, T. et al., 2003. Anti-carcinogenic activities of natural pigments from beet root and saffron. *Food Food Ingre. J. Jpn.* 208: 615–622.
17. Kapadia, G.J. et al., 2003. Chemoprevention of DMBA-induced UV-B promoted, NOR-1-induced TPA promoted skin carcinogenesis, and DEN-induced phenobarbital promoted liver tumors in mice by extract of beetroot. *Pharmacol. Res.* 47: 141–148.
18. Zhang, Q. et al., 2013. Beetroot red (betanin) inhibits vinyl carbamate- and benzo(a)pyrene-induced lung tumorigenesis through apoptosis. *Mol. Carcinogen.* 52: 686–691.
19. Reddy, M.K. et al., 2005. Relative inhibition of lipid peroxidation, cyclooxygenase enzymes, and human tumor cell proliferation by natural food colors. *J. Agri. Food Chem.* 53: 9268–9273.
20. Yi, E-Y. et al., 2012. Betaine inhibits in vitro and in vivo angiogenesis through suppression of the NF-κB and Akt signaling pathways. *Int. J. Oncol.* 41: 1879–1885.
21. Gennari, L. et al., 2011. Total extract of *Beta vulgaris* var. cicla seeds versus its purified phenolic components: Antioxidant activities and antiproliferative effects against colon cancer cells. *Phytochem. Anal.* 22: 272–279.
22. Concha, J. et al., 2013. Production of pectic extracts from sugar beet pulp with antiproliferative activity on a breast cancer cell line. *Front. Chem. Sci. Engi.* 7: 482–489.
23. Takei, T. et al., 2013. Injectable and biodegradable sugar beet pectin/gelatin hydrogels for biomedical applications. *J. Biomater. Sci. Polym. Edit.* 24: 1333–1342.
24. Haroun, A.A. et al., 2014. Cytotoxicity and antioxidant activity of *Beta vulgaris* extract released from grafted carbon nanotubes based nanocomposites. *Macromole. Symp.* 337(1, Polymers and Materials), 25–33.
25. Ustundag, U.V. et al., 2016. Effects of chard (*Beta vulgaris* L. var. cicla) on cardiac damage in valproic acid-induced toxicity. *J. Food Biochem.* 40: 132–139.

23. SWEET POTATO

Patate douce   Süßkartoffel   Batata/Boniato

甘薯   サツマイモ   고구마

Ipomoea batatas

Convolvulaceae

Sweet potato is a tuberous root vegetable with a starchy and sweet taste. Its plant is an herbaceous perennial vine *Ipomoea batatas* native to the tropical regions in America. It is now widely grown as an important food crop in tropical and subtropical regions worldwide. Sweet potato is an excellent source of β-carotene (a precursor of vitamin A), vitamin B complex, dietary fiber, polyphenols, polysaccharides, and minerals. These components were identified as strong contributors to the physiological activities of sweet potato plants. Sweet potato roots and greens not only provide considerable amounts of nutrients but also present excellent bioactivities such as antimutagenic, chemopreventive, radical-scavenging, hepatoprotective, and antidiabetic properties. Due to the importance of the crop plant as a health food, many varieties of sweet potato have been developed. Besides the edible tuberous roots, the greens (leaf, stalk, and stem) of the sweet potato plant are extensively consumed as vegetables in Asia and Africa.

SCIENTIFIC EVIDENCE OF CANCER-PREVENTIVE ACTIVITIES

In an *in vitro* assay with human NB4 histolytic lymphoma monocytes, a water extract from sweet potato veins vines (cv. Tainong 57') showed the relatively highest antiproliferative effect (EC$_{50}$ of 449.6 μg/mL) followed by water extracts of its storage roots and its leaves, ethanol extracts of the storage roots and the leaves, implying the water-soluble components to be responsible for the antitumor effect of the sweet potato plant.[1] Other *in vitro* tests also proved the antimutagenic and anticarcinogenic effects of methanolic extract from sweet potato leaves[2] and the cancer-preventing potential of the extract from baked sweet potato roots (cv. Koganesengan).[3] By gel chromatography, four fractions (I, II-a, II-b, and III) were derived from a water extract of the baked sweet potato roots. The fractions IIa and III displayed obvious suppressive and proapoptotic effects on human HL-60 leukemia cells in a dose-dependent manner. Both the fractions were also able to markedly block TPA-induced cell transformation in mouse skin JB6 C141 cell line and to scavenge radicals markedly.[3] The extracts of steamed with peeled (SP) and steamed with no peeled (SNP) of purple-fleshed sweet potato displaying anti-growth effect against MCF-7 (breast), SNU-1 (stomach), and WiDr (colon) cancer cell lines in dose- and time-dependent manner, and SP extract could elicit the MCF-7 and SNU-1 cancer cells to apoptotic death via both extrinsic and intrinsic pathways. The two extracts also exerted anti-inflammatory effects via impeding the production of NO and proinflammatory cytokines (NF-κB, TNF-α, and IL-6) in LPS-induced macrophage cells.[4]

Sweet potato green extract (SPGE) that enriched polyphenols exerted significant antiprolifera-tive activity in a panel of prostate cancer cell lines. It exhibited an ability to induce mitochondrial-mediated apoptosis of PC3 human prostate cancer cells. Oral administration of SPGE in a dose of 400 mg/kg remarkably hampered the growth of prostate tumor xenografts by ~69% in nude mice without any detectable toxicity to normal colorectal and bone marrow tissues.[5] F5, a remarkably polyphenol-enriched fraction isolated from SPGE, was ~100-fold more potent than SPGE in human prostate carcinoma cells. Daily oral administration of the F5 fraction in a dose of 400 mg/kg (body wt.) exerted ~75% inhibition against the progression of prostate tumor xenografts in nude mice.[6] According to the scientific findings, the hydrophilic nutrients in sweet potato plants were demon-strated to be able to provide cancer chemoprevention.

Scientific Evidence of Cancer-Preventive Constituents

Modern approaches in recent decades have revealed that many different types of components in the sweet potato plant, especially polyphenols (such as caffeoylquinic acids and anthocyanins), polysac-charides, peptides, proteins, and glycoproteins, play multiple roles, including cancer prevention and antioxidation.

1. Anthocyanins

Anthocyanins are flavonoid pigments that were predominant in sweet potato, especially purple sweet potato (PSP) as well as many other food plants. The chemopreventive effect of anthocya-nins has been broadly investigated by many researchers. Treatment with 800 µg/mL of anthocy-anin (PSPA) from PSP for 72 h resulted in 80% inhibition against the growth of human HepG2 hepatoma cells and promoted the HepG2 cells to apoptosis, but in low concentration slightly enhanced the proliferation of HepG2 cells.[7] Consuming anthocyanin-enriched PSP extract could reduce the size of sarcoma 180 in mice, and the highest inhibitory rate reached 69.03%.[8] In the doses of 150 mg sweet potato anthocyanins (SPA), the suppressive rates on sarcoma 180 and H22 hepatoma were 45.04% and 33.33%, respectively.[9,10] P40 is an anthocyanin-enriched purple-fleshed sweet potato extract, which has a high content of anthocyanins at 7.5–14 mg/g dry matter. In an *in vitro* treatment, the P40 extract dose-dependently restrained the survival of human SW480 colonic cancer cells due to cytostatic arrest the cell cycle at the G1 phase but not cytotoxicity. Given orally 10%–30% P40 *in vivo* significantly suppressed AOM-induced formation of ACF in the colons of CF-1 mice and elicited greater caspase-3 expression.[11] Proanthocyanidins derived from purple sweet potato in 50- and 100-mg/L concentrations exerted cytotoxic effects on HCT-116 human colorectal cancer cells but little cytotoxic to normal HF-91 fibroblast cells.[12] By HPLC/MS–MS analysis, 12 acylated anthocyanins were detected from the P40 extract, and the top 3 anthocyanins were determined as cyanidin 3-caffeoyl-p-hydroxybenz-oylsophoroside-5-glucoside (**2**), peonidin 3-caffeoylsophoroside-5-glucoside (**3**), and cyanidin 3-(6″-caffeoyl-6″-feruloylsophoroside)-5-glucoside.[13]

Furthermore, a high anthocyanin-producing purple sweet potato cell line was grown under two different media conditions, multiplication medium (MM) and high anthocyanin-producing medium (APM). The anthocyanin-rich aqueous extracts from the cell-suspension cultures at a con-centration of 1.6 mg/mL medium for 24 h suppressed the proliferation of human HL-60 leukemia cells, and the inhibitory rates were 47% for the MM extract, 21% for the APM extract, and 25% for an anthocyanin extract from the storage roots of sweet potato (cv. Ayamurasaki). Cyanidin 3-sophoroside-5-glucoside (**4**) was the dominant cyanidin-based pigment in the MM extract, which contributed the highest antiproliferative effect in the tests.[14] These anthocyanin extracts also showed dose-dependent antimutagenic and radical-scavenging activities.[10,14] However, steaming, pressure cooking, frying, and microwaving processes but not baking would significantly lessen 8%–16% of total anthocyanin contents. Relatively, monoacylated anthocyanins displayed higher resistance against the heat treatment as compared to the di- and nonacylated anthocyanins.

The stable acylated and cyanidin-predominated anthocyanins in sweet potato plants after cooking primarily provide health benefits for cancer prevention and antioxidant effects.[13]

2. Flavonoids

FSPV is flavonoids isolated from sweet potato greens (leaf, stalk, and stem) exerted marked antiproliferative effects against four tested human neoplastic cell lines such as HL-60 (promyelocytic leukemia), BGC-823 (poorly differentiated gastric adenocarcinoma), SMMC-7721 (hepatoma), and A549 (nonsmall cell lung cancer) *in vitro* in a dose-dependent manner. The inhibitory rate of FSPV at a 20-μg/mL concentration reached to 70.95% in the HL-60 cells. The *in vivo* antitumor activity was demonstrated in mouse model–implanted sarcoma 180. When the dose was 400 mg/kg, FSPV showed great anti-growth effect against sarcoma 180 cells *in vivo*.[15]

3. Caffeoylquinic acids

Sweet potato leaves contain a high content of polyphenolics that consist of caffeic acid, chlorogenic acid, 3-, 4-, or 5-caffeoylquinic acids (CQA), di-CQA (4,5-diCQA, 3,5-diCQA, and 3,4-diCQA), and 3,4,5-tri-*O*-CQA. The caffeic acid and di- and tri-caffeoylquinic acids could dose-dependently suppress the proliferation of human tumor cell lines such as Kata-III (stomach), DLD-1 (colon), and HL-60 (leukemic) *in vitro*. Among them, 3,4,5-tri-*O*-CQA (**1**) depressed the growth of these tumor cell lines effectively, and caffeic acid had an exceptionally higher effect against HL-60 cells than other di- and tri-CQAs. The growth suppression on HL-60 cells by 3,4,5-tri-*O*-CQA (**1**) was closely accompanied by the promotion of the HL-60 cells to apoptosis.[16] These CQA derivatives, in human HCT116 colorectal cancer cells, diminished β-catenin/Tcf-4 transcriptional activity and Tcf-4 transcriptional expression, wherein the di-CQAs showed stronger inhibition than mono-CQAs, suggesting that the catechol group in the caffeoyl structures plays a significant role in interfering with the β-catenin/Tcf-4 signaling in HCT116 cells. In addition, the CQAs also modulated the downstream Wnt signaling pathway in the colorectal cancer cells.[17] As the CQAs are rich components there, the evidence indicated that sweet potato leaves and greens can be a functional food for preventing some types of carcinogeneses.

4. Coumarins

Octadecyl coumarate, 7-hydroxycoumarin, and 6-methoxy-7-hydroxycoumarin were isolated from the peels of *I. batatas*, showing different potentials of antioxidant activity in a DPPH assay, which is commonly related to cancer prevention.[18]

5. Furan derivatives

Several furan derivatives such as 5-hydroxymethylfurfural and 2-acetyl-3-*O*-α-D-glucopyranosylfuran were isolated from sweet potato and were tested for the antitumor and proapoptotic effects, the results of which were patented in Japan.[19] 4-Ipomeanol (**5**) is a pneumotoxic furan derivative isolated from sweet potato, which could cause cytochrome P450–mediated conversion into DNA-binding metabolites. 4-Ipomeanol (**5**) exerted promising suppressive effects on lung carcinoma cells in preclinical studies with animal models but showed poor results on nonsmall cell lung carcinoma and advanced hepatocellular carcinoma from phase I and II clinical trials.[20,21]

6. Glycolipids

A glycolipid extract derived from sweet potato roots treated by an ion exchange chromatography produced bioactive fractions. Some of the glycolipid fractions were able to promote the differentiation of HeLa cervical cancer cells *in vitro*, which would be incorporated into food preparation being useful for cancer prevention.[22] A subfraction (IB-F002C) derived from an *n*-hexane partition fraction of sweet potato peels was active in hindering the proliferation of breast, head/neck, ovary, lung, colon-1, and colon-2 cancer cell lines with IC_{50}s of 24.75–47.91 μg/mL. Bioassay- guided separation of IB-F002C obtained a glucocerebroside (**6**), which in *in vitro* assay showed 10.51%, 12.19%, 16.14%, and 34.05% suppressive effects, respectively, on the head and neck, breast-1, colon-1, and ovarian cancer cell lines.[18]

7. Polysaccharides

Sweet potato polysaccharides demonstrated the antitumor property in *in vitro* and *in vivo* experiments. SPPS-I-Fr-II, which was composed of α-D-(1,6)-Glcp, was prepared from sweet potato. In an *in vivo* test, SPPS-I-Fr-II suppressed the growth of B16 melanoma and Lewis lung cancer cells significantly in mice.[23] A crude polysaccharide prepared from purple sweet potato had marked antitumor effect on sarcoma 180 in mice. The inhibitory rate would be 40% with a combined therapy with low-dose polysaccharide (200 mg/kg) and 5-fluorouracil (5-FU). At the same time, the polysaccharide exerted a protective effect on mouse thymus and spleen atrophy caused by 5-FU and reduced the decrease of white cells.[24] The polysaccharide derived from powdery purple sweet potato displayed both strong antioxidant and antitumor activities for inhibiting human SGC7901 gastric cancer cell lines *in vitro*.[25] Seven components, PPSP, PPSPII, PPSPIII, PPSPIV, PSPP1-1, PSPP2-1, and PSPP3-1, were separated from crude polysaccharides of purple sweet potato. PPSP II was a β-D-glucan, and PPSP III was a glycoprotein, both of which inhibited two human HeLa and HepG2 tumor cell lines in the *in vitro* assay.[26] PSPP1-1 (33.3 kDa) and PSPP3-1 (75.3 kDa) were composed of rhamnose, xylose, glucose, and galactose, whereas PSPP2-1 (17.8 kDa) was composed of rhamnose and galactose, but the three contained low proportions of proteins and uronic acids. These three polysaccharides showed antioxidant and antitumor activities *in vitro* in a dose-dependent manner. Of them, PSPP1-1 was the strongest inhibitor against growth of human SGC7901 (stomach) and SW620 (colon) cancer cell lines, and PSPP2-1 exerted the most potent power on radical-scavenging activity.[27] The findings therefore suggested that sweet potato polysaccharides have strong potential for the prevention of human carcinogenesis in colon, liver, and breast.

8. Peptide

A 16-amino acid peptide ([1]AASTPVGGGRRLDRGQ[16]) was isolated from sweet potato leaves and was designated as IbACP. *In vitro* treatment with IbACP dose-dependently inhibited the proliferation of human Panc-1 pancreatic cancer cells and promoted cell apoptosis via a mitochondrial apoptotic pathway-included activation of caspases-3/-9 and poly(ADP-ribose) polymerase (PARP).[28]

9. Proteins

The protein component prepared from sweet potato has been demonstrated to be a cancer inhibitor. A sweet potato sporamin protein (SPP) purified from fresh sweet potato roots, in an *in vitro* assay, dose-dependently restrained the proliferation and viability of human SW480 colorectal carcinoma cells (IC_{50} of 38.732 μmol/L), associated with the cell apoptosis induction and the cell migration–reduction. Either IP or i.g. administration of SPP for 9 days led to a significant inhibition against the growth of human HCT-8 colon cancer cells in nude mice by 58.0% and 43.5%, respectively. Most important, the administration of SPP IG and IP also induced significant inhibition against spontaneous pulmonary metastatic nodule formation of murine Lewis lung cancer 3LL cells in C57 BL/6 mice after 25-day treatment.[29] The observations clearly established that the sporamin protein of the sweet potato possesses prominent antiproliferative and antimetastatic properties on colorectal cancer.

Moreover, another kind of protein termed trypsin inhibitor (33 kDa) was prepared from sweet potato storage roots (cv. Tainong 57), the proteins of which contain about 60% of total water-soluble proteins. Treatment with the trypsin inhibitor (TI) for 72 h induced moderate inhibition of cellular growth in human NB4 promyelocytic leukemia cells in a time- and dose-dependent manner, showing an IC_{50} value of 57.1 μg/mL. Concurrently, TI elicited the cell-cycle G1 arrest and apoptosis, the mechanism of which was mediated by a mitochondria-dependent pathway—that is, increase of p53 and Bax expressions, decrease of Bcl-2 expression, release of cytochrome c from mitochondria, and activation of caspases-3 and -8.[30] TI also showed antioxidant activities against different radicals.[29] Therefore, the TI of sweet potato may be useful as a cancer-preventive substance. In addition, the sporamin protein as major storage protein in sweet potato root was considered as one form of trypsin inhibitor. The sporamin protein is 80% of the total proteins in the storage roots; however, its amount would decline dramatically to 2% of the original value during sprouting.[31]

10. Glycoproteins

Glycoprotein extracts prepared from two sweet potato cultivars in a dosage range of ~5000 µg/dish demonstrated significant antimutagenic activity. In the *in vitro* model, the glycoprotein extracts restrained the growth of COS-1, SHG-44, and SKOV3 tumor cell lines, and their minimum concentration was 1.5 µg/mL for anticancer effect.[32] SPG-1, a glycoprotein extracted from a cultivar Guangdong 98 of sweet potato, was evaluated in mice-implanted mouse H22 hepatoma cells. Intragastric injection of SPG-1 resulted in noticeable effects not only in growth suppression, karyokinesis reduction, and life prolongation of the tested mice against H22 hepatoma cells but also in the enhancement of spleen index, thymus index, and macrophage activity of celiac plexus *in vivo*, indicating the dual functions of antitumor and immunoregulation for the sweet potato glycoprotein.[33]

11. Fibers

Dietary fibers derived from stalks and tubers of sweet potato displayed great potential value in the prevention of colon cancer through their antioxidant and anticancer activities. In the *in vivo* experiments, both the dietary fibers resulted in obvious growth inhibitory effect against human HT-29 colon cancer cells with the upregulation of tumor suppressor p53 expression. In addition, the dietary fiber from stalks exerted 2.4 times higher DPPH radical-scavenging activity than the dietary fiber from tubers.[34]

12. Pectins

Sweet potato pomace is rich in pectin that showed inhibition of cancer cell growth and migration and induction of apoptosis. Further, both pH modification and heat treatment were found to effectively potentiate the inhibitory effect of sweet potato pectins against malignant proliferation of human neoplastic cell lines such as HT-29 (colon), Bcap-37 (breast), and SMMC-7721 (liver). The respective inhibitory rates could be augmented to 45.32% and 61.03% on the HT-29 cells and to 43.31% and 42.54% on the Bcap-37 cells.[35]

CONCLUSION AND SUGGESTION

Due to marked nutritional and functional properties, various cultivars of sweet potatoes are becoming the focus of new research. Bioactive components from different parts (tubers, leaves, stems, and stalks) of sweet potato plants such as small molecules (anthocyanins, polyphenolics, conjugated phenolic acids, glycolipids, carotenoids, and furan derivatives) and macromolecules (fibers, polysaccharides, glycoproteins, proteins, peptides, and pectins) presented versatile functions in health promotion, cancer prevention, antioxidant, hepatoprotection, anti-inflammation, and antiaging. Relatively, the purple sweet potato has higher content of anthocyanins and higher antioxidative effect, whereas sweet potato greens have enriched polyphenolics that showed great potential in lowering the risk of cancer. All the varieties of sweet potato storage roots are rich in macromolecules that are contributors for both anticarcinogensis and immunoenhancement. Some of the constituents can directly retard the proliferation and viability of some types of cancer cells such as the colon, stomach, liver, breast, and/or leukemia. Even sweet potato peel, which is usually discarded as waste, contains biological constituents that can serve as dietary components to prevent cancer development. Therefore, it is clear now that the sweet potato plant is a food treasure providing both nutritional and functional benefits for humans.

Nonetheless, postharvest storage, processing, and cooking methods would lessen the content levels of the bioactive components in sweet potatoes. Accordingly, the ways for cooking and storage of sweet potatoes should be taken seriously if the functional cancer prevention activities are preferred.

REFERENCES

1. Huang, D.J. et al., 2004. Antioxidant and antiproliferative activities of sweet potato (*Ipomoea batatas* Lam 'Tainong 57') constituents. *Botanical Bull. Acad. Sinica* 45: 179–186.
2. Kang, H.G. et al., 2010. Antimutagenic and anticarcinogenic effect of methanol extracts of sweet potato (*Ipomea batata*) leaves. *Toxicol. Res.* 26: 29–35.
3. Rabah, I. et al., 2004. Potential chemopreventive properties of extract from baked sweet potato (*Ipomoea batatas* Lam. Cv. Koganesengan). *J. Agricul. Food Chem.* 52: 7152–7157.
4. Sugata, M. et al., 2015. Anti-inflammatory and anticancer activities of taiwanese purple-fleshed sweet potatoes (*Ipomoea batatas* L. Lam) extracts. *BioMed Res. Int.* 768093/1–768093/11.
5. Karna, P. et al., 2011. Polyphenol-rich sweet potato greens extract inhibits proliferation and induces apoptosis in prostate cancer cells in vitro and in vivo. *Carcinogenesis* 32: 1872–1880.
6. Gundala, S.R. et al., 2013. Polar biophenolics in sweet potato greens extract synergize to inhibit prostate cancer cell proliferation and in vivo tumor growth. *Carcinogenesis* 34: 2039–2049.
7. Cao, D.X. et al., 2011. Effect of purple sweet potato anthocyanin on human liver cancer HepG2 cells. *Tianjin Keji Daxue Xuebao* 26: 9–12.
8. Liu, N. et al., 2008. Study on antitumor effect and its toxicity of *Ipomoea batatas* Poir Cv anthocyanins. *Weisheng Yanjiu* 37: 489–491.
9. Zhao, J.G. et al., 2013. In vivo antioxidant, hypoglycemic, and anti-tumor activities of anthocyanin extracts from purple sweet potato. *Nutri. Res. Prac.* 7: 359–365.
10. Wang, G.L. et al., 2006. Study on the antioxidant activity of sweet potato anthocyanin and its inhibiting effect on growth of cancer S180. *Yingyang Xuebao* 28: 71–74.
11. Lim, S.Y. et al., 2013. Role of anthocyanin-enriched purple-fleshed sweet potato p40 in colorectal cancer prevention. *Mol. Nutr. Food Res.* 57: 1908–1917.
12. Chen, W.L. et al., 2015. Inhibitory effect of proanthocyanidins on human colorectal carcinoma and its apoptosis-induction mechanisms. *Jilin Daxue Xuebao, Yixueban* 41: 785–789.
13. Xu, J.T. et al., 2015. Characterisation and stability of anthocyanins in purple-fleshed sweet potato P40. *Food Chem.* 186: 90–96.
14. Konczak-Islam, I. et al., 2003. Potential chemopreventive properties of anthocyanin-rich aqueous extracts from in vitro produced tissue of sweetpotato (*Ipomoea batatas* L.) *J. Agri. Food Chem.* 51: 5916–5922.
15. Luo, L.P. et al., 2006. Study on antitumor effects of flavonoids extracted from sweet potato leaf, stalk and stem. *Shipin Kexue* (Beijing, China) 27: 248–250.
16. Kurata, R. et al., 2007. Growth suppression of human cancer cells by polyphenolics from Sweet potato (*Ipomoea batatas* L.) leaves. *J. Agri. Food Chem.* 55: 185–190.
17. Taira, J. et al., 2014. Inhibition of the β-catenin/Tcf signaling by caffeoylquinic acids in sweet potato leaf through down regulation of the Tcf-4 Transcription. *J. Agri. Food Chem.* 62: 167–172.
18. Oluyori, A.P. et al., 2016. Sweet potato peels and cancer prevention. *Nutr. Cancer* 68(8): 1330–1337.
19. Fujii, M. et al., 2006. Furan derivatives as anticancer drugs and health foods. *Jpn. Kokai Tokkyo Koho* JP 2006206489 A 20060810.
20. Kasturi, V.K. et al., 1998. Phase I study of a five-day dose schedule of 4-Ipomeanol in patients with non-small cell lung cancer. *Clin. Cancer Res.* 4: 2095–2102.
21. Lakhanpal, S. et al., 2001. Phase II study of 4-ipomeanol, a naturally occurring alkylating furan, in patients with advanced hepatocellular carcinoma. *Invest. New Drugs* 19: 69–76.
22. Michioka, O. et al., 1995. Anticancer glycolipids from sweet potato. *Jpn. Kokai Tokkyo Koho* JP 07258100 A 19951009.
23. Zhao, G.H. et al., 2003. Chemical structure and antitumor activity of sweet potato polysaccharides fraction SPPS-I-Fr-II. *Zhongguo Liangyou Xuebao* 18: 59–61.

24. Ye, X.L. et al., 2005. Effect of polysaccharide in purple sweet potato on the antitumor activity of cancer bearing mice. *Xinan Shifan Daxue Xuebao, Ziran Kexueban* 30: 333–336.
25. Wu, Q.Y. et al., 2013. Method and application for extracting purple sweet potato polysaccharide by ultrasound collaborative enzymatic method. *Faming Zhuanli Shenqing* CN 103319617 A 20130925.
26. Zhao, J. et al., 2011. Antitumor activity of components isolated from purple sweet potato polysaccharides. *J. Zhejiang Univ. Med. Sci.* 40: 365–373.
27. Wu, Q.G. et al., 2015. Characterization, antioxidant and antitumor activities of polysaccharides from purple sweet potato. *Carbohydr. Polym.* 132: 31–40.
28. Chang, V.H.S. et al., 2013. IbACP, a sixteen-amino-acid peptide isolated from *Ipomoea batatas* leaves, induces carcinoma cell apoptosis. *Peptides* (NY, USA). 47: 148–156.
29. Mu, T.H. et al., 2011. Application of sweet potato sporamin protein in preparing medicine and health product for preventing and treating neoplasm. *Faming Zhuanli Shenqing* CN 102198263 A 20110928.
30. Huang, G.J. et al., 2007. Growth inhibition and induction of apoptosis in NB4 promyelocytic leukemia cells by trypsin inhibitor from sweet potato storage roots. *J. Agri. Food Chem.* 55: 2548–2553.
31. Li, P.G. et al., 2013. Anticancer effects of sweet potato protein on human colorectal cancer cells. *World J. Gastroenterol.* 19: 3300–3308.
32. Qian, J.Y. et al., 2005. Study on functional properties of sweet potato glycoprotein-an in vitro antitumor and Ames tests. *Shipin Kexue* (Beijing, China) 26: 216–218.
33. Liu, Z. et al., 2007. Experimental study of SPG-1 on antitumor and immune activity of tumor mice. *Shipin Kexue* (Beijing, China) 28: 312–316.
34. Jeong, H. et al., 2013. Antioxidant activity of dietary fibers from tubers and stalks of sweet potato and their anticancer effect in human colon cancer. *Kongop Hwahak* 24: 525–529.
35. Zhang, Y.Y. et al., 2012. Effects of modified sweet potato pectins on the proliferation of cancer cells. *Zhongguo Nongye Kexue* (Beijing, China) 45: 1798–1806.

4 Cancer-Preventive Substances in Grains and Beans

24. Adlay, Coixseed, or Job's Tears/*Coix lacryma-jobi* var. *ma-yuen*

25. Barley/*Hordeum vulgare*

26. Buckwheat/*Fagopyrum esculentum, F. tataricum*

27. Common Beans/*Phaseolus vulgaris*

28. Corn/*Zea mays*

29. Foxtail Millet/*Setaria italica*

30. Mung Bean/*Vigna radiata (= Phaseolus radiatus)*

31. Oat/*Avena sativa*

32. Soybean/*Glycine max*

Grain crops are the most necessary and basic source of food in human life and are generally divided into two main types of commercial crops: (1) cereals (wheat, rye, rice) and (2) legumes (beans, soybeans). Grains are also divided into two subgroups: (1) whole grains (which contain the entire kernel, germ, endosperm, and bran with whole nutrients) and (2) refined grains (which contain only the endosperm and kernel with little or no dietary fiber, iron, and many B vitamins). Despite dietary whole grains (including processed products of whole grain) having better nutrients and better health benefits, the fact is 95% of total grains consumption is refined grains. This chapter primarily discusses the cancer-preventive functions and constituents of six kinds of whole grains and three kinds of beans, and also introduces the anticarcinogenic activities of inedible parts in several grain plants, which may be useful for the development and improvement of food products. Most of the scientific evidences in this chapter are gained from modern research based on whole grains and beans. Thus, to obtain the entire nutritious and functional substances, whole grains and their products (such as bread, oatmeal, breakfast cereals, pasta, and flour) should be the first choice as much as possible in daily food consumption. Though not being selected in this chapter, other functional grains and dried beans such as brown rice, whole wheat, whole rye, adzuki beans, and faba beans are also highly suggested for the staple food and dietary menu. In addition, amaranth grain is a highly recommended pseudocereal with high nutritious value. It contains a superior amount of proteins when compared to most cereal grains. The cancer-preventive functions of amaranth seeds and leaves have been discussed in Chapter 1.

24. ADLAY, COIXSEED, OR JOB'S TEARS

Adlay-graine   Adlay-Samen   Cebada perlada

薏苡仁   ハトムギ   율무쌀

Coix lacryma-jobi var. *ma-yuen*

Gramineae

Adlay, or *Coix lacryma-jobi* L. var. *ma-yuen*, is a crop seed of a Gramineae plant. The seeds have been commonly used as a nutritious food in Eastern Asia and also as an herb have long been employed to treat warts, chapped skin, rheumatism, and neuralgia. Modern study evidences demonstrated that it possesses anticancer, hypoglycemic, sedative, antipyretic, diuretic, anti-inflammatory, antiallergic, antiulcer, ovulatepromoting, immunopotentiating, antipapillomas, antirheumatoid arthritic, and multiple antioxidant properties. It is also able to prevent osteoporosis and influence skeleton muscles and the cardiovascular system.

SCIENTIFIC EVIDENCE OF CANCER-INHIBITORY AND CANCER-PREVENTIVE CONSTITUENTS

By *in vitro* and *in vivo* screenings, all extracts prepared from the coixseeds, brans, and hulls have shown interesting anticarcinogenic effect and antitumor-related antioxidant activity.

1. Anticancer agents from coixseeds

Anticancer and anticarcinogenic properties: *In vivo* assay showed that the dehulled coixseeds impeded the early events of colon carcinogenesis caused by azoxymethane.[1] Feeding a diet containing 30% of powdered coixseeds to mice markedly retarded lung tumorigenesis induced by 4-(methyl-nitrosamino)-1-(3-pyridyl)-1-butanone (a tobacco-specific carcinogen) by ~50%.[2] The methanol extract of adlay significantly inhibited Epstein–Barr virus (EBV) early antigen activation against the tumor promoting effect of 12-*O*-tetra-decanoylphorbol-13-acetate (TPA).[3] The extract also exerted suppressive effect on basal and TPA-stimulated COX-2 expression of human lung cancer cells in nude mice, associated with the reduction of PGE_2 levels in serum without the influence of COX-1.[4] In an *in vitro* model, the extract exerted antiproliferative effect against human A549 lung carcinoma and Jurkat acute T-lymphoblast leukemia cells by inducing apoptosis and/or cell-cycle arrest.[2,5] After incubation with serum containing the extract, the suppressive and proapoptotic effects of coixseed extract still occurred in two human hepatoma cell lines (SMMC-7721 and HepG2).[5] A steamed whole seed extract showed antiproliferative activity in KB epidermal carcinoma cells and a roasted whole seed extract (RWSE) had proapoptotic activity in HeLa cervical carcinoma cells. Fractionation of RWSE with ethyl acetate could enhance the antiproliferative effect in HeLa (cervix), HT-29 (colon), and A549 (lung) cancer cell lines. The IC_{50}s were 0.97 µg/mL (7.82 folds of doxorubicin), 2.11 µg/mL (similar to 5FU), and 4.17 µg/mL (similar to vincristine), respectively, and the ethyl acetate fraction encloses high content of carotenoid and tannin.[6] Moreover, the proliferation of KB and HepG2 cell lines was impeded by the butanol fraction and the n-hexane fraction of RWSE, respectively, with IC_{50}s of 5.93 µg/mL (similar to doxorubicin) and 3.57 µg/mL (similar to vincristine). This butanol fraction also exerted a better free-radical scavenging effect than ascorbic acid.[6]

The obvious anti-growth effect of the coixseed extract was further substantiated in mice-burdened H22 hepatoma cells, and the inhibitory rates ranged from 33.31% to 42.46%.[1,7] The acetone extract of coixseeds showed significant inhibitory effect against Ehrlich ascites cancer, ascites sarcoma 180, ascites hepatoma, and U14 cervical carcinoma in mice.[8] Moreover, injection of the adlay extract in a high dose significantly inhibited the growth of sarcoma 180 cells *in vivo* by 46.21%. Concurrently, the expression of VEGF and bFGF were obviously downregulated, and the vascular density in the S180 tissue was lessened. In addition, human periphocyte counts could be promoted by treatment with coixseeds *in vivo*. These results indicated that the antitumor property of adlay seed was associated with both growth suppression and angiogenesis inhibition and marked activation of immunofunctions.[9]

Cancer inhibitors: The major ingredients in coixseed oil were confirmed to be monoglycerides and free fatty acids. From the coixseed extract, α-monolinolein (**1**) was separated and it exerted an inhibitory effect on tumorigenesis *in vivo* through metabolizing to α-linoleic acid.[10] α-Monoglyceride (**1**) at a dose of 50 µg/mouse displayed 60% inhibition against the carcinogenicity of DMBA in mice.[11] The ethanolic extract of dehulled coixseed presented better gastroprotective activity. Coixenolid (**2**), an oily compound derived from acetone extract, was reported to have antitumor effect against Ehrlich ascites tumor in mice.[7] An acidic fraction derived from the extract is composed of four free fatty acids: (1) palmitic acid (16.4%), (2) stearic acid (2.2%), (3) oleic acid (54.7%), and (4) linoleic acid (26.7%), exhibiting marked abilities to hinder the tumor cell growth and to prolong mouse life (163%) in the *in vivo* assay.[12] The proportion of palmitic acid and linoleic acid to oleic acid was found to display a highly positive correlation with inhibition rates of coixseed oil in human T24 bladder cancer cells.[13] The total triglyceride isolated from coixseeds (collected in six places in China) is a bioactive ingredient that in *in vitro* model hindered the proliferation of SPC-A-1 and A549 human lung carcinoma cell lines with IC_{50}s of 1.64–3.01 mg/mL and 2.33–3.24 mg/mL, respectively, though the contents of total triglyceride vary according to different places.[14] Similarly, neutral lipids that comprised glycerides and alkylacyl acetin were refined from the adlay endosperm, which exhibited multiple pharmaceutical benefits for tumor inhibition, immune enhancement, and protection from many diseases.[15]

The antiproliferative effect of adlay polyphenol components was observed in human HepG2 hepatoma cells together with significant cellular antioxidant activity. Especially, the antioxidant capacity of the bound polyphenol was markedly higher than that of free polyphenol.[16] Two phenolic agents, caffeic and chlorogenic acids isolated from the extract, were found to have notable abilities to suppress the growth of AGS gastric carcinoma cells and oxidativation.[17] Four phenolic compounds assigned as N1,N5-di-[(E)-p-coumaroyl]-spermidine (**3**), p-coumaric acid, ferulic acid, and rutin were isolated from the n-butanol fraction of acetone extract of defatted adlay. After treatment with N1,N5-di-[(E)-p-coumaroyl]-spermidine (**3**), the moderate-to-weak suppressive and proapoptotic effects were observed in human HepG2 (liver), MCF-7 (breast), and Caco-2 (colon) cancer cell lines *in vitro* with IC_{50}s of 46.34–92.69 µg/mL.[18]

A water-soluble polysaccharide (containing 1.1% glucose, 30.4% xylose, 32.4% arabinose, 0.4% galactose, and 7.0% uronic acid) was prepared from coixseeds. Daily consumption of food having 4% of this polysaccharide (arabinoxylan) for 6 months could diminish the cancer growth rate from 83% to 64%.[19] A polysaccharide fraction designated as CP-1 was extracted from coix-seeds using an ethanol-subsiding method. In an *in vitro* assay, CP-1 was able to restrain A549 cell proliferation and to elicit apoptosis via activation of an intrinsic mitochondrial pathway.[20] In addition, a bioactive peptide extract (m.w. 200–800) was prepared from coixseeds by enzyme hydrolysis, peptides of which displayed *in vivo* antitumor effect, associated with the inhibition of TNF-α and O species.[21,22]

2. Anticancer agents from adlay hull

The methanolic extract from the hulls of adlay dose-dependently inhibited the proliferation of human U937 histolytic lymphoma and HT-29 colorectal cancer cells concomitant with the induction of apoptosis.[6,23] The extract also displayed significant inhibitory effect on enzymatic oxidation of xanthine and greater capacity of scavenging superoxide anion radicals.[24] The acetone extract of adlay hulls showed potent antimutagenic activity, and six antimutagenic compounds were isolated from the extract, which were identified as *trans*-coniferylaldehyde, *p*-hydroxybenzaldehyde, vanillin, syringaldehyde, sinapaldehyde, and coixol. *trans*-Coniferylaldehyde and sinapaldehyde exerted biological activities in scavenging radicals, repressing TPA-stimulated superoxide anion generation in neutrophil-like leukocytes, and inducing Nrf2/ARE-driven luciferase activity in human HSC-3 oral neoplastic cells. *trans*-Coniferylaldehyde also exerted cytoprotective efficacy against *tert*-Bu-hydroperoxide-induced DNA double-strand breaks in cultured cells via activation of kinase signals, including p38, ERK1/2, JNK, MEK1/2, and MSK1/2. The results suggested that the *trans*-coniferylaldehyde and sinapaldehyde may have a potential for cancer chemoprevention.[25] In addition, the linoleic acid content was 8.09% (wt./wt.) in the hexane fraction of roasted hull of adlay (produced in Thailand).

3. Anticancer agents from adlay bran

Adlay bran and its ethanolic residue could significantly reduce the number of preneoplastic aberrant crypt foci (ACF) in an early stage of colon carcinogenesis in rats.[26] An ethyl acetate fraction derived from adlay bran ethanolic extract inhibited 1,2-dimethylhydrazine-induced preneoplastic lesions in rat colon, associated with downregulation of RAS and Ets2 oncogenes and reduction of COX-2 expression. Ferulic acid might be one of the active compounds in the fraction.[27] Another ethyl acetate-soluble fraction prepared from adlay bran methanolic extract exhibited a stronger antiproliferative effect against human A549 (lung) and HT-29 and Colo 205 (colorectal) carcinoma cells *in vitro*. Five lactams such as coixspirolactams-A (**4**), -B (**5**), -C (**6**), coixlactam (**7**), and methyl dioxindole-3-acetate were isolated by the fraction under bioassay-guided fractionation, and these lactams displayed moderate antiproliferative effect on the A549, HT-29 and Colo 205 cell lines.[28] At each concentration of 50 μM, coixspirolactams-A (**4**), -C (**6**), -D (**8**), -E (**9**), coixlactam (**7**), coixspiroenone (**10**), and ficusal (**11**) selectively and notably inhibited the proliferation of three human mammary cancer cell lines (MCF-7, T-47D, or MDA-MB-231).[28] Both coixspirolactam-D (**8**) and -E (**9**) are C-11 epimers that showed more potency against MCF-7 (ER-positive metastatic/wild p53) and MDA-MB-231 (ER-negative) breast adenocarcinoma cell lines than T-47D (ER-positive ductal/mutant p53) mammary carcinoma cells, where p53 DNA repair effect was found to associate with growth inhibition.[23] The most effective inhibition was achieved by ficusal (**11**) with a antitumor rate of 69% against the MDA-MB-231 cells. These findings implied that the anticancer activity of coixseed brans should be largely related to the presence of lactams and spiroenones in the brans.[29]

4. Kanglaite

Experimental investigations: Kanglaite (KLT) is a modern Chinese herbal drug made from coix-seed oil. In an *in vivo* model, intraperitoneal (i.p.) treatment of tumor-bearing mice with KLT at doses either 6.25 mL/kg or 12.5 mL/kg not only markedly deterred the growth of Lewis lung cancer cells but also remarkably enhanced spleen index and T-cell proliferation. Concurrently, it dose-dependently decreased the level of NF-κB in the nucleus and expression of IκBα, IKK, and EGFR in cytoplasm of tumor cells and significantly elevated IL-2 level in supernatant spleno-cytes.[30] When combined with gefitinib, KLT treatment exerted synergistic effects on anti-growth and antiangiogenesis in the *in vivo* Lewis tumor model.[31] Similarly, a synergistic effect was achieved by a combination of KLT and cyclophosphamide (CP) in human LoVo colon cancer cells, resulting in inhibition of cell proliferation and metastasis via downregulation of OPN (osteopon-tin), MMP-9, and uPA expressions.[32] Over 50% inhibitory rate of KLT was observed in trans-planted MDA-MB-231 breast cancer.[33] More evidences revealed the multimechanisms of KLT in the induction of cancer cell apoptosis, inhibition of angiogenesis, and reversal of multidrug resistance.[34] An *in vivo* model-transplanted human HepG2 hepatoma substantiated that KLT possesses both anti-growth and immunoregulating properties, where the immunoenhancing effect was associated with the induction of NF-κB-mediated gene transcription in CD4+ T-cells and improvement of NK cells.[35]

Clinical investigations: Clinical studies of KLT combined with therapeutic drugs were successfully processed in the treatment of nonsmall cell lung cancer (NSCLC) carried out in three hospitals in Moscow. In China, KLT has been used for the treatment of patients with advanced nonsmall cell lung carcinoma in combination with several different programs, for instance, the GP program (gemcitabine+cisplatin), NP program (vinorelbine+cisplatin), and DO program (docetaxel+oxali-platin).[36–38] KLT injections have also been clinically employed to treat advanced gastric cancer in combination with chemotherapies (such as the DCF regimen: docetaxel+cisplatin+5-fluoro-uracil) and to treat advanced colorectal cancer with the FOLFOX4 regimen (oxaliplatin+calcium folinate+5-fluorouracil).[34,39–41] These combinational treatments augmented the efficacy of chemo-therapies, lessened nausea and vomiting in patients with gastrointestinal toxicity, and improved patients' life quality with good safety. Recently, a phase-II study on the KLT injection was con-ducted in the United States for the treatment of pancreatic carcinoma. Moreover, the antitumor and immunoenhancing effects of KLT were also proved when combined with radiotherapy or surgery. More preclinical and clinical experiences have shown that KLT has a promising effect in the therapies of cancer in lung, breast, liver, esophagus, pancreas, kidney, colon and rectum, ovary, and prostate. KLT also has potential in the remedy of malignant lymphoma and acute leukemia in clinics.[33] Besides, KLT injection showed more therapeutic benefits in its capability of pro-tecting immune functions and diminishing the immune tolerance caused by chemotherapy and carcinoma, leading to improving patients' life quality, markedly relieving cancerous pain, and notably prolonging survival.[42]

FORMULATION IMPROVEMENT

A semipurified supercritical carbon dioxide fluid extract from coixseeds (S5) has been encapsulated by the liposome technique. The prepared S5-liposome (S5L) showed good physicochemical characteristics in pH stability, particle size, dispersibility, and so on, which can keep the content of linoleic acid at higher levels as compared to the free S5. In a human HT-29 colon adenocarcinoma xenografted mice model, 2 weeks' treatment with S5L and S5 achieved the tumor growth inhibition by 54.75% and 48.67%, respectively, at their high doses without toxic reactions.[43] Similarly, the coixseed-oil component has been used to prepare Coix-microemulsions (CMEs) and butyryl galac-tose ester modified coix-microemulsions (But–Gal–CMEs), respectively. The cytotoxicity of CMEs and But–Gal–CMEs was established *in vitro* with human HepG2 hepatoma cells and the IC_{50} values of CMEs and But–Gal–CMEs were 71.23 and 62.55 µg/mL, respectively. Probably due to But–Gal–CMEs that presented better qualities, for example, small particle size, good roundness, and good stability, it exerted better antihepatoma activity than CMEs.[44] These improvements indicated that coixseed has much developing potential in the formulation for the enhancement of its bioactivity and bioavailability.

CONCLUSION AND SUGGESTION

The broad anticancer spectrum of the coixseed has been disclosed by extensive scientific investigations. In the adlay, a kind of seed being used in both food and herb, the bioactive ingredients were confirmed to be a group of monoglycerides, triglycerides, free fatty acids, polyphenolics, and polysaccharides. The anticarcinogenic and anticancer activities of adlay are mostly attributed to several monoglycerides (such as α-monolinolein and coixenolid), free fatty acids (such as oleic acid, α-linoleic acid, and palmitic acid), and triglycerides. Interestingly, if the three free fatty acids in coixseed oil were in certain proportions, the growth inhibition would be positively augmented. The polyphenolics in adlay are mostly in charge of antioxidant effect though they showed certain antitumor and antitumorigenic activities, whereas the adlay polysaccharides are valuable immunostimulators. Considering coixseeds have such medical advantages (including anticancer, hypoglycemic, anti-inflammation, antiallergy, antiulcer, immunopotentiation, and antioxidation), dietary adlay as a functional food supplement should be encouraged for cancer prevention. Normally, daily intake of about 30 grams or a little more of coixseeds over an extended period would bring certain health benefits in body, skin, and body weight. However, people with constipation and pregnant women must reduce the intake of coixseeds because of its diuretic property.

Kanglaite, the first Chinese herbal drug going into clinical trials in the United States, is a promising novel anticancer agent that is patented in China, United States, Canada, Japan, and the European Union. The drug has been on top of the best selling anticancer drugs in China, though the clinical trials of Kanglaite are still being carried out.

REFERENCES

1. Lu, Y. et al., 2011. Hepatocellular carcinoma HepG2 cell apoptosis and caspase-8 and Bcl-2 expression induced by injectable seed extract of Coix lacryma-jobi. *Hepatobiliary & Pancreatic Diseases Intl.* 10: 303–307.
2. Chang, H.C. et al., 2003. Antiproliferative and chemopreventive effects of adlay seed on lung cancer in vitro and in vivo. *J. Agric. Food Chem.* 51: 3656–3660.
3. Shih, C.K. et al., 2004. Effects of adlay on azoxymethane-induced colon carcinogenesis in rats. *Food Chem. Toxicol.* 42: 1339–1347.
4. Hung, W.C. et al., 2003. Methanolic extract of Adlay seed suppresses COX-2 expression of human lung cancer cells via inhibition of gene transcription. *J. Agric. Food Chem.* 51: 7333–7337.
5. Yao, G.H. et al., 2009. Coix lacryma-jobi L. varma-yuan induces apoptosis of Jurkat cell line in acute T lymphoblast leukemia and its mechanism. *Zhongguo Shiyan Xueyexue Zazhi* 17: 879–882.
6. Manosroi, A. et al., (a) 2016. Potent in vitro anti-proliferative, apoptotic and anti-oxidative activities of semi-purified Job's tears (Coix lachryma-jobi Linn.) extracts from different preparation methods on 5 human cancer cell lines. *J. Ethnopharmacol.* 187: 281–292; (b) 2016. In vitro anticancer activities of Job's tears (Coix lachryma-jobi Linn.) extracts on human colon adenocarcinoma. *Saudi J. Biol. Sci.* 23: 248–256.
7. Gong, X.J. et al., 2012. Inhibition on H22 allografts, HepG2 and SMMC-7721 human hepatoma cells of adlay seed extracts. *Asian J. Chem.* 24: 1041–1044.
8. Ukita, T. et al., 1961. Studies on the antitumor component in the seeds of Coix lachryma-jobi variety ma-yuen. I. Isolation and antitumor activity of coixenolide. *Chem. Pharm. Bull.* 9: 43.

9. Kong, Q.Z. et al., 2003. Study on inhibiting angiogenesis in mice S180 by injections of three traditional Chinese herbs. *Zhongguo Yiyuan Yaoxue Zazhi* 23: 646–648.

10. Tokuda, M. et al., 1990. Inhibitory effects on Epstein-Barr virus activation and antitumor promoting activities of Coix seed. *Planta Med.* 56: 653–654.

11. Matsumoto, T. et al., 1990. α-Monolinolein as inhibitor against carcinogen promoters. *Jpn. Kokai Tokkyo Koho* JP 89-60535, 19890313.

12. Numata, M. et al., 1994. Antitumor components isolated from the Chinese herbal medicine Coix lachryma-jobi. *Planta Med.* 60: 356–359.

13. Xi, X.J. et al., 2016. Assessment of the genetic diversity of different Job's tears (Coix lacryma-jobi L.) accessions and the active composition and anticancer effect of its seed oil. *PLoS One* 11: e0153269.

14. Liu, C.Y. et al., 2015. Correlation analysis between content and anti-lung cancer activity of active ingredients in Coicis Semen from different areas. *Zhongguo Shiyan Fangjixue Zazhi* 21: 7–10.

15. Li, D.P. et al., 1994. Antitumor neutral lipids from endosperm of Job's tears and pharmaceuticals including them. European Patent Application EP 93-307278.

16. Wang, L.F. et al., 2013. Cytotoxicity and anti-proliferation effect on HepG2 cells and cellular antioxidant activity (CAA) of adlay polyphenols. *Zhongguo Nongye Kexue* (Beijing, China) 46: 2990–3002.

17. Chung, C.P. et al., 2011. Gastroprotective activities of Adlay (Coix lacryma-jobi L. var. ma-yuen Stapf) on the growth of the stomach cancer AGS cell line and indomethacin-induced gastric ulcers. *J. Agricult. Food Chem.* 59: 6025–6033.

18. Chen, C. et al., 2016. Identification and antitumour activities of phenolic compounds isolated from defatted adlay (Coix lacryma-jobi L. var. ma-yuen Stapf) seed meal. *J. Funct. Foods* 26: 394–405.

19. Aoe, S. et al., 1993. Colon cancer inhibitors containing water-soluble polysaccharides. Japanese Kokai Tokkyo Koho JP 91-170306, 19910617.

20. Lu, X.L. et al., 2013. A polysaccharide fraction of adlay seed (Coix lacryma-jobi L.) induces apoptosis in human non-small cell lung cancer A549 cells. *Biochem. Biophys. Res. Commun.* 430: 846–851.

21. Zou, Y.D. et al., 2002. Enzymic hydrolysis for manufacture of Coix lacryma-jobi seed peptide. Faming Zhuanli Shenqing Gongkai Shuomingshu CN 1344806 A 20020417.

22. Funatsu, I. et al., 2000. Manufacture of bioactive peptide-containing products derived from *Coix lacryma-jobi ma-yuen* and their uses. Japanese Kokai Tokkyo Koho JP 2000256394 A 20000919.

23. Chiang, W.C. et al., Novel lactams from adlay seeds and uses thereof for treating breast cancer. United States Patent Applications Publication US 20130197050 A1 20130801.

24. Kuo, C.C. et al., 2001. Antagonism of free-radical-induced damage of adlay seed and its anti-proliferative effect in human histolytic lymphoma U937 monocytic cells. *J. Agricul. Food Chem.* 49: 1564–1570.

25. Chen, H.H. et al., 2011. Antimutagenic constituents of adlay (Coix lacryma-jobi L. var. ma-yuen Stapf) with potential cancer chemopreventive activity. *J. Agricult. Food Chem.* 59: 6444–6452.

26. Li, S.C. et al., 2011. Effects of adlay bran and its ethanolic extract and residue on preneoplastic lesions of the colon in rats. *J. Sci. Food Agricult.* 91: 547–552.

27. Chung, C.P. et al., 2011. Ethyl acetate fraction of adlay bran ethanolic extract inhibits oncogene expression and suppresses DMH-induced preneoplastic lesions of the colon in F344 rats through an anti-inflammatory pathway. *J. Agricult. Food Chem.* 58: 7616–7623.

28. Lee, M.Y. et al., 2008. Isolation and characterization of new lactam compounds that inhibit lung and colon cancer cells from adlay (Coix lacryma-jobi L. var. ma-yuen Stapf) bran. *Food Chem. Toxicol.* 46: 1933–1939.

29. Chung, C.P. et al., 2011. Antiproliferative lactams and spiroenone from adlay bran in human breast cancer cell lines. *J. Agricult. Food Chem* 59: 1185–1194.

30. Pan, P. et al., 2012. Antitumor activity and immunomodulatory effects of the intraperitoneal administration of Kanglaite in vivo in Lewis lung carcinoma. *J. Ethnopharmacol.* 143: 680–685.

31. Shen, F.Q. et al., 2013. The effect of Kanglaite Injection in combination with gefitinib on angiogenesis in mice with Lewis lung cancer. *Zhongliu* 33: 1047–1053.

32. Wang, F. et al., 2011. Effect of Kanglaite injection on plasma osteopontin of human colon carcinoma liver metastasis model in nude mice. *Chin. Clin. Oncol.* 16: 282–289.

33. Home page of Zhejiang Kanglaite Pharmaceutical, CO., LTD. An introduction to Kanglaite injection, as well as basic studies and clinical studies. www.kanglaite.com and www.caca.org.cn

34. Zhan, Y.P. et al., 2012. Clinical safety and efficacy of Kanglaite® (Coix Seed Oil) injection combined with chemotherapy in treating patients with gastric cancer. *Asian Pac. J. Cancer Prev.* 13:5319–5321.

35. Huang, X.L. et al., 2014. Kanglaite stimulates anticancer immune responses and inhibits HepG2 cell transplantation-induced tumor growth. *Mol. Med. Reports* 10: 2153–2159.

36. Liang, S.M. et al., 2014. Kanglaite combined with GP for the treatment of 25 cases of senile non-small cell lung carcinoma. *Zhongyi Xuebao* 29: 11–12.
37. He, A.B. et al., 2012. Kanglaite injection combined with docetaxel and oxaliplatin in treatment of advanced NSCLC. *Shiyong Zhongliu Zazhi* 27: 653–655.
38. Yan, X.L. et al., 2013. Meta-analysis of kanglaite injection combined with NP regimen chemotherapy for advanced non-small cell lung cancer. *Zhongguo Quanke Yixue* 16: 431–435.
39. Shen, W.X. et al., 2013. A randomized controlled study on kanglaite combined with docetaxel, cisplatin, 5-fluorouracil in the treatment of patients with advanced gastric cancer. *Zhongguo Xueye Liubianxue Zazhi* 23: 451–453.
40. Wang, X.Q. et al., 2014. Clinical observation on advanced colorectal cancer treated with Kanglaite injection combined with FOLFOX4. *Liaoning Zhongyiyao Daxue Xuebao* 16: 175–177.
41. Yin, D. et al., 2012. Role of the inhibition mediated by kanglaite and molecular mechanism on metastasis of human colon cancer cells. *Weichangbingxue He Ganbingxue Zazhi* 21: 1005–1010.
42. Deng, X.N. et al., 2014. Regulatory effect of Kanglaite injection on immune function in patients with non-small cell lung cancer treated with chemotherapy. *Xiandai Zhongxiyi Jiehe Zazhi* 23: 3767–3769, 3773.
43. Sainakham, M. et al., 2016. Potent in vivo anticancer activity and stability of liposomes encapsulated with semi-purified Job's tear (Coix lacryma-jobi Linn.) extracts on human colon adenocarcinoma (HT-29) xenografted mice. *Drug Delivery* 23(9): 3399–3407.
44. Liu, M.J. et al., 2015. Preparation of butyryl galactose ester-modified Coix component microemulsions and their anticancer activity in vitro. *Zhongcaoyao* 46(18): 2696–2702.

25. BARLEY

Orge   Gerste   Cebada

大麥   大麦   보리

Hordeum vulgare

Gramineae

Barley is the fourth most important cereal crop in the world today. It is the seed of a grassy plant *Hordeum vulgare*, which is one of the traditional grains used as food, malting, and brewing sources. It is a rich source of essential nutrients such as protein, dietary fiber, B vitamins (niacin and vitamin B6), and dietary minerals (manganese and phosphorus). Barley is also used in folk remedies in China and other areas. Traditionally, powdered and parched barley grains are used in the form of gruel for treatment of painful and atonic dyspepsia. Barley and honey mixed with boiling water is prescribed for bronchial coughs, and barley and Arabic gum mixed in hot water are used for soothing irritations of the bladder and urinary passage. Barley malt was reported to enhance digestion, hypoglycemia, and mammary secretion. Its sprout juice showed antiulcerative and antiplatelet aggregation effects.

Scientific Evidence of Cancer-Inhibitory and Cancer-Preventive Components

In folk remedy, barley and its seed meal are used for the treatment of some esophageal, gastrointestinal, uterus, and lung carcinomas, other excrescences, and warts. The anticancer and anticarcinogenic effect-related approaches have provided a lot of important scientific evidences.

1. Phenolics

Total phenolics from four varieties of dehulled highland barley in *in vitro* assays showed excellent antioxidant activities and potent antiproliferative activity toward HepG2 human liver cancer cells, wherein its bound phenolics contributed not only significant content in the total phenolics but also prominent antioxidant and anticancer activities in the tests.[1] The results disclosed that the phenolics of highland barleys may serve as ingredients for health and functional foods. Tocotrienols are highly enriched in barley and other food sources such as palm oil, rice bran, oat, wheat germ, and rye, which are members of the vitamin E family. In biological studies, tocotrienols displayed potent anticarcinogenic, antioxidant, and anti-inflammatory properties. Of them, γ-tocotrienol (**1**) showed marked inhibitory effect against the proliferation of human SGC-7901 gastric adenocarcinoma cells. At a concentration of 60 μmol/L, it could cause DNA damage, cell-cycle arrest at the G0/G1-phase, and apoptosis in SGC-7901 cells. The apoptotic death induced by γ-tocotrienol was mediated by a mitochondria-dependent pathway, including activation of caspases-9 and -3.[2,3] Protocatechualdehyde (**2**, PCA), an important compound found in barley and green cavendish bananas and grapevine leaves, was able to diminish the viability of human HCT116 and SW480 (colon), MCF-7 and MDA-MB-231 (breast), and HepG2 (liver) cancer cell lines in a dose-dependent manner. The antigrowth and proapoptotic effects of PCA (**2**) in the colon cancer cells were mediated by the suppression of HDAC2-mediated cyclin-D1 and upregulation of ATF3 expression via ERK1/2 and p38-mediated transcriptional activation,[4,5] whereas the stimulation of cell-growth arrest and apoptosis in human breast cancer cells was associated with the downregulation of β-catenin expression through GSK3β and NF-κB-mediated proteosomal degradation and decrease of β-catenin-independent cyclin-D1.[6] PCA (2) also has an ability to scavenge radicals and intracellular ROS. In the oxidative cell death and apoptosis assay, PCA treatment attenuated H_2O_2-induced normal cell death and apoptotic death, suggesting that barley may exert anticarcinogenic effect by blocking H_2O_2-induced oxidative DNA damage and inducing cell death and apoptosis.[7] Similarly, PCA (2) enhanced apoptosis in human PC-9 nonsmall cell lung cancer cells by upregulation of growth arrest and DNA damage-inducible genes (GADD45 and GADD153) together with the activation of p21 and p27 and inhibition of Bcl-2, cyclin D1, CDK2, CDK4, and CDK6 genes.[8] By altering the expression of these genes, PCA (2) plays a role in the anticancer and anticarcinogenic activities. Therefore, it is now known that PCA (2) has a positive value in cancer prevention and/or treatment.

2. Polysaccharides

A prepared barley glucan was reported to have antitumor activity against sarcoma 180 in mice. A β-D-glucan purified from barley showed the inhibitory effect against endocrine-sensitive MCF-7 and endocrine-resistant LCC9 and LY2 breast cancer cell lines when dissolved in DMSO but not in water. The activities on LCC9 and LY2 cells (IC_{50}s 4.6 and 24.2 μg/mL, respectively) were much stronger than on MCF-7 cells (IC_{50}−164 μg/mL), where the gene expressions in response to 24-h treatment with 10 or 50 μg/mL β-D-glucan were different between MCF-7 and LCC9 cells, that is, β-D-glucan increased RASSF1 expression in MCF-7 cells and IGFBP-3, CTNNB1, and ERα transcript expression in LCC9 cells. In addition, the β-D-glucan was inactive to MDA-MB-231 triple negative breast cancer cells and MCF-10A normal breast epithelial cells.[9] The data suggested that the barley β-D-glucan may be useful for inhibiting endocrine-resistant breast cancer-cell proliferation.[9] After oral administration, the β-1,3-glucans were taken up by macrophages that would transport them to bone marrow, spleen, and lymph nodes. Within the bone marrow, the macrophages could degrade the large β-1,3-glucans into smaller soluble β-1,3-glucan fragments that were taken up by CR3 (an inactivated C3b receptor) of marginated granulocytes. These granulocytes with CR3-bound β-1,3-glucan-fluorescein were able to kill iC3b-opsonized tumor cells followed by their recruitment to a site of complement activation resembling a tumor coated with monoclonal antibodies (mAb).[10,11] When the glucan was modified to be its γ-propoxysulfo-derivative, the tumor-suppressive activity would be markedly potentiated.[12] Moreover, the antitumor activity of mAb could be potentiated by β-1,3- and 1,4-glucans of barley, effect of which led to increasing tumor regression and the tested mouse survival.[10,11]

BP-1 was a water-soluble polysaccharide (6.7×10^4 Da) extracted from highland barley (*H. vulgare*), composed of glucose, xylose, arabinose, and rhamnose with a relative molar ratio of 8.82:1.92:1.50:1.00. At 48.18 μg/mL for 48 h, BP-1 exerted a time- and dose-dependent antiproliferative effect against HT-29 human colon cancer cells concomitant with the induction of HT-29 apoptosis via ROS-JNK and NF-κB-mediated caspase pathways, such as enhancing c-Jun N-terminal kinase (JNK) phosphorylation and ROS formation, inhibiting NF-κB translocation from the cytoplasm into the nucleus, and activating caspase-8 and caspase-9.[13]

Barley grain from brewing contains rich insoluble fiber such as lignin and cellulose. Feeding the dietary-spent barley grain after brewing to rats in a long-term experiment resulted in significantly more protection against dimethylhydrazine (DMH)-induced intestinal cancer than wheat bran and barley bran, both of which are rich in soluble fiber (β-glucan and arabinoxylan).[14–16] However, pure cellulose and outer-layer barley bran were only moderately effective in the cancer prevention. The dietary insoluble fiber-rich barley grain could also significantly reduce plasma cholesterol concentration (down 17%) relative to wheat bran.[17–19]

3. Peptides

Polypeptide components prepared from barley presented strong tumor-inhibiting activity against Ehrlich ascites tumor and sarcoma 180 in mice.[17] A crude and partially purified lunasin (4.8 kDa

with unique 43 amino acid) from the barley seeds showed the suppressive effect on colony formation in stably *ras*-transfected mouse fibroblast cells induced by IPTG, and had an inhibitory effect
against histone acetylation in mouse NIH 3T3 fibroblast cells and human MCF-7 breast neoplastic
cells, indicating that the lunasin is a chemopreventive peptide.[18–20] As lunasin is prevalent in barley,
the consumption of barley can play an important role in cancer prevention in barley consuming
populations.

4. Ribosome-inactivating protein

Barley endosperm contains three types of ribosome-inactivating proteins (RIP) with a single polypeptide chain (30 kDa), which can be used to make immunotoxin. When the RIP was conjugated
to mAb by succinimidyl-3-(2-pyridyldithio) propionate (SPDP) or cystamine-EDAC methods, the
cross-linked hybrids showed selective toxicity to melanoma cells *in vitro* in a dose-dependent manner.[21]
The barley RIP-II constructed with antitransferrin receptor-based immunotoxins also demonstrated
comparable cytotoxicity against a human colon tumor cell line.[22]

5. Anticancer potential of germanium-enriched barley seeds

Germanium-enriched barley seeds (GEBS) at a high dosage could obviously suppress the growth of
sarcoma 180 in mice with an inhibition rate of 68.52% and potentiated the immune activity such as
increase in thymus and spleen indexes. GEBS also markedly impede the growth of mouse sarcoma
180 cells and myeloma SP-2 cells *in vitro* in a dose-dependent manner.[23]

6. Anticancer potential of germinated barley foodstuff

Germinated barley foodstuff (GBF) exhibited the potencies to attenuate mucosal inflammation and
to increase fecal butyrate production in colitis. Prebiotic treatment with the GBF could effectively
prevent colitis-related dysplasia and inflammatory change by modulating the intestinal environment, effect of which strongly related to the reduction of incidence and progression of colorectal
cancer. In the treatment, the number of ACF and β-catenin formations were markedly decreased
in the colonic mucosa, the production of slc5a8 as a tumor suppressor gene and the activity of
β-glucosidase were augmented, and the expressions of toll-like receptor-4 and cyclooxygenase-2
mRNA were reduced along with significantly lowered cecal content, leading to the diminishment of
preneoplastic lesions in a rat carcinogenic model induced by azoxymethane.[24–26] These approaches
revealed that the GBF may be useful for the treatment and prevention of colorectal carcinoma without causing the adverse effects seen in either anticancer drugs or anti-inflammatory drugs; however,
a more detailed exploration is needed.

7. Barley-PSDR

Barley-Shochu distillation is a traditional Japanese liquor distilled from fermented barley with
Saccharomyces cerevisiae. Barley-PSDR is a residual powder from barley-Shochu distillation remnants, which contains antioxidative agents such as polyphenols. Orally treated orthotopic xenograft mice-implanted HepG2 hepatoma cells with barley-PSDR (2250 mg/kg, per day) for 21 days
remarkably obstructed the tumorigenesis and prolonged survival without side effects, implying that
the barley-PSDR has both therapeutic and preventive potential on hepatocellular carcinoma.[27]

8. Anticancer activity of young barley leaves

In recent years, young barley leaves have been recommended as a dietary supplement because of
their anticancer phytochemicals and vitamin and mineral content. Dietary administration of 0.3%
young barley extract to female rats for 14 weeks moderately restrained *N*-methyl-*N*-nitrosourea-
induced mammary carcinogenesis. Incubation with the extract significantly lessened the survival
of MCF-7 human breast cancer cells *in vitro*.[28] The extract also elicited the antiproliferative and
proapoptotic effects on human B-lineage leukemia/lymphoma cell lines (Nalm-6 and BJAB) and
disrupted cell-cycle progression in the BJAB cells.[29] It inhibited TNF-α release from mononuclear

cells in human THP-1 monocyte cells. Moreover, flavone-c-glycosides, saponarin, and lutonarin have been found from young green barley leaves, which are responsible for antioxidant and anti-inflammatory activities.[29]

CONCLUSION AND SUGGESTION

The summarized laboratory experiments provided scientific evidences for barley possessing anti-carcinogenic, antioxidant, anti-inflammatory, and immunomodulating properties. Compared to the small molecules in barley, the macromolecules (such as polysaccharides, peptides, and RIP) appeared to play a more important role in cancer inhibition and prevention, especially for protection of colon, liver, and breast. Even the barley products (such as germinated barley and fermented barley), by-products (brewed barley grain), and barley leaves showed value in antioxidation and cancer prevention. Hence, these scientific data are attractive for the improvement of our dietary menu by the use of barley.

REFERENCES

1. Zhu, Y. et al., 2015. Phenolics content, antioxidant and antiproliferative activities of dehulled highland barley (Hordeum vulgare L.). *J. Functional Foods* 19 (Part-A), 439–450.
2. Sun, W.G. et al., 2009. γ-Tocotrienol induces mitochondria-mediated apoptosis in human gastric adenocarcinoma SGC-7901 cells. *J. Nutr. Biochem.* 20: 276–284.
3. Ahsan, H. et al., 2014. Pharmacological potential of tocotrienols: A review. *Nutr. Metabol.* 11: 52/1–52/44.
4. Jeong, J.B. et al., 2013. Protocatechualdehyde possesses anticancer activity through downregulating cyclin D1 and HDAC2 in human colorectal cancer cells. *Biochem. Biophys. Res. Commun.* 430: 381–386.
5. Lee, J.R. et al., 2014. The contribution of activating transcription factor 3 to apoptosis of human colorectal cancer cells by protocatechualdehyde, a naturally occurring phenolic compound. *Archiv. Biochem. Biophys.* 564: 203–210.
6. Choi, J. et al., 2014. Anticancer activity of protocatechualdehyde in human breast cancer cells. *J. Med. Food* 17: 842–848.
7. Jeong, J.B. et al., 2009. 3,4-dihydroxybenzaldehyde purified from the barley seeds (Hordeum vulgare) inhibits oxidative DNA damage and apoptosis via its antioxidant activity. *Phytomed.* 16: 85–94.
8. Patra, S. et al., 2013. Protocatechualdehyde induces apoptosis in human non-small-cell lung cancer cells by up-regulation of growth arrest and DNA damage inducible (GADD) genes. *Mol. Biol.* 2: 2, 9 pp.
9. Jafaar, Z.M.T. et al., 2014. β-D-glucan inhibits endocrine-resistant breast cancer cell proliferation and alters gene expression. *Int. J. Oncol.* 44: 1365–1375.
10. Hong, F. et al., 2004. Mechanism by which orally administered beta-1,3-glucans enhance the tumoricidal activity of antitumor monoclonal antibodies in murine tumor models. *J. Immunol.* 173: 797–806.
11. Na, C.L. et al., 2012. Advances in character and function of barley (1,3-1,4) β-glucan. *Mailei Zuowu Xuebao* 32: 579–584.
12. Hensel, A. et al., 1988. Antitumor polysaccharides. Antitumor activity of barley glucan and semisynthetic derivatives thereof. *Deutsche Apotheker Zeitung* 128: 1305–1309.
13. Cheng, D. et al., 2016. Inhibitory effect on HT-29 colon cancer cells of a water-soluble polysaccharide obtained from highland barley. *Int. J. Biol. Macromol.* 92: 88–95.
14. McIntosh, G.H. et al., 1993. Insoluble dietary fiber-rich fractions from barley protects rats from intestinal cancers. *Spec. Publ. R. Soc. Chem.* 123 (Food and Cancer Prevention: Chemical and Biological Aspects), 362–363.
15. McIntosh, G.H. et al., 1993. The potential of an insoluble dietary fiber-rich source from barley to protect from DMH-induced intestinal tumors in rats. *Nutr. Cancer* 19: 213–221.
16. Holtekjolen, A.K. et al., 2006. Contents of starch and non-starch polysaccharides in barley varieties of different origin. *Food Chem.* 94: 348–348.
17. Yoshizumi, H. et al., 1985. Polypeptide carcinostatic agent. US 81-319755, 19811109.
18. Jeong, H.J. et al., 2002. Barley lunasin suppresses ras-induced colony formation and inhibits core histone acetylation in mammalian cells. *J. Agricul. Food Chem.* 50: 5903–5908.

19. Jeong, H.J. et al., 2010. Lunasin is prevalent in barley and is bioavailable and bioactive in in vivo and in vitro studies. *Nutr. Cancer* 62: 1113–1119.

20. Jeong, J.B. et al., 2007. Cancer-preventive peptide lunasin from Solanum nigrum L. inhibits acetylation of core histones H3 and H4 and phosphorylation of retinoblastoma protein (Rb). *J. Agricul. Food Chem.* 55: 10707–10713.

21. Ebert, R.F. et al., Immunotoxin construction with a ribosome-inactivating protein from barley. *Bioconjugate Chem.* 1: 331–336.

22. Ovadia, M. et al., 1990. An antimelanoma-barley ribosome inactivating protein conjugate is cytotoxic to melanoma cells in vitro. *Anticancer Res.* 10: 671–675.

23. Du, R. et al., 2010. In vitro antitumor effect of germanium-rich barley seedling. *Shipin Kexue* (Beijing, China) 31: 371–374.

24. Komiyama, Y. et al., 2011. Prebiotic treatment in experimental colitis reduces the risk of colitic cancer. *J. Gastroenterol. Hepatol.* 26: 1298–1308.

25. Fukuda, M. et al., 2011. Prebiotic treatment reduced preneoplastic lesions through the downregulation of toll like receptor 4 in a chemo-induced carcinogenic model. *J. Clin. Biochem. Nutr.* 49: 57–61.

26. Kanauchi, O. et al., 2008. Modulation of intestinal environment by prebiotic germinated barley food-stuff prevents chemo-induced colonic carcinogenesis in rats. *Oncol. Reports* 20: 793–801.

27. Ohgidani, M. et al., 2012. Anticancer effects of residual powder from barley-Shochu distillation remnants against the orthotopic xenograft mouse models of hepatocellular carcinoma in vivo. *Biol. Pharm. Bull.* 35: 984–987.

28. Kubatka, P. et al., 2016. Young barley indicates antitumor effects in experimental breast cancer in vivo and in vitro. *Nutr. Cancer* 68: 611–621.

29. Robles-Escajeda, E. et al., 2013. Searching in mother nature for anticancer activity: Anti-proliferative and pro-apoptotic effect elicited by green barley on leukemia/lymphoma cells. *PLoS One.* 8: e73508.

26. BUCKWHEAT

Sarrasin   Buchweizen   Alforfón

蕎麥 ソバ 메밀

Fagopyrum esculentum, F. tataricum

Polygonaceae

1. R = –H
2. R = –beta-D-glucosyl(6-1)-beta-D-glucose
3. R = –beta-D-glucose

4

Common and tartary buckwheats are two varieties of pseudocereal from the fruit seeds of two Fagopyrum plants (*F. esculentum* and *F. tataricum*, respectively), which are excellent edible crops that have been widely used as a daily diet and traditional medicine for a long time. Today, buckwheat is widely consumed in numerous regions, such as Russia, Poland, China, Japan, the United States, Canada, and Europe. Buckwheat is a highly nutritious gluten-free food, which provides a rich source of dietary fiber, B vitamins, magnesium, manganese, and phosphorus but lacks vitamin C. A broad range of health benefits are shown by buckwheat, including antioxidant, anticancer, anti-inflammatory, antidiabetic, hypocholesterolemic, hypotensive, and neuroprotective properties.[1] Therefore, more and more attention has been paid in recent years for consumption of buckwheat as a raw material to prepare many types of food products, such as bread, pancakes, crepes, noodles, porridge, and tea.

SCIENTIFIC EVIDENCE OF CANCER-INHIBITORY AND CANCER-PREVENTIVE CONSTITUENTS

The investigations of phytochemical biology revealed that the presence of bioactive components such as flavonoids, phenylpropanoids, fagopyritols, and proteins may be responsible for the health beneficial effects of buckwheat and buckwheat-enriched products.[2] Among the variety of biologically active components, flavonoids are the most important substances in buckwheat to provide body protective functions.

1. Flavonoids

The natural polyphenolic flavonoids are widely distributed in the plant kingdom. They are commonly obtained from seeds, bran, flowers, leaves, and roots of *F. esculentum* and *F. tataricum*. Because of having more abundance in flavonoids such as rutin (**1**) and quercetin (**2**), tartary buckwheat has gained more attention in experimental studies for the antioxidative, hypoglycemic, hypolipemic, and anticarcinogenic activities compared to common buckwheat. HPLC analysis of the flavonoid extract from *F. tataricum* seeds exhibited the contents of rutin (**1**) and quercetin (**2**) as 1.65% and 60.12%, respectively.[3] The flavonoids from buckwheat are marked antioxidants that effectively scavenge free radicals that are responsible for as much as 90% of all human diseases, including carcinogenesis.[4] The flavonoid extract from the bran of tartary buckwheat (such as Chongqing and Sichuan cultivars) showed better oxygen radical absorbance capacity (ORAC).[5]

The NF-κB p65 nuclear factor leads to chronic inflammation and progression of lung cancer. NF-κB expression could be hindered by buckwheat flavonoids, especially rutin (1), in lung cancer cells.[6] The tartary buckwheat flavonoid extract *in vitro* obviously inhibited the proliferation of human HL-60 acute myelogenous leukemia, MGC 80-3 gastric cancer, EC9706 esophageal cancer, and HepG2 hepatoma cell lines,[4,7,8] antiproliferative activities of which were mostly contributed by their abilities in promoting apoptosis of the tumor cells and/or inducing cell cycle such as G2/M cell arrest in EC9706 and HepG2 cells.[3,9] The apoptotic mechanisms were revealed to associate with the (1) blockage of intranuclear NF-κB-DNA-binding activity, release of mitochondrial cytochrome c into cytosol, lessening of Fas expression on the cell surface, and promotion of annexin V-binding capacity and caspase 3 activation in HL-60 cells[10,11] and (2) inhibition of Bcl-2 expression and upexpression of Bax and reactive oxygen in EC9706 cells.[3] Among the three flavonoids, rutin (1), quercetin (2), and isoquercetin (3) isolated from tartary buckwheat seeds and bran, quercetin (2) was the strongest antioxidant and it showed the highest cytotoxic effects against the HepG2 cells. Quercetin (2)-induced cell apoptosis and G2/M cell arrest in HepG2 cells were mediated by upregulation of p53 and p21, downregulation of cyclin-D1, Cdk2, and Cdk7, and generation of ROS in the cells.[9] By diminution of ERK, MKK4, JNK, MKK3, and p38 phosphorylation, rutin (1) hampered UVB-induced COX-2 expression at both transcriptional and protein levels in JB6 P+ mouse epidermal cells, leading them to play a pivotal role in UVB-mediated skin carcinogenesis and skin inflammation.[12] In an *in vitro* assay, isoquercetin (3) time- and dose-dependently hindered the viability of human SGC-7901 gastric carcinoma cells and impeded the cell migration together with the induction of cell apoptosis and G2/M cell-cycle arrest. Its anti-growth rate was ≥ 35.92% at 100 µmol/L concentration for 48 h.[13,14] Likewise, red clover flavones (RCFGB) extracted from golden buckwheat (*F. dibotrys*) was found to have a capacity to deter the migration of human SGC7901 gastric cancer cells in both *in vitro* and *in vivo* models. The antimigratory effect on the SGC7901 cells should be correlated to significantly downregulating IL-6 protein expression level in the cells.[14]

In the production of tartary buckwheat sprouts, the germinating process may promote the nutritional and bioactive values of flavonoids. Ethanolic extract of buckwheat sprouts is rich in flavonoids and the ratio of rutin–quercetin is 0.92:1 in the ethanol extract from tartary buckwheat sprouts germinated for 3 days.[15,16] The extract in the *in vitro* tests showed obvious suppressive effect on the growth of human breast and lung carcinoma cell lines. An ethyl acetate fraction of the buckwheat sprout ethanol extract at 1.0 mg/mL concentration showed greater cytotoxic effects against human A549 (lung), AGS (stomach), MCF-7 (breast), Hep3B (liver), and Colo 205 (colon) neoplastic cell lines with inhibitory rates of 70.3%, 94.8%, 79.6%, 82.3%, and 73.2%, respectively.[15–17] The antimutagenic activity was also observed in the *in vitro* experiments, wherein an ethyl acetate fraction from the ethanol extract exhibited greater suppressive effect against the mutagenesis.[18]

2. Phenylpropanoid glycosides

The root of tartary buckwheat is a folk medicine used in China for its antioxidant, hypotensive, hypoglycemic, hypolipidemic, and antitumor properties. From an ethyl acetate fraction from the roots, eight phenylpropanoid glycosides designated as tatarisides-A–G and diboside-A were separated. Most of the eight compounds showed moderate-to-weak suppressive effect against the four *in vitro* tested human carcinoma cell lines. Of them, tatariside-C (4) was the most active compound with IC_{50}s of 6.44–7.49 µg/mL against the A549 (lung), HCT-116 (colon), ZR-75-30 (breast), and HL-60 (leukemic) cancer cell lines. Tatarisides-B, -F, and -G selectively hindered the growth of ZR-75-30 and HL-60 cell lines with IC_{50}s ranging from 5.09–6.33 µg/mL. The most potent inhibitory effect was exerted by tatariside-C (4) on A549 cells (IC_{50} of 2.83 µg/mL) and by diboside-A on HL-60 cells (IC_{50} of 4.61 µg/mL).[19] In both *in vitro* and *in vivo* models, tatariside-F showed notable antitumor effect against H22 hepatoma cells, and it also exhibited protective effects against cyclophosphamide-induced liver damage in cotreatment.[20] These findings revealed the potential of buckwheat roots in cancer inhibition, showing the usage of buckwheat waste portion.

3. Buckwheat trypsin inhibitors

Protease inhibitors are broadly distributed in nature to play an important role in animals, plants, and microorganisms to maintain the balance of proteolytic enzymes. A buckwheat protease inhibitor labeled as BWI-1 and a buckwheat protease inhibitor assigned as BWI-2a prominently hindered the growth of T-acute lymphoblastic leukemia (T-ALL) cell lines, such as Jurkat and CCRF–CEM in the *in vitro* test system.[21] Tartary buckwheat trypsin inhibitor (TBTI) and buckwheat trypsin inhibitor (BTI) are serine protease inhibitors belonging to members of the potato inhibitor I family similar to BWI-1. TBTI showed obvious antiproliferative effect against human HL-60 acute myelogenous leukemia cells in a dose- and time-dependent manner, and showed less effect on normal human peripheral blood mononuclear cells (PBMCs) with IC_{50}s of 0.29 and 1.01 mg/mL, respectively.[22] Modern recombinant techniques have been used to produce recombinant buckwheat trypsin inhibitor (rBTI). The yielded rBTIs have been extensively evaluated in a variety of cancer cell lines. The results disclosed that the rBTIs were effective in suppressing the proliferation of many types of carcinoma cell lines such as EC9706 (esophagus), MCF-7 (breast), HeLa (cervix), H22, and HepG2 (liver) cancer cells, HL-60 and K562 leukemia, and IM-9 B-lymphoblastoid cells, and in inducting apoptosis and/or cell-cycle arrest.[23–32] The *in vivo* anticancer activity of rBTI was confirmed in mouse model-implanted H22 hepatoma.[33] All the results from the experimental studies suggested that BTI may have a potential to be developed as a therapeutic drug for the treatment of various carcinomas.

4. Tatary buckwheat lectin

A tatary buckwheat lectin (TBL) protein with a molecular mass of 65 kDa was obtained from the fractionation of tartary buckwheat seeds; it is stable in both acid and alkali conditions and is active at up to 60°C. The dose-dependent growth inhibition of TBL was achieved in human DLD-1, HCT-116, and SW480 colon cancer cell lines *in vitro* but not in normal cells and other types of tested cancer cell lines.[34] More evidences indicated that TBL acted as a type-II ribosome-inactivating protein (II-RIP) with a *N*-glycosidase activity. The antiproliferative activity of TBL on the HCT-116 colon cancer cells might be mediated by repressing miRNA expressions (e.g., miR-135a and b) and attaching to HCT-116 cell surface via competing with the galectin-3 receptor on the cell membrane in a dose- and time-dependent manner.[35,36] At a dose range between 12.5 and 100 µg/mL, TBL treatment dose-dependently prompted the apoptosis of human U937 leukemia cells *in vitro*.[35] In addition, tartary buckwheat and the TBL were also able to exert immunopotentiating activity, leading to promoting maturation and proliferation of peripheral blood dendritic cells and immune responses in humans to help in cancer prevention.[35]

5. Proteins and peptides

An antitumor protein fraction termed TBWSP31 was isolated from a water-soluble extract of tartary buckwheat, which was composed of a single polypeptide with a molecular weight of about 57 kDa.[37] In an *in vitro* assay, TBWSP31 dose- and time-dependently suppressed the proliferation of human Bcap37 mammary cancer cells with IC_{50}s of 19.75 µg/mL (72 h).[38] After treatment with TBWSP31 for 48 h, the cell apoptosis and G0/G1 cell-cycle arrest were elicited in Bcap37 cells in association with upregulation of Fas expression and downregulation of Bcl-2 expression.[39,40] Similarly, BWP, a buckwheat protein product, showed anticarcinogenic activity in an *in vivo* model. Fed diets of BMP (200 g/kg) for 124 days markedly deterred the colon carcinogenesis caused by 1,2-dimethylhydrazine (DMH) in rats and lessened the incidence of colon adenocarcinoma by 47%. The intake of BWP significantly reduced the proliferation together with downregulated c-myc and c-fos proteins in the colonic epithelium cells.[41] Taken together, the findings revealed the protective potential of tartary buckwheat proteins from buckwheat against the carcinogenesis of breast and/or colon.

Moreover, an antifungal peptide (4 kDa) isolated from buckwheat seeds is stable at 0°C–70°C and pH 1.0/2.0–13. Its antiproliferative effect was observed in mouse L1210 leukemia, human MCF-7 breast cancer, HepG2 hepatoma cells, and WRL 68 liver embryonic cells with IC_{50}s of 4, 25, 33, and 37 μM, respectively, showing obvious anticancer activity. It was also able to repress HIV-1 reverse transcriptase (IC_{50} of 5.5 μM).[42]

6. RNase

A ribonuclease (22.5 kDa) with an *N*-terminal sequence was purified from Japanese large brown buckwheat seeds, which in the *in vitro* models hampered the proliferation of human HepG2 hepatoma and MCF-7 breast cancer cell lines with IC_{50}s of 79.2 and 63.8 μM, respectively, in addition to its inhibitory effect on HIV-1 reverse transcriptase activity (IC_{50} of 48 μM).[43]

7. Polysaccharides

The antitumor activity of buckwheat polysaccharides (BWPS) has been evaluated in an *in vitro* model with human THP-1 acute monocytic leukemia cells. The observation displayed that BWPS directly elicited the differentiation and maturity of THP-1 leukemia cells in a dose-dependent manner after treatment for five days and indirectly stimulated cytokine secretion (differentiation inducer) in monocytes from PBMCs followed by one-day treatment, indicating the potential of BWPS in leukemia chemotherapy by the induction of differentiation.[44]

CONCLUSION AND SUGGESTION

The comprehensive phytochemical and pharmacological explorations provided a scientific basis for both edible and medicinal uses of the buckwheats in the human diet. The seeds of *F. esculentum* and *F. tataricum* are consumed widely in many areas due to health beneficial ingredients such as flavonoids, phenolics, and several types of macromolecules. Two flavonoid constituents, rutin (**1**) and quercetin (**2**), as the major bioactive small molecules in buckwheat pseudocereals were confirmed to play prominent roles in anticancer and antioxidant effects. Because of having much greater content of the flavonoids, tartary buckwheat is getting more popular as a functional food than common buckwheat. The macromolecules derived from buckwheat, including trypsin inhibitors/protease inhibitors, lectins, proteins/peptides, and polysaccharides, also displayed convincing potentials for cancer prevention. In addition, phenylpropanoid glycosides were designated as the major anticancer constituents in *F. tataricum* roots. Besides, the buckwheats have been shown to possess antioxidant, anti-inflammatory, antiallergic, hepatoprotective, cardiocerebral vascular protective, and anti-diabetic properties. Therefore, these considerable scientific evidences clearly validated that the consumption of buckwheats is beneficial for lessening the risk of cancer especially in blood, colon, stomach, breast, and liver, as well as lessening the incidence of other diseases.

REFERENCES

1. a) Zhao, F. et al., 2008. Progress on bioactive compounds in buckwheat. *Shipin Yu Yaopin* 10: 58–61; b) Jing, R. et al., 2016. Phytochemical and pharmacological profiles of three Fagopyrum buckwheats. *Int. J. Mol. Sci.* 17: 589.
2. Gimenez-Bastida, J.A. et al., 2015. Buckwheat as a functional food and its effects on health. *J. Agricul. Food Chem.* 63: 7896–7913.
3. Yan, F.Y. et al., 2010. Effect of buckwheat flavonoids on proliferation of esophageal cancer cells EC9706. *Zhongcaoyao* 41: 1142–1145.
4. Kishore, K. et al., 2010. Rutin (natural bioflavonoid): Traditional and medicinal uses. *Pharmacologyonline* (1, Newsletter), 931–937.
5. Li, F.H. et al., 2014. Cellular antioxidant and antiproliferative activities of flavonoids extracted from tartary buckwheat (Fagopyrum tartaricum (L.) Gaertn) bran. *Shipin Kexue* (Beijing, China) 35: 58–63.
6. Revathi Mani, B. et al., 2014. Insilico analysis on the effect of rutin bioflavonoid and chemotherapeutic drug cyclophosphamide on nuclear factor kappa-b protein expression. *Int. J. Pharm. Biol. Sci.* 5: 560–569.

7. Tan, Y.R. et al., 2012. Research status and prospect of flavonoids from tartary buckwheat. *Shipin Gongye Keji* 33: 377–381.
8. Zhou, X.L. et al., 2013. Comparative antitumor activity study of tartary buckwheat flavonoids and amphibian peptides. *Advanced Materials Research* (Durnten-Zurich, Switzerland) 781–784. (Advances in Chemical Engineering III), 1270–1274,
9. Li, Y.Y. et al., 2014. Flavonoids from tartary buckwheat induce G2/M cell cycle arrest and apoptosis in human hepatoma HepG2 cells. *Acta Biochimica et Biophysica Sinica* 46: 460–470.
10. Ren, W. et al., 2003. Molecular basis of fas and cytochrome c pathways of apoptosis induced by tartary buckwheat flavonoid in HL-60 cells. *Methods and Findings in Experim. Clin. Pharmacol.* 25: 431–436.
11. Ren, W. 2001. Tartary buckwheat flavonoid activates caspase 3 and induces HL-60 cell apoptosis. *Methods and Findings in Experim. Clin. Pharmacol.* 23: 427–432.
12. Kim, J.H. et al., 2013. Protective effect of rutin against ultraviolet b-induced cyclooxygenase-2 expression in mouse epidermal cells. *Food Sci. Biotechnol.* 22: 1–6.
13. Li, Y.Y. et al., 2014. Effect of isoquercetin from Fagopyrum tataricum on the proliferation and apoptosis of human gastric carcinoma cell line SGC-7901. *Shipin Kexue* (Beijing, China) 35(3): 193–197.
14. Zhang, H.X. et al., 2013. Inhibitory effect of red clover flavone from golden buckwheat on migration ability of human gastric cancer cell line SGC7901 and its mechanism. *Jilin Daxue Xuebao, Yixueban* 39: 78–81.
15. Zhou, X.L. 2012. Anti-infection effects of buckwheat flavonoid extracts (BWFEs) from germinated sprouts. *J. Med. Plants Res.* 6: 24–29.
16. Zhou, X.L. et al., 2011. Toward a novel understanding of buckwheat self-defensive strategies during seed germination and preliminary investigation on the potential pharmacological application of its malting products. *J. Med. Plants Res.* 5: 6946–6954.
17. Zhou, X.L. et al., 2011. Inhibitory effect of flavonoids from tartary buckwheat sprouts on proliferation of human breast cancer cells. *Shipin Kexue* (Beijing, China) 32: 225–228.
18. Cui, C.B. et al., 2008. Antimutagenic and cytotoxic effects of an ethanol extract of buckwheat sprout. *Han'guk Eungyong Sangmyong Hwahakhoeji* 51: 212–218.
19. Zheng, C.J. et al., 2012. Cytotoxic phenylpropanoid glycosides from Fagopyrum tataricum (L.) Gaertn. *Food Chem.* 132: 433–438.
20. Peng, W. et al., 2015. Antitumor activity of tatariside F isolated from roots of Fagopyrum tataricum (L.) Gaertn against H22 hepatocellular carcinoma via up-regulation of p53. *Phytomed.* 22(7–8): 730–736.
21. Park, S.S. et al., 2004. Suppressive activity of protease inhibitors from buckwheat seeds against human T-acute lymphoblastic leukemia cell lines. *Applied Biochem. Biotechnol.* 117: 65–73.
22. Wang, H.W. et al., 2002. Antiproliferative effect of tartary buckwheat trypsin inhibitor on HL-60 cells. *Shanxi Yike Daxue Xuebao* 33: 3–5.
23. Li, Y.Y. et al., 2010. buckwheat trypsin inhibitor (BTI) transfection induced apoptosis and G1 arrest in EC9706 cells. *Zhongguo Shengwu Huaxue Yu Fenzi Shengwu Xuebao* 26: 362–368.
24. Zhang, Z. et al., 2007. Expression of a buckwheat trypsin inhibitor gene in Escherichia coli and its effect on multiple myeloma IM-9 cell proliferation. *Acta Biochimica et Biophysica Sinica* 39: 701–707.
25. Li, Y.Y. et al., 2015. NFκB/p65 activation is involved in regulation of rBTI-induced glucocorticoid receptor expression in MCF-7 cell lines. *J. Functional Foods* 15: 376–388.
26. Cui, X.D. et al., 2013. Buckwheat trypsin inhibitor enters HepG2 cells by clathrin-dependent endocytosis. *Food Chem.* 141: 2625–2633.
27. Li, Y.Y. et al., 2009. rBTI induces apoptosis in human solid tumor cell lines by loss in mitochondrial transmembrane potential and caspase activation. *Toxicol. Lett.* 189: 166–175.
28. Li, F. et al., 2009. Effect of recombinant buckwheat trypsin inhibitor on apoptosis and caspases activity in human hepatoma (HepG2) cells. *Zhongguo Shengwu Huaxue Yu Fenzi Shengwu Xuebao* 25: 182–187.
29. Li, J.S. et al., 2011. Expression and purification of truncated rBTI and its inhibitory effect on EC9706 cell proliferation. *Zhongguo Shengwu Huaxue Yu Fenzi Shengwu Xuebao* 27: 467–472.
30. Cui, X.D. et al., 2012. Expression, purification and activity of the wild and mutants of potato I type protease inhibitor rBTI. *Zhongguo Shengwu Huaxue Yu Fenzi Shengwu Xuebao* 28: 346–351.
31. Li, Y.Y. et al., 2011. Expression of rBTI-2 of buckwheat and its inhibition on proliferation activity of tumor cells. *Zhongguo Xibao Shengwuxue Xuebao* 33: 759–765.
32. Wang, Z.H. et al., 2007. Induction of apoptosis by buckwheat trypsin inhibitor in chronic myeloid leukemia K562 cells. *Biol. Pharm. Bull.* 30: 783–786.
33. Bai, C.Z. et al., 2015. Anti-tumoral effects of a trypsin inhibitor derived from buckwheat in vitro and in vivo. *Mol. Med. Reports* 12(2, Pt. A): 1777–1782.

34. Jia, Q.J. et al., 2015. Proliferative inhibition of tatary buckwheat lectin in colon cancer cells. *Zhongguo Shengwu Huaxue Yu Fenzi Shengwu Xuebao*, 31: 383–390.

35. Bai, C.Z. et al., 2015. Stimulation of dendritic cell maturation and induction of apoptosis in lymphoma cells by a stable lectin from buckwheat seeds. *GMR,Genetics and Mol. Res.* 14: 2162–2175.

36. Guo, P.Y. et al., 2017. Mechanism of tartary buckwheat lectin-targeted inhibition of HCT116 colon cancer cell proliferation. *Zhongguo Shengwu Huaxue Yu Fenzi Shengwu Xuebao* 33(1): 73–80.

37. Guo, X.N. et al., 2007. Purification and characterization of the antitumor protein from Chinese tartary buckwheat (Fagopyrum tataricum Gaertn.) water-soluble extracts. *J. Agricul. Food Chem.* 55: 6958–6961.

38. Guo, X.N. et al., 2010. Anti-proliferative effect of tartary buckwheat protein fraction tbwsp31 on breast cancer cells. *Shipin Kexue* (Beijing, China) 31: 317–320.

39. Guo, X.N. et al., 2011. Study on the mechanism of Tartary buckwheat protein on breast cancer cells. *Shipin Yu Shengwu Jishu Xuebao* 30: 55–59.

40. Guo, X.N. et al., 2010. Antitumor activity of a novel protein obtained from tartary buckwheat. *Int. J. Mol. Sci.* 11: 5201–5211.

41. Liu, Z.H. et al., 2001. A buckwheat protein product suppresses 1,2-dimethylhydrazine-induced colon carcinogenesis in rats by reducing cell proliferation. *J. Nutr.* 131: 1850–1853.

42. Leung E.H.W. et al., 2007. A relatively stable antifungal peptide from buckwheat seeds with antiproliferative activity toward cancer cells. *J. Peptide Sci.* 13: 762–767.

43. Yuan, S.S. et al., 2015. Isolation of a ribonuclease with antiproliferative and HIV-1 reverse transcriptase inhibitory activities from Japanese large brown buckwheat seeds. *Applied Biochem. Biotechnol.* 175: 2456–2467.

44. Wu, S.C. et al., 2011. Buckwheat polysaccharide exerts antiproliferative effects in THP-1 human leukemia cells by inducing differentiation. *J. Med. Food* 14: 26–33.

27. COMMON BEANS

菜豆 インゲンマメ 강낭콩

Phaseolus vulgaris

Fabaceae

Similar to soybean, the common beans (*Phaseolus vulgaris*) are widely consumed throughout the world and showed outstanding importance for human nutrition. However, owing to the long history of cultivation, various well-known bean cultivars/varieties are generated from this species, such as kidney bean, wax bean, pinto bean, black bean/dark bean, white bean, flageolet bean, calypso bean, yellow bean, red/pink bean, and so on, with a wide range of colors and shapes of pods and seeds. The common beans present a high nutritional value, being a significant source of plant proteins, fibers, some minerals, and certain vitamins, and also contain substantial amounts of bioactive substances, for example, phenolic acids, flavonoids, anthocyanins, saponins, peptides, lectins, and oligosaccharides, that contribute overall to the antioxidant, radical scavenging, antiradical, anticarcinogenic, and anti-diabetic properties. Hence, increasing the daily consumption of a broad variety of common beans has gained more and more attention in order to optimize human health and to minimize the risk of some chronic diseases. In addition to common beans, the beans produced from other *Phaseolus* plants, for example, runner bean (*P. coccineus*), lima bean (*P. lunatus*), and tepary bean (*P. acutifolius*) are also used as nutritional foods. These inexpensive beans are an important food source in the diets of Central and South America, the Mediterranean, and southern and eastern Africa.

SCIENTIFIC EVIDENCE OF CANCER PREVENTION

The studies of chemical biology and phytochemistry disclosed that the rich micronutrients and macronutrients and a number of bioactive constituents in the common beans are contributors to the anticarcinogenic and antioxidant activities. However, the different varieties of common beans contain quite varied quantities of bioactive substances, which would largely influence the potencies of inhibitory effects against oxidative stress and cancer-cell proliferation.

1. Hydrophilic extracts and their bioactive substances

Generally, the hydrophilic extracts of common beans are rich in polyphenolics, such as phenolic acids, flavonoids/isoflavonoids, and/or anthocyanins. The polyphenols are essentially present in the seed coats and husks in the common beans. The extracts of two types of common beans (pinto and black beans) and two types of soybeans (yellow and black) displayed cellular antioxidant activities and antiproliferative capacities against human colorectal (SW480) and gastric (AGS) cancer cell lines in dose-dependent manners, but the yellow soybean had weak-to-no inhibition in AGS cells. Of them, black soybean, black beans, and pinto beans presented higher cellular antioxidant activities in AGS cells (IC_{50}s of 0.61–0.64 mg/mL) and the extracts of pinto bean and black bean achieved better anticancer effects with IC_{50}s of 0.66 and 0.74 mg/mL in AGS cells and 0.83 and 0.93 mg/mL in SW480 cells, respectively. However, the investigation further found that thermal processing would significantly decrease the capacities of these hydrophilic extracts in the antioxida-tive, antiproliferative, and other health-promoting effects, implying that the food cooking process caused complex changes in the hydrophilic chemical compositions, especially degradation of the polyphenols and reduction of saponins and phytic acids.[1] The methanolic extract of Jamapa bean (a black variety of *P. vulgaris*) was a better DPPH radical scavenger than butylated hydroxytoluene (an antioxidant used as a food additive), showing 45.6% and 33.9% antiradical capacity at 400 μM concentrations, respectively. Treatment of HeLa cervical cancer cells with the extract in a dose of 35 μg/mL for 24 h elicited cell apoptosis concomitant with the upregulation of Bax and caspase-3 proapoptotic proteins. The antioxidant, antiradical, and anticancer activities were further found to be closely correlated to the high concentration of proanthocyanidins in the Jamapa bean.[2]

The aqueous acetone extracts of 12 ecotypes of common beans have been evaluated for their antioxidant and antiproliferative activities. These extracts showed different degrees of DPPH radical-scavenging activities, and the extracts except those derived from white beans (nonpigment) exerted suppressive effects against human A549 (lung), MCF-7 (breast), and Caco-2 (colorectal) carcinoma cell lines. Among them, the stronger antiproliferative effects occurred after treatment with the extracts of three types of black beans, where the ED_{50}s were 49.4–67.64 µg(GAE)/mL for nero acerra (NR) dark beans, 35.79–63.75 µg(GAE)/mL for nero frigento (NF) dark beans, and 73.53–119.02 µg(GAE)/mL for nero caposele (NC) dark beans. Nonetheless, the strongest anticancer effect was established by the extract of cannellino rosso (CR) red beans with ED_{50}s of 28.52–31.32 µg(GAE)/mL. After the cooking process, the anticancer potencies of most of the common bean extracts were slightly lessened. However, the effects of NF and NC dark beans on the three cancer cell lines were impressively enhanced by cooking, and the effects of speckled beans one some tested cancer cells were reinforced by cooking.[3] An 80% methanolic extract of a Spain-produced dark beans (*P. vulgaris* c.v. Tolosana) was effective in deterring oxidation and cancer proliferation and protecting neurons. More impressively, the boiling process and germination dramatically amplified the antiproliferative potencies of tolosana beans on MCF-7 breast cancer cells from ED_{50} of 31.5 µg/mL to 0.80 and 0.57 µg/mL and on UACC-62 melanoma cells from ED_{50} of 137 µg/mL to 0.22 and 0.07 µg/mL, respectively, but the cooked beans lost the inhibition against TK-10 renal adenocarcinoma cells.[4] Likewise, an 80% ethanolic extract of Korean kidney bean husk triggered a series of antitumor and proapoptotic responses in HT-29 colon cancer cells to show that its antitumor potentials were mediated by the activation of anti-growth proteins p53 and p21 and stimulation of p-AMP-activated protein kinase (p-AMPK) and p-acetyle coenzyme-A carboxylase (p-Acc).[5] In addition, an *in vitro* assay showed weak cytotoxic effects of kidney bean hydrophilic extract on Caco-2 colon cancer cells.[6]

Furthermore, the *in vitro* anticancer activities of the bean extracts were also supported by the *in vivo* experiments. In three male murine models, fed with 20% beans (kidney bean, pinto bean, black-eyed pea, or soybean) to male rats hindered azoxymethane (AOM)-induced formation of ACF in the colon by 46%, 64%, 77%, and 56%, respectively,[6–8] whereas cooked navy beans, 60% ethanol insoluble extract, or soluble extract to male obese mice attenuated AOM-caused colon carcinogenesis by 56%, 67%, and 87%, respectively, compared with those of control groups fed an AIN-93G diet.[9] The results revealed that both 60% ethanolic soluble and insoluble extracts (i.e., micromolecules and macromolecules) contributed to the cancer-protection activity of cooked navy beans.[10] Similarly, a diet containing small red dry beans could decline the incidence of mammary cancer prompted by 1-methyl-1-nitrosourea (MNU) in a dose-dependent manner in rats along with the induction of apoptosis via a mitochondrial pathway.[10] Six diverse market classes of dry beans (*P. vulgaris*) in the United States were evaluated for the polyphenol contents, oxygen radical absorbance capacity, and anticancer activity. The cooked dry bean powder from two crop years were fed to rats in the diet resulted in the lessening of MNU-induced mammary carcinogenic rates.[11] The dose-dependent inhibitory activities of these dry beans on breast carcinogenesis were associated with reducing insulin, insulin-like growth factor (IGF), and C-reactive protein, but were not correlated with their flavonoid contents. Overall, the dietary intake of common beans has a potential to decline the breast cancer incidences, tumor multiplicity, and tumor mass.[12]

In addition, the methanolic extracts derived from the seed coats of *P. vulgaris* and *P. coccineus* black cultivars exhibited antioxidant activity that correlated with phenolic content. Comparatively, *P. coccineus* had higher content of phenolics and *P. vulgaris* showed higher values of anthocyanins. The antimutagenicity of phenolic-rich extract from *P. coccineus* (cv. Ayocote Negro) was higher against aflatoxin B1 than that of *P. vulgaris* (cv. Negro Jamapa).[13] The polyphenols such as the flavonoids (kaempferol and quercetin) and condensed and hydrolysable tannins have been found to play an effective role in the antioxidant, anticarcinogenic, antimutagenic, and anti-inflammatory actions. Their antiproliferative activities were lower than those of oleanane-type saponins (one kind of component of the common beans) on human HepG2 (liver), Caco-2 (colon), and MCF-7 (breast) cancer cell lines but better than the free triterpene and sterol components.[14,15] In addition, other micromolecules such as phytate and 1,2-di-O-α-linolenoyl-3-O-β-D-galactopyranosyl-sn-glycerol (DLGG) were found to exert antitumor, anti-inflammatory and/or antioxidant effects besides their important nutritional values.[15,16]

2. Fibers and polysaccharides

Colon/colorectal carcinoma is one of the most common causes of morbidity and mortality in western countries. The *in vitro* and *in vivo* experiments clearly evidenced the remarkable inverse relationship between consumption of the common beans and the incidences of colon/colorectal cancers owing to the beans providing rich polysaccharides and a nondigestible fraction, which is the proximate composition of fibers (~77%) and proteins/peptides (~17%). Either common bean polysaccharide extract or nondigested fibers in cooked common beans (*P. vulgaris*) were fermented with human gut flora for 24 h, leading to production of short-chain fatty acids (SCFAs) by metabolic degradation. In an *in vitro* model, the SCFAs could have hampered the growth of human HT-29 colon adenocarcinoma cells in association with modulation of the protein/gene expression profiles related to apoptotic death, cell-cycle arrest, and proliferation, such as upregulation of apoptotic genes (SIAH1, PRKCA) and cell-cycle gene (MSH2), marked downregulation of cell-cycle genes (CHEK1 and GADD45A), and increase in p53 activity.[17,18] The findings demonstrated that the fibers and polysaccharides of common beans are able to be biotransformed to micromolecular fatty acids that play a chemopreventive role in colon/colorectal carcinogenesis. In the *in vivo* systems, fed diets containing the nondigestible fraction of cooked common beans (cultivar Bayo Madero) to rats repressed the early stage of AOM-induced colon cancer through the modulation of a series of signaling pathways involved in apoptosis, cell-cycle G1/S, and G2/M arrest, antiproliferation and anti-inflammation, and DNA repair, such as upregulation of Tp53, Bax, Gadd45a, and Cdkn1a expressions and downregulation of Cdc25c, Ccne2, E2f1,and Bcl-2expressions.[19] Likewise, the fermentation of a polysaccharide extract from cooked common beans (*P. vulgaris* cv. Negro 8025) induced SCFAs production, which were rich in butyrates. The SCFAs in the large intestine amplified the Bax and caspase-3 transcriptional expressions, leading to declining numbers of ACF caused by AOM in rats.[20] Accordingly, the current results acclaimed that the dietary intake of common beans is feasible for chemoprotection from colon/colorectal cancers.

3. Peptides

AH-PE and BM-PE, two peptide extracts were isolated from the nondigestible fractions of two common bean cultivars: Azufrado Higuera and Bayo Madero (*P. vulgaris*), respectively. Treatment with 0.5 mg/mL AH-PE or BM-PE for 24 h deterred the proliferation of human HCT-116 and RKO colon cancer cell lines through different pathways, that is, AH-PE modulated the expression of cell-cycle regulation proteins (p21 and cyclin-B1) and BM-PE modulated the expression of mitochondria-activated apoptotic proteins (BAD, cytC, c-casp3, survivin, and BIRC7), but both amplified the expression of p53 in HCT-116 cells by 76% and 68%, respectively.[21,22] Compared to their antiproliferative effects, the RKO cells were sensitive to BM-PE (IC$_{50}$ of 0.51 mg/mL) and the HCT-116 and RKO cells to AH-PE (IC$_{50}$s of 0.53 and 0.59 mg/mL) and to N8-PE (Negro 8025 cultivar peptide extract, IC$_{50}$s of 0.8 and 0.79 mg/mL), but all of them were inactive to human KM20L4 colorectal cancer cells. Further, five peptides whose sequences were GLTSK (12.05%–14.59%), GEGSGA (5.31%–7.8%), MTEEY (10.85%–14.01%), LSGNK (4.18%–9.56%), and MPACGSS (29.94%–35.23%) were identified in 70% of the total peptide extract in four common bean cultivars (Azufrado Higuera, Bayo Madero, Negro 8025, and Pinto Durango).[22] The weak suppressive effects of GLTSK and GEGSGA were observed in the HCT-116 cells with IC$_{50}$s of 134.6 and 156.7 μM, respectively, and those of LSGNK, MTEEY, and MPACGSS were less active, but all the five were nontoxic to human

CCD-33Co normal colon cells. To inhibit the HCT-116 cell proliferation, GLTSK elicited mitochondrial membrane disruption via significantly increasing intracellular ROS and loss of mitochondrial potential, whereas GEGSGA caused cell cycle G1 arrest, PARP cleavage, and DNA damage.[23] In a combined treatment, both GLTSK and GEGSGA could synergistically enhance the effects of oxaliplatin (a clinical drug for the inhibition of colorectal cancer) against the HCT-116 cells.[23] In addition, a 7.3 kDa peptide was purified from dried red kidney beans and its N-terminal sequence of the peptide was elucidated as DGVCFGGLANGDRT. Besides possessing antifungal and anti-HIV HIV-1 reverse transcriptase activities, the anti-growth activity of this 7.3 kDa peptide was observed in an *in vitro* assay against MBL2 lymphoma and L1210 leukemia cell lines with IC_{50}s of 5.2 and 7.6 µM, respectively.[24] Hence, the emerging evidences indicate that the peptide component in common beans is one of the contributors to lower cancer risk in human populations.

4. Defensin

Defensins are small cysteine-rich cationic proteins/peptides that play a defense role not only in animals but also in plants, including legumes. Because molecules of plant defensins included 6–8 cysteine residues, these cysteine residues formed stable intramolecular disulfide bonds, resulting in strong stabilities of plant defensins to temperature, pH degree, and proteases. The defensins prepared from the cultivars of *P. vulgaris* usually exhibit antifungal, anti-HIV reverse transcriptase, antimicrobial, and antitumor activities. White kidney bean defensin presented a marked effect on restraining the proliferation and viability of human A549 lung cancer cells via an apoptosis pathway by the upexpression of p53 and caspase-3.[25] Two antifungal peptides with a defensin-like sequence and similar molecular mass of 7.3 kDa were purified from dried seeds of cloud bean and spotted bean cultivars (*P. vulgaris*), respectively. By suppressing thymidine incorporation, the peptides of cloud bean and spotted bean exerted antiproliferative effects against L1210 leukemia cells with IC_{50}s of 10 and 4.0 µM and against MBL2 leukemia cells with IC_{50}s of 40 and 9.0 µM, respectively.[26,27] A 5443 Da peptide with sequence homology to defensin was separated from extra-long purple pole bean (*P. vulgaris*), the peptide of which obviously deterred the proliferation of HepG2 hepatoma (IC_{50} of 4.1 µM), MCF-7 breast cancer (IC_{50} of 8.3 µM), HT-29 colon cancer (IC_{50} of 71.4 µM) and SiHa cervical cancer (IC_{50} of < 30.7 µM) cell lines but no inhibition on human WRL68 embryonic liver cells,[28] whereas a 7458 Da peptide with defensin characteristic isolated from white cloud beans (*P. vulgaris*) showed a better inhibitory effect on the MCF-7 cells (IC_{50} of 5.7 µM).[29]

Likewise, a peptide designated coccinin (7 kDa) and a protein assigned phaseococcin (5422 Da) were purified from large scarlet runner beans (*P. coccineus* cv. Major) and small scarlet runner beans (*P. coccineus* cv. Minor), respectively. Their molecules hold a N-terminal sequence resembling those of defensins and displayed the inhibitory effects against the proliferation of HL-60 and L1210 leukemia cell lines with the respective IC_{50} values of 30 µM and 40 µM for coccinin.[30,31] From the seeds of shelf beans of *P. limensis*, a defensin-like peptide (6.5 kDa) named limenin was separated. The antiproliferative effect of limenin occurred *in vitro* toward L1210 leukemia and M1 myeloma cell lines concomitant with the blockage of thymidine incorporation into the tumor cells.[32] Besides, both coccinin and phaseococcin did not affect the proliferation of mouse splenocytes, though some of the common bean defensins (including limenin) were able to elicit a mitogenic response from mouse splenocytes and to stimulate thymidine incorporation into mouse splenocytes.

5. Lectins

Lectins/hemagglutinins are defined as a class of sugar-binding proteins that agglutinate cells and/or precipitate glycol conjugates and have ubiquitous distribution in plants, animals, and fungi. Lectins/hemagglutinins are well characterized to have various biological properties, including anticancer, anti-HIV, and/or antifungal effects. Many types of lectins/hemagglutinins have been discovered from the seeds of *Phaseolus vulgaris* varieties and showed varied anticancer potencies. Significantly, the most potent antiproliferative activity was achieved by a dimeric hemagglutinin (LSH) purified from the seeds of *P. vularis* cultivar *Legumi secchi* (a product of Italy) against

MCF-7 breast cancer cells (IC_{50} of 0.2 µM). The molecule of LSH (relative molecular mass: 62000) has a N-terminal amino acid sequence elucidated as ANDISFNFVRFNETNLILGG. The LSH treatment elicited the cell-cycle arrest in G2/M phase and apoptosis of MCF-7 cells through a death receptor-mediated pathway involving Fas ligands, caspases-8 and 9 activation, p53 release, BID truncation, and lamin A/C truncation.[33] Other potent lectins/hemagglutinins were effective in deterring the MCF-7 cells, for instance, FBH-1 and FBH-2, two hemagglutinin (64 and 60 kDa) from French beans of *P. vularis*, which showed IC_{50}s of 2.0 and 6.6 µM, respectively.[34,35] The IC_{50} of LPBH, a hemagglutinin (60 kDa) from Hokkaido large pinto beans of *P. vularis* was 6.07 µM and the IC_{50} of BKL, a dimeric glucosamine-specific lectin (64 kDa) from brown kidney beans of *P. vularis* was 4.8 µM.[36,37]

Among these lectins/hemagglutinins, NRBH, a hemagglutinin (64 kDa) from red beans of *P. vularis* (produced in northeast China) and BKL showed the best inhibition against CNE-1 nasopharyngeal carcinoma cells with IC_{50}s of 1.63 and 3.12 µM, respectively.[36,37] The strongest antileukemia activity was shown by DRKH, a hemagglutinin (67 kDa) derived from dark red kidney beans of *P. vulgaris* against L1210 cells with IC_{50} of 1.6 µM.[38] Table 4.1 summarized the anticancer activities and stability required conditions of the lectins/hemagglutinins isolated from diverse cultivars of *Phaseolus vulgaris*. It is noticeable that most of the lectins /hemagglutinins are sensitive to temperature and pH conditions; thus, their anticancer properties would be significantly decreased in the cooking process. However, these scientific evidences can provide a comprehensive perspective for further elucidating the potentials of lectins and hemagglutinins from *P. vulgaris* cultivars in the suppression of cancer proliferation and the induction of apoptosis.

6. Trypsin inhibitors

Several trypsin inhibitors were obtained from the separation of *P. vulgaris* beans, which exerted some degree of anticancer activities in the *in vitro* models. From brown kidney beans, a Bowman–Birk trypsin inhibitor ($\approx$17 kDa) was purified, which displayed prominent thermostability up to 90°C and pH stability (0–14). It was a weak inhibitor on human MCF-7 breast cancer cells (IC_{50} of 71.52 µM). At > 110 µM concentration, it only slightly deterred the proliferation of HepG2 hepatoma cells and WRL68 embryonic liver cells.[46] Two trypsin inhibitors (16 kDa) with an intact disulfide were separated from white cloud beans (*P. vulgaris*), both of which were able to block thymidine incorporation by L1210 leukemia cells with IC_{50} values of 28.8 and 21.5 µM, respectively. Even the concentrations increased to 100 µM, the inhibition on MBL2 lymphoma cells failed but on HIV-1 reverse transcription inhibition occurred.[47] A 16 kDa trypsin inhibitor with disulfide bonds and a blocked N-terminus was prepared from small pinto beans (*P. vulgaris*), which was stable at 100°C and pH 2–10. Nonetheless, at 125 µM concentration, it only slightly hindered the viability of MCF-7 breast cancer and HepG2 hepatoma cells.[48] Besides, a 26 kDa storage protein-like trypsin inhibitor was isolated from moth beans (*P. acutifolius*), which could restrain thymidine incorporation by MBL2 lymphoma cells (IC_{50} of 20 µM).[49]

7. Leguminous peroxidase

Limlin, a leguminous peroxidase (34 kDa) was isolated from *P. limensis* seeds, which exerted anticancer, antifungal, and antibacterial effects on the experimental models. Its antiproliferative effect occurred toward human Bel-7402 hepatoma and SHSY5Y neuroblastoma cell lines *in vitro* with IC_{50} values of 106.2 and 75.8 µM, respectively.[50]

CONCLUSION AND SUGGESTION

Numerous investigations based on phytochemistry and chemical biology have clearly demonstrated that the various cultivars of common beans (*Phaseolus vulgaris*) provided an inexpensive but functional food source rich in macronutrients, important micronutrients, and a variety of other stored bioactive components (i.e., phytates, polyphenols, anthocyanins, triterpenoids, saponins, tannins, steroids,

TABLE 4.1

Anticancer Activities and Stability Conditions of the Lectins/Hemagglutinins Purified from *Phaseolus vulgaris* Cultivars

Lectins/Hemagglutinins	Molecular Weights	*P. vulgaris* Cultivars	Stabilities	Antiproliferative Activities on Cancer Cell Lines (IC$_{50}$ μM)[a]
Lectin (EAPL) [39]	60 kDa	Extra-long autumn purple beans	0°C–50°C pH 4–11	HepG2 (34.8); HNG-2 (160.2); MCF-7 (171.6); CNE-2 (253.2) and CNE-1 (420.7). Induction of HepG2 cell apoptosis.
Mg^{2+}-dependent Lectin (CPBL) [44]	58 kDa	Chinese Pinto beans	60°C pH 7–8	HONE-1 (17.3); inactive to MCF-7.
Dimeric galacturonic acid-specific lectin (BTKL) [45]	60 kDa	Blue tiger king seeds		HepG2 (7.9); weakly active to HNE-2, CNE-1, L1210; and inactive to CNE-2, MCF-7, SUME-α. Triggering of HepG2 cell apoptosis and necrosis
Heterotetrameric lectin (PVAL) [40]	136 ku	Small white kidney beans	Stable in HCl, NaOH	Active to MDA-MB-435s
Dimeric lectin (JBL) [41]	60.8 kDa	Jade beans	30°C–70°C pH 4.5–9.4	MCF-7 (174)
Dimeric glucosamine-specific lectin (BKL) [37]	64 kDa	Brown kidney beans	20°C–60°C pH 3–12	MCF-7 (4.80, 48 h); CNE-1 (3.12, 24 h); CNE-2 (6.64, 48 h); HepG2 (32.85, 24 h). Induction of MCF-7 cell apoptosis-involved ER stress.
Hemagglutinin [42]	30 kDa	Hokkaido red beans	0°C–80°C pH 4–11	Active to HepG2 in 36–320 μg/mL
Hemagglutinin (DRKH) [38]	67 kDa	Dark red kidney beans	25°C–70°C pH 4–11	L1210 (1.6)
Hemagglutinin (LSH) [33]	62,000	Legumi secchi seeds	0°C–60°C pH 4–11	MCF-7 (0.2). Promotion of MCF-7 cell apoptosis.
Hemagglutinin (NRBH) [43]	64 kDa	Red beans from northeast China	65°C pH 2–12	CNE-1 (1.63); MCF-7 (11.66); CNE-2 (35); HepG2 (50).
Dimeric hemagglutinin (LPBH) [36] (in large yield)	60 kDa	Large Pinto beans from Hokkaido, Japan		MCF-7 (6.07); HepG2 (8.10); CHE-2 (7.99, 48 h).
Hemagglutinin (FBH-1) [44]	64 kDa	French beans cv. 35	0°–50°C pH 6–8	MCF-7 (2.0); HepG2 (100). Induction of MCF-7 cell apoptosis and cell-cycle arrest at G0/G1 and G2/M phases.
Hemagglutinin (FBH-2) [35]	60 kDa	French beans	10°C–80°C pH 1–12	MCF-7 (6.6); L1210 (7); HepG2 (13); but normal WRL-68 cells (15).

a Human nasopharyngeal cancer cell lines: HONE-1, CNE-1, CNE-2, HNE-2, and SUME-α; human breast cancer cell line: MCF-7; human hepatoma cell line: HepG2; mouse leukemia cell line: L1210; and human normal embryonic hepatocyte line: WRL-68.

vitamins, polysaccharides, fibers, lectins/hemagglutinins, defensins, α-amylase inhibitors, peroxidase, and some minerals). They endowed positive health benefits through their antioxidant, anticarcinogenic, anticancer, antidiabetic, antifungal, antibacterial, phytoestrogenic, and neuroprotective properties. Especially, the micromolecules (such as phytates, polyphenols, anthocyanins, and saponins) and the macromolecules (such as fibers, polysaccharides, lectins/hemagglutinins, defensins, and peroxidase) in the common beans have been elucidated to be bioactive substances responsible for the prevention of colorectal, colon, breast, liver, and blood cancers. The antioxidant and radical-scavenging activities of the common beans are primarily attributed to their polyphenols, anthocyanins, and phytates; these components are essentially present in the common bean coats but their contents varied depending on the common bean varieties/cultivars and the coat colors, resulting in different potencies of antioxidant and anticarcinogenic effects. In addition, there is no question that these micro- and macromolecules play a modulating role in immunity. The experimental evidences also revealed that polyphenols, anthocyanins, and lectins/hemagglutinins are weak to thermal treatment in general cases. According to the impressive scientific data, the common beans are definitely important nutraceutical and functional food. On high consumption, the common beans can obviously contribute to lessening the risk of some cancers and other diseases and promoting health.

REFERENCES

1. Xu, B.J. et al., 2011. Reduction of antiproliferative capacities, cell-based antioxidant capacities and phytochemical contents of common beans and soybeans upon thermal processing. *Food Chem.* 129(3): 974–981.
2. Aparicio-Fernandez, X. et al., 2008. Antiradical capacity and induction of apoptosis on HeLa cells by a Phaseolus vulgaris extract. *Plant Foods Hum Nutr* (Dordrecht, Netherlands) 63(1): 35–40.
3. Ombra, M.N. et al., 2016. Phenolic composition and antioxidant and antiproliferative activities of the extracts of twelve common bean (Phaseolus vulgaris L.) endemic ecotypes of southern Italy before and after cooking. *Oxid. Med. Cell. Longevity* 2016, Article ID 1398298.
4. Lopez, A. et al., 2013. Effect of cooking and germination on phenolic composition and biological properties of dark beans (Phaseolus vulgaris L.). *Food Chem.* 138(1): 547–555.
5. Lee Y.K. et al., 2009. Kidney bean husk extracts exert antitumor effect by inducing apoptosis involving AMP-activated protein kinase signaling pathway. *Annals of the New York Academy of Sci.* 1171: 484–488.
6. Boateng, J. et al., 2008. Antitumor and cytotoxic properties of dry beans (Phaseolus sp. L.): An in vitro and in vivo model. *Int. J. Cancer Res.* 4(2): 41–51.
7. Boateng, J.A. et al., 2007. Inhibitory effects of selected dry beans (Phaseolus spp L) on azoxymethane-induced formation of aberrant crypt foci in Fisher 344 male rats. *Nutr. Res.* (NY, NY, U.S.) 27(10): 640–646.
8. Hughes, J.S. et al., 1997. Dry beans inhibit azoxymethane-induced colon carcinogenesis in F344 rats. *J. Nutr.* 127(12): 2328–2333.
9. Bobe, G. et al., 2008. Dietary cooked navy beans and their fractions attenuate colon carcinogenesis in azoxymethane-induced ob/ob mice. *Nutr. Cancer* 60(3): 373–381.
10. Thompson, M.D. et al., 2008. Mechanisms associated with dose-dependent inhibition of rat mammary carcinogenesis by dry bean (Phaseolus vulgaris, L.). *J. Nutr.*138: 2091–2097.
11. Thompson, M.D. et al., 2009. Chemical composition and mammary cancer inhibitory activity of dry bean. *Crop Sci.* 49(1): 179–186.
12. Thompson, M.D. et al., 2012. Physiological effects of bean (Phaseolus vulgaris L.) consumption on cellular signaling in cancer. *Cell Cycle* 11(5): 835–836.
13. Loarca-Pina, G. et al., 2007. Chemical parameters and biological activity of phenolic compounds in Phaseolus vulgaris and Phaseolus coccineus beans. *ACS Symp. Ser.* 946 (Hispanic Foods): 89–101.
14. Dong, M. et al., 2007. Phytochemicals of black bean seed coats: Isolation, structure elucidation, and their antiproliferative and antioxidative activities. *J. Food Chem.* 55(15): 6044–6051.
15. Doria, E. et al., 2012. Anti-nutrient components and metabolites with health implications in seeds of 10 common bean (Phaseolus vulgaris L. and Phaseolus lunatus L.) landraces cultivated in southern Italy. *Agricul. J. Food Composit. Anal.* 26(1–2): 72–80.

16. Larsen, E. et al., 2007. Common vegetables and fruits as a source of 1,2-di-O-α-linolenoyl-3-O-β-D-galactopyranosyl-sn-glycerol, a potential anti-inflammatory and antitumor agent. *J. Food Lipids* 14(3): 272–279.

17. Campos-Vega, R. et al., 2012. Human gut flora-fermented nondigestible fraction from cooked bean (Phaseolus vulgaris L.) modifies protein expression associated with apoptosis, cell cycle arrest, and proliferation in human adenocarcinoma colon cancer cells. *J. Agricul. Food Chem.* 60(51): 12443–12450; 2014. The fermented non-digestible fraction of common bean (Phaseolus vulgaris L.) triggers cell cycle arrest and apoptosis in human colon adenocarcinoma cells. *Genes Nutr.* 9(1): 1–12.

18. Campos-Vega, R. et al., 2010. Bean (Phaseolus vulgaris L.) polysaccharides modulate gene expression in human colon cancer cells (HT-29). *Food Res. Int.* 43(4): 1057–1064.

19. Hayde, V.C. et al., 2012. Non-digestible fraction of beans (Phaseolus vulgaris L.) modulates signalling pathway genes at an early stage of colon cancer in Sprague-Dawley rats. *British J. Nutr.* 108(S1): S145–S154.

20. Feregrino-Perez, A.A. et al., 2008. Composition and chemopreventive effect of polysaccharides from common beans (Phaseolus vulgaris L.) on azoxymethane-induced colon cancer. *J. Agricul. Food Chem.* 56(18): 8737–8744.

21. Vital, D.A.L. et al., 2014. Peptides extracted from common bean (Phaseolus vulgaris L.) non-digestible fraction caused differential gene expression of HCT116 and RKO human colorectal cancer cells. *Food Res. Int.* 62: 193–204.

22. Vital, D.A.L. et al., 2014. Peptides in common bean fractions inhibit human colorectal cancer cells. *Food Chem.* 157: 347–355.

23. Vital, D.A.L. et al., 2016. Selective mechanism of action of dietary peptides from common bean on HCT116 human colorectal cancer cells through loss of mitochondrial membrane potential and DNA damage. *J. Functional Foods* 23: 24–39.

24. Li, M. et al., 2011. An antifungal peptide with antiproliferative activity toward tumor cells from red kidney beans. *Protein Pept Lett.* 18(6): 594–600.

25. Liu, G. et al., 2014. Efficiency of white kidney bean defensin in promoting apoptosis and inhibiting proliferation of lung cancer cell line A549. *Jiangsu Yiyao* 40(8): 884–886.

26. Wu, X.L. et al., 2011. An antifungal defensin from Phaseolus vulgaris cv. 'Cloud Bean'. *Phytomed.* 18: 104–109.

27. Wang, H.X. et al., 2007. Isolation and characterization of an antifungal peptide with antiproliferative activity from seeds of Phaseolus vulgaris cv. 'Spotted Bean'. *Applied Microbial. Biotechnol.* 74(1): 125–130.

28. Lin, P. et al., 2010. A defensin with highly potent antipathogenic activities from the seeds of purple pole bean. *Biosci. Reports* 30(2): 101–109.

29. Wong, J.H. et al., 2006. A mitogenic defensin from white cloud beans (Phaseolus vulgaris). *Peptides* 27, 2075–2081.

30. Ngai, P.H.K. et al., 2004. Coccinin, an antifungal peptide with antiproliferative and HIV-1 reverse transcriptase inhibitory activities from large scarlet runner beans. *Peptides* (NY, NY, US) 25(12): 2063–2068.

31. Ngai P.H.K. et al., 2005. Phaseococcin, an antifungal protein with antiproliferative and anti-HIV-1 reverse transcriptase activities from small scarlet runner beans. *Biochem. Cell Biol.* (Biochimie et biologie cellulaire) 83(2): 212–220.

32. Wong, J.H. et al., 2006. Limenin, a defensin-like peptide with multiple exploitable activities from shelf beans. *J. Peptide Sci.* 12(5): 341–346.

33. Lam, S.K. et al., 2011. Apoptosis of human breast cancer cells induced by hemagglutinin from Phaseolus vulgaris cv. Legumi secchi. *Food Chem.* 126(2), 595–602.

34. Lam, S.K. et al., 2010. First report of a haemagglutinin-induced apoptotic pathway in breast cancer cells. *Biosci. Reports* 30(5): 307–317; 2010. Isolation and characterization of a French bean hemagglutinin with antitumor, antifungal, and anti-HIV-1 reverse transcriptase activities and an exceptionally high yield. *Phytomedicine* 17(6): 457–62.

35. Leung, E.H. et al., 2008. Concurrent purification of two defense proteins from french bean seeds: A defensin-like antifungal peptide and a hemagglutinin. *J. Peptide Sci.* 14(3): 349–353.

36. Yin, C.M. et al., 2015. Isolation of a hemagglutinin with potent antiproliferative activity and a large antifungal defensin from Phaseolus vulgaris cv. Hokkaido large pinto beans. *J. Agricul. Food Chem.* 63(22): 5439–5448.

37. Chan. Y.S. et al., 2012. Isolation of a glucosamine binding leguminous lectin with mitogenic activity towards splenocytes and anti-proliferative activity towards tumor cells. *Plos One* 7(6): e38961.

38. Xia, L.X. et al., 2006. A hemagglutinin with mitogenic activity from dark red kidney beans. *J. Chromatography* B: 844(2): 213–216.

39. Fang, E.F. et al., 2010. A Lectin with anti-HIV-1 reverse transcriptase, antitumor, and nitric oxide inducing activities from seeds of Phaseolus vulgaris cv. extralong autumn purple bean. *J. Agricul. Food Chem.* 58(4): 2221–2229.

40. Li, F. et al., 2010. Purification and properties of a novel lectin from seeds of Phaseolus vulgaris var. albus. *J. Zhengzhou Univ.* 42(1): 120–124.

41. Cheung, C.F. et al., 2013. A calcium ion-dependent dimeric bean lectin with antiproliferative activity toward human breast cancer MCF-7 cells. *Protein J.* 32(3): 208–215.

42. Wong, J.H. et al., 2010. Characterisation of a haemagglutinin from hokkaido red bean (Phaseolus vulgaris cv. Hokkaido red bean). *J. Sci. Food Agricul.* 90(1): 70–77.

43. Chan, Y.S. et al., 2013. A hemagglutinin from northeast red beans with immunomodulatory activity and anti-proliferative and apoptosis-inducing activities toward tumor cells. *Protein Pept. Lett.* 20(10): 1159–1169.

44. Ang, A.S.W. et al., 2014. Purification and characterization of a glucosamine-binding antifungal lectin from Phaseolus vulgaris cv. Chinese pinto beans with antiproliferative activity towards nasopharyngeal carcinoma cells. *Applied Biochem. Biotech.* 172(2): 672–686.

45. Fang, E.F. et al., 2011. A new Phaseolus vulgaris lectin induces selective toxicity on human liver carcinoma HepG2 cells. *Archiv. Toxicol.* 85(12): 1551–1563.

46. Chan, Y.S. et al., 2013. Brown kidney bean Bowman-Birk trypsin inhibitor is heat and pH stable and exhibits anti-proliferative activity. *Applied Biochem. Biotech.* 169(4): 1306–1314.

47. Sun, J. et al., 2010. Trypsin inhibitors with antiproliferative activity toward leukemia cells from Phaseolus vulgaris cv "White Cloud Bean". *J. Biomed. Biotech.* 2010: Article ID 219793.

48. Chan, Y.S. et al., 2014. A thermostable trypsin inhibitor with antiproliferative activity from small pinto beans. *J. Enzyme Inhib. Med. Chem.* 29(4): 485–490.

49. Ma, D.Z. et al., 2010. A storage protein-like trypsin inhibitor from the moth bean (Phaseolus acutifolius) with antiproliferative activity toward lymphoma cells. *Protein & Peptide Lett.* 17(6): 782–788.

50. Wang, S.Y. et al., 2011. Limlin, a novel leguminous peroxidase with antifungal activity from Phaseolus limensis. *J. Food Biochem.* 35(4): 1206–1222.

28. CORN

Blé   Mais   Maiz

玉米 トウモロコシ 옥수수

Zea mays

Gramineae

Corn is the seed of an herbaceous plant *Zea mays* L. (Gramineae), which was domesticated in Central America as a major cultivated grain crop for American Indians. After the fifteenth century, corn was spread to Europe and Asia. Now, corn is one of people's favorable health foods for having good contents of vitamins B5, B1, B5, B9, and C. Corn oil is one of the common vegetable oils mainly utilized for cooking. Besides its consumption as a fresh food, dried corn is a very important source for the food industry, industrial production of starch, and fermentative material in pharmaceuticals. It is sometimes used as a carrier for drug formulation. In China, other portions of corn such as leaves, flowers, corncob, cornsilk, cornstalk, and cornhusk are still useful for Chinese folk medicines.

SCIENTIFIC EVIDENCE OF CANCER-INHIBITORY AND CANCER-PREVENTIVE COMPONENTS

1. Activity of corn oil

Corn oil is rich in 18:2 *n*-6 fatty acids. Diet plus 6% of corn oil to mice-implanted lung alveolar carcinoma resulted in a higher count of apoptosis, an increase of lipoxygenase (LOX), and a decrease of cyclooxygenase (COX). After the treatment, arachidonic acid and eicosanoids have been found in high levels in tumor cells, implying the fatty acids were involved in the induction of tumor cell apoptosis.[1] However, the *n*-6 fatty acids-rich corn oil had been reported to promote the formation of preneoplastic lesions in rat hepatocellular carcinogenesis caused by an oncogene, diethylnitrosamine (DEN).[2]

2. Anticancer activity of corn seeds

Corn tortillas, which were processed with lime-cooked blue, red, yellow, and white corn grains, were administered into the diet (27% wt/wt) of male Sprague–Dawley rats preinoculated with 1,2-dimethylhydrazine (a colon carcinogen). The corn tortillas, particularly made of white and blue corn, significantly lessened the incidences of adenocarcinoma by ~77.5%. Simultaneously, the corn tortillas restrained β-glucuronidase activity, downregulation of two most important proliferative proteins (K-ras and β-catenin), and stimulated detoxifying enzymes in the liver and colon.[3] The results indicated that the consumption of corn and corn products may have a potential for cancer prevention.

3. Anticancer activity of corn silk

The tested corn silks were derived from six cultivars of corn (Denghai6702, Delinong988, Tunyu808, Zhongdan909, Liangyu208, and Jingke968) in China. In a panel of *in vitro* assays, Zhongdan909 corn silk possessing the highest total phenolic content exerted the highest DPPH radical-scavenging activity and strongest cytotoxicity against human MCF-7 breast carcinoma cells.[4] Different concentrations of corn tassel extracts (CTTs) inhibited the proliferation of human MGC-803 gastric adenocarcinoma cells in a dose-dependent manner, concomitant with remarkable antioxidant and antigenotoxic activities.[5]

4. Anticancer activity of corncob

Incubation of corncob with the fungus *Pleurotus ostreatus* could increase the dietary fiber content up to 78%. The fermented corncob fiber could significantly diminish the incidence of colon carcinogenesis caused by DMH in rats, accompanied with the promotion of apoptotic death and the activation of proliferating cell nuclear antigen (PCNA) and p53.[6] When the protein- and starch-removed corncob was hydrolyzed partially by xylanase, the degraded hemicellulose also demonstrated anti-colon neoplastic activity in mice.[7]

SCIENTIFIC EVIDENCE OF CANCER-INHIBITORY AND CANCER-PREVENTIVE CONSTITUENTS

1. Alkaloids

Several antitumor and anticarcinogenic components were discovered from corn and corn oil. Methyl-substituted diindolylmethanes (DIM, **1**) prepared from corn oil exhibited significant suppressive effects against the formation and growth of human T47D breast carcinoma caused by estrogen *in vivo* without any changes in organ/body weight and/or histopathology. Of them, the most bioactive DIMs are 1,1′-, 2,2′-, or 5,5′-dimethyl-DIMs and 1,1′, 2,2′-tetramethyl-DIM. Administration of the DIM (**1**) analogs (by gavage in corn oil) at a dose of 1 mg/kg/day for 10 days caused antitumorigenic effect in rat mammary tumor model induced by 7,12-dimethylbenz[a]anthracene (DMBA), the effect of which was correlated with selective blockage of hydrocarbon receptor (AhR)-estrogen cross talk.[8] Several hydroxylcinnamic acid derivatives were isolated from corn bran. One of them, diferuloylputrescine (**2**, DFP) dose-dependently exerted the strongest cytotoxic and proapoptotic effects on human U937 leukemic monocyte lymphoma cells. The DFP-induced apoptosis was associated with downregulation of antiapoptotic proteins (XIAP and cIAP2, Bcl-2, and Mcl-1), release of cytochrome c, and activation of caspase-3.[9]

2. Pigments

Maize yellow pigment (MYP) was extracted from corn protein powder. MYP in the *in vitro* experiments specifically inhibited the viability of human MDA-MB-231 (breast), PC3 (prostate), ES-2 (clear cell ovary), and A549 (lung) cancer cell lines, especially on ES-2 cells. At 100 μg/mL concentration, MYP could induce apoptosis, arrest cell cycle at the G1 stage, and hamper the cell proliferation and migration of ES-2 cells.[10] SBCP was a pigment derived from super black glutinous corncob, which showed inhibitory effect on the proliferation of human BEL-7402 (liver) and SGC-7901 (stomach) cancer cell lines *in vitro*, though the potencies were low (IC_{50}s 4.13 and 3.83 mg/mL). SBCP also showed obvious antioxidant effect for scavenging radicals.[11] Zeaxanthin, one of the most common carotenoid alcohols found in nature, was derived from corn gluten meal as well. It obviously suppressed the growth curve of human KB oral squamous carcinoma cells at a concentration of 20 μM and disturbed the KB cell-cycle progression in addition to its eye-improving function.[12]

3. Flavonoid

Maysin (**3**), as a major flavonoid in corn silk, was isolated from a Korean hybrid corn (Kwangpyeongok). Maysin (**3**) dose-dependently reduced the viability of human PC3 prostate cancer cells by 87% at a concentration of 200 μg/mL and significantly induced cell apoptosis via stimulation of a mitochondria-dependent pathway and attenuation of Akt and ERK phosphorylation. A combined treatment with maysin and anticancer agents, such as etoposide, 5-FU, cisplatin, and camptothecin, synergistically enhanced the PC3 cell death. More findings revealed a strong therapeutic potential of maysin (**3**) for treatment of either chemoresistant or androgen-independent human prostate carcinoma.[13] In addition, pretreatment with maysin (**3**) suppressed H_2O_2-induced apoptosis and DNA damage in human neuroblastoma SK-N-MC cells, the effect of which was associated with diminishing oxidative stress via (1) dose-dependent reduction of intracellular ROS level and (2) dose-dependent increases of mRNA levels of antioxidant enzymes (CAT, SOD-1, SOD-2, GPx-1, and HO-1) and restraining PARP cleavage, leading to the neuroprotection from the risk of cancer.[14]

4. Glycoprotein

A glycoprotein (m.w. 30×10^4) obtained from corn displayed some cancer prevention-related multiple biological activities including interferon-inducing, B-cell-activating, IgE production-inhibiting, macrophage-activating, mitogenic, antitumor, and immunostimulating effects in experimental animals.[15]

5. Peptides

Corn peptides (CP) were prepared from corn gluten meal by proteolysis with alkali protease. Dietary 10% CP for 10 weeks markedly lowered the incidence of mammary tumor progression induced by DMBA in female rats together with obvious reduction of total number and total weight of tumors.[16] *In vitro* assay showed that CP elicited apoptosis of HepG2 hepatoma cells via increase of intracellular Ca^{2+} concentration and chromatin condensation and accumulation of cytoplasmic condensation. I.p. injection of the CP at different dosages to mice for 10 days significantly suppressed the growth of H22 murine hepatoma cells. Concurrently, the CP augmented the spleen index and improved SOD activity in serum and MDA content in the liver of H22-bearing mice.[17] Therefore, the corn peptides can be considered a safe and effective antitumor and anticarcinogenic agent for cancer prevention.

6. Polysaccharides

A water-extracted polysaccharide from corn bran showed an obvious suppressive effect on the proliferation of HT-29 human colon cancer cells in a dose-dependent manner *in vitro*. At a 0.02 g/L concentration for 48 h, its suppressive rate reached 60.62%.[18] Corn pectic polysaccharide (COPP) is an arabinogalactan with methyl/ethyl esters that is composed of 54% galactose, 20% arabinose, 4% mannose, 3% xylose, 1% rhamnose, and 10% uronic acid. COPP at 20 μg/mL effectively obstructed the growth of B16F10 melanoma cells by 60%, hindered cell invasion by 63% via inhibition of galectin-3 activity, and diminished cell adhesion by 65% in the *in vitro* assays.[19] The antimetastatic activity of COPP has been proven in an *in vivo* mouse model-implanted B16F10 melanoma. Administration of COPP 200 mg/kg per mouse as basal diet for 21 days resulted in significant suppression of the lung tumor nodule formation, representing 75% reduction in metastatic nodules. The anti-invasive and antimetastatic effect of COPP was largely mediated by downregulation of MMPs-2 and -9 expressions.[19] Xylooligosaccharides (XOS) derived from corncob demonstrated protective effect on DMH-induced colon cancer in rats. Dietary XOS alleviated the incidence and multiplicity of ACF formation in the colon of DMH-treated animals *in vivo*, concomitant with the amelioration of lipid peroxidation and stimulation of glutathione-S-transferase and catalase activities in colonic mucosa and liver, whose interactions might contribute to deterring colon carcinogenesis.[20]

Corn silk polysaccharides (CSP) possess multiple biological potentials, including antitumor and immunoelevating activities. In a mouse model with H22 hepatocarcinoma, CSP at a dose of 50 mg/kg for 10 days not only obstructed the tumor growth by 47.44% and extended the survival time of tumor-bearing mice but also augmented the body weight, peripheral white blood cell (WBC) count, thymus and spleen indexes, and serum cytokine production. When the dose was increased to 200 g/kg for 60 days, the CSP prolonged the survival time of ascites H22-bearing mice by three times more than that of the model control group,[21] effect of which was associated with the promotion of serum hemolysin level, carbon particle clearance rate, and IL-2 and TNF-α contents.[22] After combined CSP with cyclophosphamide (CP), the tumor-inhibitory ratio was enhanced to 68.71%, and the survival time of ascites tumor-burdened mice was significantly extended to 72.07% compared with the CP group. Simultaneously, thymus and spleen indexes, WBC, and nucleated cells of marrow, which all were decreased by CP, were ameliorated significantly and the levels of ALT and AST, which were increased by CP, were reduced, leading to a synergetic anticancer effect and an attenuated toxic effect.[23] The findings indicated that CSP is a safe and effective component for the treatment of hepatoma, the cancer inhibitory effect of which are achieved by regulating immune function of tumor-bearing mice.

CONCLUSION AND SUGGESTION

The experimental investigations disclosed the potential of corn in the inhibition of cancer cells and the prevention of carcinogenesis in addition to its nutritional values. Some small molecules (such as alkaloids and pigments) and macromolecules (such as glycoproteins, peptides, and polysaccharides) were demonstrated to be responsible for the moderate-to-weak properties of corn in the suppression of cancer-cell proliferation, invasion, and adhesion. These evidences suggested that dietary corn may help humans safely prevent certain carcinogenesis to lower the risk of cancer.

REFERENCES

1. Pasqualini, M.E. et al., 2005. Dietary lipids modulate eicosanoid release and apoptosis of cells of a murine lung alveolar carcinoma. *Prostaglandins, Leukot Essent Fatty Acids* 72: 235–240.
2. Kim, S. et al., 2005. Effects of dietary levels of corn and tuna oils on the formation of preneoplastic lesions in rat hepatocellular carcinogenesis. *Hanguk Yongyang Hakhoechi* 38: 20–29.
3. Reynoso-Camacho, R. et al., 2015. Anticarcinogenic effect of corn tortilla against 1,2-dimethylhydrazine (DMH)-induced colon carcinogenesis in Sprague-Dawley rats. *Plant Foods Hum Nutr* (NY, NY, USA) 70: 146–152.
4. Tian, J.G. et al., 2013. Comparative studies on the constituents, antioxidant and anticancer activities of extracts from different varieties of corn silk. *Food Function* 4: 1526–1534.
5. Wang, L.C. et al., 2014. Antioxidant and antigenotoxic activity of bioactive extracts from corn tassel. *J. Huazhong Univ. Sci./Technol, Med. Sci* 34: 131–136.
6. Zusman, I. et al., 1997. Role of apoptosis, proliferating cell nuclear antigen and p53 protein in chemically induced colon cancer in rats fed corncob fiber treated with the fungus Pleurotus ostreatus. *Anticancer Res.* 17: 2105–2113.
7. Takeuchi, M. et al., 2002. Antitumor agents from maize rind extracts. Japanese Kokai Tokkyo Koho JP 2001-143025.
8. McDougal, A. et al., 2001. Methyl-substituted diindolylmethanes as inhibitors of estrogen-induced growth of T47D cells and mammary tumors in rats. *Breast Cancer Res. Treat.* 66: 147–157.
9. Kim, E.-O. et al., 2014. Diferuloylputrescine, a predominant phenolic amide in corn bran, potently induces apoptosis in human leukemia U937 cells. *J. Med. Food* 17: 519–526.

10. Li, X.L. et al., 2014. Effect of maize yellow pigment on invasion, migration, proliferation and cell cycle of ovarian carcinoma cell line ES-2. *Xiandai Shipin Keji* 30: 1–5.
11. Ran, Y.X. et al., 2012. Anticancer effect and antioxidant activity of super black glutinous corncob pigment. *Anhui Shifan Daxue Xuebao, Ziran Kexueban* 35: 351–354, 359.
12. Sun, Z. et al., 2005. Inhibitory effects of zeaxanthin from corn gluten meal on human oral squamous cell carcinoma. *Shipin Yu Shengwu Jishu Xuebao* 24: 34–7.
13. Lee, J.S. et al., 2014. Corn silk maysin induces apoptotic cell death in PC3 prostate cancer cells via mitochondria-dependent pathway. *Life Sci.* 119: 47–55.
14. Choi, D.J. et al., 2014. Neuroprotective effects of corn silk maysin via inhibition of H2O2-induced apoptotic cell death in SK-N-MC cells. *Life Sci.* 109: 57–64.
15. Kojima, Y. et al., 1987. Interferon-inducing glycoprotein from *Zea mays* and pharmaceutical containing the substance. Japanese Kokai Tokkyo Koho 13 pp, JP 85-157843.
16. Yamaguchi, M. et al., 1997. Inhibitory effect of peptide prepared from corn gluten meal on 7,12-dimethylbenz[a]anthracene-induced mammary tumor progression in rats. *Nutr. Res.* (NY, USA) 17: 1121–1130.
17. Li, J.T. et al., 2013. Antitumor activity of corn peptides in vitro and in vivo. *Shipin Kexue* (Beijing, China) 34: 223–227.
18. Xu, W.L. et al., 2015. Inhibition effect of proliferation on human cancer HT-29 cells by polysaccharides extracted from corn bran. *Harbin Gongye Daxue Xuebao* 47: 62–66.
19. Jayaram, S. et al., 2015. Pectic polysaccharide from corn (Zea mays L.) effectively inhibited multi-step mediated cancer cell growth and metastasis. *Chemico-Biological Interactions* 235: 63–75.
20. Aachary, A.A. et al., 2015. Protective effect of xylooligosaccharides from corncob on 1,2-dimethylhydrazine induced colon cancer in rats. *Bioact. Carbohydr. Dietary Fibre* 5: 146–1452.
21. Yang, J.Y. et al., 2014. Anti-hepatoma activity and mechanism of corn silk polysaccharides in H22 tumor-bearing mice. *Int. J. Biol. Macromol.* 64: 276–280.
22. Wu, X.C. et al., 2015. Effects of polysaccharides extracts from corn silk on growth of H22 liver cancer and immune function. *Huaxi Yaoxue Zazhi* 30: 26–29.
23. Wu, X.C. et al., 2014. Protective effect of polysaccharides extracts from corn silk against cyclophosphamide induced host damages in mice bearing H22 tumors. *Zhongyaocai* 37: 1833–1836.

29. FOXTAIL MILLET

Miller   Hirse   Mijo

小米 キビ 기장

Setaria italica

Poaceae

Foxtail millet (*Setaria italica*) is one of the oldest grains of the semiarid tropics, subtropics, and south temperate regions. The first cultivation of foxtail millet occurred in China since about 8000 years ago, had been the most important food source in ancient north China, and still is a major food staple grain growing in the regions of hot and dry climates, such as in northern Africa and parts of northern China. The millet is a gluten-free grain with rich vitamin B1 and phosphorus, also affording a good source of iron, manganese, and tryptophan. Due to the well-balanced amino-acid profile in millet protein, and the special nature of its carbohydrates and high content of fiber, dietary millet may slowly release glucose in the bloodstream during digestion, reducing the level of blood cholesterol and preventing constipation. It is especially available for heart, gastric, and diabetic patients because of its least allergenic and easily digestible nature. As a healthier diet, it has been increasing in popularity in Europe and North America in recent years, though it is used largely for cattle and bird feed.

SCIENTIFIC EVIDENCE OF CANCER-PREVENTIVE CONSTITUENTS

Besides millet grain as a nutritional food in its growing areas, millet bran has been used extensively as an animal feed for long time, which is obtained in the millet-decladding process as a by-product. However, the *in vitro* experiments in recent years interestingly disclosed that the polyphenols and a peroxidase protein extracted from both millet grain and bran showed antiproliferative and proapoptotic effects against human neoplastic cell lines. However, these bioactive components are in much higher content and with more potent functions in millet bran.

1. Polyphenols

A bound polyphenol component (BPIS) was extracted by ethyl acetate from the inner shell of millet bran after the removal of soluble-free polyphenols by using 80% acetone. *In vitro* assay showed that BPIS hindered the proliferation and the clonogenic survival of human HepG2 (liver), HeLa (cervix), MCF-7 (breast), and HCT-116 (colon) carcinoma cell lines. After long-term exposure to BPIS, cell apoptosis would be observed.[1] The proapoptotic activity in HCT-116 cells was mainly mediated by promoting reactive oxygen species (ROS) generation, activation of mitochondria-mediated intrinsic pathways, and blockage of the NF-κB signaling pathway downstream of ROS. The anticolon cancer effect was further proved in a nude mice model-implanted HCT-116 tumor.[2] In addition, the bound polyphenols of millet bran also exhibit higher activities, including antioxidant, immunomodulation, antifungal, and antihyperglycemic effects.

2. Peroxidase protein

FMBP, a highly homologous peroxidase protein (35 kDa) with cancer-cell proliferation inhibitory activity was purified from foxtail millet bran, the yield of which was 16.87 μg/100 mg of dry foxtail millet bran. Three human colon cancer cell lines (HT-29, DLD1, and SW480) and cervical cancer cells (HeLa) have been assayed for FMBP in *in vitro* models, resulting in the antiproliferative effect with IC_{50}s of 0.10–0.13 mg/mL. Notably, FMBP showed lower toxicity in human normal HL-7702 liver cells and FHC colon epithelial cells (IC_{50}s of 0.65–0.72 mg/mL). The suppressive effect of FMBP against colon cancer cell growth was associated with the induction of G1 phase arrest and caspase-dependent apoptosis. The proapoptotic mechanism was revealed to be correlated with the accumulation of ROS via blockage of STAT3 signaling pathway, loss of mitochondrial transmembrane potential, activation of caspases-8 and -3, downregulation of NF-E2-related factor 2 (Nrf2) expression, and decline of catalase activity and glutathione content. *In vivo* antitumor tests evidenced that FMBP was able to inhibit xenografted DLD1 cell tumor growth in nude mice.[3–5] FMBP also displayed antimigration effect on human DLD1 colon carcinoma cells together with deterring JAK1 phosphorylation and its downstream STAT3 signaling and antagonizing epithelial–mesenchymal transition (EMT) via downregulation of c-Myc and Snail1 expressions.[6] The findings established that the millet bran-derived peroxidase has both therapeutic and preventive potentials in the inhibition of certain carcinomas and carcinogenesis, especially colon neoplasm.

OTHER BIOACTIVITIES

The bound polyphenols usually possess higher antioxidant and radical-scavenging capacities compared to free polyphenols. The bound polyphenols from foxtail millet bran are also responsible for antidiabetic and antihypertensive properties.

CONCLUSION AND SUGGESTION

These interesting findings released the new value of foxtail millet bran in cancer prevention and in particular discovered the millet-derived active components, bound polyphenols and peroxidase protein, playing important roles in colon cancer prevention and suppression. Significantly, these evidences have provided more support of further investigations of foxtail millet grain and of the development of inedible foxtail millet bran to produce a dietary supplement, exerting the cancer risk lowering and antioxidant benefits.

REFERENCES

1. Shi, J.Y. et al., 2015. Inhibitory effects of bound polyphenols from foxtail millet bran on proliferation of four tumor cell lines. *Yingyang Xuebao* 37: 178–184.
2. Shi, J.Y. et al., 2015. Bound polyphenol from foxtail millet bran induces apoptosis in HCT-116 cell through ROS generation. *J. Functional Foods* 17: 958–968.
3. Shan, S.H. et al., 2013. Isolation and purification of a protein from foxtail millet bran and its anti-proliferation activities against cancer cells. *Shipin Kexue* (Beijing, China) 34: 296–300.
4. Shan, S.H. et al., 2014. A novel protein extracted from foxtail millet bran displays anti-carcinogenic effects in human colon cancer cells. *Toxicol. Lett.* 227: 129–138.
5. Shan, S.H. et al., 2015. Targeted anti-colon cancer activities of a millet bran-derived peroxidase were mediated by elevated ROS generation. *Food & Function* 6: 2331–2338.
6. Shan, S.H. et al., 2014. A millet bran-derived peroxidase inhibits cell migration by antagonizing STAT3-mediated epithelial-mesenchymal transition in human colon cancer. *J. Functional Foods* 10: 444–455.

30. MUNG BEAN

Haricot mungo   Mungbohne   Frijol mungo

绿豆   サヤインゲン   녹두

Vigna radiata (= *Phaseolus radiatus*)

Leguminosae

Mung bean is the dried seed of a Leguminosae plant *Vigna radiata* (= *Phaseolus radiatus*). Its seeds are one of the common food crops in Eastern Asia and its sprouts are widely used traditionally as a vegetable for fresh salad and sauté in East Asia. It is now known that mung beans contain abundant nutrients with various biological activities. Mung bean affords excellent sources of vitamins B9, B1, B5, and other B-vitamins and minerals (iron, magnesium, manganese, and phosphorus). In pharmacological investigations, mung bean exerted antiatheroschlerosis and hypolipidemic effects. In the past few decades, many types of constituents have been isolated from mung bean and its sprouts, such as flavonoids, phenolic acids, organic acids, amino acids, carbohydrates, and lipids. Especially, the sprouts of mung bean have gained more recognition owing to their marked biological activities, including antioxidant, anti-inflammatory, antidiabetic, antihypertensive, anti-hyperlipidemia, antimicrobial, and antitumor effects.

SCIENTIFIC EVIDENCE OF CANCER-INHIBITORY AND CANCER-PREVENTIVE ACTIVITIES

Mung bean contains various nutrients and phytochemicals that play various health-promoting functions. A boiling water extract of mung beans showed antitumor-promoter and alkyl peroxide radical-scavenging activities. It restrained the tumor-promoting potential of EBV/B-lymphocyte system *in vitro* and hindered the carcinogenesis of oxygen-related radicals, whereas its cold-water extract showed activities > 90% lower than its hot-water extract.[1,2] Dietary mung bean powder given to mice markedly obstructed the reaction of sodium nitrite with morphine, the reaction of which was known to correlate with carcinogenesis in lung and liver, and the powder also reduced the number and size of the carcinomas in initial stages.[3] All extracts from the seeds and its sprouts displayed certain antiproliferative activity on human Calu-6 (lung) and SNU-601 (stomach) cancer cells *in vitro*, but the sprout extracts, especially the sprouts ethyl acetate (EtOAc) extract, presented relatively higher activity than the seed extracts.[4] Interestingly, the sprouts extract could dose- and time-dependently promote the apoptosis of HepG2 hepatoma and HeLa cervical cancer cells and caused G0/G1 cell-cycle arrest in HeLa cells and G0 arrest in HepG2 cells. Concurrently, the expressions of CDK inhibitors (such as p21, p53, and p27) were upregulated in the HeLa cells, but only p53 was activated in the HepG2 cells after the treatment. The levels of two anticancer cytokines (TNF-α and IFN-β) were increased in both the cell lines, and two immunological cytokines (IL-4 and IFN-γ) were also affected by the extract, then leading to triggering cell-mediated immunity and cellular cytotoxicity.[5] A 70% acidic acetone extract of mung beans exerted antiproliferative effects against various human cancer cells such as HepG2 (liver), SW480 and Caco (colon), HL-60 (leukemic), AGS (stomach), SKOV3 (ovary), CAL27 (tongue), and MCF-7 (breast) lines with IC_{50}s of 0.36–0.86 mg/mL but DU145 prostate cancer cells were relatively less sensitive to the extract (IC_{50} of 1.98 mg/mL) in addition to the radical-scavenging activity.[6] On the basis of many pharmaceutical evidences, it is clear that a group of bioactive flavonoids and phenolics (such as chlorogenic acid, neohesperidin, vanillin, vanillic acid, gallic acid, shikimic acid, rhamnetin, kaempferol, and rutin) in common vegetables play a remarkable role in the radical-scavenging effect. Some of these valuable compounds were shown in the hot-water extracts of mung bean sprouts and mung bean in higher percentages.[7,8] Vitexin and isovitexin were found to be the major constituents having antioxidant property in the mung bean.[8]

Significantly, mung beans are composed of about 20%–24% protein, and globulin and albumin are the major storage proteins found in mung bean seeds. The bean sprouts are a rich source of phenylalanine ammonium-lyase (PAA), and a nuclease (PhA). The PAA-lyase demonstrated dose- and time-dependent suppressive effect against the growth of mouse L1210 leukemia cells. The PhA nuclease displayed significant antitumor effect on human ML-2 melanoma cells after intratumoral or i.p. administration into athymic mice, but was almost noneffective in the ML-2 cells *in vitro*.[9,10] A novel protease inhibitor termed mungoin (10 kDa) was isolated from the mung bean seeds, which was proved to possess antiproliferative activity toward tumor cells and antifungal and antibacterial properties.[11] MPH, a hydrolysate of mung bean protein derived from tropic hydrolysis exhibited antioxidant capacity. It could act as a carrier to deliver the anticancer efficacy of asiatic acid (a pentacyclic triterpene) against HepG2 hepatoblastoma.[12] A Bowman–Birk trypsin inhibitor (BBI) extracted from mung bean could hinder the proliferation of human nonsmall cell lung adenocarcinoma cells *in vitro*, associated with the induction of cell apoptosis and caspase-3 activation.[13] Likewise, some mung bean trypsin inhibitor fragments (e.g., LysGP33 and GST-LysGP33) were found to have potential in the inhibition of metastasis and proliferation of human SW480 colon cancer cells.[14] Due to their cytotoxicity and high efficiency, these macromolecules in mung bean appear to have some biological potentials, including tumor cytostatics.

Two acid heteropolysaccharides labeled as MP1 and MP2 were isolated from an extract of mung bean water. MP1 (83 kDa) was mainly composed of mannose with 9.9% uronic acid, whereas MP2 (45 kDa) consisted of rhamnose and galactose with 36.4% uronic acid. In the antioxidant assays, MP1 exhibited higher reduction power and stronger DPPH radical-scavenging capacities and MP2 had higher hydroxyl radical-scavenging activity. In addition, MP1 showed greater inhibition against self-oxidation of 1,2,3-phentriol than MP2.[14]

CONCLUSION AND SUGGESTION

From these research results, it is demonstrated that mung beans and sprouts contain high levels of nutritive and functional components. Both, particularly mung bean sprouts, can play multiple roles in the anticarcinogenesis-related actions such as antiproliferation, DPPH radical scavenging, immunoenhancing, and tyrosinase and alcohol dehydrogenase (ADH)-inhibiting effects, leading to lessening of the incidence of certain carcinogenesis such as in stomach, liver, lung, and cervix and for the protection of liver and kidney. The anticarcinogenic and antioxidant activities of mung bean and its sprouts were primarily contributed by their constituents such as polyphenolic and some special enzymes/proteins. The mung-seed sprouting process usually augments the suppressive potencies against cancer and oxidation. According to these evidences, mung beans and sprouts are recommended as excellent nutritional and functional foods defined for lowering the risk of carcinomas and exerting health-promoting effects. As mung bean sprouts showed more health-promoting effects, in addition to nutritive value, the sprouting of seeds are paid more attention in western countries today as a superior functional food.

OTHER BIOACTIVITIES OF THE COMPONENTS

The PhA nuclease in mung bean also exhibited low immunosuppressive activity on human lymphocyte but strong aspermatogenic effect on the width of spermatogenic layers.

REFERENCES

1. Maeda, H. et al., 1992. High correlation between lipid peroxide radical and tumor-promoter effect: Suppression of tumor promotion in the Epstein-Barr virus/B-lymphocyte system and scavenging of alkyl peroxide radicals by various vegetable extracts. *Jpn. J. Cancer Res.: Gann* 83: 923–928.
2. Sawa, T. et al., 1999. Alkylperoxyl radical-scavenging activity of various flavonoids and other phenolic compounds: Implications for the anti-tumor-promoter effect of vegetables. *J. Agricul. Food Chem.* 47: 397–402.

3. Chen, H.Y. et al., 1989. Preventive effect of mungbean on tumorigensis in experimental mice. *Diyi Junyi Daxue Xuebao* 9: 231–234.

4. Kim, D.K. et al., 2012. Total polyphenols, antioxidant and antiproliferative activities of different extracts in mungbean seeds and sprouts. *Plant Foods Hum. Nutr.* 67: 71–75.

5. Hafidh, R.R. et al., 2012. Novel molecular, cytotoxical, and immunological study on promising and selective anticancer activity of Mung bean sprouts. *BMC Complem. Altern. Med.* 12: 208.

6. Xu, B. et al., 2012. Comparative study on antiproliferation properties and cellular antioxidant activities of commonly consumed food legumes against nine human cancer cells. *Food Chem.* 134(3): 1287–1296.

7. Sawa, T. et al., 1999. Alkylperoxyl radical-scavenging activity of various flavonoids and other phenolic compounds: Implications for the antitumor-promoter effect of vegetables. *J. Agricul. Food Chem.* 47: 397–402.

8. Cao, D. et al., 2011. Antioxidant properties of the mungbean flavonoids on alleviating heat stress. *PLoS One* 6: e21070.

9. Niu, S.Y. et al., 1992. Isolation and purification of phenylalanine ammonium-lyase from Mung bean and its antitumor activity. *J. Lanzhou Med. College* 18: 148–151.

10. Soucek, J. et al., 2006. Mung bean sprout (Phaseolus radiatus) nuclease and its biological and antitumor effects. *Neoplasma* 53: 402–409.

11. Wang, S.Y. et al., 2006. Isolation and characterization of a novel mung bean protease inhibitor with anti-pathogenic and anti-proliferative activities. *Peptides* 27: 3129–3136.

12. Wongekalak, L.D. et al., 2011. Potential use of antioxidative mungbean protein hydrolysate as an anti-cancer asiatic acid carrier. *Food Res. Intl.* 44: 812–817.

13. Wang, S.S. et al., 2013. Apoptosis of human lung adenocarcinoma cell line A549 induced by mung bean trypsin inhibitor BBI. *Huanan Shifan Daxue Xuebao, Ziran Kexueban* 45: 91–94.

14. Tang, D.Y. et al., 2014. A review of phytochemistry, metabolite changes, and medicinal uses of the common food mung bean and its sprouts (Vigna radiata). *Chem. Central J.* 8: 4/1–4/9.

31. OAT

Avoine   Hafer   Avena

燕麥   エンバク   귀리

Avena sativa

Poaceae

1. $R_1 = R_2 = -H$
2. $R_1 = -OCH_3$, $R_2 = -H$
3. $R_1 = -OH$, $R_2 = -H$
4. $R_1 = -OH$, $R_2 = -CH_3$

Oat is the seeds of a species of cereal grain (*Avena sativa*). Since ancient times, oats have been commonly used as foods for humans and livestock, and are usually presented as oatmeal and rolled oats in food markets. As one of the important dietary staples for the people in many countries, oats are now cultivated over the world to form several varieties. Oats are rich in proteins, dietary fiber, carbohydrates, vitamin B complex, and are a source of dietary minerals (such as manganese, phosphorus, magnesium, calcium, and potassium). Due to high nutritional values, oats have received considerable attention for producing a variety of oat-based food products such as breads, cookies, breakfast cereals, biscuits, flakes, probiotic drinks, and infant food. Oats were also revealed to contain various phytochemicals such as avenanthramides, flavonoids, flavonolignans, triterpenoid saponins, sterols, tocols, and β-glucan. Oats have been traditionally considered as stimulant, antispasmodic, antitumor, diuretic, and neurotonic. Modern studies further showed that dietary intake of oats is beneficial for the induction of cholesterol-lowering, anti-inflammatory, wound healing, antioxidant, anticolon cancer, immunomodulatory, nerve restorative, and antidiabetic activities. Oats are recently suggested to be a suitable diet for celiac patients.[1]

SCIENTIFIC EVIDENCE OF CANCER-PREVENTIVE CONSTITUENTS

The chemopreventive activity of oats was demonstrated in two *in vivo* experiments. Whole oat diets in middle and high doses notably lessened 1,2-dimethylhydrazine- and dextran sodium sulfate-triggered ACF and colon tumors in an inflammation-related mouse colon cancer model, and in the same doses reduced the tumor volumes by 17%–43% and the tumor weights by 38%–54% in nude mice-implanted human colon carcinoma.[2] The findings revealed the property of oats in suppression of colon cancer development and recommended oats as a daily nutrient and health-promoting food for cancer chemoprevention. The oat phytochemicals such as β-glucan, avenanthramides, and polyphenols have been found to be responsible for fighting the risk of cancer.

1. β-Glucan

Oat β-glucan is composed of D-glucose only with β-1,3 and β-1,4 linkages and its molecular weight is in a range of $1.56–6.87 \times 10^5$ g/mol.[3] The broken β-1,3-glucan unit is soluble and flexible but the broken β-1,4-glucan unit is insoluble and indigestible. The (1,3)(1,4)-β-D-glucan from oat after 24 h incubation with human melanoma HTB-140 cells resulted in the elicitation of cell apoptosis and cell-cycle arrest at the G1 phase through a dose-dependent activation of caspases-3, -7, and appearance of phosphatidylserine on the external surface of cellular membranes, leading to the suppressive effect on HTB-140 cells with LD_{50} of 194.6 μg/mL.[4] Low molecular weight oat (1,3)

(1,4)-β-glucan (LMW β-glucan) has high water solubility and low viscosity. Treatment with LMW β-glucan in a concentration of 400 μg/mL for 5 days attenuated the viabilities of human A431 epidermoid carcinoma cells by 51% and human Me45 pigmented malignant melanoma cells by 53%.[5] Feeding soluble oat fiber β-glucan (OβG) contained drinking water plus moderate exercise for 10 days diminished lung tumor foci from B16 melanoma cells and enhanced the cytotoxic effect of macrophages in mice, implying that the OβG has an ability to retard lung metastatic spread from melanoma, the effect of which can be mediated, in part, by enhanced macrophage cytotoxicity.[6] All these data evidenced that oat β-glucan showed a potential in the treatment of human dermal carcinomas. Research further pointed out that the molecular weight of β-glucan in a range of $2.42–1.61 \times 10^5$ g/mol is optimum for both the hypocholesterolemic and antitumor activities *in vitro*, MW range of which was the most water soluble.[3]

2. Protein-bound polysaccharide

Two Korean patents reported that protein-bound polysaccharides derived from oat powder could inhibit the growth of large-intestine tumor and ascites tumor.[7,8]

3. Lunasin

Lunasin is a unique peptide with 43 amino acids, which has been isolated from oat-containing cereals and soybean. Both *in vitro* and *in vivo* investigations demonstrated the chemopreventive activities of lunasin. Treatment with the lunasin obviously restrained the foci formation of mouse C3H10T1/2 fibroblasts cells induced by DMBA and MCA (two chemical carcinogens) at nanomolar concentrations and retarded the colony formation of NIH3T3 cells, effect of which was 4-fold more effective than Bowman–Birk inhibitor, a known cancer-preventive agent from soy. Lunasin was also capable of preventing viral oncogenes-induced transformation of mammalian cells, dose-dependently inhibiting an oncogene E1A-elicited foci formation of C3H and NIH3T3 tumors, and repressing ras-oncogene-caused colony formation of MCF-7 cells. In an *in vivo* mouse model, dermal administration of lunasin in a dose of 250 μg per week resulted in 70% reduction of skin tumor incidence caused by DMBA (a tumor initiator) and TPA (a tumor promoter) and then delayed the appearance of papilloma after 2 weeks' treatment. Lunasin also deterred the epidermal cell proliferation of mouse skin either in absence or presence of DMBA *in vivo*.[9,10] These evidences have proven the benefits of lunasin in the skin cancer prevention. It was also reported to have anti-inflammatory and cholesterol-reducing properties.

4. Avenanthramides

Avenanthramides (Avns) are unique polyphenolic alkaloids extracted from oats with anti-inflammatory property. Three Avns, (1) Avn-A (**1**), (2) Avn-B (**2**), and (3) Avn-C (**3**), and a methylated derivative (Me-Avn-C, **4**) in an *in vitro* model hindered the proliferation of COX-2-positive HT-29, Caco-2, and LS174T human colon cancer cell lines and COX-2-negative HCT-116 human colon cancer cells, wherein Me-Avn-C (**4**) was the most potent. But these Avns exerted no effect on the cell viability of confluence-induced differentiated Caco-2 cells. The findings indicated that the cancer risk-reducing effect of oats and oat bran is contributed by not only the high fiber content but also by the Avns.[11]

CONCLUSION AND SUGGESTION

These scientific observations demonstrated that the major constituents in oats are Avns, β-glucan, and lunasin, which can contribute to cancer prevention synergically. The daily consumption of oats and oat products should be encouraged for safely lowering the risk of cancer in colon and skin, in addition to their nutritional advantages and biological benefits. Consequently, according to the favorable health attributes and functions of dietary oats and oat-based products, eating at least three servings of these grains every day would be an effective menu.

REFERENCES

1. Singh, R. et al., 2013. Avena sativa (Oat), a potential neutraceutical and therapeutic agent: An overview. *Critical Reviews in Food Sci. Nutr.* 53: 126–144.
2. Wang, H.C. et al., 2011. Inhibitory effect of whole oat on aberrant crypt foci formation and colon tumor growth in ICR and BALB/c mice. *J. Cereal Sci* 53: 73–77.
3. Kim, H.J. et al., 2011. Optimizing the molecular weight of oat β-glucan for in vitro bile acid binding and fermentation. *J. Agricul. Food Chem.* 59: 10322–10328.
4. Parzonko, A. et al., 2015. Pro-apoptotic properties of (1,3)(1,4)-β-D-glucan from Avena sativa on human melanoma HTB-140 cells in vitro. *Int. J. Biol. Macromol.* 72: 757–763.
5. Choromanska, A. et al., 2015. Anticancer properties of low molecular weight oat beta-glucan – An in vitro study. *Int. J. Biol. Macromol.* 2015. 80: 23–28.
6. Murphy, E.A. et al., 2004. Effects of moderate exercise and oat β-glucan on lung tumor metastases and macrophage antitumor cytotoxicity. *J. Applied Physiol.* 97: 955–959.
7. Kang, T.S. et al., 2005. Method for inhibiting large intestines tumor using oat protein-bound polysaccharide. Republic of Korean Kongkae Taeho Kongbo KR 2005112221 A 20051130.
8. Kang, T.S. et al., 2005. Method for inhibiting ascites tumor using oat protein-bound polysaccharide. Republic of Korean Kongkae Taeho Kongbo KR 2005112220 A 20051130.
9. Hernández-Ledesma, B. et al., 2008. Lunasin: A novel cancer preventive seed peptide. *Perspect Medicin Chem.* 2: 75–80.
10. Nakurte, I. et al., 2013. Detection of the lunasin peptide in oats (Avena sativa L). *J. Cereal Sci.* 57: 319–324.
11. Guo, W.M. et al., 2010. Avenanthramides inhibit proliferation of human colon cancer cell lines in vitro. *Nutr. cancer* 62: 1007–1016.

32. SOYBEAN

Soja   Sojabohne   La soja

黄豆/黑豆   大豆   콩

Glycine max

Leguminosae

3. $R_1 = R_2 = -H.$
4. $R_1 = -H, R_2 = -OH.$
5. $R_1 = -beta\text{-}D\text{-}glucose$
   $R_2 = -OH.$

Soybean is the dried seeds of an annual plant *Glycine max* native to East Asia, which has been used as a nutritional food for 5000 years. Today, soybean is an important source of cooking oil and vegetable protein as well as the primary ingredient in many processed foods and dairy substitutes worldwide. Nutritionally, soybean affords exceptional amounts of vitamins B9, B1, B2, phytoproteins, dietary fiber, and minerals such as iron, manganese, phosphorus, high contents of vitamin K, magnesium, and zinc, and is a good source of chlorine, potassium, and calcium. In chemical biology, soybean is rich in isoflavones, a valuable group of phytoestrogens that serves as estrogens in the body to play many protective functions and positive effects on metabolism, osteoporosis, menopausal symptoms, free-radical scavenging, atherosclerosis, and cardiovascular diseases. Pharmacological studies have proven that soybean and its isoflavones possess remarkable properties such as hypolipidemic, antiatheroschlerotic, lipotropic, hepatoprotective, antioxidant, anti-fatty liver, cardiac flow increasing, and antiaging activities. In addition, some soybean triterpenoid saponins exert an antivirus effect.

Soybean and its products highly represent the traditional East-Asian diet. Numerous epidemiological studies commended that East Asians (especially Chinese, Japanese, Korean, and Vietnamese) who consume traditional diets high in soybean products as well as unrefined grain products have low incidences of certain carcinomas, particularly steroid hormone-dependent, for example, breast and prostate carcinomas. According to the comparison of the related cancer rates between eastern Asia and western populations, soybean consumption is considered to have a capability to lower the hormone levels in breast, ovary, and prostate. Thus, in the past 20 years, soybean and its products have being paid extensive attention in cancer prevention, leading to numerous scientific investigations focused on the anticancer and anticarcinogenesis properties of soybean.[1]

Scientific Evidence of Antitumorigenic Activities

Antitumor activities of soybean: *In vitro* and *in vivo* studies demonstrated that dietary soybean hypocotyls are capable of hampering breast carcinogenesis induced by *N*-methyl-*n*-nitrosourea,[2] repressing both spontaneous and DL-ethionine-induced liver carcinogenesis, and inhibiting melanoma promotion caused by DMBA and TPA.[3–5] The soybean hypocotyls could diminish the incidence of colon carcinogenesis by decreasing CYP24 expression and increasing cytochrome P450 hydroxylase CYP27B1.[6] A 60% methanolic fraction of soybean hypocotyls was found to be able to attenuate the activity of matrix metalloproteinase (MMP), which especially is related with cancer-cell metastasis and nascent vessel formation.[7] A chloroform-soluble fraction derived from vinegar- treated small black soybean showed antiproliferative and proapoptotic activities against human myeloid leukemia HL-60 cells. From the fraction, genistein and daidzein were separated as active principles.[8]

Antitumor activities of fermented soybean: Fermented soybean pastes are also traditionally popular in East-Asian countries as cooking materials. Two Korean-type fermented soybean pastes (Chungkookjang and doenjang) have been found to exert noticeable antimutagenic and cytotoxic effects against tumor cells.[9] Chunggookjang (similar to Japanese Natto) and its butanolic extract significantly retarded the growth of three *in vitro* human cancer cell lines, HL-60 (leukemia), MCF-7 (breast), and SNU-638 (stomach), and also displayed *in vivo* antitumorigenic effect in a rat model with DMBA-induced breast tumor.[9] The anti-breast cancer mechanism of Chungkookjang in MCF-7 cells was found to be mediated by the activation of the TGFβ1/Smad3 pathway and downregulation of inflammation-related CSF2, CSF2RA, and CSF3.[10] Soybean doenjang (SD) and black soybean doenjang (BD) exerted the anticancer effects by inhibiting human HT-29 colon cancer cells together with the induction of apoptosis and regulation of proinflammatory cytokines, cell cycling related genes, and so on, but showed no toxicity on normal RAW 264.7 cells at 0.1 to 0.5 mg/mL concentrations. Probably due to higher levels of polyphenolics content, including anthocyanins, BD showed more potent antioxidative and anticancer effects than SD.[11]

ES is another kind of fermented soybean product, which exerted the anti-growth effect against human Caco-2 colon cancer cells by 65.5% together with the induction of G2/M cell-cycle arrest at 10 µL/mL concentration.[12] Soybean-dongchunghacho (SDC) was produced by the cultivation of a fungus *Paecilomyces tenuipes* on soybean. In a rat model, dietary SDC could lessen dimethylhydrazine (DMH)-induced DNA damage in colon and reduce oxidative stress and plasma lipid peroxidation, showing a potential for inhibition of early-stage colon carcinogenesis.[13]

Antitumor activity of transgenic soybean: In the *in vivo* models, the oil produced from transgenic soybean demonstrated marked inhibitory effect against the growth of carcinoma cells. The anti-growth rates ranged from 31.91% to 34.34% in mice-implanted hepatoma H22, sarcoma 180, or Ehrlich carcinoma after oral administration of transgenic soybean oil. Interestingly, the activities were much better than those of normal soybean oil.[14]

Scientific Evidence of Antitumorigenic Constituents

The extensive investigations on the chemical biology of soybean have revealed that soybean components, such as isoflavones, anthocyanin, saponins, peptides/proteins, and polysaccharides, could contribute to the chemopreventive activity. By attenuating steroid hormones and enhancing antioxidative effect, the soybean phytochemicals were able to lessen the growth rate of tumor cells and the risk of carcinogenesis.

1. Isoflavones

The major components of soybean are assigned as isoflavones, including genistein (**1**), daidzein (**2**), biochanin-A, and genistin, the content of which are > 80% in the soybean hypocotyl. The isoflavones serve as therapeutic phytoestrogens in response to steroid hormone modulation. The accumulated evidences from experimental animal models and clinical trials suggest that the phytoestrogens may potentially confer health benefits related to the inhibition of steroid hormone-dependent carcinomas.[15] Soybean isoflavones even at a low concentration deterred the proliferation of MCF-7 breast cancer cells and hindered the cell mitosis *in vitro* with IC_{50} 32.0 μmol/L.[22] Genistein (**1**) was effective in hindering human DU145 prostate cancer cells (IC_{50}–20 μM) and breast carcinoma development induced by dimethylbenzo[a]anthracene, and was also active in repressing TPA-promoted phospholipid synthesis.[15–18] The antiproliferative effect on DU145 prostate cancer cells was found to be associated with (1) early activation of cell cycle-related genes such as p53, p53-dependent growth regulator CGR19, and MDM2-like p53-binding protein RBQ-3, and (2) downregulation of Efp (estrogen-responsive finger protein) expression.[18–20] The inactivation of Efp was found to be partially involved in the prevention and inhibition of prostate and breast cancers.[21,22]

Besides the breast and prostate cancer cells, the soy isoflavones were also proven to be sensitive to various types of carcinoma cells.[16] Genistein (**1**) potently restrained the anticancer effect on human HL-60 leukemia cells, in terms of induction of proliferative inhibition and apoptosis.[8] Treatment of HCT-116 colon cancer cells with genistein (**1**, 2 μM) and lunasin (2 μM) individually hindered the cell viability and colonosphere formation concomitant with proapoptosis.[23] In ~75 μmol/L concentrations, genistein (**1**) dose-dependently impeded the proliferation and invasion of pancreatic carcinoma cell lines (IA8-ARCaP and LNCaP/HIF-1a), antiinvasive effect of which was associated with the reversal of epithelial–mesenchymal transition (EMT).[24] Due to the fact that genistein (**1**) is also a nontoxic inactivator of miRNA (such as miR27a), the growth and migration of human SKOV3 ovarian cancer cells were retarded by genistein (**1**) by downregulation of miR-27a expression and upregulation of Sprouty2 expression.[25] The *in vitro* and/or *in vivo* tests showed that genistein (**1**) exerted significantly both growth inhibition and metastasis suppression against K1 sex gland cancer and A549 and H358 lung cancer cell lines, antimetastatic effect of which in A549 and H358 cells was mediated by modulation of MMP-2 and FLT4.[24,26] More experiments reported multiple antitumor effects of genistein (**1**) such as inhibiting growth and metastasis in pancreatic cancer, hepatoma, and colorectal carcinoma.[27]

In vitro approaches have shown that genistein (**1**), daidzein (**2**), genistin, and biochanin-A dose-dependently restrained the growth of murine (MB49 and MBT-2) and human (HT-1376, UM-UC-3, RT-4, J82, and TCCSUP) bladder cancer cell lines *in vitro*, together with elicitation of G2/M cell-cycle arrest.[28] Genistein (**1**) was the most effective isoflavonoid found in soybean to have suppressive effect against HL-60 promyelocytic leukemia cell line.[29] In rat B35 neuroblastoma cells, genistein (**1**) was also able to promote the G2/M cell-cycle arrest and apoptosis via upregulation of p21waf1/cip1 and Bax and downregulation of Bcl-2 expression.[14] In addition to enhancing apoptosis and inhibiting tumor cell proliferation, these isoflavonoids also played an antiangiogenetic role in the blockage and destruction of tumor neovasculature, but showed no histopathological effects on normal bladder mucosa.[30]

Moreover, genistein (**1**) and daidzein (**2**) are the most valuable isoflavones in soybean for anticarcinogenesis. The genistin and daidzin and their aglucones genistein (**1**) and daidzein (**2**) could also repress covalent binding of oncogen benzo[a]pyrene (BAP) metabolites to DNA via blockage of CYP1A1 enzyme activity in mouse hepatoma cells in terms of exerting the inhibition of liver carcinogenesis.[31] When soybean milk is fermented with lactic acid bacteria, the isoflavone glycosides can be 100% decomposed to their aglycons, leading to increasing genistein (**1**) and daidzein (**2**).[16,32–34] The aglycons also played various roles in obstructing carcinogenesis in colon, gastric, liver, lung, breast, and so on, and in enhancing NK cell activity, indicating both their capacities in anticarcinogeneis and immunostimulation. Furthermore, their beneficial effects also showed in restoring the enervated immunity caused by cancer radio- and chemotherapies.[32–35] When soybean isoflavones (40 mg/L) was combined with vinorelbine (8–32 mg/L), the growth inhibition on A549 lung carcinoma cells was synergistically enhanced to 71%–93%.[36]

According to the investigations, the anticancer and anticarcinogenic mechanism of soybean isoflavones could be summarized to be primarily accompanied with the (1) regulation of sex hormones action; (2) induction of cellular apoptosis and/or cell-cycle arrest; (3) specific inhibition of tyrosine protein kinase and repression of topoisomerase; (4) antioxidation antiangiogenesis, and (5) improvement in efficacy of anticancer drugs.

2. Anthocyanins

Several anthocyanins isolated from the seed coats of black soybean exerted marked suppressive activity against the proliferation of colon carcinoma cells and colonic inflammation *in vitro* and *in vivo*. Cyanidin (3) and delphinidin (4) as the major anthocyanins in black soybean markedly impeded the proliferation of human HT-29 colon adenocarcinoma cells *in vitro* at concentrations of 1 μM, and also repressed cyclooxygenase-2 (COX-2) activity and TPA-stimulated inducible nitric oxide synthase mRNA in the HT-29 cells.[37] Cyanidin 3-O-β-D-glucoside (5) showed obvious anti-growth effects against human Molt-4B leukemia cells *in vitro* through production of active oxygen and induction of apoptosis. Likewise, these anthocyanins were isolated from the skin of red grapes as well.[38]

3. Phytoalexins

Glyceollins are one of the primary groups of phytoalexins produced in soybean fermentation but are only trace levels in unfermented soybean and are also not in soy food products. A mixture of three phytoalexin-type constituents, which contains glyceollin-I (68%, 6), glyceollin-II (21%, 7), and glyceollin-III (11%, 8) were prepared from soybean fermented with *Aspergillus sojae*. The glyceollins showed marked antiestrogenic activity on estrogen receptor (ER) function, leading to the growth inhibition of estrogen-dependent tumor *in vivo*. The antiestrogenic glyceollins in per injection dose of 20 mg/kg/day for 20 days were markedly effective in lowering ER-induced progesterone receptor expression in the tumors and thereby suppressing the growth of ER-positive MCF-7 breast cancer and BG-1 ovarian cancer cells in nude mice. The inhibitory rates on the MCF-7 and BG-1 cell lines were 53.4% and 73.1%, respectively, being better than that of tamoxifen (a clinically used ER antagonist). Concurrently, the uterotropic effect of estrogen in the treatment was partially antagonized.[19]

Coumestrol (9) is a major representative phytoestrogen naturally found in soybeans as well as brussel sprouts, legumes, and spinach. Coumestrol (9) exerted strong cancer-preventive effects on estrogen-responsive carcinomas. In human ES2 epithelial ovarian cancer cells, coumestrol (9) hampered cell viability, proliferation, and invasion and elicited cell apoptosis via blockage of PI3K and ERK1/2 MAPK pathways, such as inhibiting PI3K, inactivating Akt, p70S6K, ERK1/2, JNK1/2, and p90RSK, and lessening phosphorylation levels of Akt, ERK1/2, p70S6K, and S6.[39] Accordingly, the findings proposed that glyceollins as antiestrogenic agents have potential to improve the prevention and treatment of hormone-dependent cancers, especially breast and ovarian neoplasms.

4. Soysaponins

Soysaponins are another major constituent in soybean, which have important time-dependent anticarcinogenic and antitumor promoting activities. When HT-29 colon cancer cells were treated with soysaponins for 72 h, the COX-2 expression and PKC activity were diminished remarkably in the PMA-stimulated HT-29 cells.[30] B-group soysaponins selectively inhibited the proliferation of human HCT-15 colon carcinoma, amplified a nonapoptotic programmed cell death (PCD), and arrested cell cycle at S-phase via reduction of cyclin-dependent kinase-2 (CDK-2) activity and induction of macroautophagy, but had no such effects on normal human NCM460 colon epithelial cells.[40] Treatment with the B-group soysaponins also resulted in a greater growth inhibition against

MCF-7 and MDA-MB-231 human breast cancer cell lines.[40,41] The cancer-suppressive and cancer-preventive effects clearly indicated that the soysaponins are capable of decreasing the risk of colon and breast tumorigenesis.

Some soysaponins such as soyasapogenol-B glycosides not only promoted the apoptosis of human SNB19 glioblastoma cells by stimulating cytochrome c release and activating caspases-9, -3, but also restrained the invasion of SNB19 cells by 45% *in vitro*. Two pure saponins designated as soyasaponins-αg and -βg displayed significant inhibitory effect against matrix metalloproteinase (MMP), known to be involved in tumor invasion/metastasis and angiogenesis.[42,43] Similarly, by diminishing MMPs-2, -9 levels and stimulating TIMP-2 secretion, the soybean saponins notably inhibited the invasion of HT-1080 fibrosarcoma cells. The antimetastatic potential of soysaponins was further confirmed by *in vivo* mice assay. Feeding mice with dietary soybean saponins for 2 weeks moderately lessened the incidence of metastatic tumor colonization in lungs from implanted CT-26 colon cancer, signifying the chemopreventive potential of soybean saponin on cancer metastasis.[44] The soysaponins also exerted significant effects in repressing the mutagenicity of aflatoxin B1 (AFB1) by 52 ~ 81% at concentrations of 600 ~ 1,200 μg per plate and inhibiting AFB1-induced DNA damages by 50.1% at a concentration of 30 μg/mL in HepG2 hepatoma cells.[45,46] These positive results suggest that the soybean saponins are useful to block the initiation stages of carcinogenesis and metastasis, leading to the benefit for cancer chemotherapy.

In addition, soyasapogenols as the aglycones of soybean saponins were able to hinder the activation of STAT3 in both macrophages and tumor cells probably through inhibiting M2 polarization and increasing IL-12 secretion. In an *in vitro* assay, soyasapogenols obstructed the proliferation of U373 glioma, SaOS2, and LM8 osteosarcoma cell lines. Oral administration of soyasapogenol-B obviously resulted in both antitumor and antimetastatic (lung) effects against LM8 mouse osteosarcoma together with amplification of an antitumor immune response in mice. These findings represent the usefulness of the aglycones of soysaponins in cancer chemotherapy and/or chemoprevention.[47]

5. Polysaccharides

A unique polysaccharide (PSBS) component was prepared from black soybean, the structure of which was assigned as a (1,6)-α-D-glucan with molecular of weight about 480,000. After injection of PSBS to mice, the immune response of mononuclear cells (MNCs) in blood serum was distinctly activated. The PSBS-treated serum termed PSBS–MNC–CM was used to treat human U937 leukemia cells *in vitro*, showing significant suppression against the proliferation of U937 leukemia cells for 98.5%. PSBS–MNC–CM could also provoke the U937 cells to differentiation into mature monocytes/macrophages by 83%–90%. The U937 cell differentiation was triggered by the activation of MNCs.[48]

A special polysaccharide was produced by soybean fermentation with fungi, either *Agrocybe cylindracea* or *Phellinus igniarius*. The polysaccharides showed chemopreventive activity for protecting organs from carcinogenesis. Intragastric administration of the polysacchrides to mice for 14 days notably activated phase-II and antioxidant enzymes in various organs; for instance, glutathione S-transferase (GST) and quinone reductase (QR) in liver and kidney, glutathione (GSH), and superoxide dismutase (SOD) in liver, kidney, lung, and stomach, and glutathione peroxidase (GPx) in liver, lung, and kidney. All the activated enzymes can help to effectively protect organs from carcinogenesis and mutation.[49]

GCP, a genistein-combined polysaccharide, was prepared by the fermentation of soybean with basidiomycetes, the product of which was rich in bioactive genistein. *In vitro* and *in vivo* studies confirmed that GCP has potential as an effective chemopreventive agent against the growth of prostate carcinoma cells. The suppressive rates of GCP significantly reached 78% in androgen-independent PC3 prostate cancer cells and 89% in androgen-sensitive LNCaP prostate cancer cells at a dose of 10 μg/mL over 72 h treatment. But the induction of apoptosis and the activation of p27 and p53 proteins were observed only in the treated LNCap cells.[50] Similarly, oral administration of GCP to mice for 28 days notably obstructed the growth of human MDA-MB-231 breast cancer cells and promoted cell apoptosis in association with activation of cleavage of poly(ADP-ribose) polymerase and p21 protein expression and reduction of cyclin-B1 expression in the breast tumor tissues.[51]

6. Peptide and protein

The bioactive peptides/small proteins, lunasin, BBI, and bikunin were isolated from soybean and proved to be effective in anticarcinogenesis in both *in vitro* and *in vivo* model systems.[52] The soybean protein hydrolates described below may be used in dietary and soybean products as bioactive ingredients of functional food.

Soybean Peptides: A peptide was prepared from soybean by hydrolyzation and fractionation, which inhibited PC3 prostate cancer-cell proliferation, arrested G2/M cell cycle, and induced cell apoptosis at middle and late stages after treatment with the peptide in 5–20 μmol/L concentration range for 24–72 h.[53] A peptide fraction (>10 kDa) was obtained from a germinated soybean protein hydrolysate with digestive enzymes, the peptide fraction of which was effective in impeding the growth of HeLa cervical cancer cells and inducing cell apoptosis by downregulation of PTTG1 and TOP2A expressions, activation of caspase cascade, and induction of DNA fragmentation.[54]

Lunasin: Lunasin (5 kDa) was initially isolated from soybean cotyledon and also found in wheat, barley, and others. It was identified as a peptide with 43 amino acid residues that contain a RGD-cell adhesion motif followed by eight aspartic acid residues at the carboxyl end and a structurally conserved helix region. Due to the anti-inflammatory and anticancer activities, lunasin has received extensive attention. The chemopreventive efficacy of lunasin was demonstrated by oral administration in mouse models. Lunasin exogenously reduced foci formation in mouse fibroblast cells treated with chemical carcinogens and obstructed skin tumorigenesis induced by chemical carcinogens in mice.[55,56] Lunasin applied to cell culture suppresses foci formation in oncogene E1A-transfected mouse fibroblast NIH 3T3 cells. Concurrently, lunasin increased p21 protein levels 5-fold in the cells transfected with E1A but not in untransfected cells. However, lunasin did not inhibit the growth of immortalized and established cancer cell lines.[57] In MCF-7 breast cancer cells, lunasin elicited p53-independent cellular apoptotic death via (1) upregulation of a tumor-suppressor PTEN activity, increased PTEN transcript and protein levels, and enhanced nuclear PTEN localization and (2) promotion of E-cadherin and β-catenin nonnuclear localization.[58] In addition, lunasin was also capable of significantly hindering the proliferation and enhancing the apoptosis of rheumatoid arthritis synovial fibroblasts via downregulation of MMP expression and proinflammatory cytokines (IL-6, IL-8, and NF-κB).[59]

BBI: Bowman–Birk protease inhibitor (BBI) is a universal cancer-preventive protein (m.w. 8000), which has a well-characterized ability to restrain chymotrypsin and trypsin. BBI significantly obstructed carcinogenic process induced by various chemical and physical carcinogens in a variety of *in vivo* (mice, rats, and hamsters) and *in vitro* (colon, liver, esophagus, lung, oral epithelium, and cells of hematopoietic origin) systems without toxicity.[60] The soybean BBI showed remarkable inhibitory effects on the proliferation and metastasis of both AGS gastric adenocarcinoma and HT-29 colorectal adenocarcinoma cell lines concomitant with the repression of MMPs-2, -9, and VEGF secretion, implying that antimetastatic and antiangiogenic effects were also involved in the anticancer activity of soybean BBI.[61] In addition, BBI appears particularly effective against malignant transformation in different routes of administration, including diet, oral, and injection, leading to obstruction of different types of neoplastic cells (e.g., adenocarcinomas, angiosarcomas, and squamous cell carcinomas) but only moderate effects against breast and prostate carcinomas.[60] In addition, the researchers also found that the BBI is able to protect soybean lunasin from proteolytic attack of digestive enzymes in gastrointestinal tract. Then the remained lunasin and BBI as well as their released peptides exert the anticancer activity.[62]

Bikunin: A Kunitz-type protease inhibitor termed bikunin exhibits anti-inflammatory activity in the protection against neoplasm and inflammation. Once-daily oral administration of soybean bikunin to female nude mice at 30 mg/kg dose for incessant 7 days could diminish the proliferation of human ovarian carcinoma by 40% without toxicity.[63] The soybean bikunin could specifically inhibit the invasion and metastasis of HRA ovarian cancer cells with IC_{50} value of about 3 μM. The anti-invasive and antimetastatic activities were found to be mediated by blocking urokinase upregulation, reducing transforming growth factor-β1 (TGF-β1)-induced ERK1/2 activation, and deterring ERK1/2 and p38 kinase-mediated NF-κB activation.[64]

7. Other active agents

Three other soybean constituents were also found to have anticarcinogenic activity. Myoinositol (**10**) and tocotrienol (**11**) were effective in suppressing spontaneous liver carcinogenesis in mice. Both compounds also repressed lung tumorigenesis initiated by 4-nitroquinoline-1-oxide and promoted by glycerol in mice.[15] A sphingolipid-type soy glucosylceramide (GlcCer) consists predominantly of a 4,8-sphingadiene backbone and α-hydroxypalmitic acid. The soy GlcCer at 0.025% and 0.1% of the diet (wt./wt.) reduced the number of aberrant colonic crypt foci (an early marker of colon carcinogenesis) by 38% and 52%, and inhibited colon tumorigenesis by 50% and 56%, respectively, in mice treated with a colon carcinogen, DMH.[65]

SCIENTIFIC EVIDENCE FROM CLINICAL TRIAL

A clinical trial of using soy isoflavones (Novasoy) on patients suffering from prostate cancer was been conducted. In the trial, 100 mg of soy isoflavone was orally administrated to patients twice daily for 3–6 months. Thirty-nine patients completed the course of treatment. The result showed that the levels of serum prostate-specific antigen (PSA) were stabilized in 83% of hormone-sensitive patients and in 35% of hormone-refractory patients, inferring that the soy isoflavones (Novasoy) are more suitable for treatment of hormone-dependent prostate cancer patients compared to hormone-refractory patients as a supplement agent.[65]

CONCLUSION AND SUGGESTION

The extensive scientific investigations in chemical biology have confirmed the cancer-preventive advantages of soybean, soybean products, and fermented soybean products in addition to their rich nutrients. The anticancer, anticarcinogenic, and immunoenhancing properties of soybean were found to be attributed to the abundant contents of isoflavonoids (such as genistein and daidzein), soysaponins, polysaccharides, and peptides/proteins. Especially in the past 15 years, the soybean isoflavonoids that present phytoestrogen nature have been paid more attention in the prevention of hormone-dependent urogenital carcinogenesis and gastrointestinal carcinogenesis. The major constituents in soybean are able to affect the key events occurring in cancer cells such as DNA repair, cell-signaling cascades including Wnt-signaling, induction of apoptosis and cell-cycle arrest, cell proliferation–inhibition, EMT, and blockage of invasion and metastasis, thus displaying cancer-preventive functions. Overall, the research results highlighted great health benefits and functions of soybean and further pointed out a wide prospect of dietary soybean in promoting human health and lowering cancer incidences.

REFERENCES

1. Lu, L.J.W. et al., 2000. Decreased ovarian hormones during a soya diet: Implications for breast cancer prevention. *Cancer Res.* 60: 4112–4121.
2. Zaizen, Y. et al., 2000. Antitumor effects of soybean hypocotyls and soybeans on the mammary tumor induction by N-methyl-n-nitrosourea in F344 rats. *Anticancer Res.* 20: 1439–1444.
3. Nishino, H. et al., 1999. Liver cancer inhibitors comprising heated soybean hypocotyls and food containing them. Japanese Kokai Tokkyo Koho Application: JP 97-208742 19970804.

4. Yasuhara, T. et al., 1999. Anti-carcinogenic effect of soybean hypocotyl. *Daizu Tanpakushitsu Kenkyu* 2: 94–98.
5. Aiad, F. et al., 2004. Protective effect of soybean against hepatocarcinogenesis induced by DL-ethionine. *J. Biochem. Mol. Biol.* 37: 370–375.
6. Kallay, E. et al., 2002. Phytoestrogens regulate vitamin D metabolism in the mouse colon: Relevance for colon tumor prevention and therapy. *J. Nutrition* 132(11S): 3490S–3493S.
7. Takeshita, M. et al., 1998. Inhibitory effect of soybean hypocotyls on tumor promotion: Effect of dietary hypocotyls on N-nitroso-N-methylurea-induced rat tumorigenesis. *Daizu Tanpakushitsu Kenkyu* 1: 124–128.
8. Oh, C.H. et al., 2006. Antiproliferative constituents from the vinegar treated small black soybean (Glycine max Merr.). *Nat. Prod. Sci.* 12: 109–112.
9. Kwak, C.S. et al., 2006. Cytotoxicity on human cancer cells and antitumorigenesis of Chungkookjang, a fermented soybean product, in DMBA-treated rats. *Hanguk Yongyang Hakhoechi* 39: 347–356.
10. Hwang, J.S. et al., 2011. Inflammation-related signaling pathways implicating TGFβ are revealed in the expression profiling of MCF7 cell treated with fermented soybean, Chungkookjang. *Nutr Cancer* 63: 645–652.
11. Park, E. et al., 2015. Seong; Anticancer effects of black soybean doenjang in HT-29 human colon cancer cells. *Han'guk Sikp'um Yongyang Kwahak Hoechi* 44: 1270–1278.
12. Han, J.K. et al., 2006. Effects of ES soybean fermentation products on human intestinal cancer cells. *Gekkan Fudo Kemikaru* 22: 100–103.
13. Park, E.J. et al., 2007. Antigenotoxic effect of Paecilomyces tenuipes cultivated on soybeans in a rat model of 1,2-dimethylhydrazine-induced colon carcinogenesis. *Food Sci. Biotechnol.* 16: 1064–1068.
14. Bu, Y.P. et al., 2005. Antitumor effect of the oil of transgenic soybeans. *Zhongguo Shengwu Zhongguo Shengwu Gongcheng Zazhi* 25: 92–97.
15. a) Wietrzyk, J. et al., 2005. Phytoestrogens in cancer prevention and therapy-mechanisms of their biological activity. *Anticancer Res.* 25: 2357–2366; b) Ismail, I.A. et al., 2006. Genistein induces G2/M cell cycle arrest and apoptosis in rat neuroblastoma B35 cells; Involvement of p21waf1/cip1, Bax and Bcl-2. *Kor. J. Pathol.* 40: 339–347.
16. Nishino, H. et al., 1998. Anticarcinogenic effect of isoflavonoids in soybeans. *Daizu Tanpakushitsu Kenkyu* 1: 129–132.
17. Nishino, H. et al., 2000. Study on cancer preventive substances in soybeans. *Daizu Tanpaku-shitsu Kenkyu* 3: 59–62.
18. Fritz, W.A. et al., 1998. Dietary genistein: Perinatal mammary cancer prevention, bioavailability and toxicity testing in the rat. *Carcinogenesis* 19: 2151–2158.
19. Lamartiniere, C.A. et al., 1998. Genistein studies in rats: Potential for breast cancer prevention and reproductive and developmental toxicity. *Am. J. Clin. Nutr* 68(6, Suppl.): 1400S–1405S.
20. Salvo, V.A. et al., 2006. Antiestrogenic glyceollins suppress human breast and ovarian carcinoma tumorigenesis. *Clin. Cancer Res.* 12: 7159–7164.
21. Urano, T. et al., 2008. The role of genistein in breast and prostate cancer prevention through the protein modification and degradation pathway. *Daizu Tanpakushitsu Kenkyu* 11: 88–94.
22. Chen, J. et al., 2009. Studies on antitumor effect of soybean isoflavone in vitro. *Zhonghua Shiyong Yiyao Zazhi* 9: 161–163.
23. Montales, M.T.E. et al., 2015. Metformin and soybean-derived bioactive molecules attenuate the expansion of stem cell-like epithelial subpopulation and confer apoptotic sensitivity in human colon cancer cells. *Genes Nutr.* 10: 1–14.
24. Zhang, L.L. et al., 2008. A novel anti-cancer effect of genistein: Reversal of epithelial mesenchymal transition in prostate cancer cells. *Acta Pharmacologica Sinica* 29: 1060–1068.
25. Xu, L.L. et al., 2013. Oncogenic microRNA-27a is a target for genistein in ovarian cancer cells. *Anti-Cancer Agents in Med. Chem.* 13: 1126–1132.
26. Schleicher, R.L. et al., 1999. The inhibitory effect of genistein on the growth and metastasis of a transplantable rat accessory sex gland carcinoma. *Cancer Lett.* 136: 195–201.
27. Xing, X.L. et al., 2015. Genistein inhibits lung cancer cell growth, migration and invasion by regulating MMP2 and FLT4. *Biomed. Pharmacother.* 6(5): 3225–3239.
28. Zhou, J.R. et al., 1998. Inhibition of murine bladder tumorigenesis by soy isoflavones via alterations in the cell cycle, apoptosis, and angiogenesis. *Cancer Res.* 58: 5231–5238.
29. Gowri, A.M. et al., 2006. Antiproliferative activity of Soybean on mitogen stimulated bone marrow cells. *Biosci. Biotech. Res. Asia* 3: 399–401.

30. Kim, H.Y. et al., 2004. Antiproliferative crude soy saponin extract modulates the expression of IκBα, protein kinase C, and cyclooxygenase-2 in human colon cancer cells. *Cancer Lett.* 210: 1–6.

31. Shertzer, H.G. et al., 1999. Inhibition of CYP1A1 enzyme activity in mouse hepatoma cell culture by soybean isoflavones. *Chemico-Biol. Interactions* 123: 31–49.

32. Lu, K.M. et al., 2003. Method of using fermented Glycine max (L) extract for enhancing natural killer cell activity. U.S. Patent Application Publication US2002-178364 20020625.

33. Fujino, T. et al., a) 2002. Antitumor health food preparation from ferment soybean milk extract. Japanese Kokai Tokkyo Koho JP 2001-51683 20010227; b) 2005. *Gongcheng Zazhi* 25: 92–97.

34. Sakaguchi, Y. et al., 2001. Manufacture of isoflavone aglycon-rich fermented soybean milk useful for cancer prevention. Japanese Kokai Tokkyo Koho JP 2000-154586 20000525.

35. Nishino, H. et al., 1997. Anticarcinogenic effect of isoflavonoids in soybeans. *Daizu Tanpakushitsu Kenkyukai Kaishi* 18: 130–134.

36. Yin, X.Z. et al., 2012. Synergistic antitumor effect of soybean isoflavones combined with chemotherapy on A549 cells. *Zhongguo Gonggong Weisheng* 28: 1465–1467.

37. Kim, J.M. et al., 2008. Effects of black soybean [Glycine max (L.) Merr.] seed coats and its anthocyanidins on colonic inflammation and cell proliferation in vitro and in vivo. *J. Agricul. Food Chem.* 56: 8427–8433.

38. Katsuzaki, H. et al., 2003. Cyanidin 3-O-β-D-glucoside isolated from skin of black Glycine max and other anthocyanins isolated from skin of red grape induce apoptosis in human lymphoid leukemia Molt 4B cells. *Oncol. Reports* 10: 297–300.

39. Lim, W.S. et al., 2016. Coumestrol suppresses proliferation of ES2 human epithelial ovarian cancer cells. *J. Endocrinol.* 228: 149–160.

40. Allison, A.E. et al., 2005. Induction of macroautophagy in human colon cancer cells by soybean B-group triterpenoid saponins. *Carcinogenesis* 26: 159–167.

41. Rowlands, J.C. et al., 2002. Estrogenic and antiproliferative properties of soy sapogenols in human breast cancer cells in vitro. *Food Chem. Toxicol.* 40: 1767–1774.

42. Sugimoto, A. et al., 2000. Studies on the anti-carcinogenic effects of soybean hypocotyls. *Seitai Zairyo Kogaku Kenkyusho Hokoku* (Tokyo Ika Shika Daigaku) 34: 37–41.

43. Yanamandra, N. et al., 2003. Triterpenoids from Glycine max decrease invasiveness and induce caspase-mediated cell death in human SNB19 glioma cells. *Clin. Experim. Metastasis* 20: 375–383.

44. Kang, J.H. et al., 2008. Soybean saponin inhibits tumor cell metastasis by modulating expressions of MMP-2, MMP-9 and TIMP- 2. *Cancer Lett.* (Amsterdam, the Netherlands) 261: 84–92.

45. Jun, H.S. et al., 2002. Protective effect of soybean saponins and major antioxidants against aflatoxin B1-induced mutagenicity and DNA-adduct formation. *J. Med. Food* 5: 235–240.

46. Kerwin, S.M. et al., 2004. Soy saponins and the anticancer effects of soybeans and soy-based foods. *Current Med. Chem.* 4: 263–272.

47. Fujiwara, Y. et al., 2015. Soyasapogenols contained in soybeans suppress tumor progression by regulating macrophage differentiation into the protumoural phenotype. *J. Functional Foods* 19(Part-A): 594–605.

48. Liao, H.F. et al., 2001. Isolation and characterization of an active compound from black soybean [Glycine max (L.) Merr.] and its effect on proliferation and differentiation of human leukemic U937 cells. *Anti-Cancer Drug.* 12: 841–846.

49. Shon, Y.H. et al., 2000. Enhancement of phase II and antioxidant enzymes in mice by soybeans fermented with basidiomycetes. *J. Microbiol. Biotechnol.* 10: 851–857.

50. Bemis, D.L. et al., 2004. A concentrated aglycone isoflavone preparation (GCP) that demonstrates potent anti-prostate cancer activity in vitro and in vivo. *Clin. Cancer Res.* 10: 5282–5292.

51. Yuan, L. et al., 2003. Inhibition of human breast cancer growth by GCP (genistein combined polysaccharide) in xenogeneic athymic mice: Involvement of genistein biotransformation by β-glucuronidase from tumor tissues. *Mutat. Res. Fund. Mol Mech Mut* 523–524, 55–62.

52. Park, J.H. et al., 2007. In vitro digestibility of the cancer-preventive soy peptides lunasin and BBI. *J. Agricul. Food Chem.* 55: 10703–10706.

53. Hu, K.B. et al., 2014. Effect of soybean peptide on proliferation and apoptosis of prostate cancer PC3 cells. *Zhongguo Shengwu Zhipinxue Zazhi* 27: 1176–1180.

54. Robles-Ramirez, M.C. et al., 2012. A peptide fraction from germinated soybean protein down-regulates PTTG1 and TOP2A mRNA expression, inducing apoptosis in cervical cancer cells. *J. Exper. Therap. Oncol.* 9: 255–263.

55. Hernandez-Ledesma, B. et al., 2009. Lunasin, a novel seed peptide for cancer prevention. *Peptides* (Amsterdam, the Netherlands) 30: 426–30.
56. Jeong, H.J. et al., 2007. Inhibition of core histone acetylation by the cancer preventive peptide lunasin. *J. Agricult. Food Chem.* 55: 632–637.
57. Lam, Y. et al., 2003. Lunasin suppresses E1A-mediated transformation of mammalian cells but does not inhibit growth of immortalized and established cancer cell lines. *Nutr. Cancer* 47: 88–94.
58. Pabona, J.M.P. et al., 2013. The soybean peptide lunasin promotes apoptosis of mammary epithelial cells via induction of tumor suppressor PTEN: Similarities and distinct actions from soy isoflavone genistein. *Genes Nutr.* 8: 79–90.
59. Jia, S.H. et al., 2015. Lunasin inhibits cell proliferation via apoptosis and reduces the production of proinflammatory cytokines in cultured rheumatoid arthritis synovial fibroblasts. *BioMed Res. Int.* 346839/1–346839/9.
60. Kennedy, A.R. 1998. The Bowman-Birk inhibitor from soybeans as an anticarcinogenic agent. *Am. J. Clin. Nutr.* 68(6, Suppl.): 1406S–1412S.
61. Fereidunian, A. et al., 2014. Soybean Bowman-Birk protease inhibitor (BBI): Identification of the mechanisms of BBI suppressive effect on growth of two adenocarcinoma cell lines: AGS and HT29. *Arch. Med. Res.* 45: 455–461.
62. Cruz-Huerta, E. et al., 2015. The protective role of the Bowman-Birk protease inhibitor in soybean lunasin digestion: The effect of released peptides on colon cancer growth. *Food & Function* 6: 2626–2635.
63. Kobayashi, H. et al., 2004. A soybean Kunitz trypsin inhibitor suppresses ovarian cancer cell invasion by blocking urokinase upregulation. *Clin. Experim. Metastasis* 21: 159–166.
64. Kobayashi, H. et al., 2004. (a) Therapeutic efficacy of once-daily oral administration of a Kunitz-type protease inhibitor, bikunin, in a mouse model and in human cancer. *Cancer* (NY, NY, USA) 100: 869–877.
65. Symolon, H. et al., 2004. Dietary soy sphingolipids suppress tumorigenesis and gene expression in 1,2-dimethylhydrazine-treated CF1 mice and ApcMin/+ mice. *J. Nutr.* 134: 1157–1161; (b) Hussain, M. et al., 2003. Soy isoflavones in the treatment of prostate cancer. *Nutr. Cancer* 47: 111–117.

5 Cancer-Preventive Substances in Fruits

33. Avocado/*Persea americana*

34. Cherry/*Prunus avium, P. cerasus*

35. Chestnut Rose/*Rosa roxburghii, R. roxburghii* f. *normalis*

36. Citrus Fruits/*Citrus*

37. Cranberry/*Vaccinium macrocarpon*

38. Fig Fruit/*Ficus carica*

39. Grape/*Vitis vinifera*

40. Guava/*Psidium guajava*

41. Hawthorn Berry/*Crataegus monogyna, C. laevigata, C. pinnatifida, C. azarolus*

42. Jujube (Chinese date)/*Ziziphus jujuba*

43. Kiwi Fruit/*Actinidia chinensis*

44. Mango/*Mangifera indica*

45. Papaya/*Carica papaya*

46. Persimmon/*Diospyros kaki*

47. Pomegranate/*Punica granatum*

48. Ume, Chinese Plum, or Japanese Apricot/*Prunus mume*

The health benefits of common fruits are widely recognized and emphasized in recent years, signifying that diversity of bioactive phytochemicals such as polyphenolics, vitamins, minerals, dietary fibers, and macronutrients make fruits very advantageous for human health without increasing any unnecessary fats. For the reason of the phytochemicals presented, the properties in potent antioxidative, conspicuous anticarcinogenic, anti-inflammatory, cardiovascular improving, and so on, daily intake of fresh fruits is beneficial not only for the proper functioning of the body but also in lowering of the risks of cancerous formation and some chronic diseases. It is definitely right that, by keeping the habit of regularly eating dietary fruits for over 10 years, a great deal of health improvement and body function promotion would be achieved. In this Chapter, 16 botanical fruits common in Western or Eastern markets are selected as examples to introduce the latest research discoveries concerning their potentials in cancer prevention and anticarcinogenesis. Most common fruits such as plum, melon, honeymelon, blueberry, waxberry, strawberry, banana, carambola, apple, pear, apricot, and so on, display significant health stimulating and antioxidant activities that are good for cancer prevention. However, their anticarcinogenic and anticancer potentials are less active and/or less investigated compared to the fruits described here, according to the research results.

33. AVOCADO

Avocat   Avocado   Aguacate

鳄梨   アボカド   악어없음

Persea americana

Lauraceae

Avocado (*Persea americana*), a fruit from a Lauraceae tree native to South Central Mexico, is a favorable healthy food consumed popularly in human diet today. Generally, a typical serving of avocado (100 g) can afford prominent amounts of vitamin B complex and vitamin K and good amounts of vitamins C, E, potassium and heart-healthy fats including omega-3s. This nutrition-rich fruit has been demonstrated to possess health benefits such as antioxidant cardiovascular protection, anti-inflammation, and arthritis-risk reduction. Several phytochemicals and phytonutrients have been discovered from avocado fruit and other parts of the plant. Some of them presented cancer-impeding and cancer-preventing potentials. Especially, the avocado plant is an important source of a folk medicine in some areas.

Scientific Evidence of Anticarcinogenic Activity and Constituents

Avocado contains numerous bioactive alkanols (also termed aliphatic acetogenins) and significant quantities of vitamins E and B6. An acetone extract from avocado displayed the antiproliferative effect against both androgen-independent (PC3) and androgen-dependent (LNCaP) prostate cancer cell lines *in vitro*. Concurrently, the extract elicited G2/M cell cycle arrest in PC3 cells in association with p27 activation.[2] Four extracts prepared from avocado fruits with ethanol, chloroform, ethyl acetate, and petroleum, respectively, were effective in the inhibition of colon adenocarcinoma and esophageal squamous cell carcinoma cell lines but not in normal peripheral blood mononuclear cells. After the treatment of esophageal and colon cancer cell lines for 48 h, its ethanol extract reduced the survival rates to 42% and 70.3%, respectively; its chloroform extract reduced to 32.7% and 56%, respectively; ethyl acetate extract reduced to 7% and 56%, respectively; and its petroleum extract reduced to 33% and 52%, respectively.[3] Its chloroform extract (D003) retarded the proliferation of human normal (TE1177), premalignant (SCC83-01-82), and malignant (SCC83-01-82CA) oral cell lines *in vitro*. In the treatments, the apoptosis of human oral epithelial cancer cells was elicited by D003 extract by augmenting the levels of reactive oxygen species (ROS) and p21WAF1/Cip1 and diminishing the levels of cyclins-D, -A, and cdk2. The GI_{50} values of D003 were 14 µg/mL in SCC83-01-82CA cancer cells and 38 µg/mL in TE1177 normal cells.[4,5] D003 also obviously deterred 7,12-dimethylbenz[a]anthracene (DMBA)-induced tumorigenesis in hamster cheek pouches *in vivo* and suppressed the cell proliferation in DMBA-initiated mucosa together with amplifying ROS level.[6]

Treatment with water extract (100 µg/mL) of avocado fruit for 48 h resulted in 93.3%, 98.3%, 97.8%, and 91.7% mortality, respectively, in human A549 (lung), HepG2 (liver), HT-29 (colon), and MCF-7 (breast) cancer cell lines. The 50% lethal concentrations (LC_{50}) of the water extract were 13.3, 22, 35.4, and 54.5 µg/mL, respectively, in HepG2, HT-29, A549, and MCF-7 cell lines.[7] The methanol extracts isolated from avocado seed, sarcocarp, and peel showed 2,2′-diphenyl-1-picrylhydrazyl (DPPH) and ABTS radical-scavenging activities and the proapoptotic effect in human MDA-MB-231 breast cancer cells in association with activation of caspase-3 and poly(ADP-ribose) polymerase (PARP). Due to less content of polyphenolics, avocado sarcocarp was lesser effective than avocado peel and seeds.[7] On the other hand, the phytochemicals extracted from avocado fruits with 50% methanol were able to enhance the proliferation of human lymphocytes and to diminish chromosomal aberrations induced by an anticancer drug cyclophosphamide. The avocado chemicals also can attenuate the side effect of cancer chemotherapy.[8] Moreover, two aliphatic acetogenins separated from D003 extract were elucidated as (2S,4S)-2,4-dihydroxyheptadec-16-enyl acetate (**1**) and (2S,4S)-2,4-dihydroxyheptadec-16-ynyl acetate (**2**). Either acetogenins **1** or **2** hindered the growth of premalignant and malignant human oral cell lines (83-01-82CA and MEK-overexpressing 83-01-82CA/MEKCA) through blockage of EGFR/RAS/RAF/MEK/ERK1/2 pathways.[5] Acetogenins (**1** and **2**) together synergistically inhibited the proliferation of human oral carcinoma cells together with block of c-RAF (Ser338) and ERK1/2 (Thr202/Tyr204) phosphorylation.[10]

Compared with the matured fruits, avocado unripe fruits exhibited more cytotoxic and pesticide activities. As avocado ripens, the activities could be lessened 10-fold, indicating that the cytotoxic constituent is degraded when the fruit ripened.[11] In addition, the constituent separated from avocado fruit peel, seed, leaf, and bark demonstrated cytotoxicity that was more potent. Persin isolated from the leaves of the avocado tree is a toxin for lactating livestock, especially to animals, but it showed the cytotoxicity on some cancer cell lines.[5]

CONCLUSION AND SUGGESTION

These scientific examinations evidenced the antiproliferative and proapoptotic properties of avocado fruit and the better cytotoxic activity of avocado leaf, bark, fruit peel, and seed. As an advantageous dietary program, consumption of avocado fruit is recommended for cancer prevention, especially for the protection of esophageal, oral, lung, colon, prostate, and breast cancer, as well as helpful in protection from heart disease and age-related macular degeneration. Although its antioxidant and cancer inhibitory potencies are lower than those of other tropical fruits such as papaya, carambola, mangostan, mango, pineapple, wax apple, coconut, pitaya, and durian, avocado fruit still is a nutrition-enriched food favorite of the people due to its multiple health-promoting benefits.[12,13] However, the leaves and bark of the avocado plant are a rich source of cancer inhibitors. Avocado leaves can be used to make a great tea that helps to prevent cancer and to treat various health problems.

REFERENCES

1. (a) Kunnumakkara, A.B. et al., 2014. *Anticancer Properties of Fruits and Vegetables*. Toh Tuck Link, Singapore, World Scientific Publishing; (b) Terry, L.A. et al., 2011. *Health-promoting Properties of Fruits and Vegetables*. Boston, MA: CABI.
2. Lu, Q.Y. et al., 2005. Inhibition of prostate cancer cell growth by an avocado extract: Role of lipid-soluble bioactive substances. *J. Nutr. Biochem.* 16: 23–30.

3. Vahedi, L.L. et al., 2014. Evaluating the effect of four extracts of avocado fruit on esophageal squamous carcinoma and colon adenocarcinoma cell lines in comparison with peripheral blood mononuclear cells. *Acta Medica Iranica*. 52: 201–205.

4. Ding, H. et al., 2009. Selective induction of apoptosis of human cancer cell lines by avocado extract via a ROS-mediated mechanism. *Nutr Cancer* 61: 348–356.

5. Ding, H.M. et al., 2007. Chemopreventive characteristics of avocado fruit. *Seminars in Cancer Biol.* 17: 386–394.

6. Ding, H.M. et al., 2014. Avocado extract inhibits 7,12-dimethylbenz[a]anthracene (DMBA)-induced carcinogenesis in hamster cheek pouches. *Med. Chem.* S1: 008.

7. Lee, S.G. et al., 2008. Antioxidant activities and induction of apoptosis by methanol extracts from avocado. *Han'guk Sikp'um Yongyang Kwahak Hoechi* 37: 269–275.

8. Paul, R. et al., 2011. Avocado fruit (Persea americana Mill) exhibits chemo-protective potentiality against cyclophosphamide induced genotoxicity in human lymphocyte culture. *J. Exper. Therap. Oncol.* 9: 221–230.

9. Khalifa, N.S. et al., 2013. Effect of the water extracts of avocado fruit and cherimoya leaf on four human cancer cell lines and vicia faba root tip cells. *J. Agric. Sci.* 5: 245–254.

10. D'Ambrosio, S.M. et al., 2011. Aliphatic acetogenin constituents of avocado fruits inhibit human oral cancer cell proliferation by targeting the EGFR/RAS/RAF/MEK/ERK1/2 pathway. *Biochem. Biophys. Res. Commun.* 409: 465–469.

11. Oberlies, N.H. et al., 1998. Cytotoxic and insecticidal constituents of the unripe fruit of Persea americana. *J. Nat. Prod.* 61: 781–785.

12. Li, W. et al., 2013. Antioxidant and antiproliferative activities of polyphenol extract from 12 tropical fruits. *Xiandai Shipin Keji* 29: 2383–2387.

13. Garcia-Solis, P. et al., 2009. Screening of antiproliferative effect of aqueous extracts of plant foods consumed in Mexico on the breast cancer cell line MCF-7. *Intl. J. Food Scie. Nutr.* 60(Suppl. 6): 32–46.

34. CHERRY

Cerise   Kirsche   Cereza

櫻桃　サクランボ　벗나무

Prunus avium, P. cerasus

Rosaceae

Cherry is a kind of popular fruit commercially that is mostly derived from two cultivated species, that is, sweet cherry (*Prunus avium*) and sour cherry (*Prunus cerasus*). Both species are native to Europe and western Asia. Sweet cherry is commonly used for directly eating and production of fruit juice and fruit cocktails, whereas sour cherry is often used for cooking. Some other species of *Prunus* have edible fruits, which are not grown extensively for consumption, except *Prunus pseudocerasus* (= *Cerasus pseudocerasus*), which is the major species in China used for providing the cherry fruits to market. Each 100 g raw sweet or sour cherry contains vitamin C (8% versus 12%), vitamin B complex (total 15% versus 17%), vitamin K (2% versus 2%), and vitamin A (0% versus 8%), implying sour cherries provide much higher levels of nutrients in vitamins despite the taste of sweet cherries being more favorable. The pharmacological tests demonstrated that cherries could afford multiple health supports including improvement of digestive tract and cardiovascular system, antioxidation, anti-inflammation, and anticarcinogenesis.

Scientific Evidence of Cancer Prevention

Cherries are a rich source of polyphenols, carotenoids, vitamins, and melatonin, and these constituents display multiple health-promoting advantages, especially marked antioxidative and radical-scavenging activities. However, the cultivars, UV concentration, degree of ripeness, and postharvest storage condition and time may remarkably influence the contents of bioactive phytochemicals and nutrients.

1. Polyphenolics

Polyphenolics are known to be associated with anticarcinogenic, antioxidant, antimutagenic, and anti-inflammatory potentials that are able to reduce the occurrence of carcinogenesis and mutation. At 250 μg/mL concentrations, the water extracts of the red sweet cultivars (Skeena, Glacier, Regina, and Kordia) suppressed lipid peroxidation (LPO) by 70%–89%, while two extracts of the red sour cultivars (Balaton and Montmorency) and yellow sweet cultivars (Rainier and Gold) deterred LPO by 48%–63%. The extracts from these red cultivars at the same concentration were also effective in repressing the activities of cyclooxygenases (COX)-1 and -2 with reducing rates of 76%–99%, but the extracts from the yellow cultivars showed low and no inhibition on COX-2 and COX-1 enzymes.[1]

HPLC analysis revealed that the water extracts contain cyanidin-3-rutinoside as a major compound that was 185 mg/100 g (fresh weight [FW]) in Kordia, 159 mg/100 g in Regina, and 134 mg/100 g in Skeena red sweet cherries, indicating a relationship between the higher antioxidant activities and the dominant quantities of cyanidin-3-rutinoside in the water extracts.[1] Normally, red sweet cherry cultivars contain higher cyanidin-3-O-rutinoside as a major anthocyanin, whose amounts in the cultivars were in the order Kordia > Regina > Skeena.[2]

The methanol extracts of yellow sweet cherry cultivars (Rainier and Gold) primarily contain β-carotene, coumaric, ursolic, ferulic, and caffeic acids. They demonstrated anti-LPO and anti-COX effects at 250 μg/mL with 77%–78% and 79%–94% inhibitory rates, respectively.[1] The ethyl acetate extracts of Rainier and Gold cultivars showed good inhibition of COX-1 and -2 enzyme but less inhibition on LPO,[1] while the CO_2-EtOH supercritical fluid extract of sweet cherry Saco cultivar exerted significant antioxidant activity. The prominent antioxidant activities were certainly associated with the anticarcinogenic activity. A CO_2-EtOH (9:1) extract impeded the proliferation of HT-29 human colon cancer cells (ED_{50} of 0.20 mg/mL, in 96 h) in addition to potent antioxidant activity. Three polyphenols, cyanidin-3-rutinoside, sakuranin, and cyanidin-3-glucoside, were detected in higher quantities in this extract.[2] Although there was no effect in human MCF-7 (breast), HeLa (cervix), NCI-H460 (lung), and HepG2 (liver) carcinoma cell lines, an 80% methanol extract of *P. avium* fruits selectively hindered the proliferation of human HCT-15 colon carcinoma cells (GI_{50} 73.51 μg/mL) *in vitro*. This extract contains total phenolic acids and total flavonols (1.58 and 3.96 mg/g, respectively), wherein cyanidin-3-O-rutinoside (14.5 μg/g) and cyanidin-3-O-glucoside (2.19 μg/g) were the major anthocyanins in the extract.[3]

In four sweet cherry cultivars (Van, Noir de Guben, Larian, and 0-900 Ziraat) grown in Turkey, the content of cyanidin-3-rutinoside (43.57–128.28 mg/100 g, FW) was greater than the content of hydroxycinnamic acids (27.23–93.22 mg/100 g, FW), flavan-3-ols (10.84–22.01 mg/100 g, FW), and rutin (3.55–5.78 mg/100 g, FW). By ABTS and DPPH assays, the orders of antioxidant potencies in the components were found as anthocyanins > total phenolics >> flavan-3-ols > hydroxycinnamic acids, and those in these cultivars were Noir de Guben > 0-900 Ziraat > Larian > Van.[4] Due to the marked antioxidant property, cyanidin-3-O-rutinoside (1) was able to induce oxidative stress in HL-60 human leukemic cells and then elicit the cell apoptosis in a dose- and time-dependent manner in association with ROS-dependent activation of p38 MAPK/JNK and stimulation of Bim-mediated mitochondrial pathways.[5] However, it did not lead to ROS accumulation and cytotoxicity in normal human peripheral blood mononuclear cells and A549 human lung carcinoma cells.[5] By downregulation of u-PA and MMP-2 expressions and inactivation of NF-κB and c-Jun, cyanidin-3-O-rutinoside (1) and cyanidin-3-O-glucoside hindered the invasion and motility of the A549 tumor cells.[6] In concentrations of 20–100 μM, cyaniding-3-O-glucoside deterred the viability of HS578T human breast cancer cells by 82%–90% concomitantly with induction of G2/M cell arrest and apoptosis.[7] According to the experimental data, it is recognized that the anthocyanins in cherries, especially cyanidin-3-O-rutinoside (1), were the important contributors to afford the protective effects against oxidative stress and cancer initiation, disclosing that diet of cherry with high amounts of anthocyanins (either sweet or sour cherries) is helpful for antioxidation and cancer prevention.

2. Monoterpenes

Perillyl alcohol (POH, 2) occurs naturally in the essential oils of plants including cherry fruits, citrus fruits, spearmint, sage, lavender, peppermint, and lemongrass. Owing to cancer-fighting properties, POH (2) has received extensive attention in the preclinical and clinical investigations. POH (2) at 25 μg/mL concentration exhibited high cytotoxic effect in human OVCAR-8 (ovary), HCT-116 (colon), and SF-295 (brain) cancer cell lines, with anti-growth rates of 90.92%–95.82%.[8] At 1.707 mg/L, POH exerted 93.97% and 95.45% growth inhibition against human NCI-H1299 and A549 lung carcinoma cell lines, respectively.[8,9] Moreover, POH (2) and its metabolite perillic acid (PA, 3) were able to elicit the dose-dependent cytotoxic effect in human nonsmall cell lung cancer (NSCLC) (A549 and H520) cell lines, associated with induction of cell cycle arrest and apoptosis via upregulating Bax and p21 expressions and activating caspase-3.[10] Both monoterpenes also could sensitize the lung cancer cells to cisplatin and radiation in a dose-dependent manner and act as radiosensitizers in glioma, head/neck cancer, and prostate carcinoma cell lines,[10–12] showing the values in the combination therapies. The antiproliferative, proapoptotic, and/or cell cycle arrest-inducing effects of POH (2) were also observed in *in vitro* models against a variety of human cell lines: colon cancer (HT-29, SW620), pancreatic cancer (MIA PaCa-2, BXPC3), glioblastoma (U87, U251, A172), prostate cancer (LNCap), lung cancer (H322 and H838), ER⁺ breast cancer (KPL-1, MCF-7), ER⁻ breast cancer (MKL-F, MDA-MB-231, MDA-MB-435), leukemia (K562), lymphoma (U937), B-lymphoma (WEHI-231), and head/neck cancer (HTB-43, SCC-25, BroTo) and against murine C6 glioma and TM6 mammary transformed tumor cell lines.[11–20] In *in vivo* tests, POH (2) retarded UVB-induced skin carcinogenesis[21] and hindered various chemical oncogenes-caused carcinogenesis, such as 4-methylnitrosamino-1-(3-pyridyl)-1-butanone-caused lung carcinogenesis, DMBA-elicited breast carcinogenesis, azoxymethane (AOM)-caused colon carcinogenesis, DMBA-elicited and TPA-promoted skin tumorigenesis, aflatoxin B1-triggered hepatocarcinogenesis, and diethyl-nitrosamine-initiated and 2-acetylamino-fluorine (2-AAF)-promoted hepatocarcinogenesis.[22–28] The *in vivo* assays further demonstrated the antigrowth effect of POH (2) against HCT-116 colon carcinoma cells and temozolomide-resistant U251 glioma cells in xenograft nude mouse models.[30,31] Co-treatment with POH (2) and chemotherapeutic drugs, pentoxifylline or STI571 (gleevec), promoted the sensitivities of U937 myelomonocytic leukemia cells or K562 chronic myelogenous leukemia cells, respectively, and synergistically potentiated the anticancer efficacies.[32,33] Coupling POH with adenovirus-mediated mda-7/IL-24 gene therapy effectively retarded human pancreatic cancer xenografts and obviously amplified the survival period of tested nude mice.[34] Even hyperthermia (43°C) could additively augment the cytotoxicity of POH (2) against SCK mammary carcinoma cells *in vivo*.[35] Nevertheless, nitrosamine-caused esophageal tumorigenesis was weakly promoted POH (2) *in vivo*.[29]

The mechanisms of POH (2) have been revealed to be mediated characteristically by (1) inducing G1 cell arrest through impeding cyclin-D1, c-Myc, and Skp2 expressions and enhancing p53 and p21 expression and inhibiting HIF protein expression and synthesis via blockage of mTOR/4E-BP1 signaling pathways in HCT-116 cells;[30] (2) causing G1 arrest via induction of p15INK4b and p21WAF1/Cip1 pathways in HT-29 and SW620 cells;[36] (3) rapidly restraining NF-κB-DNA-binding activity and repressing a calcium-dependent constitutive NF-κB pathway in WEHI-231 cells;[37] (4) inducing the cell apoptosis via activation of caspase-3 and cleavage of PARP in H322 and H838 cells;[38] (5) markedly amplifying proapoptotic protein Bak expression in BxPC3 cells;[39] (6) activating p38 and/or JNK1/2 and suppressing Na/K-ATPase in U87 and U251 cells;[40] (7) lessening ROS level and inhibiting Ras signaling pathway in DMBA-induced melanoma cells;[41] and obstructing oxidative stress and lowering tumor incidences through repression of ornithine decarboxylase (ODC), thymidine phosphorylase, and proliferating cell nuclear antigen (PCNA) protein in 2-AAF caused hepatoma.[42] Moreover, POH (2) expressed its anti-invasive and antimigratory effects in human hepatoma cell lines (SMMC-7721, MHCC97H, and HepG2) via limiting Notch signaling pathway and amplifying Snail-regulated E-cadherin expression.[43] At a noncytotoxic concentration of 0.5 mmol/L, POH (2) inhibited the migration of MDA-MB-435 breast carcinoma cells besides the growth inhibition of the malignant cells.[44] The i.p. administration of POH at a dose of 75 mg/kg (3 times per week) for 6 weeks to nude mice arrested the growth of orthotopically transplanted estrogen receptor-positive KPL-1 breast cancer cells and limited the regional lymph node metastasis.[45] The anti-angiogenic potential of POH (2) was evidenced by a decrease in VEGF expression in cancer cells and suppression of the vessels via upregulation of Ang2 protein in endothelial cells, events that would lead to the obstruction of new vessel formation.[46] Also, by blocking Mek and Raf-Mek-Erk cascade signaling, POH (2) prompted G0/G1 cell cycle arrest and c-Myc-dependent apoptosis in Bcr/Abl transformed leukemia and myeloid cells, thereby hindering the cell growth.[47,48]

On the basis of the excellent scientific observations, POH (2) has been extensively studied in clinical trials of phases II and I. Intranasal administration of POH (440 mg, per day) temporarily retarded the tumor growth and extended the overall survival of patients with recurrent glioblastoma by more than eight months, with almost nonexistent side effects even in the patients treated by POH for over 4 years.[49,50] However, the phase-II trials with oral administration of POH did not appear to have any clinical effect in patients suffering with advanced colorectal cancer or advanced hormone refractory prostate cancer, but appeared to have adverse effects of POH, especially causing gastro-intestinal symptoms.[51,52]

Consequently, the antitumor activity of perillyl alcohol (2) has been shown in both *in vitro* and/or *in vivo* studies against a range of cancer types including pancreatic, lung, colon, liver, breast, prostate, and brain cancers. It is better to translate more into clinical cancer therapies in humans. An inhaled formulation of POH has shown preliminary evidence of safety and effectiveness in patients burdened with recurrent gliomas.

CONCLUSION AND SUGGESTION

The two dominant compounds, cyanidin-3-O-rutinoside (1) and perillyl alcohol (2), from cherry fruits have been demonstrated to possess antioxidant, anticarcinogenic, and/or anticancer activities by scientific explorations. Especially, perillyl alcohol (2) demonstrated marked and broad anticancer spectrum *in vitro* and *in vivo*. The facts indicated dietary consumption of cherry fruits benefits the cancer chemoprevention and retards the progress of certain types of cancers. However, up to now, there are no reports regarding the quantity of perillyl alcohol (2) in cherry fruits, but it is detectable by TLC examination. Considering the adverse side effects can be caused by perillyl alcohol (2), the diet amount of cherries must be limited. Hence, the best is daily intake of not more than 20 cherries. By the means, cherry fruits not only lower the risk of cancer safely but also cut the risk of heart attack by 30%.

REFERENCES

1. Serra, A.T. et al., 2010. Processing cherries (Prunus avium) using supercritical fluid technology. Part 1: Recovery of extract fractions rich in bioactive compounds. *J. Supercrit Fluids* 55: 184–191.
2. Mulabagal, V. et al., 2009. Anthocyanin content, lipid peroxidation and cyclooxygenase enzyme inhibitory activities of sweet and sour cherries. *J. Agricult. Food Chem.* 57: 1239–1246.
3. Bastos, C. et al., 2015. Chemical characterisation and bioactive properties of Prunus avium L.: The widely studied fruits and the unexplored stems. *Food Chem.* 173: 1045–1053.
4. Kelebek, H. et al., 2011. Evaluation of chemical constituents and antioxidant activity of sweet cherry (Prunus avium L.) cultivars. *Int. J. Food Sci. Technol.* 46: 2530–2537.
5. Feng, R.T. et al., 2007. Cyanidin-3-rutinoside, a natural polyphenol antioxidant, selectively kills leukemic cells by induction of oxidative stress. *J. Biol. Chem.* 282: 13468–13476.
6. Chen, P.N. et al., 2006. Mulberry anthocyanins, cyanidin 3-rutinoside and cyanidin 3-glucoside, exhibited an inhibitory effect on the migration and invasion of a human lung cancer cell line. *Cancer Lett.* 235: 248–259.
7. Chen, P.N. et al., 2005. Cyanidin 3-glucoside and peonidin 3-glucoside inhibit tumor cell growth and induce apoptosis in vitro and suppress tumor growth in vivo. *Nutr Cancer.* 53: 232–243.
8. Andrade, L. N. et al., 2015. Evaluation of the cytotoxicity of structurally correlated p-methane derivatives. *Molecules* 20: 13264–13280.
9. Li, X. et al., 2010. Inhibitory effect of perillyl alcohol on human lung cancer cell lines NCI-H1299 and A549 in vitro and toxicology evaluation of perillyl alcohol. *Guangdong Yaoxueyuan Xuebao* 26: 287–291.
10. Yeruva, L. et al., 2007. Perillyl alcohol and perillic acid induced cell cycle arrest and apoptosis in non-small cell lung cancer cells. *Cancer Lett.* 257: 216–226.
11. Samaila, D. et al., 2004. Monoterpenes enhanced the sensitivity of head and neck cancer cells to radiation treatment in vitro. *Anticancer Res.* 24(5A): 3089–3095.
12. Rajesh, D. et al., 2003. Perillyl alcohol mediated radiosensitization via augmentation of the fas pathway in prostate cancer cells. *Prostate* (NY, NY, US) 57: 14–23; 2003. Perillyl alcohol as a radio-/chemosensitizer in malignant glioma. *J. Biol. Chem.* 278: 35968–35978.

13. Chung, B.H. et al., 2006. Perillyl alcohol inhibits the expression and function of the androgen receptor in human prostate cancer cells. *Cancer Lett.* 236: 222–228.

14. Yuri, T. et al., 2005. Suppression of breast cancer cell proliferation by perillyl alcohol. *Nyugan Kiso Kenkyu* 14: 17–21.

15. (a) Fernandes, J. et al., Perillyl alcohol induces apoptosis in human glioblastoma multiforme cells. *Oncol. Reports* 13: 943–947; (b) de Fischer, J.S.G. et al., 2011. Chemo-resistant protein expression pattern of glioblastoma cells (A172) to perillyl alcohol. *J. Proteome Res.* 10: 153–160.

16. Elegbede, J.A. et al., 2003. Perillyl alcohol and perillaldehyde induced cell cycle arrest and cell death in BroTo and A549 cells cultured in vitro. *Life Sci.* 73: 2831–2840.

17. Brooks, J.D. et al., 2002. Identification of potential prostate cancer preventive agents through induction of quinone reductase in vitro. *Cancer Epidemiol. Biomark. Prev.* 11: 868–875.

18. Satomi, Y. et al., 1999. Induction of AP-1 activity by perillyl alcohol in breast cancer cells. *Carcinogenesis* 20: 1957–1961.

19. Shi, W.G. et al., 2002. Induction of cytostasis in mammary carcinoma cells treated with the anticancer agent perillyl alcohol. *Carcinogenesis* 23: 131–142.

20. Balassiano, I.T. et al., 2002. Effects of perillyl alcohol in glial C6 cell line in vitro and anti-metastatic activity in chorioallantoic membrane model. *Int. J. Mol. Med.* 10: 785–788.

21. Stratton, S.P. et al., 2008. Phase 1 study of topical perillyl alcohol cream for chemoprevention of skin cancer. *Nutr. Cancer* 60: 325–330.

22. Sultana, S. et al., 2013. Perillyl alcohol as a protective modulator against rat hepatocarcinogenesis via amelioration of oxidative damage and cell proliferation. *Human Exp. Toxicol.* 32: 1179–1192.

23. Stratton, S.P. et al., 2010. A phase 2a study of topical perillyl alcohol cream for chemoprevention of skin cancer. *Cancer Prev. Res.* 3: 160–169.

24. Chaudhary, S.C. et al., 2009. Perillyl alcohol attenuates Ras-ERK signaling to inhibit murine skin inflammation and tumorigenesis. *Chemico-Biol. Interactions* 179: 145–153.

25. Lantry, L.E. et al., 1998. Chemopreventive effect of perillyl alcohol on 4-(methylnitrosamino)-1-(3-pyridyl)-1-butanone induced tumorigenesis in (C3H/HeJ X A/J)F1 mouse lung. *J. Cell. Biochem.* 67(Suppl. 27): 20–25.

26. Reddy, B.S. et al., 1997. Chemoprevention of colon carcinogenesis by dietary perillyl alcohol. *Cancer Res.* 57: 420–425.

27. Haag, J.D. 1994. Mammary carcinoma regression induced by perillyl alcohol, a hydroxylated analog of limonene. *Cancer Chemother. Pharmacol.* 34: 477–483.

28. Elegbede, J.A. et al., 2002. Monoterpenes reduced adducts formation in rats exposed to aflatoxin B1. *Afr. J. Biotechnol.* 1: 46–49.

29. Liston, B.W. et al., 2003. Perillyl alcohol as a chemopreventive agent in N-nitrosomethylbenzylamine-induced rat esophageal tumorigenesis. *Cancer Res.* 63: 2399–2403.

30. Ma, J. et al., 2016. Perillyl alcohol efficiently scavenges activity of cellular ROS and inhibits the translational expression of hypoxia-inducible factor-1α via mTOR/4E-BP1 signaling pathways. *Int. Immunopharmacol.* 39: 1–9.

31. Cho, H.Y. 2012. Perillyl alcohol for the treatment of temozolomide-resistant gliomas. *Mol. Cancer Therapeutics* 11: 2462–2472.

32. Gomez-Contreras, P.C. et al., 2006. In vitro induction of apoptosis in U937 cells by perillyl alcohol with sensitization by pentoxifylline: Increased Bcl-2 and Bax protein expression. *Chemotherapy* (Basel, Switzerland) 52: 308–315.

33. Chen, Y. et al., 2004. Effects of POH in combination with STI571 on the proliferation and apoptosis of K562 cells. *J. Huazhong Univ. Sci. Technol. Med. Sci.* 24: 41–44.

34. Lebedeva, I.V. et al., 2008. Chemoprevention by perillyl alcohol coupled with viral gene therapy reduces pancreatic cancer pathogenesis. *Mol.Cancer Ther.* 7: 2042–2050.

35. Ahn, K.J. et al., 2003. Cytotoxicity of perillyl alcohol against cancer cells is potentiated by hyperthermia. *Int. J. Radiat. Oncol. Biol. Physics* 57: 813–819.

36. Koyama, M. et al., 2013. Perillyl alcohol causes G1 arrest through p15INK4b and p21WAF1/Cip1 induction. *Oncol. Reports* 29: 779–784.

37. Berchtold, C.M. et al., 2005. Perillyl alcohol inhibits a calcium-dependent constitutive nuclear factor-κB pathway. *Cancer Res.* 65: 8558–8566.

38. Xu, M. et al., 2004. Perillyl alcohol-mediated inhibition of lung cancer cell line proliferation: Potential mechanisms for its chemotherapeutic effects. *Toxicol. Applied Pharmacol.* 195: 232–246.

39. Burke, Y.D. et al., 2002. Effects of the isoprenoids perillyl alcohol and farnesol on apoptosis biomarkers in pancreatic cancer chemoprevention. *Anticancer Res.* 22(6A): 3127–3134.

40. Garcia, D.G. et al., 2015. Na/K-ATPase as a target for anticancer drugs: Studies with perillyl alcohol. *Mol. Cancer* 14: 1–14.

41. Lluria-Prevatt, M. et al., 2002. Effects of perillyl alcohol on melanoma in the TPras mouse model. *Cancer Epidemiol. Biomark. Prevention* 11: 573–579.

42. Sultana, S. et al., 2013. Perillyl alcohol as a protective modulator against rat hepatocarcinogenesis via amelioration of oxidative damage and cell proliferation. *Human Experim. Toxicol.* 32: 1179–1192.

43. Ma, Y. et al., 2016. Inhibition of perillyl alcohol on cell invasion and migration depends on the notch signaling pathway in hepatoma cells. *Mol. Cell. Biochem.* 411(1–2): 307–315.

44. Wagner, J.E. et al., 2002. Perillyl alcohol inhibits breast cell migration without affecting cell adhesion. *J. Biomed. Biotechnol.* 2: 136–140.

45. Yuri, T. et al., 2004. Perillyl alcohol inhibits human breast cancer cell growth in vitro and in vivo. *Breast Cancer Res. Treat.* 84: 251–260.

46. Loutrari, H. et al., 2004. Perillyl alcohol is an angiogenesis inhibitor. *J. Pharmacol. Experim. Ther.* 311: 568–575.

47. Clark, S.S. et al., 2003. Anti-leukemia effect of perillyl alcohol in Bcr/Abl-transformed cells indirectly inhibits signaling through Mek in a Ras- and Raf-independent fashion. *Clinical Cancer Res.* 9: 4494–4504; 2006. Perillyl alcohol induces c-Myc-dependent apoptosis in Bcr/Abl-transformed leukemia cells. *Oncol.* 70: 13–18.

48. Sahin, M.B. et al., 1999. Perillyl alcohol selectively induces G0/G1 arrest and apoptosis in Bcr/Abl-transformed myeloid cell lines. *Leukemia* 13: 1581–1591.

49. da Fonseca, C.O. et al., 2011. Efficacy of monoterpene perillyl alcohol upon survival rate of patients with recurrent glioblastoma. *J. Cancer Res. Clin. Oncol.* 137: 287–293.

50. da Fonseca, C.O. et al., 2011. Case of advanced recurrent glioblastoma successfully treated with monoterpene perillyl alcohol by intranasal administration: Intranasal POH promotes long-term survival of recurrent glioma. *J. Cancer Ther.* 2: 16–21.

51. Liu, G., 2003. Phase II trial of perillyl alcohol (NSC 641066) administered daily in patients with metastatic androgen independent prostate cancer. *Invest. New Drugs.* 21: 367–372.

52. Meadows, S.M. et al., 2002. Phase II trial of perillyl alcohol in patients with metastatic colorectal cancer. *Int. J. Gastrointestinal Cancer* 32: 125–128.

35. CHESTNUT ROSE

刺梨

Rosa roxburghii, R. roxburghii f. *normalis*

Rosaceae

Chestnut rose (= Burr rose) is the fruit of two Rosaceae plants *Rosa roxburghii* and *R. roxburghii* f. *normalis*. The edible fruits are full of vitamin C, whose content is much greater than that in other kinds of fruits such as grape, apple, pear, and dahurian rose fruit. Its content of vitamin P also is higher than that in general vegetables and fruits. Chestnut rose fruits are widely used in health supplements and medicine due to multiple health benefits such as digestive, antioxidation, hypotensive, antiatherosclerosis, immunoincremental, hepatoprotective, anti-inflammation, antivirus, detoxification, sedation, antiaging, and antilipemic effects.

SCIENTIFIC EVIDENCE OF ANTIMUTAGENIC ACTIVITY

Probably in part due to the high contents of vitamin C and superoxide dismutase (SOD), chestnut rose fruit displayed attractive cancer-preventing effect together with effective blocking of synthesis of nitrite-type mutagen *in vivo*. A 0.5 mL of the fruit juice could obstruct the formation of *N*-nitrosoproline from a reaction between proline and sodium nitrite by 78.7% in rats, in whom the effect was stronger than that of 20 μM vitamin C.[1] Importantly, the inhibition of *N*-nitrosoproline synthesis by the fruit juice was demonstrated in peoples who are lived in highly incident region of gastric carcinoma.[2] The fruit juice not only repressed the formation of nitrite in normal persons, but also inhibited the synthesis of endogenous *N*-nitrosoproline in patients having gastric cancer.[3] Oral administration of 8 mL/kg of the fruit juice retarded the formation of ethylcarbamide *N*-nitrite in pregnant mice and reduced the possibility of carcinogenesis mainly in the nervous system in the mice of the next generation.[2]

Both *in vitro* and *in vivo* experiments demonstrated that the fruit extract has obvious antitumor activity. The extract exerted the antiproliferative effect on human JEC endometrial adenocarcinoma cells in a concentration- and time-dependent manner, with IC_{50} of 0.05 μg/mL in 96 h. At a concentration of 10 μg/mL, the extract arrested G2/M cell cycle and promoted 25.59% of JEC cells to apoptosis.[4] In a combined treatment, chestnut rose fruit extract could synergistically reinforce the cytotoxicity of 5-FU on the JEC cells, induce the cell differentiation and apoptosis, and inhibit the cell proliferation and division.[5] Co-treatment with the fruit extract and matrine (an alkaloid from the *Sophora* plant) at the respective doses of 40–160 mg/L and 60–240 mg/L resulted in 84.2%–94.8% inhibition against human endothelial EVC-304 cells derived from human SGC-7901 gastric cancer cells, together with significant decreases in Ki-67 level and Bcl-2 expression.[6] Likewise, the synergistic antitumor and proapoptotic effects of combination of *R. roxburghii* and *Fagopyrum cymosum* (a folk herb) obviously appeared in human CaEs-17 esophageal squamous cell carcinoma, SGC-7901 gastric cancer, and A549 pulmonary cancer cell lines.[7]

1. Triterpenoids

An ethanolic extract of the fruit and its triterpene components were effective in inducing the growth inhibition and apoptotic death in human SMMC-7721 hepatoma cells but not affecting the differentiation of CD34+ hematopoietic progenitor cells.[8] The triterpenes of chestnut rose fruits in the treatment also triggered the SMMC-7721 cells to differentiation.[9] The *in vivo* anti-neoplastic effect of chestnut rose fruit mainly presented in the life span prolongation in mouse bearing Ehrlich ascetic cancer (EAC) tumor and the increase in thymus and spleen indexes, implying the effects were largely in relation to enhancing immune function in the EAC mice.[4]

2. Polysaccharides

Polysaccharides prepared from chestnut rose fruit in an *in vitro* assay displayed the suppressive effects against the viability, migration, and invasion of human A2780 ovarian cancer cells. The anti-invasive effect occurred in parallel with downregulation of MMP-9 expression, showing an anti-metastatic potential for the therapy of ovarian cancer.[10]

CONCLUSION AND SUGGESTION

From the current scientific findings, it is recognized that chestnut rose fruit and the fruit juice are capable of blocking *N*-nitrosoproline synthesis to exert the anticarcinogenic activity in the stomach and additively augmenting the anticancer effect of chemo drugs and herbs. The triterpenoid components from chestnut rose fruit could effectively protect the liver against carcinogenesis together with immune potentiation. The rich polysaccharide component in chestnut rose fruit should be helpful for hindering ovarian cancer development and metastasis. Accordingly, the consumption of chestnut rose fruit and the fruit juice should be encouraged not only for the cancer prevention but also for the rich vitamins C and P supplement. However, more explorations of the anticancer activity of chestnut rose fruit are still expected.

REFERENCES

1. Lin, D.X. et al., 1987. Cancer prevention of Rosa roxburghii, I and II. *J. Beijing Med. Univ.* 19: 231; 19: 305.
2. Lin, D.X. et al., 1987. Cancer prevention of Rosa roxburghii, III. *J. Beijing Med. Univ.* 19: 383.
3. Xu, G.P. et al., 1993. The Cili juice blocked the synthesis of N-nitrosoproline in peoples at highly incident region of gastric carcinoma. *Beijing Yike Daxue Xuebao* 25: 445.
4. Dai, Z.K. et al., 2007. Anticancer effect of CL extract of Rosa roxburghii. *Zhongguo Zhongyao Zazhi* 32: 1453–1457.
5. Dai, Z.K. et al., 2011. Anticancer effect of 5-florouracil combined with extract of Rosa roxburghii Tratt on human endometrial adenocarcinoma. *Zhongguo Zhongxiyi Jiehe Zazhi* 31: 1108–1112, 1117.
6. Guo, J. et al., 2009. Effects of Rosa roxburghii Tratt extract and matrine on proliferation and apoptosis of human endothelial cells cultured with supernatant of gastric cancer cells. *Shiyong Zhongliu Zazhi* 24: 547–552.
7. Liu, W. et al., 2012. Inhibition of tumor growth in vitro by a combination of extracts from Rosa roxburghii Tratt and Fagopyrum cymosum. *Asian Pacific J. Cancer Prev.* 13: 2409–2014.
8. Yu, L.M. et al., 2007. Effects of Rosa roxburghii extract on proliferation and differentiation in human hepatoma SMMC-7721 cells and CD34+ hematopoietic cells. *J. Health Sci.* 53: 10–15.
9. Huang, J.E. et al., 2013. Effect of Rosa roxburghii tratt triterpene on proliferation of human hepatoma SMMC-7721 cells. *Shipin Kexue* (Beijing, China) 34: 275–279.
10. Chen Y. et al., 2014. Inhibition of metastasis and invasion of ovarian cancer cells by crude polysaccharides from rosa roxburghii tratt in vitro. *Asian Pacific J. Cancer Prev.* 15: 10351–10354.

36. CITRUS FRUITS

Les agrumes   Zitrusfrüchte   Frutas cítricas

柑橘水果　かんきつ類の果実　감귤류

Citrus

Rutaceae

4. $R_1 = -H$, $R_2 = -CH_3$, $R_3 = -glucose-(6)-rhamnose$
5. $R_1 = -glucose-(6)-rhamnose$, $R_2 = R_3 = -H$
6. $R_1 = -H$, $R_2 = -CH_3$, $R_3 = -glucose-(2)-rhamnose$

7. $R = -H$
8. $R = -OCH_3$

Citrus plants have presented many types of favorable citrus fruits to humans since ancient times. Various natural and cultivated citrus hybrids are produced commercially for the common citrus fruits such as oranges, tangerines, lemons, limes, grapefruits, and citrons. Today, these fruits and their juices are popular as a group of the most important fruits and fruit juice beverages in the world. All citrus fruits display higher acidity indicated by rich content of vitamin C. Vitamin C in addition to other vitamins and other bioactive phytochemicals such as flavonoids, limonoids, volatile organics, dietary fibers, and/or carotenoids in the citrus fruits makes the fruits a beneficial addition to a healthy diet. A variety of tests demonstrated that the fruits also help to prevent diabetes, constipation, high blood pressure, indigestion, and other problems and to augment antioxidant ability and the immune system, as well as improving the skin, hair, and teeth.

SCIENTIFIC EVIDENCE OF CANCER PREVENTION

The cancer preventive potential of citrus fruits is revealed to be primarily attributed to two types of constituents in citrus, that is, limonoids and monoterpenes. The flavonoids and polyphenolics in the fruits showed certain potentials in anticarcinogenesis, but the effect was believed to tightly correlate with their significant antioxidant properties. A total phenolic extract derived from tangerine pulp and orange pulp that was produced in China was weakly effective in inhibiting human hepatoma HepG2 cells (EC_{50} of 33.32 and 208.6 mg/mL, respectively) but not active in human colon cancer Caco-2 cells.[1] The free phenolic content extracted from fruits of lemon, grapefruit, and orange displayed antioxidant effect in an assay for total oxyradical-scavenging capacity and showed antiproliferative effect in HepG2 cells *in vitro*. The ED_{50} values were 30.56 mg/mL for lemon and 130.09 mg/mL for grapefruit but n/b for orange.[2] A lemon fruit methanolic extract retarded the proliferation of MCF-7 human breast cancer cells in association with the induction of apoptosis via upregulation of p53 and Bax expressions, downregulation of Bcl-2 expression, and activation of caspase-3.[3] All extracts of chloroform, acetone, methanol, and methanol/water (8:2) from the juice of Mexican lime (*C. aurantifolia*) deterred the growth of Panc-28 human pancreatic cancer cells, wherein the methanol extract showed the maximum activity (IC_{50} of 81.20 μg/mL, 72 h).[4] In radical-scavenging tests, the chloroform extract elicited the greatest activity, whereas the methanol/water extract showed the lowest activity.[4] The fruit juice from *C. bergamia* exerted marked inhibitory effects on the proliferation, invasion, and adhesion of human LAN-1 and SK-N-SH neuroblastoma cells *in vitro* and on the pulmonary metastases of LAN-1 tumor in a nude mouse model without any apparent toxicity.[5] In addition, the dietary fibers from citrus fruits were reported to be good for the protection from the risk of colon cancer.

Here, the anticancer and anticarcinogenic activities of limonoids, flavonoids, sterols, and mono-terpenes from the citrus fruits were evidenced for their application in the cancer prevention.

1. Limonoids

Contents of limonoids: Limonoids are unique highly oxygenated triterpenoids long recognized to have marked biological activities. Limonoids are found in high levels in the citrus fruits, especially in the fruit seeds (such as orange seeds and lemon seeds). Currently, 44 limonoid aglycones and 18 limonoid glucosides have been identified from citrus plants. The limonoids appear in large amounts in the seeds as a water-insoluble aglycone form, which gives a bitter taste, but appears in citrus juices and citrus pulps as a water-soluble glucoside form that is not bitter. During fruit maturation, the bitter aglycones in the pulps are converted into the nonbitter limonoid glucosides, affording the unpleasant taste and flavor. Limonin (**1**) is a representative limonoid aglycone in citrus fruit seeds, while limonin 17-O-β-D-glucopyranoside (**2**) constitutes over 50% of the total limonoid glucosides in the juices. According to the latest analysis, it is recognized that the concentrations of limonoid glucosides reach levels of 204.3–123.8 mg/L in sweet orange juices, 119.2 mg/L in Ruby red grape-fruit, and 100.0–68.4 mg/L in tangerine juices. Nonetheless, in lime and lemon varieties, the con-tents of limonoid glucosides were lowest, namely 30.2 mg/L in lime and 3.9 mg/L in Meyer lemon.[6] When the citrus juice or citrus fruits are consumed, the human digestive system separates the sugar part from the limonoids and the limonoid glycosides biologically transfer to the aglycones, which then would be absorbed into the blood stream to play remarkable roles in antioxidant, anticarcino-genic, and anticancer activities.

Limonin (**1**) and nomilin (**3**) are two predominant limonoids found in Rutaceous plants such as lemon, lime, orange, and grapefruit, whereas limonexic acid and isolimonexic acid are the most prominent limonoids of lime juice. As a major glucoside in citrus juices, limonin 17-O-β-D-glucoside (**2**) constitutes over 50% of the total limonoid glucosides in the juices. Obacunone and obacunone glucoside occur in the different parts of citrus fruits in very low concentrations (7.2–60 ppm).[6]

Anticancer effects: *In vitro* assays have revealed that the citrus limonoids have the capacities of scav-enging free radicals and eliciting growth arrest and apoptosis in various human cancer cell lines, such as MDA-MB-435, MDA-MB-231, and MCF-7 (breast), SW480, Caco-2, and HT-29 (colon), Panc-28 (pancreas), CCRF-CEM (leukemic), and SH-SY5Y (brain) lines.[7,8] Deacetylnomilin, oba-cunone, and methyl nomilinate presented devastating effects toward estrogen receptor (ER)-positive MCF-7 cells with IC_{50} values of 0.005, 0.009, and 0.01 μg/mL, respectively, and diacetylnomilin was the most effective inhibitor on ER-negative MDA-MB-435 cells (IC_{50} of 0.07 μg/mL). The anti-proliferative effects were not related to their antiaromatase activity but correlated with caspase-7 activation pathway in MCF-7 cells.[9] In human LNCaP androgen-dependent prostate cancer cells, obacunone and obacunone glucoside exerted time- and dose-dependent inhibition against the cell proliferation and achieved more than 60% inhibition of the cell viability at 100 μM concentration after 24 and 48 h, together with the activation of programmed cell death.[10] Incubation of limonin (**1**) impeded the proliferation of SW480 cells by 67.0%–67.8% in 25–50 μM concentrations at 72 h, whereas limonin glucoside (**2**) inhibited SW480 cells by 61% in 6.25 µM at 24 h and by 77% in 100 µM at 72 h.[11] The IC_{50} in SW480 cells (72 h) were in a range of 37.39–60.47 µM for limonin (**1**), limonin glucoside (**2**), obacunone, and obacunone glucoside, and limonin glucoside (**2**) was the most potent inhibitor among them.[11] Other limonins such as methyl nomilinate, isolimonexic acid, limonexic acid, and isoobacunoic acid exerted much lower suppressive effect on SW480 cells in 50 µM but elicited cell cycle arrest at G1 phase via inactivation of CDK4/6 and cyclin-D3 and downregulation of CDK inhibitors.[12] Combined with the limonoids with curcumin, the proliferative suppression of SW480 cells could have reached 96% along with 3.5–4.0-fold elevation in total cellular caspase-3 activity and 2–4-fold increase in Bax/Bcl-2 ratio, implying that consumption of curcumin and limonoids together may offer better protection against colon carcinoma.[13] Also, the IC_{50}s (72 h) of isolimonexic acid, limonexic acid, limonin glucoside (**2**), and limonin (**1**) were 18.01, 20.49, 21.91, and 42.40 µM, respectively, in Panc-28 pancreatic cancer cells.[14]

Compared to Caco-2 colon cancer cells, SH-SY5Y neuroblastoma cells were more sensitive to the limonoids. The aglycones (such as limonin, obacunone, nomilin, and deacetylnomilin) showed similar 72% inhibition of SH-SY5Y cells at 50 µmol/L (48 h), and four limonoid glucosides (such as obacunone 17-β-D-glucoside, nomilinic acid 17-β-D-glucoside, limonin 17-β-D-glucoside, and diacetylnomilinic acid 17-β-D-glucoside) were effective in hindering SH-SY5Y cancer cells and activating caspases-3 and -7 in a dose- and time-dependent manner, indicating that the glucosides were capable of inducing apoptotic death.[15] Significant arrest of the growth of HT-29 colon cancer cells was achieved by isolimonoic acid at 5.0 µM, ichanexic acid at 10.0 µM, and limonexic acid at 50 µM within 24 h of treatment, concomitant with induction of G2/M phase cell cycle arrest.[16,17] However, Caco-2 colon cancer cells were less sensitive to the aglycones, wherein nomilin (**1**) was the most effective cytotoxic agent and deacetylnomilin was the least effective on Caco-2 cells.[18] Treatments of IOMM-Lee and CH157MN meningioma cell lines with limonin (**1**) triggered the antitumor and proapoptotic activities via repression of Wnt/β-catenin signaling pathway.[19]

Importantly, limonin (**1**) and deacetylnomilin were inhibitors of *P*-glycoprotein (*P*-gp), a membrane transporter encoded by MDR1 gene in human cells, which could obstruct the efflux of *P*-gp substrate rhodamine 123 in a dose-dependent manner, leading to the antiproliferation of multidrug-resistant human leukemia CEM/ADR5000 cells (IC_{50} of 159.44 and 73.83 µM, respectively). At a nontoxic concentration of 20 µM, limonin (**1**) potentiated the cytotoxicity of doxorubicin by 2.98-fold in the Caco2 cells and 2.2-fold in the CEM/ADR5000 cells, revealing that the citrus limonoids are capable of augmenting the accumulation and efficacy of chemo drugs in the leukemia cells.[20] Exposure of obacunone to human MCF-7 breast cancer cells elicited the cell apoptosis and G1 cell cycle arrest and then hampered the proliferation of MCF-7 cells without affecting nonmalignant breast cells. During the treatment, obacunone hampered inflammatory pathways and aromatase as well, effects that may be helpful in preventing estrogen-responsive breast carcinogenesis.[21] In addition, both *in vitro* and *in vivo* results showed that limonin (**1**) had no reversal influences on chemo drugs (camptothecin or cyclophosphamide)-induced proapoptosis and tumor regression against human breast cancer cells.[31] Nevertheless, no obvious antiproliferative effects were observed in human HL-60 (leukemic), SKOV-3 (ovary), NCI-SNU-1 (stomach), HeLa (cervix), and HepG2 (liver) cancer cell lines cultured with the four limonoids (obacunone 17β-D-glucoside, nomilinic acid 17β-D-glucoside, limonin, and nomilin) individually at 100 µg/mL.[22] Also, the citrus limonoids were ineffective on noncancerous cell lines such as mammalian epithelial Chinese hamster ovary cells and COS-1 African green monkey kidney cells.

Anticarcinogenic effects: The anticarcinogenic activities of citrus limonoids were further demonstrated in *in vivo* tests. In rat models, feeding of 0.02 or 0.05% limonin (**1**) or obacunone and consumption of limonin (200 mg/kg) or grapefruit pulp powder (13.7 g/kg) obviously impeded (AOM)-induced aberrant crypt foci (ACF) in colon and diminished the incidence of colon carcinogenesis by hampering the proliferation and elevating the apoptosis through anti-inflammatory activities (such as decline in levels of both iNOS and COX-2) and reducing PCNA-labeling index in crypts.[23-25] Topically giving 2.5%–3.5% deacetyl nomilin, limonin 17-β-D-glucoside, or obacunone 17-β-D-glucoside to hamster cheek pouch hindered the development of DMBA-caused oral tumorigenesis,[26,27] but 2.5% deoxylimonic acid was ineffective in the same model.[28] Similarly, addition of nomilin or limonin to the diet in various concentrations inhibited benzo[a]pyrene (BAP)-induced lung tumor formation and BAP-DNA adduct formation in A/J mice, and gavage of nomilin to ICR/Ha mice or rat reduced the incidences of forestomach tumors and gastric tumors caused by BAP.[29,30] During these treatments, the functions of glutathione S-transferase and quinone reductase were enhanced in small intestine, liver, stomach, or colon mucosa, events that might contribute to the anticarcinogenic effects. Also, both initiation and promotion phases of carcinogenesis could be impeded by the topical application of nomilin and limonin to the skin of SENCAR mice, wherein nomilin (3) was more effective during the initiation stage, while limonin (1) was more potent during the promotion phase in the skin carcinogenesis.[30]

2. Flavonoids

Flavonoids are one of the important components in citrus fruits responsible for lowering the risk of cancer. The content of flavonoids in citrus fruit or fruit juice is about 10%, and hesperidin (4) is the most observable flavonoid in many citrus fruits. Besides the flavonoids from citrus fruit peels that displayed obvious anticancer activities related to proliferation, invasion, metastasis, and apoptosis, the flavonoids and their glycosides from the fruit pulp and juice were also valuable in the cancer prevention.

Flavonone glycosides: Hesperidin (4) and rutin (5) are the major flavonoids and limonin (1) and its glucoside (2) are the prominent limonoids in lime juice (*C. aurantifolia*). Treatment with hesperidin (4) and rutin (5), respectively, resulted in the antiproliferative and proapoptotic effects against Panc-28 pancreatic cancer cells with IC_{50}s of 16.70 and 41.73 μg/mL. The hesperidin activities were greater than those of limonin (IC_{50} of 89.3 μg/mL) and limonin glucoside (IC_{50} of 31.7 μg/mL) in the same assay.[4] Hesperidin (4) and neohesperidin (6) as the major flavonoids in fruit peel of rough lemon (*C. jambhiri*) were effective in inhibiting CCRF-CEM leukemia cells (IC_{50} of 95.09 versus 122.16 μM) and Caco-2 colon carcinoma cells (IC_{50} of 194.89 versus 174.13 μM). Similar to diacetylnomilin and limonin (1), both flavonoids (4 and 5) could act as *P*-gp inhibitors to repress the proliferation of MDR-CEM/ADR 5000 leukemia cells (IC_{50} of 229.77 versus 168.71 μM).[20] In an *in vitro* assay with HeLa cervical cancer cells, hesperidin (4) induced the cell apoptosis via endoplasmic reticulum stress pathways and elicited G0/G1 cell cycle arrest via downexpression of cyclin-D1, cyclin-E1, and cyclin-dependent kinase-2, thereby inhibiting the cell proliferation.[32]

Naringin is a major flavonoid in grapefruit and other citrus fruits, in which aglycone moiety is naringenin. Treatment of HeLa cervical cancer cells and triple-negative breast cancer cells with naringin triggered the growth inhibition and apoptosis, but the effects were mediated by different mechanisms, that is, by inhibition of NF-κB/COX-2-caspase-1 pathway in the HeLa cells and by modulation of β-catenin pathway, activation of p21, and lessening survivin expression in the breast cancer cells.[33,34] Correspondingly, the antitumor potential was further proved in naringin-treated MDA-MB-231 breast cancer xenograft mice.[34] Also, naringin was found to be able to suppress chondrosarcoma cell viability and migration, the antimigratory effect that was associated with downregulation of vascular adhesion molecule (VCAM)-1 expression by increasing miR-126.[35] Poncirin is a bitter flavanone glycoside abundantly present in many species of citrus fruits. In an *in vitro* model, it provoked the apoptosis of AGS gastric cancer cells via an extrinsic pathway, that is, upregulation of Fas ligand protein, activation of caspases-8 and -3, and subsequent cleavage of PARP.[36]

Free flavonones: Tangeritin (7) and nobiletin (8) were isolated from tangerine (*C. tangerina*) and Shiikuwasha (*C. depressa*), respectively, the two hindered cell cycle progression at G1 phase in human HT-29 (colon), MDA-MB-435, and MCF-7 (breast) cancer cell lines and then inhibited the cell proliferation in a dose- and time-dependent manner, but did not cause the cell apoptosis or cell death. If the treatments lasted for four days, the inhibitory rates could be up to 80%.[37] Tangeritin (7) and nobiletin (8) also exerted the inhibitory effects on human SKOV-3 ovarian cancer cell migration.[38] Moreover, tangeritin (7) could promote the apoptosis of human meningioma cell lines (IOMM-Lee and CH157MN) and did not induce normal human neurons to apoptosis. The proapoptotic mechanism was revealed to be associated with increase in GSK3β phosphorylation via blockage of a Wnt5/β-catenin pathway, upregulation of apoptotic factors (Bax and caspase-3) expressions, and inhibition of survival proteins (Bcl-xL and Mcl-1) and tetraspanin protein (TSPAN12).[19] Despite less-effective chemotherapies for treatment of recurrent meningioma, tangeritin (7) as well as limonin (1) showed therapeutic potential for the treatment of malignant meningioma. Nobiletin (8) was more effective in arresting the proliferation of p53-mutated SNU-16 human gastric cancer cells than other flavonoids. Nobiletin (8) also prompted the apoptosis of SNU-16 cells by multiple pathways involving intracellular ER stress-elicited protective autophagy, activation of caspases-9 and -3, and degradation of PARP.[39] In human HL-60 acute myeloid leukemia cells, nobiletin (8) treatment induced the cell cycle arrest at G0/G1 phase via deterrence of extracellular signal-regulated kinase activity and provoked the cell apoptosis via activation of caspases-8, -9, -3 and upexpression of p38 mitogen-activated protein kinase, thereby restraining the HL-60 cell proliferation.[40] Similarly, nobiletin (8) was able to diminish mitogen-activated protein and extracellular signal-regulated kinase activities directly and to deter MMP expression, then exerting the anti-metastatic effect in human HT-1080 fibrosarcoma cells.[41]

When used in co-treatment with chloroquine (an autophagy inhibitor) or 5-FU (a chemo drug), the anticancer effect was synergistically enhanced against the SNU-16 tumor in a concentration-dependent manner, implying a promising co-therapy for gastric cancer patients.[39] Combination of nobiletin (8) with *cis*-diamminedichloride platinum or doxorubicin resulted in synergistic effects to obstruct the growth of gastric cancer cell lines (MKN-45, MKN-74, KATO-III, and TMK-1) and MCF-7 breast cancer cell but not T47D breast cancer cells *in vitro*.[42,43] Similarly, the proliferation of human nonsmall-cell lung carcinoma cell lines (A549 and H460) could be retarded concomitant with elicitation of G1 cell arrest when used in combination with nobiletin (8) and either carboplatin or paclitaxel in the treatments. After the co-treatments, the synergistic inhibitory effect was further demonstrated in nude mice transplanted A549 lung cancer xenografts.[44]

Another important flavanone in citrus fruits as well as tomatoes is naringenin, which frequently occurs in human diet. In the last few years, it has gained an increasing attention due to its health-improving and health-protecting properties, including its antioxidant, anti-inflammatory, anti-mutagenic, and anticarcinogenic activities. The molecular biology studies revealed the ability of naringenin to elicit apoptosis and growth suppression in HepG2 hepatoma cells and A431 epidermoid carcinoma cells concomitant with the induction of ROS generation and cell cycle arrest.[45,46] In the rat models, administration of naringenin repressed the proliferation of C6 glioma and obstructed *N*-methyl-*N'*-nitro-*N*-nitrosoguanidine-caused gastric carcinogenesis.[47,48] In an *in vivo* mouse 4T1 breast cancer resection model, oral administration of naringenin obviously prolonged the survival of tested mice and retarded the lung metastasis concomitantly with the promotion of T-cell activation and restoration of T-cell function. The observation revealed that the anti-metastatic effect of naringenin was mainly contributed by the upregulated host antitumor immunity.[49] Therefore, naringenin may be developed as a surgical adjuvant agent for breast cancer patients because it showed both anti-metastatic and immunoregulating activities. Moreover, in a co-treatment, naringenin could enhance curcumin (a cancer inhibitor)-triggered apoptosis and cell cycle arrest in THP-1 acute myeloid leukemia cells through blocking Akt and ERK pathways and promoting JNK and p53 pathways, leading to the cell viability inhibition additively.[50]

3. Phytosterols

β-Sitosterol glucoside and stigmasterol are the predominant naturally occurring sterols commonly found in a variety of foods and plants. The phytosterols were also reported from the isolation of fruit peels of rough lemon (*C. jambhiri*) and poudersa lemon (*C. pyriformis*) and fruit seeds of lime (*C. aurantifolia*) and sour orange (*C. aurantium*), but very small amounts of phytosterols are present in the fruit pulps. In the *in vitro* assays, β-sitosterol glucoside at 40 μM retarded the proliferation of HT-29 colon cancer cells by 38.4% after 24 h treatment, accompanied by the induction of cell cycle arrest at G2/M phase.[18] β-Sitosterol glucoside and stigmasterol exerted a certain degree of suppressive effects against human cancer cell lines. The IC_{50}s (72 h) were 66.60 versus 80.97 μM in CCRF-CEM leukemia cells, 133.81 versus 209.87 μM in multidrug-resistant CEM/ADR5000 leukemic cells and 337.77 versus 387.06 μM in Caco colon cancer cells for β-sitosterol glucoside and stigmasterol, respectively. The most active inhibition by β-sitosterol glucoside (IC_{50} of 32.32 μM in 72 h) was observed in Panc-28 pancreatic cancer cells. The data implied that the phytosterols presented the lowest activity to colon cancer cells and lower inhibitory effect to multidrug-resistant leukemia cells.[14,18,20]

4. Coumarins

Three coumarins, 8-geranyloxypsolaren, 5-geranyloxypsolaren, and 5-geranyloxy-7-methoxycoumarin, were isolated from lemon (*C. limon*) fruit peel as inhibitors of tumor promoter TPA-elicited Epstein–Barr virus activation in Raji cells. The coumarins were also able to hinder TPA-caused superoxide (O^{2-}) generation in differentiated human HL-60 pro-myelocytic leukemia cells and to restrain both lipopolysaccharide and interferon-induced nitric oxide (NO) generation in mouse macrophage RAW 264.7 cells, indicating that the inhibition of radical generation might be correlated to the antitumor-promoting activity of the lemon coumarins.[51] A coumarin identified as 7-methoxy-5-prenyloxycoumarin was found from Meyer lemon (*C. meyeri*). It similarly exerted the inhibitory effects on tumor promotion in the Epstein–Barr virus early antigen test and in an *in vivo* two-stage mouse skin carcinogenic test[52]; therefore, the antitumor promoting property clearly designated the chemopreventive value of lemon coumarins. In addition, auraptene, another citrus fruit-derived coumarin, could hinder CD3/CD28-activated lymphocyte proliferation in a dose-dependent manner in an *in vivo* mouse model, indicating its anti-inflammatory property via inhibiting T-cell proliferation and the inflammatory cytokine secretion.[53]

5. Essential oil and monoterpenes

The cytotoxicity of essential oil (OE) extracted from citrus fruit peels was explored widely by the *in vitro* assays. D-Limonene (**9**) was assigned to be an important and a major compound in the citrus essential oil, which is primarily responsible for the anticancer effect of citrus EO. The peel EOs from Iranian *C. limon* and *C. sinensis* contain about 98.4% and 98.8% limonene (**9**), respectively, showing the suppressive activities against MCF-7 breast cancer and HeLa cervical cancer cell lines. The IC_{50}s of EOs (72 h) in MCF-7 and HeLa cells were 10 and 17 μg/mL for *C. limon* and 0.5 and 3 μg/mL for *C. sinensis*, respectively. The EO from Iranian *C. medica* var. *cedrate* showed more potent inhibitory effect on the two cell lines with the same IC_{50}s (72 h) of 1 μg/mL. Interestingly, the EO from *C. medica* contained only 56.6% limonene (**9**) but showed better inhibition of the MCF-7 and HeLa cells than the EO from *C. limon* with a much higher percentage of limonene.[54] The EOs from Syrian *C. limon* peels collected in three places, which contain 61.8%–73.8% of limonene (**9**), were effective in inhibiting LIM1863 colorectal cancer cells with IC_{50}s of 5.75–7.92 μg/mL.[55] The EO extracted from lemon produced in Yancheng, China, exerted 39% inhibition against HeLa cancer cell growth in a concentration of 60 μg/mL, wherein the main constituents in this EO were assigned as propylphosphonic acid-fluoroanhydride-octyl ester (15.72%), decanoic anhydride (12.63%), 2,4-difluoro-1-isocyanatobenzene (11.72%), 1,1′-hexadecylidenebiscyclopentane (9.98%), and limonene (4.25%).[56] The facts implied that the synergistic action of the compounds in citrus fruit peels plays an important role in impeding the cancer cells, though limonene (**9**) is the most predominant cancer inhibitor in many citrus EOs.

Three other EOs extracted from sweet orange (*C. aurantium* var. *dulcis*), grapefruit (*C. paradisi*), and lemon (*C. limon*) collected in Japan could induce human HL-60 leukemia cells to apoptotic death. The proapoptotic activities of sweet orange EO and grapefruit EO were largely attributed to the limonene content in these EOs, but the effect of lemon EO was also contributed by other constituents such as decanal, octanal, and citral.[57] These results indicated that other monoterpenes in the EOs besides limonene also possess the anticancer activities and the monoterpenes exerted synergistic effects with limonene. An *in vivo* experiment showed that D-limonene (**9**) pronouncedly obstructed the formation of pulmonary adenoma and the occurrence of forestomach tumor when administrated orally to mice 1 h prior to incubation of 4-(methylnitrosamino)-1-(3-pyridyl)-1-butanone (a carcinogen).[58] Moreover, a limonene-rich volatile oil was prepared from blood oranges (*C. sinensis*) and formulated into an emulsion (BVOE). Besides inducing growth suppression and apoptosis in HT-29 and SW480 human colon cancer cell lines in a dose-dependent manner, BVOE was also able to inhibit vascular endothelial growth factor (VEGF) and block VEGF receptor-1 binding and matrix metalloproteinases (MMP-9) expression at a concentration of 100 g/mL, exerting the antiangiogenic and anti-metastatic potentials.[59]

NANOFORMULATION

For ameliorating the applicability in the cancer therapy and prevention, hesperetin (**4**) has been formulated in nanoparticles and liposomes. Hesperetin was encapsulated in Eudragit-E 100 nanoparticles in the presence of polyvinyl alcohol as a stabilizer. The hesperetin-loaded nanoparticles (size: 55–180 nm) revealed higher cytotoxic efficacy than free hesperetin (**4**) in KB oral carcinoma cells together with more effectivity in inducing ROS generation, DNA damage, and apoptotic indexes.[60] The hesperetin-loaded liposomes exerted anticancer efficacy in both H441 lung cancer cells and MDA-MB-231 breast cancer cells.[61] The two types of modern formulation significantly improved the stable periods and conditions in serum and notably amplified the bioavailability and delivery efficacy of hesperetin,[60,61] showing a further potential for clinical use in the treatment and prevention of cancers.

OTHER NEWLY DISCOVERED BIOACTIVITIES

According to recent research reports, hesperidin and naringenin were demonstrated to have the abilities to deter neuroinflammatory responses and improve immunological responses.[62,63] These findings might disclose a new possible application for the two flavonoids in the prevention of brain cancer.

CONCLUSION AND SUGGESTION

These scientific research results have revealed that intake of citrus fruits and fruit juices can provide a functional protection against a wide range of cancer risk in pancreas, breast, colon, lung, stomach, brain, skin, and/or blood. It is believable that the citrus fruits can give us the calm, present, and effective cancer prevention in a safer and healthier manner. The flavonoids, limonoids, monoterpenes, and phytosterols in citrus fruit pulps have been confirmed to contribute to cancer prevention. The integration of these active agents may offer great chemoprevention against carcinomas and carcinogenesis by eliciting cell cycle arrest and apoptosis, limiting cell proliferation and metastasis, deterring angiogenesis and inflammation, and inducing phase II detoxifying enzymes and antioxidant enzymes. However, the commercial citrus juices tend to have low levels of bioactive components; thus, fresh citrus fruit and freshly squeezed fruit juices with pulps are recommended for consumption due to high levels of antioxidant and cancer inhibitors. However, overconsumption of citrus fruits and juices, especially lemon and lime, should be avoided as the high acidic content may trigger heartburn and dental problems.

Interestingly, the citrus fruit wasters such as a large amount of citrus peels are utilized in bioethanol production by enzyme hydrolysis. The hydrolyzed citrus residues have been proven to exert not only similar degrees of antioxidant activity but also suppressive effect against the proliferation of carcinoma cells (such as human melanoma A375 and colon cancer HCT-116 cells) due to good quantity of flavonoids (such as naringin, naringenin, hesperetin, and neohesperidin) and co-products (such as limonoids, D-limonene, and galacturonic acid) in the hydrolyzed residues.[64] The findings excited an attention in comprehensive application of the hydrolyzed citrus residues in the production of functional supplements.

REFERENCES

1. Liu, D. et al., 2015. Evaluation of antiproliferative activities of main fruit species in China on HepG2 human liver and Caco colon cancer cells. *Xiandai Shipin Keji* 31: 23–28.
2. Sun, J. et al., 2002. Antioxidant and antiproliferative activities of common fruits. *J. Agric. Food Chem.* 50: 7449–7454.
3. Alshatwi, A.A. et al., 2011. Apoptosis-mediated inhibition of human breast cancer cell proliferation by lemon citrus extract. *Asian Pac. J. Cancer Prev.* 12: 1555–1559.
4. Patil, J.R. et al., 2009. Bioactive compounds from Mexican lime (Citrus aurantifolia) juice induce apoptosis in human pancreatic cells. *J. Agric. Food Chem.* 57: 10933–10942.
5. Navarra, M. et al., 2014. Effect of Citrus bergamia juice on human neuroblastoma cells in vitro and in metastatic xenograft models. *Fitoterapia* 95: 83–92.
6. Breksa, A.P. et al., 2015. Determination of Citrus limonoid glucosides by high performance liquid chromatography coupled to post-column reaction with Ehrlich's reagent. *Beverages* 1: 70–81.
7. Zhou, Y.F. et al., 2011. Anticancer activities of Citrus limonoids. *Zhongguo Xibao Shengwuxue Xuebao* 33: 548–553.
8. Kim, J.H. et al., 2012. Cancer chemopreventive properties of citrus limonoids. *ACS Symp Ser.* 1093(Emerging Trends in Dietary Components for Preventing and Combating Disease): 37–50.
9. (a) Guthrie, N. et al., 2000. Inhibition of human breast cancer cells by citrus limonoids. *ACS Symp. Ser.*, 758 (Citrus Limonoids): 164–174; (b) Kim, J.H. et al., 2013. Limonoids and their anti-proliferative and antiaromatase properties in human breast cancer cells. *Food Funct.* 4: 258.
10. Murthy, K.N. et al., 2015. Cytotoxicity of obacunone and obacunone glucoside in human prostate cancer cells involves Akt-mediated programmed cell death. *Toxicol.* 329: 88–97.
11. (a) Murthy, K.N. et al., 2009. Limonin and its glucoside from citrus can inhibit colon cancer: Evidence from in vitro studies. *Acta Horticulturae* 841 (Proceedings of the 2nd International Symposium on Human Health Effects of Fruits and Vegetables, 2007): 145–150; (b) Chidambara, M.K.N. et al., 2011. Citrus limonin and its glucoside inhibit colon adenocarcinoma cell proliferation through apoptosis. *J. Agricul. Food Chem.* 59: 2314–2323.
12. Kim, J.H. et al., 2012. Methyl nomilinate from citrus can modulate cell cycle regulators to induce cytotoxicity in human colon cancer (SW480) cells in vitro. *Toxicol. In Vitro* 26: 1216–1223.
13. Chidambara, M.K.N. et al., 2013. Citrus limonoids and curcumin additively inhibit human colon cancer cells. *Food Funct* 4: 803–810.
14. Patil, J.R. et al., 2010. Characterization of Citrus aurantifolia bioactive compounds and their inhibition of human pancreatic cancer cells through apoptosis. *Microchem. J.* 94: 108–117.
15. Poulose, S.M. et al., 2005. Citrus limonoids induce apoptosis in human neuroblastoma cells and have radical scavenging activity. *J. Nutr.* 135: 870–877.
16. Jayaprakasha, G.K. et al., 2008. Novel triterpenoid from Citrus aurantium L. possesses chemopreventive properties against human colon cancer cells. *Bioorg. Med. Chem.* 16: 5939–5951.
17. Jayaprakasha, G.K. et al., 2010. Bioactive compounds from sour orange inhibit colon cancer cell proliferation and Induce cell cycle arrest. *J. Agricul. Food Chem.* 58: 180–186.
18. Poulose, S.M. et al., 2006. Antiproliferative effects of citrus limonoids against human neuroblastoma and colonic adenocarcinoma cells. *Nutr. Cancer* 56: 103–112.
19. Das, A. et al., 2015. A novel component from citrus, ginger, and mushroom family exhibits antitumor activity on human meningioma cells through suppressing the Wnt/β-catenin signaling pathway. *Tumor Biol.* 36: 7027–7034.
20. El-Readi, M.Z. et al., 2010. Inhibition of P-glycoprotein activity by limonin and other secondary metabolites from citrus species in human colon and leukaemia cell lines. *Eur. J. Pharmacol.* 626: 139–145.

21. Kim, J.H. et al., 2014. Obacunone exhibits anti-proliferative and anti-aromatase activity in vitro by inhibiting the p38 MAPK signaling pathway in MCF-7 human breast adenocarcinoma cells. *Biochimie* 105: 36–44.

22. Tian, Q. et al., 2001. Differential inhibition of human cancer cell proliferation by citrus limonoids. *Nutr. Cancer*, 40: 180–184.

23. Tanaka, T. et al., 2000. Citrus limonoids obacunone and limonin inhibit azoxymethane-induced colon carcinogenesis in rats. *BioFactors* 13: 213–218.

24. Vanamala, J. et al., 2006. Suppression of colon carcinogenesis by bioactive compounds in grapefruit. *Carcinogenesis* 27: 1257–1265.

25. Tanaka, T. et al., 2000. Citrus limonoids obacunone and limonin inhibit the development of a precursor lesion, aberrant crypt foci, for colon cancer in rats. *ACS Symp. Ser.* 758(Citrus Limonoids): 145–163.

26. Miller, E.G. et al., 2006. Further studies on the anticancer activity of citrus limonoids. *Abstracts of Papers, 232nd ACS National Meeting*, San Francisco, CA: AGFD-097, September 10–14.

27. Miller, E.G. et al., 2004. Further studies on the anticancer activity of citrus limonoids. *J. Agricul. Food Chem.* 52: 4908–4912.

28. Miller, E.G. et al., 1994. Citrus limonoids as inhibitors of oral carcinogenesis. *Food Technol.* (Chicago, IL) 48: 110–112, 114.

29. Hasegawa, S. et al., 1990. Limonoids as antitumor agents. *Ger. Offen. DE* 3922666 A1 19900322.

30. Lam, L.K.T. et al., 1994. Inhibition of chemically induced carcinogenesis by citrus limonoids. *ACS Symp. Ser.* 546 (Food Phytochemicals for Cancer Prevention I): 209–219.

31. Somasundaram, S. et al., 2012. Citrus limonin lacks the antichemotherapeutic effect in human models of breast cancer. *J. Nutrigenet. Nutrigen.* 5: 106–114.

32. Wang, Y.X. et al., 2015. Hesperidin inhibits HeLa cell proliferation through apoptosis mediated by endoplasmic reticulum stress pathways and cell cycle arrest. *BMC Cancer* 15: 682/1–682/11.

33. Zeng, L. et al., 2014. Naringin inhibits growth and induces apoptosis by a mechanism dependent on reduced activation of NF-κB/COX-2-caspase-1 pathway in HeLa cervical cancer cells. *Int. J. Oncol.* 45(5): 1929–1936.

34. Li, H.Z. et al., 2013. Naringin inhibits growth potential of human triple-negative breast cancer cells by targeting β-catenin signaling pathway. *Toxicol. Lett.* 220(3): 219–228.

35. Tan, T.W. et al., 2014. Naringin suppress chondrosarcoma migration through inhibition vascular adhesion molecule-1 expression by modulating miR-126. *Int. Immunopharmacol.* 22(1): 107–114.

36. Saralamma, V.V.G. et al., 2015. Poncirin induces apoptosis in AGS human gastric cancer cells through extrinsic apoptotic pathway by up-regulation of fas ligand. *Int. J. Mol. Sci.* 16(9): 22676–22691.

37. Morley, K.L. et al., 2007. Tangeretin and nobiletin induce G1 cell cycle arrest but not apoptosis in human breast and colon cancer cells. *Cancer Lett.* 251: 168–78.

38. Zhang, J.K. et al., 2014. Chemopreventive effect of flavonoids from Ougan (Citrus reticulata cv. Suavissima) fruit against cancer cell proliferation and migration. *J. Funct. Foods* 10: 511–519.

39. Moon, J.Y. et al., 2013. Nobiletin induces apoptosis and potentiates the effects of the anticancer drug 5-fluorouracil in p53-mutated SNU-16 human gastric cancer cells. *Nutr. Cancer* 65(2): 286–295; 2016. Nobiletin induces protective autophagy accompanied by ER-stress mediated apoptosis in human gastric cancer SNU-16 cells. *Molecules* 21(7): 914/1–914/13.

40. Hsiao, P.C. et al., 2014. Nobiletin suppresses the proliferation and induces apoptosis involving MAPKs and caspase-8/-9/-3 signals in human acute myeloid leukemia cells. *Tumor Biol.* 35(12): 11903–11911.

41. Miyata, Y. et al., 2008. A citrus polymethoxyflavonoid, nobiletin, is a novel MEK inhibitor that exhibits antitumor metastasis in human fibrosarcoma HT-1080 cells. *Biochem. Biophys. Res. Commun.* 366: 168–173.

42. Meiyanto, E. et al., 2011. Nobiletin increased cytotoxic activity of doxorubicin on Mcf-7 cells but not on T47d cells. *Int. J. Phytomed.* 3: 129–137.

43. Yoshimizu, N. et al., 2004. Combination effects of nobiletin with CDDP on gastric cancer cells. *American Association for Cancer Research Meeting. Proceedings of the American Association for Cancer Research 45*: Abstract #838; 2004. Antitumour effects of nobiletin, a Citrus flavonoid, on gastric cancer include: Antiproliferative effects, induction of apoptosis and cell cycle deregulation, *Aliment Pharmacol Ther.* 1: 95–101.

44. Uesato, S. et al., 2014. Synergistic antitumor effect of a combination of paclitaxel and carboplatin with nobiletin from citrus depressa on non-small-cell lung cancer cell lines. *Planta Med.* 80: 452–457.

45. Ahamad, M.S. et al., 2014. Induction of apoptosis and antiproliferative activity of naringenin in human epidermoid carcinoma cell through ROS generation and cell cycle arrest. *PLoS One.* 9: e1100032014.
46. Arul, D. et al., 2013. Naringenin (citrus flavonone) induces growth inhibition, cell cycle arrest and apoptosis in human hepatocellular carcinoma cells. *Pathol Oncol Res.* 19: 763–770.
47. Sabarinathan, D. et al., 2011. Naringenin, a flavanone inhibits the proliferation of cerebrally implanted C6 glioma cells in rats. *Chem Biol Interact.* 189: 26–36.
48. Ekambaram, G. et al., 2008. Naringenin reduces tumor size and weight loss in N-methyl-N'-nitro-N-nitrosoguanidine-induced gastric carcinogenesis in rats. *Nutr Res.* 28: 106–112.
49. (a) Qin, L. et al., 2011. Naringenin reduces lung metastasis in a breast cancer resection model. *Protein Cell.* 2: 507–516; (b) Mir, I.A. et al., 2015. Chemo-preventive and therapeutic potential of "Naringenin," a flavanone present in citrus fruits. *Nutr. Cancer* 67(1): 27–42.
50. Shi, D.Y. et al., 2015. Co-treatment of THP-1 cells with naringenin and curcumin induces cell cycle arrest and apoptosis via numerous pathways. *Mol. Med. Reports* 12(6): 8223–8228.
53. Niu, X.L. et al., 2015. Auraptene has the inhibitory property on murine T lymphocyte activation. *Eur. J. Pharmacol.* 750: 8–13.
51. Miyake, Y. et al., 1999. Identification of coumarins from lemon fruit (Citrus limon) as inhibitors of in vitro tumor promotion and superoxide and nitric oxide generation. *J. Agricul. Food Chem.* 47: 3151–3157.
52. Miyake, Y. et al., 2015. Evaluation for antitumor-promoting activity of meyerin and 7-methoxy-5-prenyloxycoumarin in Meyer lemon. *Sci. Technol. Res.* 21: 879–882.
54. Monajemi, R. et al., 2005. Cytotoxic effects of essential oils of some Iranian Citrus peels. *Iranian J. Pharm. Res.* 4: 183–187.
55. Samer, J. et al., 2012. The cytotoxic effect of essential oil of Syrian citrus limon peel on human colorectal carcinoma cell line (Lim1863). *Middle East J. Cancer* 3: 15–21.
56. Huang, C.Y. et al., 2010. Evaluation of antioxidant and antitumor activities of lemon essential oil. *J. Med. Plants Res.* 4: 1910–1915.
57. Hata, T. et al., 2003. Induction of apoptosis by Citrus paradisi essential oil in human leukemic (HL-60) cells. *In Vivo* 17: 553–559.
58. Wattenberg, L.W. et al., 1991. Inhibition of 4-(methylnitrosamino)-1-(3-pyridyl)-1-butanone carcinogenesis in mice by D-limonene and citrus fruit oils. *Carcinogenesis* 12: 115–117.
59. Chidambara, M.K.N. et al., 2012. D-limonene rich volatile oil from blood oranges inhibits angiogenesis, metastasis and cell death in human colon cancer cells. *Life Sci.* 91: 429–439.
60. Gurushankar, K. et al., 2014. Synthesis, characterization and in vitro anticancer evaluation of hesperetin-loaded nanoparticles in human oral carcinoma (KB) cells. *Adv. Nat. Sci.: Nanosci. Nanotechnol.* 5(1): 015006/1–015006/10.
61. Wolfram, J. et al., 2016. Hesperetin liposomes for cancer therapy. *Curr. Drug Del.* 13(5): 711–719.
62. Wu, L.H. et al., 2016. Naringenin suppresses neuroinflammatory responses through inducing suppressor of cytokine signaling 3 expression. *Mol. Neurobiol.* 53(2): 1080–1091.
63. Haghmorad, D. 2017. Hesperidin ameliorates immunological outcome and reduces neuroinflammation in the mouse model of multiple sclerosis. *J. Neuro- immunol.* 302: 23–33.
64. Im, S.J. et al., 2014. Evaluation of bioactive components and antioxidant and anticancer properties of citrus wastes generated during bioethanol production. *Nat. Prod. Commun.* 9: 483–486.

37. CRANBERRY

Canneberge   Cranberry   Arándano

蔓越莓　クランベリー　크랜베리

Vaccinium macrocarpon

Ericaceae

2. R = –H
3. R = –A

Cranberry (*Vaccinium macrocarpon*) is a major commercial crop that is cultivated throughout the northern United States, Canada, and Chile. The cranberry juice is a health beverage popular in North American region. It can provide rich antioxidants, moderate levels of vitamin C, dietary fiber, and three dietary minerals (manganese, calcium, and magnesium) as well as vitamin B complex, E and K. In addition to the nutritional values, cranberry is also beneficial to fight inflammation and oxidation, amplify the immune system, and promote cardiovascular and digestive tract functions; cranberry juice is effective in treating urinary tract infections. In the past decade, dietary cranberry for lowering cancer occurrence has received more attention.

SCIENTIFIC EVIDENCE OF CANCER-PREVENTIVE CONSTITUENTS

In the *in vitro* models, cranberry juice suppressed the proliferation of human PC3 prostate cancer and MDA-MB-231 breast cancer cell lines with IC_{50}s of 25 and 46 μL/mL, respectively,[1] and the juice extract inhibited the growth of human HSC-2 oral carcinoma cells with midpoint cytotoxicity at 200 μg/mL.[2] After treatment with a 6.7% cranberry juice for 20 h, human MCF-7, MDA-MB-231, and MDA-MB-435 breast cancer cells were killed over 20%.[3] *In vitro* treatment with 25 and 50 μg/mL of whole cranberry extract for 6 h significantly diminished the cellular viability of human DU-145 prostate cancer cells together with elicitation of cell cycle arrest via increase in p27 activity and decrease in CDK4, cyclins-A, -B1, -D1, and -E expressions.[4] Cranberry methanolic extract in a range of 16–125 μg/mL exerted the antiproliferative effect on K562 leukemia and HT-29 colon cancer cells.[5] A cranberry extract with chilled 80% acetone showed the inhibitory effect on human HepG2 (liver), MCF-7 (breast), and SGC-7901 (stomach) carcinoma cell lines, and the ED_{50}s were 14.5, 28.6, and 37.12 mg/mL, respectively, whose suppression on SGC-7901 cells was partly mediated by lessening of PCNA expression and induction of apoptosis.[6] The acetone extract at 50 mg/mL could arrest the MCF-7 cell cycle at G0/G1 phase and trigger the cell apoptosis and, at 30 mg/mL, obstruct the proliferation of MCF-7 cells by 52.3%.[7] Exposure to a 0.1% HCl contained methanol extract of cranberry led to increased antiproliferative effect against human oral (KB, CAL27), breast (MCF-7), colon (HT-29, HCT-116), and prostate (LNCaP) tumor cell lines, and the IC_{50}s were in a range of 100.00–180.61 μg/mL, wherein the order of sensitivities to the acidified methanol extract was LNCaP > HCT-116 > HT-29 > CAL27 > MCF-7 >> KB.[8] Treatment with 200 μg/mL total cranberry extract for 48 h showed the antiproliferative effect against HT-29 colon cancer cells (78%) and metastatic SW620 colon cancer cells (35%) but no activity on SW480 primary colon neoplastic cells.[9] 2-CME, a chloroform/methanol fraction derived from the acidic methanol extract, was effective in retarding human K562 leukemic cells in concentrations of 16–63 µg/mL, HT-29 tumor cells in 31–125 µg/mL, and other cancer cell lines (such as BALB/c3T3, H460, ME-180, DU-145, MCF-7, and PC3) in 63–250 µg/mL.[5]

The anticancer potential of cranberry was also demonstrated by *in vivo* experiments. The *N*-butyl-*N*-(4-hydroxy-butyl)-nitrosamine-triggered urinary bladder cancer could be reduced by 38% *in vivo* after oral administration of cranberry juice concentration at a daily dose of 1.0 mL per rat.[10] The growth and metastasis of human MDA-MB-435 breast cancer cells were lessened when the tested mice were fed cranberry press-cake.[11] The antigrowth effect of the 80% chilled acetone extract also presented in nude mice transplanted human SGC-7901 gastric cancer. In its dose of 20 mg/mL, the diameter, weight, and volume of SGC-7901 tumor xenografts were reduced by 47.2, 48.9, and 44.0%, respectively. The growth of SGC-7901 cells was restrained by 31.7% at 20 mg/mL dose and by 45.1% at 40 mg/mL dose.[5] Feeding either meal or juice of cranberry to Fisher 344 male rats obstructed AOM-induced colon cancer concomitantly with activation of hepatic enzymes phase 1 (CYP2E1) and phase 11 (GST).[12] In addition, the cranberry extract limited COX-2 expression and IκBα degradation in both unstimulated and PMA-stimulated HT-29 colon adenocarcinoma cells, playing a role in the prevention of colon cancer by hindering inflammatory responses.[13] The cranberry extracts also are inhibitors of quinone reductase (a phase II xenobiotic detoxification enzyme) and ODC.[7,14] All the findings demonstrated the potentials of dietary cranberry in preventing the carcinogenesis and lowering the risk of cancer development, and may act synergistically with other functional foods.

SCIENTIFIC EVIDENCE OF CANCER PREVENTERS

Like grapes and other dark berries, cranberry is an excellent dietary source of polyphenolics that includes flavonoids (such as flavonols, anthocyanins, and proanthocyanidins (PACs)), caffeic acid derivatives, catechins, substituted cinnamic acids, as well as triterpenoids (such as ursolic acid and its esters). The polyphenolics-rich cranberry and other Vaccinium berries have been demonstrated to have multiple health benefits such as radical-scavenging and oxidative stress-counteracting effects, limitation of some cancer initiation/development, inhibition of inflammation as well as lessening of the severity of atherosclerosis, ischemic stroke, and neurodegeneration of aging. The phytochemicals of cranberry fruits have been reported to impede the growth fractions and proliferation of breast, colon, prostate, and other carcinoma cell lines.

In the chilled 80% acetone extract, the total phenolic content is 570.4 mg (gallic acid equivalent)/100 g fresh cranberries (FC), the total flavonoid content is 161.6 mg (catechin equivalent)/100 g FC, and the total monomeric anthocyanins is 92.0 mg (cyaniding-3-glucoside equivalent)/100 g FC.[7] Unripened cranberries have lower content of anthocyanin but high content of flavonoids and phenolic acids in comparison to ripened cranberries.[15] The findings evidenced that the polyphenolics including flavonoids and anthocyanins are the major components in cranberries, which are primarily responsible for the health-improving benefits of cranberries.

1. Polyphenolics

Compared to apple, red grape, strawberry, peach, lemon, pear, banana, orange, grapefruit, and pineapple, cranberry fruits showed greater total antioxidant activity (177.0 µmol of vitamin C equivalent/g of fruit). The soluble free form of phenolic extract from cranberry displayed the highest antiproliferative effect on HepG2 hepatoma cells with EC_{50} of 14.5 mg/mL, followed by lemon (30.6 mg/mL), apple (49.4 mg/mL), strawberry (56.3 mg/mL), red grape (71.0 mg/mL), banana (110.1 mg/mL), grapefruit (130.1 mg/mL), and peach (156.3 mg/mL).[16] A total polyphenolics-enriched fraction derived from cranberries at a dose of 200 µg/mL exerted significant suppressive effect on oral cancer cell lines (KB and CAL27) for 95%–96.1% and prostate neoplastic cell lines

(RWPE-1, RWPE-2, and 22Rv1) for 95%–99.6%.[9] In four colon cancer cell lines, the fraction exerted greater antiproliferative activity against HCT-116 (92.1%) than against HT-29 (61.1%), SW480 (60%), and SW620 (63%).[9]

Flavonoids: Fr6 was a flavonoid-rich fraction derived from cranberry press-cake extract in C18 Flash 40M cartridge column eluted with methanol plus 1% acetic acid. In the *in vitro* assay, Fr6 retarded the proliferation of eight tested human cancer cell lines of multiple origins, wherein LNCaP androgen-dependent prostate cells and DMS lung cancer cells were most sensitive to Fr6 (respective IC_{50} of 9.9 and 21.1 mg/L), and DU-145 androgen-independent prostate cancer cells and MDA-MB-435 estrogen-independent breast cancer cells were least sensitive to Fr6 (respective IC_{50} of 234 and 212 mg/L). Other human tumor lines originating from brain (U87) breast (MCF-7), skin (SK-MEL-5), and colon (HT-29) had intermediate sensitivity to Fr6 (IC_{50} of 128–168 mg/L). In a range of 100–400 mg/L concentrations, treatment with Fr6 for 48 h blocked cell cycle progression and induced the MDA-MB-435 cells to undergo apoptotic death in a dose-dependent manner, thereby hindering the cell proliferation.[11,17] Similarly, within 24–48 h of exposure to the U87 cells, Fr6 arrested cell cycle at G1 phase and elicited apoptosis.[17] The antineoplastic effect has been further proved in nude mice model implanted U87 glioblastoma multiform. Intraperitoneal administration of Fr6 in the tested animals in a dose of 250 mg/kg notably delayed the growth of implanted U87 tumors *in vivo*.[17]

Bioactivity-guided fractionation led to the identification of the major cancer prevention-related constituents to be quercetin (**1**) and its glycosides in the flavonoid extract of cranberries. The antiproliferative activities were observed for quercetin (**1**) with moderate to low degrees in the *in vitro* assays. The IC_{50}s of quercetin (**1**) were 10 μM in A549 lung and B16-4A5 skin cancer cells, 6.5 μM in TGB-11TKB gastric cancer cells, 7.9 μM in CCRF-HSB-2 T-cell leukemia cells, 40 or 62 μM in HT-29 colon cancer cells, 37.5 or 73 μM in MCF-7 breast cancer cells, and 86 μM in DU-145 prostate cancer cells, as well as its EC_{50} values were 40.9 μM in HepG2 hepatoma cells and 137.5 μM in MCF-7 breast cancer cells.[18–21] Quercetin-3-O-β-glucoside showed the growth inhibitory effect against the HepG2 and MCF-7 cells (respective EC_{50} of 49.22 and 23.90 μM), whereas quercetin 3-O-β-galactoside showed no such activity. However, the observation also pointed out no cytotoxic effect on the HepG2 and MCF-7 cells for quercetin (**1**) and quercetin-3-O-β-glucoside.[18–20] In another *in vitro* assay, quercetin (**1**) was effective in suppressing human ovarian cancer cell lines: OVCAR-8 cells (IC_{50} of 61 μg/mL) and SKOV-3 cells (IC_{50} of 83 μg/mL), while myricetin-3-galactoside and quercetin-3-arabinopyranoside demonstrated low cytotoxicity (IC_{50} of 130 and 212 μg/ml).[22] By activation of caspase-3 and deactivation of PARP, quercetin (**1**) induced the apoptosis of SKOV-3 and OVCAR-8 ovarian cancer cells; by blockage of MAPK/ERK pathway, upregulation of p21 and downregulation of cyclin-D1, DNA-PK, and phosphohistone H3, quercetin (**1**) arrested cell cycle progression in the ovarian cancer cells. This flavonol was also capable of lessening EGFR activity and expressing and augmenting the sensitivity of SKOV-3 cells to cisplatin.[22] In addition, most of the flavonol glycosides from cranberries showed the antioxidant activity and radical-scavenging ability being comparable or superior to that of vitamin E.[5]

Anthocyanins: An anthocyanin-enriched fraction was derived from the fractionation of cranberry polyphenolic extract by a Sephadex LH-20 column chromatography, whose fraction in an *in vitro* assay restrained the proliferation of human oral cancer cell lines (KB and CAL) by 21%–22%, human prostate cancer cell lines (RWPE-1, RWPE-2, and 22RV-1) by 55%–69%, and human SW620 colon cancer cells by 14% at 7.1 μg/mL concentration, but did not influence the proliferation of SW480 colon cancer cells.[9] Cyanidin-3-galactoside is one of the most powerful antioxidants in cranberries, with antioxidant activity superior to that of vitamin E and Trolox. However, it was weakly effective in restraining the growth of cancer cell lines (BALB/3T3, MCF-7, ME-180, PC3, H460, DU-145, K562, HT-29, and M-14) with GI_{50}s greater than 250 μM.[21]

Proanthocyanidins: PACs are a diverse group of polymeric structures made up of flavan-3-ols (primarily epicatechin) and their polymer ranged greatly in size and structure. PAC are termed condensed tannins as well. The content of PAC is only 1.2% in the total polyphenolic extract of cranberries. Dissimilar to most fruits, a structural feature identified in cranberry PAC is the prominence of A-type linkages between units; these types of linkages strongly impact the biological properties. Normally, the A-type linkage-containing dimers and trimers of PAC are more cytotoxic than only B-type linkage-containing dimers and trimers. A PAC-enriched fraction (PACf) derived from cranberry in 6.5 μg/mL concentration exerted the growth suppression against oral cancer cell lines (KB and CAL27) for 41% and 37.6%, prostate cancer cell lines (RWPE-1, RWPE-2, and 22RV-1) for 80%, 88%, and 70%, and colon cancer cell lines (SW620 and SW480) for 10% and 0%, respectively.[9] The IC_{50}s of PACf were 48 mg/L in U87 glioblastoma cells, 79 mg/L in HT-29 colon cancer cells, and 96 mg/L in DU-145 androgen-independent prostate cancer cells;[17] the GI_{50}s of PACf were 20 μg/mL in NCI-H460 lung cancer cells, 30 μg/mL in ME-180 cervical cancer cells, 70 μg/mL in K562 leukemia cells, 110 μg/mL in HT-29 cells, and >125 μg/mL in MCF-7, DU-145, BALB/c3T3, and M14 tumor cell lines.[23] At 25 μg/mL concentration for 6 h exposure, the PACf markedly diminished the viability of DU-145 cells by approximately 30%.[11] The i.p. injection of the PACf in a dose of 100 mg/kg to the tested mice could delay the growth of U87 tumor and inhibit the growth of HT-29 and DU-145 tumors *in vivo*.[17] Following 48 h of the PACf treatment (50 μg/mL), the acid-induced cell proliferation of SEG-1 esophageal cancer cells was obviously hindered, and the proliferation of BIC-1 esophageal cancer cells was restrained by 49.8% at 48 h and 64.5% at 72 h.[24] During the suppressive effects, PACf induced cell cycle arrest at G1 checkpoint via p21 activation in the cancer cell lines of U87, SEG-1, and NCI-H460.[23–25] The suppressive effect in DU-145 cells by the PACf at 100 μg/mL was also found to be accompanied with decline in MMPs-2 and -9 expression via alterations in multiple cellular signaling pathways, such as inhibition of PI-3 kinase and Akt proteins, decrease in NF-κB and AP-1 translocation, and increase in MAP kinase expression and both p38 and ERK1/2 phosphorylation.[26] By the PACf treatment, the autophagic death of esophageal adenocarcinoma cell lines (JHAD1, OE33, and OE19) was elicited via a caspase-independent and Beclin-1-independent but LC3-II-dependent pathway, wherein autophagic LC3-II was induced by the PACf following siRNA suppression of Beclin-1 in these tumor cell lines.[27]

A fine separation of the PACf by Sephadex LH-20 column chromatography let to two subfractions PAC-1 and PAC-2. Both were selectively cytotoxic to SKOV-3 ovarian epithelial adenocarcinoma, PC3 prostate adenocarcinoma, and SMS-KCNR neuroblastoma cell lines. The IC_{50} values were 0.40 and 0.48 mg/mL for PAC-1 and 0.25 and 0.53 mg/mL for PAC-2 in SMS-KCNR and PC3 cell lines, respectively, but much less cytotoxic to normal human lung fibroblasts ($IC_{50} \geq 1$ mg/mL). Compared to PAC-2, the SKOV-3 cells were more sensitive to PAC-1.[28] The inhibition on SKOV-3 cells by PAC-1 was associated with block of cell cycle progression at G2/M phase and increase in ROS generation and activation of intrinsic and extrinsic pathway to apoptosis.[29] The SKOV-3 cell viability and proliferation were diminished by 39.1% and 64.5% by PAC-1 at 50 μg/mL, 66% and 84.9% at 75 μg/mL, and 81.8% and 92.4% at 100 μg/mL, respectively.[29]

Moreover, co-treatment of SKOV-3 cells with PAC-1 and paraplatin could hamper the cell proliferation at lower concentrations than with either individually,[28] indicating that the synergic activity may warrant for the cancer chemotherapies and reversal of paraplatin resistance. PAC-1A (97% purity of PAC-1) was effective in suppressing the viability and proliferation of neuroblastoma cell lines (IMR-32, SMSKCNR, SKNSH, and SHSY5Y) *in vitro* and the IC_{50} values were ~12.5 μg/mL in SH-SY5Y and IMR-32 cell lines and 25 μg/mL in SMS-KCNR and SK-N-SH cell lines. Correlating to the antineuroblastoma effect, PAC-1A promoted the ROS increase-triggered apoptosis together with loss of mitochondrial transmembrane depolarization potential, downregulation of prosurvival (Bcl-2, Bcl-xL, Mcl-1) proteins, upregulation of proapoptotic (Bax, Bad, Bid) proteins, activation of SAPK/JNK MAPK pathway, and lessening of PI3K/Akt/mTOR pathway; it disturbed the cell cycle progression at G2/M stage via upregulation of cyclin-D1 and downregulation of CDK6 and p27 expression. When combined with cyclophosphamide (CP), PAC-1A amplified the cellular uptake/retention of CP in the neuroblastoma cells and synergistically augmented the cytotoxicity and proapoptosis, as well as reducing cellular glutathione (GSH) and SOD levels.[30] In addition, the *in vitro* assay with human umbilical vein endothelial cells (HUVEC) further showed that PAC-1 might have antiangiogenic property to block VEGF function and endothelial tube formation.[29] These results revealed the chemotherapeutic and chemopreventive potentials of PAC to treat a broad spectrum of carcinomas including highly malignant tumors and drug-resistant tumors.

Phenolic acids: By a C-18 cartridge column chromatography, fractionation of the total cranberry extract gave an organic/phenolic acids-enriched fraction, which contains caffeic acid derivatives with substituted cinnamic acids. The fraction at 60 µg/mL concentration demonstrated the obvious growth inhibitory effect in human prostate cancer cell lines: RWPE-1 (95%), RWPE-2 (88%), and 22RV-1 (61%); and the lower effect in human oral cancer cell lines: KB (26.7%) and CAL27 (29%) *in vitro*.[9]

2. Triterpenoids

Ursolic acid (**2**) is a presentative triterpenoid in the cranberry that has the highest content of 0.460–1.090 g/kg (FW) and its esters 0.040–0.160 g/kg (FW). Compared to other berries, cranberry is the best source of ursolic acid and its *cis*- and *trans*-3-O-*p*-hydroxycinnamoyl esters. Ursolic acid (**2**) exerted the antiproliferative effects against HepG2 hepatoma (EC_{50} of 87.4 µM) and MCF-7 breast cancer cells (EC_{50} of 14.35 µM) besides its antioxidant activity.[32] In human HT-29 and HCT-116 colon cancer cell lines, the percentage of proapoptosis in the cancer cells was amplified by ursolic acid (**2**) in a dose-dependent manner.[33] At micromolar concentrations, ursolic acid (**2**) and its esters suppressed the growth of human DU-145 prostate cancer cells and limited prostate carcinogenesis, the cell invasion, and metastasis through inhibition of MMPs-2 and -9.[31] The *cis*-3-O-*p*-hydroxycinnamoyl ursolic acid (**3**) showed greater tumor cell growth inhibition *in vitro* than ursolic acid (**2**) and *trans*-3-O-*p*-hydroxycinnamoyl esters. The GI_{50} of *cis*-3-O-*p*-hydroxycinnamoyl ursolic acid (**3**) were 18.8 µM in MCF-7 cells, 21.6–24.3 µM in BALB/3T3 fibroblast, ME-180 cervical cancer, and PC3 prostate cancer cells, 27.1–28.9 µM in H460 large cell lung cancer, DU-145 prostate cancer and K562 leukemia cells, 32.9 µM in HT-29 colon cancer cells, and 46.4 µM in M14 melanoma cells, whereas the GI_{50} was 93–230 µM for ursolic acid (**2**) and 25–100 µM for *trans*-3-O-*p*-hydroxycinnamoyl ursolic acid in these cells.[21] These data indicated that the ursolic acid (**2**) and its esters may contribute to cranberry's role in chemoprevention.

3. Macromolecules

In addition to the cancer preventive and inhibitory constituents as described earlier, a nondialyzable material (NDM), with a molecular weight in the range of 12–13K, prepared from cranberry juice was found to exert the antigrowth and anti-invasive effect to impair Rev-2-T-6 murine lymphoma cells *in vitro*. Intraperitoneal injection of NDM to tested mice at nontoxic doses not only inhibited the growth of Rev-2-T-6 lymphoma cells but also augmented the generation of antilymphoma antibodies in an *in vivo* model. The discovery delivered more evidences to demonstrate the efficacy of cranberries for the cancer prevention in immune-competent hosts.[34]

Conclusion and Suggestion

The wide number of laboratory observations has highlighted that the cancer inhibitory and antioxidant properties of cranberries are attributed to the high contents of a diverse range of polyphenolics (such as flavonoids, anthocyanins, phenolic acids, and PACs) and a group of ursolic acid and its esters, providing the scientific supports for dietary cranberry to protect human against the damages from carcinogens and oxidation. Compared to the treatment with the individual phytochemicals, the combination of bioactive components from intake of cranberries may achieve more additive or synergistic functions for lowering the risk of carcinogenesis and partially delaying the cancer development, especially for protecting brain, prostate, colon, ovarian, lung, and blood system. Likewise, the cranberry extract has been found to have another protective effect on doxorubicin (a chemo drug)-caused cardiotoxicity.[35] Therefore, consumption of cranberries is encouraged as it may impart the greatest benefit to help us keep away from the cancer threat and prevent agonizing chemotherapy-induced toxicity/side effects. However, large quantities of cranberry juice and cranberry products in diet in a short period could cause some troubles in human such as stomach inflammation, sugar over intake, or kidney stone formation.

REFERENCES

1. Boivin, D. et al., 2007. Inhibition of cancer cell proliferation and suppression of TNF-induced activation of NF-κB by edible berry juice. *Anticancer Res.* 27: 937–948.
2. Babich, H. et al., 2012. Cranberry juice extract, a mild prooxidant with cytotoxic properties independent of reactive oxygen species. *Phytother. Res.* 26: 1358–1365.
3. Zuo, Y.G. et al., 2003. Antioxidant and anti-breast-cancer capacity of American cranberry and other fruits. *Abstracts of Papers, 225th ACS National Meeting*, New Orleans, LA: AGFD-05, March 23–27, 1.
4. Deziel, B. et al., 2012. American cranberry (Vaccinium macrocarpon) extract affects human prostate cancer cell growth via cell cycle arrest by modulating expression of cell cycle regulators. *Food & Funct.* 3: 556–564.
5. Yan, X.J. et al., 2002. Antioxidant activities and antitumor screening of extracts from cranberry fruit (Vaccinium macrocarpon). *J. Agricult. Food Chem.* 50: 5844–5849.
6. Liu, M. et al., 2009. Cranberry phytochemical extract inhibits SGC-7901 cell growth and human tumor xenografts in Balb/c nu/nu mice. *J. Agricul. Food Chem.* 57: 762–768.
7. Sun, J. et al., 2006. Cranberry phytochemical extracts induce cell cycle arrest and apoptosis in human MCF-7 breast cancer cells. *Cancer Lett.* 241: 124–134.
8. Seeram, N.P. et al., 2006. Blackberry, black raspberry, blueberry, cranberry, red raspberry, and strawberry extracts inhibit growth and stimulate apoptosis of human cancer cells in vitro. *J. Agricul. Food Chem.* 54: 9329–9339.
9. Seeram, N.P. et al., 2004. Total cranberry extract versus its phytochemical constituents: Antiproliferative and synergistic effects against human tumor cell lines. *J. Agricul. Food Chem.* 52: 2512–2517.
10. Prasain, J.K. et al., 2008. Effect of cranberry juice concentrate on chemically-induced urinary bladder cancers. *Oncol. Rep.* 19: 1565–1570.
11. Ferguson, P.J. et al., 2004. A flavonoid fraction from cranberry extract inhibits proliferation of human tumor cell lines. *J. Nutr.* 134: 1529–1535.
12. Sunkara, R. 2009. Suppression of colon cancer development in an azoxymethane-fisher 344 rat model by cranberry. *Res. J. Phytochem.* 3: 25–34.
13. Narayansingh, R. et al., 2009. Cranberry extract and quercetin modulate the expression of cyclooxygenase-2 (COX-2) and IκBα in human colon cancer cells. *J. Sci. Food Agricul.* 89: 542–547.
14. Caillet, S. et al., 2011. Effect of juice processing on the cancer chemopreventive effect of cranberry. *Food Res. Int.* 44: 902–910.
15. Liberty, A.M. et al., 2002. Antioxidant properties and composition of extracts from cranberry (Vaccinium macrocarpon). *Abstracts of Papers, 224th ACS National Meeting*, Boston, MA: AGFD-080, August 18–22.
16. Sun, J. et al., 2002. Antioxidant and antiproliferative activities of common fruits. *J. Agricult. Food Chem.* 50: 7449–7454.
17. Ferguson, P.J. et al., 2006. In vivo inhibition of growth of human tumor lines by flavonoid fractions from cranberry extract. *Nutr. Cancer* 56: 86–94.
18. He, X.J. et al., 2006. Cranberry phytochemicals: Isolation, structure elucidation, and their antiproliferative and antioxidant activities. *J. Agricult. Food Chem.* 54: 7069–7074.
19. Manthey, J.A. et al., 2002. Antiproliferative activities of citrus flavonoids against six human cancer cell lines. *J. Agric. Food Chem.* 50: 5837–5843.
20. Kawaii, S. et al., 1999. Antiproliferative activity of flavonoids on several cancer cell lines. *Biosci. Biotechnol. Biochem.* 63: 896–899.
21. Murphy, B.T. et al., 2003. Identification of triterpene hydroxycinnamates with in vitro antitumor activity from whole cranberry fruit (Vaccinium macrocarpon). *J. Agricult. Food Chem.* 51: 3541–3545.
22. Wang, Y.F. et al., 2015. The cranberry flavonoids PAC DP-9 and quercetin aglycone induce cytotoxicity and cell cycle arrest and increase cisplatin sensitivity in ovarian cancer cells. *J. Oncol.* 46: 1924–1934.
23. Neto, C.C. et al., 2005. MALDI-TOF MS characterization of proanthocyanidins from cranberry fruit (Vaccinium macrocarpon) that inhibit tumor cell growth and matrix metalloproteinase expression in vitro. *J. Sci. Food Agricul.* 86: 18–25.

24. Kresty, L.A. et al., 2008. Cranberry proanthocyanidins induce apoptosis and inhibit acid-Induced proliferation of human esophageal adenocarcinoma cells. *J. Agricult. Food Chem.* 56: 676–680.

25. Kresty, L.A. et al., 2011. Cranberry proanthocyanidins mediate growth arrest of lung cancer cells through modulation of gene expression and rapid induction of apoptosis. *Mol.* 16: 2375–2390.

26. Deziel, B.A. et al., 2010. Proanthocyanidins from the American cranberry (Vaccinium macrocarpon) inhibit matrix metalloproteinase-2 and matrix metalloproteinase-9 activity in human prostate cancer cells via alterations in multiple cellular signalling pathways. *J. Cell. Biochem.* 111: 742–754.

27. Weh, K.M. et al., 2016. Expression, modulation, and clinical correlates of the autophagy protein Beclin-1 in esophageal adenocarcinoma. *Mol. Carcinogen.* 55: 1876–1885.

28. Singh, A.P. et al., 2009. Cranberry proanthocyanidins are cytotoxic to human cancer cells and sensitize platinum-resistant ovarian cancer cells to paraplatin. *Phytother. Res.* 23: 1066–1074.

29. Kim, K.K. et al., 2012. Anti-angiogenic activity of cranberry proanthocyanidins and cytotoxic properties in ovarian cancer cells. *Int. J. Oncol.* 40: 227–235.

30. Singh, A.P. et al., 2012. Purified cranberry proanthocyanidines (PAC-1A) cause pro-apoptotic signaling, ROS generation, cyclophosphamide retention and cytotoxicity in high-risk neuroblastoma cells. *Int. J. Oncol.* 40: 99–108.

31. Kondo, M. et al., 2011. Ursolic acid and its esters: occurrence in cranberries and other Vaccinium fruit and effects on matrix metalloproteinase activity in DU-145 prostate tumor cells. *J. Sci. Food Agricult.* 91: 789–796.

32. He, X.J. et al., 2006. Cranberry phytochemicals: isolation, structure elucidation, and their antiproliferative and antioxidant activities. *J. Agricul. Food Chem.* 54: 7069–7074.

33. Liberty, A.M. et al., 2009. Cranberry PACs and triterpenoids: Anticancer activities in colon tumor cell lines. *Acta Horticult.* 841 (Proceedings of the 2nd International Symposium on Human Health Effects of Fruits and Vegetables, 2007): 61–66.

34. Hochman, N. et al., 2008. Cranberry juice constituents impair lymphoma growth and augment the generation of antilymphoma antibodies in syngeneic mice. *Nutr. Cancer* 60: 511–517.

35. Elberry, A.A. et al., 2010. Cranberry (Vaccinium macrocarpon) protects against doxorubicin-induced cardiotoxicity in rats. *Food Chem. Toxicol.* 48: 1178–1184.

38. FIG FRUIT

Figue   Feige   Higo

無花果 イチジク 무화과

Ficus carica

Moreaceae

Fig is a famous fruit tree *Ficus carica* (Moreaceae) native to the Middle East and western Asia. The fig tree has been cultivated since ancient times, and it is now grown worldwide as a fruit crop and ornamental plant. Fig fruits are a good source of dietary fiber, vitamin B complex (especially B6), copper, potassium, manganese, and pantothenic acid. The approaches for its biological properties evidenced that the aqueous extract of fig fruits can enhance immune functions of erythrocytes, diminish blood pressure, induce laxation, and exert antitumor effect. The fig fruit extract also showed significant analgesic activity by suppression of lecithin enzyme in brain and no toxicity after oral administration.

SCIENTIFIC EVIDENCE OF ANTITUMOR ACTIVITIES

Fig fruit milk obtained from the unripe fruits showed notable suppressive effect on the growth of sarcoma implanted in rat and spontaneous breast carcinoma in mouse. It also retarded the development of transplanting lymphosarcoma, marrow leukemia, and adenoma *in vivo* due to its ability to elicit tumor cell degeneration and tumor necrosis.[1] The milk from fig plant stems also presented antisarcoma effect.[2] The antigrowth effects against sarcoma 180, Ehrlich entity cancer, hepatoma HepA, and Lewis lung carcinoma were shown after oral administration of the water extract of fig fruits to tumor-bearing mice in a dose of 250 mg/kg per day continuously for 6 days, and the inhibitory rates ranged 41.82%–53.81%.[3] Fig fruit latex which contains rich polyphenols plays a marked role in antioxidant and cytotoxic activities on human glioblastoma and hepatoma. The mechanism of antiproliferation and anticolony formation was revealed to be attributable to block of DNA synthesis and induction of cell cycle arrest and apoptosis.[4] Fig fruit extract also displayed antimutagenic activities, that is, it could antagonize the mutagenesis evoked by mitomycin C and radiation, and suppress the formation of spontaneous micronuclei in the cancer patients and the aged people.[5] Moreover, fig fruit latex showed the best antiradiative effect (IC$_{50}$ of 0.05 mg/mL) on the UVA irradiation at a dose of 1.08 J/cm, while fig leaf latex exerted marked antiproliferative activity on human A375 melanoma cells (IC_{50} of 1.5 µg/mL).[2,6] Also, the bioactive components yielded from fig fruit residue by CO_2-extracting technique exhibited the notable antiproliferative effect against U937 lymphoma, 95D highly metastatic lung cancer, and AGS gastric cancer cell lines *in vitro* and against a transplanted hepatoma in mice with 49.3% inhibitory rate.[7]

SCIENTIFIC EVIDENCE OF ANTITUMOR CONSTITUENTS AND ACTIVITIES

1. Coumarins

Some less potent antitumor coumarins were isolated from the fruits and leaves of fig. Bergapten (**1**) and psoralen (**2**) isolated from fig as anticancer compounds. 6-(2-Methoxy-Z-vinyl)-7-methyl pyranocoumarin (**3**) derived from a EtOAc extract of fig fruits displayed *in vitro* suppressive effect toward human BGC-823 (stomach), A431 (epidermis), and HCT (colon) cancer lines.[8]

2. Sterols

From a petroleum ether extract of fig fruits, 9,19-cyclopropane-24,25-ethyl-eneoxide-5-en-3-spirostol was separated, which exerted the inhibitory effect on the BGC-823 and HTC tumor cells *in vitro* by 48.49% and 37.48%, respectively.[9] 6'-O-Acyl-β-D-glucosyl- β-sitosterols (**4**, 6-AGS) from fig fruits presented the inhibitory effects against various human cancer cell lines such as leukemia, lymphoma, and prostate epithelial cancer and mammary cancer. Treatment with 6-AGS (**4**) in a dose of 50 µg/mL triggered the growth inhibitory effect by 69% and 87% against Burkitt B-cell lymphoma Raji and DG-75 cells; by 81% and 66% against T-cell leukemia Jurkat and HD-MAR cells; and by 75% and 66% against DU-145 prostate cancer and MCF-7 breast cancer cells, respectively.[8] Interestingly, unfermented soybean products (tofu, soymilk) contain 6-AGS (**4**) in large amounts as well. The findings designated that 6-AGS (**4**) might contribute to the lower incidences of breast, colon, and prostate cancers in the regions where soybean products are used in the common diet.[10] As another sterol from fit fruit, 5,22-cyclopentyloxy-22-deisopentyl-3β-hydroxyfurostanol (**5**) was effective in BGC-823 (stomach) and HCT (colon) cancer cell lines with respective suppressive rates of 37.66% and 32.64%.[11] Likewise, β-sitosteryl 3β-glucoside-6'-O-palmitate, which was isolated from a dichloromethane extract of *F. odorata* leaves, exhibited the cytotoxicity against human gastric adenocarcinoma cell line (AGS), with 60.28% growth inhibition, and against A549, HT-29, and PC3 cancer cell lines, with 22%–28% growth inhibition at its 100 µM concentration.[12]

3. Triterpenoids

Nine tirucallane-type triterpenoids assigned as ficutirucins A-I (1-9) were isolated from *F. carica* fruit. Ficutirucins-A–C, -F, G, and -I exhibited moderate inhibitory effect against the proliferation of human MCF-7 (breast), HepG2 (liver), and U-2 OS (bone) carcinoma cell lines with IC_{50}s of 11.67–45.61 µM. The highest activity was shown by ficutirucin-A (**6**) in HepG2 cells (IC_{50} 11.67 µM) and the second levels of suppressive effects were shown by ficutirucin-B (**7**) in HepG2 and MCF-7 cells (respective IC_{50}s 17.76 and 17.94 µM). The IC_{50} value of ficutirucin-F (**8**) was 20.70 µM, which was the best activity in U-2 OS cells among the ficutirucins.[13] In addition, a triterpenoid assigned as ficusonolide (**9**) was discovered from a dichloromethane fraction of *F. faveolata* stems (collected in Pakistan), which displayed selective activity to deter human H116 (colon) and H125 (lung) cancer cell lines with respective IC_{50}s of 7.8 and 11.0 µg/mL.[14]

4. Polyphenolics

Figs contain diverse polyphenolics such as gallic acid, chlorogenic acid, syringic acid, (+)-catechin, (−)-epicatechin, and rutin. The different concentrations of anthocyanins influenced the fruit color in the different cultivars of fig trees. In the fig anthocyanins, cyanidin-3-O-rutinoside is particularly in high content. All these polyphenolics commonly exist in many fruits, which were always reported having the marked antioxidant activities and anticarcinogenic potentials.[15]

5. Polysaccharides

A polysaccharide (FCPS) component derived from fig fruits was reported showing antitumor-related properties such as enhancement of SOD activity and diminution of glutathione peroxidase (GPx) level in mice implanted sarcoma 180.[16] FCPS could effectively stimulate dendritic cells (DCs) partially through a dectin-1/Syk pathway and promote their maturation by upregulation of CD40, CD80, CD86, and major histocompatibility complex II (MHCII). FCPS also potentiated DCs to produce cytokines (IL-12, IFN-γ, IL-6, and IL-23) and to promote T-cell responses, thereby upregulating the immunostimulatory capacity of DCs.[17] FCPS-1, -2, and -3 were homogeneous polysaccharides purified from FCPS; all three exhibited dose-dependent antioxidant activities *in vitro*, but FCPS-3 presented relatively stronger antioxidant and inhibitory activities against HepG2 (liver) and 7901 (stomach) cancer cell lines. At a concentration of 2.0 mg/mL, the inhibition rates of FCPS-3 on HepG2 and 7901 cell lines were 57.30% and 54.49%, respectively.[18] In addition, a group of cationic polypeptides was prepared as pectinesterase inhibitors (PEIs) from jelly fig (*F. awkeotsang*), a similar fig plant. The PEI exerted remarkable growth inhibition against human U937 leukemic monocyte lymphoma cells in a dose- and time-dependent manner together with induction of apoptotic death and G2/M cell cycle arrest. By exposure of the PEI in 50 μg/mL concentration to U937 cells, the cell growth inhibition reached 90% *in vitro*.[19]

Conclusion and Suggestion

The observations in chemical biology studies have signified that the components in the fig fruits such as phytosterols, triterpenoids, coumarins, polyphenolics, and polysaccharides are primarily and synergically in charge of biological activities of fig fruits, including anti-inflammatory, anticarcinogenic, antioxidant, and cholesterol-lowering effects. The cancer inhibitory potencies of these phytochemicals were weak to moderate in the *in vitro* assayed carcinoma cells, but without influences on normal cells. The antioxidant properties of fig polyphenolics are conducive to the cancer prevention. Accordingly, the research results have afforded a helpful recognition to encourage people to frequently intake fig fruits to exert the antioxidant activity and lessen the incidence of carcinogenesis.

Other Bioactivities

Cysteine proteinases from fig fruits and latex are a group of enzymes leading to apoptosis of some cancer cells.[15] An isolated dihydrofuryl-β-D-lactose from fig fruits showed obvious immunoenhancing properties.[11]

REFERENCES

1. Ullman, S.B. et al., 1952. The inhibitory and necrosis-inducing effects of the latex of Ficus carica on transplanted and spontaneous tumors. *Experim. Med. Surgery* 10: 26–49; The effects of the fraction R3 of the latex of Ficus carica on the tissues of mice bearing spontaneous mammary tumors. *Experim. Med. Surgery* 10: 287–305.
2. (a) State Administration of Medicines of China, 1999. *Chinese Materia Medica*, Vol. 2, 2–1033, p. 484–486. Published by Shanghai Science and Technology express. China; (b) Loizzo, M.R. et al., 2014. Chemical composition and bioactivity of dried fruits and honey of Ficus carica cultivars Dottato, San Francesco and Citrullara. *Sci Food Agric.* 94(11): 2179–86.
3. Wang, Y.X. et al., 1990. The studies on the anticancer activity of fig. *Aizheng* 9: 223.
4. Wang, J. et al., 2008. Cytotoxicity of fig fruit latex against human cancer cells. *Food Chem. Toxicol.* 46: 1025–1033.
5. Ma, J.G. et al., 2002. The studies on the mutagenic and anti-mutagenic effects of fig extract. *Carcinogen. Teratogen. Mutagen.* 14: 177–180.

6. Menichini, G. et al., 2012. Fig latex (Ficus carica L. cultivar Dottato) in combination with UV irradiation decreases the viability of A375 melanoma cells in vitro. *Anti-Cancer Agents in Med. Chem.* 12: 959–965.

7. Wang, Z.B. et al., 2005. Study on anticancer components of fig residues with super-critical fluid carbon dioxide extracting technique. *Zhongguo Zhongyao Zazhi* 30: 1443–1447.

8. Yin, W.P. et al., 1997. A new coumarin compound with anticancer activity. *Zhongcaoyao* 28: 3–4.

9. Yin, W.P. et al., 1997. Research on the chemical structure and anticancer activity of 9, 19-Cyclopropane-24, 25 ethyleneoxide-5-en-3β-spirostol (sic). *Zhongguo Yaowu Huaxue Zazhi* 7: 46–47.

10. Rubnov, S. et al., 2001. Suppressors of cancer cell proliferation from fig (Ficus carica) resin: Isolation and structure elucidation. *J. Nat. Prods.* 64: 993–996.

11. Yin, W.P. et al., 1998. Structures and antitumor activities of two new compounds isolated from fig (Ficus carica). *Zhongcaoyao* 29: 505–507.

12. Tsai, P.W. et al., 2012. Chemical constituents of Ficus odorata. *Pharm. Chem. J.* 46: 225–227.

13. Jing, L. et al., 2015. Tirucallane-type triterpenoids from the fruit of Ficus carica and their cytotoxic activity. *Chem. Pharm. Bull.* 63: 237–243.

14. Din, A. et al., 2013. Bioassay-guided isolation of new antitumor agent from Ficus faveolata (Wall. ex Miq.). *J. Cancer Sci. Ther.* 5: 404–408.

15. Hashemi, S.A. et al., 2011. The effect of fig tree latex (Ficus carica) on stomach cancer line. *Iran Red Crescent Med. J.* 13: 272–275.

16. Dai, W.J. et al., 2002. The influence of Fit polysaccharide on MDASOD and GSH-PX in S180 bearing mice. *J. Jining Med. College* 25(1): 20–21.

17. Tian, J. et al., 2014. Ficus carica polysaccharides promote the maturation and function of dendritic cells. *Intl. J. Mol. Sci.* 15: 12469–12479.

18. Guo, R.N. et al., 2015. Antioxidant and antitumor activities of polysaccharides from Ficus carica L. in vitro. *Huaxue Yu Shengwu Gongcheng* 32: 49–52.

19. Chang, J. et al., 2005. Pectinesterase inhibitor from jelly fig (Ficus awkeotsang Makino) achene induces apoptosis of human leukemic U937 cells. *Annals of the New York Academy of Sciences* 1042 (Role of the Mitochondria in Human Aging and Disease): 506–515.

39. GRAPE

Grain de raisin   Traube Uva

葡萄　グレープ　포도

Vitis vinifera

Vitaceae

1. $R_1 = R_2 = -H$
2. $R_1 = -H$, $R_2 = -bata$-O-D-glucoside
3. $R_1 = R_2 = -OCH_3$

Grape berries (*Vitis vinifera*) are one of the world's most valued conventional fruits, having many cultivars with diversity of colors such as crimson, black, dark blue, yellow, green, orange, and pink, as well as seedless grapes. The grape cultivation is believed to have started in the Mediterranean region 6,000–8,000 years ago. Today, the grape is one of the top four most common fruits in the world, and is usually consumed as fresh fruit for tables and processed fruits such as wine, grape juice, jam, jelly, raisin, molasses, and grape seed oil. In the last two decades, numerous studies have disclosed that grapes might not only afford rich nutrients and polyphenolics but also possess antioxidative, cancer-preventive, kidney-improving, and liver-protecting properties.[1] The consumption of grapes, wine, and grape juice provides various health-promoting effects, particularly lessening risks of certain types of cancers, cardiovascular diseases, type II diabetes, and other chronic complications. Therefore, fresh grapes, wine, and grape products have attracted more and more increasing interest in recent years for their health benefits and possible anticancer effects.

Scientific Evidence in Cancer Prevention

The approaches of chemical biology revealed that the most important phytochemicals in grapefruit were designated as polyphenolics (including phenolic acids, stibenoids, anthocyanins, and PACs) and isoprenoid monoterpens that are mostly in charge of biological functions of grape berries. A 100 g of fresh grapes contain 63–182 mg of the polyphenolics, which include 65%–76% flavonoids. The distribution of polyphenolics is in the order grape seeds > peels > pulps, except for anthocyanins, which are rich in the peels of only red grapes. Relatively, the grape skin contains more resveratrols, catechins, and/or anthocyanins, grape seeds have large contents of procyanidins and proanthocyanidins, and grape pulps have higher hydroxycinnamic acids. However, the substantial amount of polyphenolics in grape skins is free- and sugar-bonded phenolic acids such as caffeic acid, gallic acid, ferulic acid, syringic acid, and *p*-coumaric acid, whereas resveratrol, one of the most prominent bioactive compounds in grapes, is only 0.21 mg/g in the grape extract and 0.2–5.8 mg/L in red wine depending on the grape variety.[1,2]

1. Polyphenolic-enriched grape extracts

Antioxidant activities: The antioxidant properties of grape seed extract (GSE) primarily are presented in scavenging free radicals, preventing ROS-induced DNA damage, and reducing LPO. In a test for the capacities in scavenging a standard antioxidant (Trolox), the extracts demonstrated greater antioxidant capacities than vitamins C and E. All the polyphenolics in grapes serve as prominent antioxidants and radical-scavenging agents when dietary intake of grapes with seeds. The different polyphenolic-rich

GSEs at a concentration of 100 ppm diminished the radical-scavenging rates by 65%–90% in a β-carotene-linoleate model system and a linoleic acid peroxidation model. The ethanolic extracts of red grape seeds and peels exerted a high antioxidative effect against primary and secondary lipid oxidation in sunflower and conjugated sunflower oils after six-day treatment. Even at the concentration as low as 0.1%, the GSE was obviously effective in impeding the primary and secondary oxidation in various muscle systems, being more potent than gallic acid in inhibiting oxidation. Furthermore, by activation of a transcription factor nuclear factor, erythroid-2 p45 (NF-E2)-related factor (Nrf2), the polyphenolics in the seed extract augmented the activities of several antioxidant enzymes (such as glutathione, SOD, catalase) and other detoxifying enzymes and activated many types of phase II antioxidant/detoxifying enzymes. The protection of normal rat colonic mucosa from ROS injury by dietary GSE was in parallel with strong lessening of mucosal apoptosis via modulation of both mitochondrial and cytosolic antioxidant enzyme systems and increase in cellular glutathione, but the protective antioxidant effect in normal cells by the extract in another test was mediated by lessening of catalase activity and/or glutathione level, indicating that polyphenolics have an ability to modulate intracellular peroxide production. Eight-week dietary intake of grape juice (480 mL/day) led to 15% reduction in lymphocyte DNA damage caused by the ROS formation.[1-5] These discoveries may provide basic information about health-beneficial advantages of grapes and reveal that the activities are closely correlated to the radical scavenging and antioxidant capacities.

Anticancer activities: A number of *in vitro* and *in vivo* investigations confirmed that consumption of large quantities of grape with antioxidant polyphenolics lessens the risk of some cancers such as those of breast, colon, prostate, and skin, and pointed out that their apparent effects against cancer initiation and development is largely mediated by the antioxidant actions. Both *in vitro* and *in vivo* experiments showed that the growth of Detroit 562 pharynx cancer cells and FaDu head/neck squamous cell carcinoma (HNSCC) cells was impeded by GSE together with the induction of cell cycle arrest and apoptosis by the activation of DNA damage checkpoint cascade and caspases-8, -9, -3, wherein intracellular ROS amplification was elicited by GSE to trigger cell death and DNA damage.[1-7] The growth of MDA-MB-468 breast carcinoma cells was irreversibly deterred by blockage of MAPK/ERK1/2 and MAPK/p38 signaling pathways, and a cell cycle in G1 arrest was caused by the promotion of CDKI Cip1/p21 and decrease in CDK4 after MDA-MB-468 cells were treated with the seed polyphenolics. Both extracts of grapefruits and leaves were moderately effective in hindering the MDA-MB-231 breast cancer cells. GSE treatment could restrain histone acetyltransferases in human LNCaP prostate cancer cells and then block androgen-receptor-mediated transcription, thereby limiting the cancer cell viability.[3-7] GSE elicited both antiproliferative and proapoptotic effects against human colon cancer cells (Caco-2 and HCT-8), which inhibitory effects were superior to the isolated procyanidins, while GSE induced G1 cell cycle arrest in HT-29 human colon carcinoma cells, which effect was associated with up-regulation of p21 (Cip1) by redox-mediated activation of ERK1/2 pathway and post-transcriptional regulation.[8,9] The anticancer efficacy of GSE was also shown in human lung (A427, A549, and H1299), gastric (CRL-1739), leukemic (U937, Jurkat, and HL-60), and oral squamous cell (CAL27 and SCC25) cancer cell lines.[5,10] Two kinds of red wines produced from the red grapes of muscadine (*V. rotundifolia*) and cabernet sauvignon (*V. vinifera*) reduced the cell viability and induced the cell death of MOLT-4 leukemia cells with G2/M cycle arrest.[11] A peel extract of muscadine grape, which contained no resveratrol, has been shown to selectively suppress the growth of RWPE-1, WPE1-NA22, WPE1-NB14, and WPE1-NB26 prostate tumorigenic cells.[12] Only weak cytotoxicity was observed (IC$_{50}$ of 480 μg/mL) for GSE in A4321 skin carcinoma cells.[13]

Moreover, intake of GSE or red wine markedly lessened the number of metastatic nodules on lung surface in mice inoculated with B16F10 melanoma cells.[10] Giving 0.25% or 0.5% (w/w) GSE in diet to rats repressed AOM-elicited ACF formation, leading to 60% decrease in ACF numbers and 60% reduction in crypt multiplicity. During the consumption of purple grape juice extract, the juice phenolics inhibited carcinogen DMBA-induced mammary tumorigenesis in rats along with blockage of DMBA-DNA adduct formation.[14] Concord grape juice (*V. labrusca*) constituents could inhibit the promotion stage of DMBA-induced rat mammary tumorigenesis *in vivo* and partly hamper the cell proliferation.[15] The grape antioxidants also could downregulate EGFR expression and restrain the EGFR downstream pathways in HNSCC cells.[7] Similarly, in both human MDA-MB-231 breast cancer and U251 glioma cells, GSE inhibited VEGF expression by reducing HIF-1α protein synthesis via blockage of Akt activation and then exerted an antiangiogenic potential.[16] Muscadine grape skin extract could antagonize Snail-cathepsin L-mediated invasion and migration of human prostate (LNCaP, ARCaP-E) and breast (MCF-7) cancer cells to block osteoclastogenesis.[17] The antitumor promoting effect of grape seed polyphenolics was observed in CD-1 mouse skin epidermis. At doses of 5–20 mg of the polyphenolics per mouse, the tumor promotion was impeded by 51%–94%.[10] In addition, these grape antioxidants also exerted immuno-enhancing activities through the enhancements of lymphocyte proliferation, NK cell cytotoxicity, CD4+/CD8+ ratio, IL-2, and IFN-γ productions.[5] Taken together, the scientific experiments give the overall perception about the importance of grapes and grape polyphenolics in the cancer chemoprevention and human health improvement, suggesting that the anticarcinogenic role of grape polyphenolics is largely attributed to their antioxidant protection and immunoprotection. Hence, the grape polyphenolics/antioxidants have drawn an increased attention for their anticancer potentials.

2. Resveratrol

Anticancer activities: Resveratrol (**1**) is found in large quantities as a natural phytoalexin in grape peels, peanuts, red wine, and other food sources. Numerous studies have revealed that resveratrol has remarkable ability to suppress a wide variety of tumor cells, including lymphoid and myeloid cancers, multiple myeloma, head and neck squamous cell cancer, and the carcinomas in breast, ovary, prostate, cervix, thyroid, stomach, colon, pancreas, and skin.[18–20] Consuming 1.2% or 3.6% crude resveratrol extract in a diet for 27 weeks significantly lowered AOM-induced formation of ACF by 40%–42%. Dietary intake of 1.2% resveratrol extract to mice for 37 weeks lessened the numbers of AOM-induced tumors per colon by 61% and diminished the percentage of mice bearing colon tumor by 49%. Similarly, the percentage of mammary carcinogenesis caused by DMBA in rats was attenuated by 44% when 1% resveratrol extract was given in the diet to female rats for 23 weeks.[21]

In *in vitro* experiments, resveratrol (**1**) has been shown to inhibit growth of human MDA-MB-231 (breast), PANC-1 and AsPC-1 (pancreas), Caco-2 (colon), and LNCaP, DU-145, and PC3 (prostate) cancer cell lines.[12] Resveratrol (**1**) hampered the proliferation of human MCF-7 breast cancer cells at S/G2/M phase[22] and reversed multidrug resistance to exert obvious suppression of adriamycin-resistant MCF-7 cells.[20] The proliferation of human SGC-7901 gastric cancer cells could be hindered by resveratrol (**1**) concomitantly with dose-dependent induction of the cell apoptosis through a PI3K/Akt signal pathway including downregulated Bcl-2 expression and p-Akt protein and upregulated Bax and caspase-3.[23] The mitochondrial respiration and apoptosis of SW620 colon cancer cells was triggered by resveratrol (**1**) concomitant with hyperpolarization of mitochondrial membrane and increase in ROS production, thereby exerting the cancer inhibitory effect.[24] The antitumor effects of resveratrol on human colorectal cancer cells (HCT-116 and LoVo) were associated with blockage of Wnt/β-catenin signaling and MALAT1 expression and inhibition of its target genes such as c-myc and MMP-7. These elicited events then led to the suppression of colorectal cancer cell proliferation, invasion, and metastasis.[25] By strongly blocking DNA synthesis and promotion of apoptosis, resveratrol (**1**) in doses of 2.5 and 10 mg/kg notably obstructed the tumor volume, size, and the metastasis to lung by 42%–56% in mice bearing highly metastatic Lewis lung cancer.[26–28]

Besides the anticancer and anticarcinogenic activities, resveratrol (**1**) also was able to hamper the angiogenesis of HUVEC *in vitro*, associated with blockage of VEGF binding to HUVEC at 10–100 μmol/L concentrations and blockage of neovascularization in tumor at doses of 2.5 and 10 mg/kg in an animal model.[26–28] Moreover, a combined treatment with resveratrol (**1**) and curcumin was found to exert a synergistic antiproliferative effect on colon carcinoma and hepatoma cells. The apoptosis of Hepal-6 hepatoma cells promoted by resveratrol plus curcumin was mediated by the elevation of intracellular ROS level, downregulation of XIAP and survivin expressions, and activation of caspase-3, -8, and -9.[29] By deterring Bcl-2 expression, disrupting mitochondrial membrane potential, and activating caspase-3, resveratrol (1) induced the cell apoptosis of human Mum2c choroidal malignant melanoma and inhibited the cell proliferation.[30] Accordingly, these findings provided important preclinical evidences supporting the uses of resveratrol (1) in chemoprevention, chemotherapy, antiangiogenesis, and anti-metastasis toward the malignant tumor diseases. In addition, a modern technique of magnetic orcinol-imprinted poly(ethylene-co-vinyl alcohol) composite particles (MOIPs) not only improved the extraction of resveratrol (1) but also enhanced the delivery of resveratrol to its targeted human osteogenic sarcoma cells, resulting in an efficient suppressive effect.[31]

Other stilbenes: Resveratrol-3-O-β-D-glucoside (2) was markedly effective in terms of antiadhesive and anti-invasive effects on four colorectal cancer cell lines (HR8348, Hce8693, HT-29, and LoVo) *in vitro* at a concentration of 3.2 mmol/L. The adhesion inhibitory rates were 67.6%–78.8% and the invasion inhibitory rates were 82.7%–92.7%. In addition, PKC activity was diminished by 2 at the same concentration with suppressive rates of 35.1%–49.6%. The results implied that the antiadhesive and anti-invasive effects of resveratrol-3-O-β-D-glucoside are probably mediated through the inhibition of PKC activity in the colorectal carcinoma cells.[32] 3,4′-Dimethoxy-5-hydroxystilbene (3), which was derived from a structural modification of resveratrol-3-O-glucoside (2), could enhance the expressions of Bax and caspases and then promote human HL-60 promyelocytic leukemia cells to apoptotic death.[33]

Mechanism exploration: The antitumor and anticarcinogenic mechanism of resveratrol (1) has been deeply explored to show the following events primarily involved: (1) upregulation of p21Cip/WAF1, p53, Bax, and caspases activities; (2) downregulation of cyclins-D1 and -E, survivin, Bcl-2, Bcl-xL, and cIAPs expressions; (3) inhibition of transcription factors including NF-κB, AP-1, and Egr-1; (4) inhibition of protein kinases including IαBa kinase, JNK, MAPK, Akt, PKC, PKD, and casein kinase-II; and (5) reduction of gene products such as COX-2, 5-LOX, VEGF, IL-1, IL-6, IL-8, AR, and PSA.[18] Various cancer cells provoked by resveratrol (1) to apoptotic death could be also mediated by some characteristic multiple modulations. For instance, the apoptosis of resveratrol in human U251 glioma cells and primary gastric cancer cells was associated with the decrease in Bcl-2 activity, increase in Bax expression, cleavage of PARP, release of cytochrome c from mitochondria to cytoplasm, and activation of caspases-3 and -9.[34,35] However, in human HL-60 leukemia cells, the FasL-related apoptosis elicited by resveratrol (1) was mainly mediated by Cdc42 activation in ASK1/JNK-dependent signaling cascade.[36] The inhibitory effect of resveratrol (1) in human MCF-10A breast epithelial cells was characteristically accompanied with decrease in aryl hydrocarbon receptor (AhR)-DNA binding activity, decline in 2-hydroxyestradiol and 4-hydroxyestradiol formation, and induction of cytochrome P450 1A1 and 1B1 expressions.[37] Also, resveratrol (1) obviously limited the intracellular ROS formation and oxidative DNA damage and reduced catechol estrogens-induced cytotoxicity, thereby obstructing the neoplastic transformation in human breast epithelial cells.[37] Further, the breast cancer cell metastasis obstructed by resveratrol (1) was found to correlate with rapidly inducing global array of filopodia, retarding focal adhesions and focal adhesion kinase (FAK) activity and altering the cytoskeleton.[37,38]

Moreover, resveratrol (1) was capable of blocking NF-κB activation induced by an inflammatory agent TNF via blockage of NF-κB-dependent reporter gene transcription and repression of phosphorylation and nuclear translocation of p65 subunit in NF-κB, events that coincided with the inhibition of AP-1. Resveratrol (1) also restrained the TNF-induced activations of MAPK, JNK, and downregulated HER-2/neu gene expression.[39–41] Resveratrol (1), by the inhibition of COX-2 and MMP-9 activities, impeded generation of reactive oxygen intermediate and TNF-induced LPO. The resveratrol-provoked multi-interactions were reported also to complicatedly involve in the growth inhibition and apoptosis induction in many carcinoma cell lines, such as in MCF-7 (breast cancer), U937 (lymphoma), Jurkat (lymphoid leukemia), H4 (hepatoma), HeLa (cervical cancer), and melanoma.[42,43]

3. Proanthocyanidins

In grape berries, PACs are predominantly located in seeds as oligomers and polymers of flavan-3-ol with an average molecular mass ranging between 578 and >5,000 Da. The grape varieties and the extraction processes prominently affect the content of PACs in the extract products. Generally, the major PACs in grape seeds present higher polymerization, which are important pigments for the color stability of red wines. Numerous chemical biological studies have established a large number of health and medical advantages of grape seed proanthocyanidins (GSPs), such as hindering the carcinogenesis and neoplastic processes in different stages, detoxifying carcinogenic metabolites, as well as obstructing degeneration and many types of acute and chronic oxidative stress in cardiovascular system, gastrointestinal tract, neurons, pancreas, and so on.[4,7,10]

In a mouse skin two-stage carcinogenic model, GSP at doses of 0.5 and 1.5 mg/mouse/application suppressed the tumor promotion elicited by DMBA and 12-O-tetradecanoylphorbol-13-acetate, where the tumor incidences were lowered by 35% and 60%, the tumor multiplicities were reduced by 61% and 83%, and the tumor volumes were diminished by 67% and 87%, respectively. In an *in vitro* assay, GSP was sensitive to NSCLC cells. It obviously influenced the growth of NSCLC cell lines (A549, H1299, H460, H226, and H157) and stimulated the cell apoptosis. The proapoptosis in the NSCLC cells was found to be mediated by downregulation of Bcl-2 and Bcl-xL expression, increase in Bax expression, disruption of mitochondrial membrane potential, and activation of caspases-9, -3, and PARP. The invasion of NSCLC cells also could be hindered in a concentration-dependent manner by GSP treatment, an effect that was associated with decrease in EGFR levels and ERK1/2 phosphorylation, reversal of epithelial–mesenchymal transition (EMT) process, increase in epithelial biomarker (E-cadherin) level, and loss of mesenchymal biomarkers (vimentin, fibronectin, and N-cadherin) in the cells. The anti-NSCLC activity of GSP has been further demonstrated in *in vivo* models. Oral administration of GSP in doses of 50, 100, or 200 mg/kg (5 days per week) or dietary 0.5% GSP noticeably inhibited the growth of A549 and H1299 lung tumor xenografts in athymic nude mice. During the treatment, GSP simultaneously inhibited COX-2, PGE2, and PGE2 receptors (EP1, EP3, and EP4) in the tumors. Similarly, under the marked reduction of COX-2 expression and PGE2 production, treatment with GSP resulted in concentration-dependent anti-invasive and/or antimigratory effects in human melanoma A375 and Hs294t cells.[2–7,10]

Likewise, concentration- and/or time-dependent cytotoxic effects of GSP were observed in human A-427 (lung), MCF-7 (breast), CRL-1739 (stomach), K562 (chronic myelogenous leukemia), and CNE (brain) cancer cell lines *in vitro*. After the GSP treatment, SCC-25 human tongue squamous cell carcinoma cells were induced in both G1 cell cycle arrest and mitochondria-mediated apoptosis in a dose-dependent manner, thereby repressing the SCC-25 cell proliferation, whereas OEC-M1 human oral squamous carcinoma cells were elicited in cell cycle arrest only by upregulation of p21(Cip1)/p27(Kip1) protein but did not influence the cell apoptosis. However, GSP also was able to limit the migration and invasion of both SCC-25 and OEC-M1 cells along with inhibition of MMPs-2 and -9. By suppressing urokinase-type plasminogen activator (u-PA) and DNA-binding activity of NF-κB transcription, GSP treatment deterred the invasion of highly metastatic androgen-independent PC3 prostate cancer cells. In addition, GSP was also effective in synergistically promoting the proapoptotic and suppressive effects of doxorubicin in K562, A549, and CNE carcinoma cells by amplifying intracellular doxorubicin and concentrations of Ca^{2+} and Mg^{2+} and diminishing pH value and mitochondrial membrane potential.[2–7,10] In addition to amplification of cisplatin-induced A549 lung cancer cell death, the extract of grape seed oligomeric PACs at 16 mg/L also obviously protected cisplatin-induced nephron toxicity in human embryonic kidney HEK239 cells.[44]

These observations from the scientific investigations recommend a potential for grape seed PACs to hamper the viability, growth, invasion, and metastasis of certain neoplastic cells such as the carcinomas of lung, skin, prostate, breast, oral, and/or brain and to lower the toxicity of chemo drugs.

4. Procyanidins

In addition to the antioxidant and high oxygen radical absorbance capacities, procyanidins are also able to play a role in the cancer prevention. The chemical biology studies disclosed that grape seed procyanidins in oral cancer and MDA-MB-468 breast cancer cells elicited cell cycle G1-phase arrest by enhancing p21(Cip1)/p27(Kip1) protein and inactivating MAPK/ERK1/2 and MAPK/p38, thereby repressing some levels of the cancer cell proliferation. In HepG2 hepatoma cells, the grape seed procyanidins induced Nrf2/ARE-mediated phase II detoxifying/antioxidant enzymes via a p38 and PI3K/Akt pathway, showing a potential in the cancer chemoprevention.[2–7] By blocking COX-2/prostaglandin E2 (PGE2) eicosanoid pathways, this procyanidin extract exerted antiproliferative and proapoptotic effects against A549 lung carcinoma cells.[45] Among the procyanidins, procyanidin B5-3′-gallate showed the highest antioxidant activity (IC_{50} of 20 µM) in an epidermal LPO assay and procyanidin-B2 3,3″-di-O-gallate presented the most potent effects in promoting cell apoptosis and cell cycle arrest and restraining the cell growth and clonogenicity in various human prostate cancer cell lines.[2–7,10]

5. Anthocyanins

Red cultivars of grapes are rich in anthocyanins that impart red color to the berry peels. An anthocyanin-rich extract from Concord grapes (*V. labrusca*) deterred the formation of carcinogen–DNA adduct in noncancerous immortalized human normal breast epithelial MCF-10F cells, implying certain preventive potential against the cancer initiation.[12] An anthocyanin fraction of muscadine grapes (*V. rotundifolia*) at concentrations of ~200 µg/mL showed 50% inhibition against HT-29 colon cancer cells and at 100–300 µg/mL against Caco-2 colon cancer cells, along with 2–4 times increase in DNA fragmentation.[46] Also, a report disclosed that the extracts of grape pomace and strawberry are rich in malvidin-glucoside and pelargonidin-glucoside, respectively. The anthocyanins-rich grape and strawberry extracts and their generated metabolites such as hydroxyphenylacetic acid showed proapoptotic effects in HT-29 colon cancer cells, having the possible contribution to the anticarcinogenesis.[47]

6. Phenolic acids

The phenolic acid fractions derived from muscadine grapes (*V. rotundifolia*) exerted 50% growth inhibition against HT-29 and Caco-2 colon cancer cells at 0.5–3 mg/mL concentrations and against HepG2 hepatoma cells at 1–2 mg/mL.[46] Gallic acid is a very common phenolic acid present in a wide range of vegetables and fruits including various varieties of grapes; isolated from grape seeds in an *in vitro* assay, it dose-dependently diminished the viabilities of androgen-independent DU-145 and androgen-dependent-22Rv1 human prostate cancer cells largely via apoptosis induction and reduced microvessel density in the prostate tumor xenografts (DU-145 and 22Rv1).[48] The ellagic acid-rich fractions from red muscadine grape juice could elicit the apoptotic death and disturb cell cycle progression in Caco-2 colon cancer cells in a concentration-dependent manner.[49] The anticancer activity of ellagic acid was also showed in other types of cancers such as leukemia and oral and esophageal tumors. In addition, ellagic acid has been known to participate in various biological actions.

NANOFORMULATION

A green synthesis route created the gold nanoparticles (VV-AuNPs) with Vitis vinifera peel/seed. In an *in vivo* mouse model, topical application with VV-AuNPs enhanced abilities to stimulate antioxidant enzymes within the cells and to suppress abnormal skin cell proliferation against skin papillomagenesis initiated by DMBA and promoted by 12-O-tetradecanoylphorbol-13-acetate. During the treatment, VV-AuNPs also facilitated the tumor cell apoptotic death through downregulation of mutant p53, Bcl-2, and pan-cytokeratins.[50] Likewise, the grape peel polyphenols have been utilized for biosynthesis of gold nanoparticles. The produced grape peel AuNPs (GP-AuNPs) were cytotoxic to A431 melanoma cells concomitant with ROS-elicited apoptosis and had potential to damage membrane significantly. Its IC_{50} (in 24 h) value was 23.6 μM in the A431 melanoma cell line.[51] On the basis of these studies, the AuNPs with grape bioactive component can be considered beneficial in the field of biomedicine for the chemotherapy and chemoprevention.

CONCLUSION AND SUGGESTION

On the basis of the extensive investigations by various scientific groups, we can definitely conclude that grapes and grape-based products are excellent sources of various antioxidants and anticarcinogenic agents, and that the cancer preventive and inhibitory properties of grapes should be largely associated by the prominent antioxidant and radical-scavenging activities. Hence, the regular consumption of grapes and grape products is no doubt beneficial to the health of the population in terms of lessening the risk of cancer. Various polyphenolics (viz., resveratrols, PACs, procyanidines, phenolic acids, and/or anthocyanins) in the grape berries, especially in grape peels and grape seeds, can be designated as the most important contributors in their antioxidant and anticarcinogenic activities. Consequently, the scientific approaches have proved that the healthy phytochemical contents in the grapes enriched in pulps < peels < seeds, despite seedless grape cultivars, were developed to appeal to customs. Besides fresh red grapes, red grape juices, and red wines, GSE is also extensively marketed as a functional supplement today. All the intakes are recommended for potentiating human body protection against carcinogenesis in lung, colon, stomach, breast, prostate, skin, and so on, as well as against some other diseases.

REFERENCES

1. Marjan, N.A. et al., 2016. Review of the pharmacological effects of *Vitis vinifera* (Grape) and its bioactive constituents: An update. *Phytother. Res.* 30: 1392–1403.
2. Georgiev, V. et al., 2014. Recent advances and uses of grape flavonoids as nutraceuticals. *Nutrients* 6: 391–415.
3. Xia, E.Q. et al., 2010. Biological activities of polyphenols from grapes. *Int. J. Mol. Sci.* 11: 622–646.
4. Zhu, F. M. et al., 2015. Recent advance on the antitumor and antioxidant activity of grape seed extracts. *Int. J. Wine Res.* 7: 63–67.
5. Zhou, K.Q. et al., 2012. Potential anticancer properties of grape antioxidants. *J. Oncol.* 2012: Article ID 803294.
6. Zahra, E. et al., 2013. Evaluation of anticancer activity of fruit and leave extracts from Virus infected and healthy cultivars of Vitis vinifera. *Cell J.* 15: 116–23.
7. Dinicola, S. et al., 2014. Anticancer effects of grape seed extract on human cancers: A review. *J. Carcinogen. Mutagen.* S8-005: 14.
8. Kaur, M. et al., 2011. Grape seed extract upregulates p21 (Cip1) through redox-mediated activation of ERK1/2 and posttranscriptional regulation leading to cell cycle arrest in colon carcinoma HT29 cells. *Mol. Carcinog.* 50: 553–562.
9. Dinicola, S. et al., 2010. Apoptosis-inducing factor and caspase-dependent apoptotic pathways triggered by different grape seed extracts on human colon cancer cell line Caco-2. *Brit. J. Nutr.* 104: 824–832.
10. Kaur, M. et al., 2009. Anticancer and cancer chemopreventive potential of grape seed extract and other grape-based products. *J. Nutr.* 139: 1806S–1812S.
11. Mertens-Talcott, S.U. et al., 2008. Extracts from red muscadine and cabernet sauvignon wines induce cell death in Molt-4 human leukemia cells. *Food Chem.* 108: 824–832.
12. Hudson, T.S. et al., 2007. Inhibition of prostate cancer growth by muscadine grape skin extract and resveratrol through distinct mechanisms. *Cancer Res.* 67: 8396–8405.
13. Mohansrinivasan, V. et al., 2015. Exploring the anticancer activity of grape seed extract on skin cancer cell lines A431. *Braz. Arch. Biol. Technol.* 58: 540–546.
14. Jung, K.J. et al., 2006. Purple grape juice inhibits 7,12-dimethylbenz[a]anthracene (DMBA)-induced rat mammary tumorigenesis and in vivo DMBA-DNA adduct formation. *Cancer Lett.* (Amsterdam, Netherlands) 233: 279–288.

15. Singletary, K.W. et al., 2003. Inhibition of rat mammary tumorigenesis by Concord grape juice constituents. *J. Agricul. Food Chem.* 51: 7280–7286.

16. Lu, J.M. et al., 2009. Grape seed extract inhibits VEGF expression via reducing HIF-1α protein expression. *Carcinogen.* 30: 636–644.

17. Burton, L.J. et al., 2015. Muscadine grape skin extract can antagonize snail-cathepsin-L-mediated invasion, migration and osteoclastogenesis in prostate and breast cancer cells. *Carcinogen.* 36: 1019–1027.

18. Aggarwal, B.B. et al., 2004. Role of resveratrol in prevention and therapy of cancer: Preclinical and clinical studies. *Anticancer Res.* 24: 2783–2840.

19. Li, T. et al., 2008. Anti-leukemia effect of resveratrol of *Polygonum cuspidatum* exerts and possible molecular mechanism. *J. Xi'an Jiaotong Univ.* (*Med. Edit.*), 29: 340–345.

20. (a) Feng, L. et al., 2006. Active substance of anticancer effect in *Polygonum cuspidatum. Zhongyaocai* 29: 689–691; (b) Sinha, D. et al., 2016. Resveratrol for breast cancer prevention and therapy: Preclinical evidence and molecular mechanisms. *Seminars in Cancer Biol.* 40–41: 209–232.

21. Huang, M.T. et al., 2001. Inhibitory effect of an extract of the root of the Chinese plant Polygonum cuspidatum on chemically-induced several biomarker changes and tumorigenesis in mice. *Abst. Paper 221st ACS National Meeting,* San Diego, CA, U.S. April 1–5, AGFD-023.

22. Banerjee, S. et al., 2002. Suppression of 7,12-dimethylbenz(a)anthracene-induced mammary carcinogenesis in rats by resveratrol: role of nuclear factor-κB, cyclooxygenase 2, and matrix metalloprotease 9. *Cancer Res.* 62: 4945–4954.

23. Liu, J. et al., 2013. Effect of Polygonum cuspidatum extract resveratrol on human gastric cancer 7901 cell proliferation and apoptosis. *Shizhen Guoyi Guoyao* 24: 1627–1629.

24. Blanquer-Rossello, M.M. et al., 2017. Resveratrol induces mitochondrial respiration and apoptosis in SW620 colon cancer cells. *Biochimica et Biophysica Acta,* 1861(2): 431–440.

25. Ji, Q. et al., 2013. Resveratrol inhibits invasion and metastasis of colorectal cancer cells via MALAT1 mediated Wnt/β-catenin signal pathway. *Plos One* 8: e78700.

26. Kimura, Y. et al., 2001. Resveratrol isolated from Polygonum cuspidatum root prevents tumor growth and metastasis to lung and tumor-induced neovascularization in Lewis lung carcinoma-bearing mice. *J. Nat. Prod.* 131: 1844–1849.

27. Wang, S.S. et al., 2004. Angiogenesis and anti-angiogenesis activity of Chinese medicinal herbal extracts. *Life Sci.* 74: 2467–2478.

28. Cao, Y. et al., 2005. Anti-angiogenic activity of resveratrol, a natural compound from medicinal plants. *J. Asian Nat. Prods. Res.* 7: 205–213.

29. Du, Q. et al., 2013. Synergistic anticancer effects of curcumin and resveratrol in Hepa1-6 hepatocellular carcinoma cells. *Oncol. Reports* 29: 1851–1858.

30. Li, M.X. et al., 2012. Effects of resveratrol on cell apoptosis of human choroidal melanoma Mum2c cells. *Zhonghua Shiyan Waike Zazhi* 29: 2566–2568.

31. Lee, M.W. et al., 2012. Extraction of resveratrol from Polygonum cuspidatum with magnetic orcinol-imprinted poly(ethylene-co-vinyl alcohol) composite particles and their in vitro suppression of human osteogenic sarcoma (HOS) cell line. *J. Mat. Chem.* 22: 24644–24651.

32. Li, X.N. et al., 2001. Inhibition of protein kinase C by 3,4',5,-trihydroxystibene-3-β-mono-D-glucoside in human colorectal carcinoma cell lines. *Shijie Huaren Xiaohua Zazhi* 9: 198–201.

33. Lee, S.H. et al., 2002. Induction of apoptosis by 3,4'-dimethoxy-5-hydroxystilbene in human promyeloid leukemic HL-60 cells. *Planta Med.* 68: 123–127.

34. Jiang, H. et al., 2005. Resveratrol-induced apoptotic death in human U251 glioma cells. *Mol. Cancer Therap.* 4: 554–561.

35. Zhou, H.B. et al., 2005. Anticancer activity of resveratrol on implanted human primary gastric carcinoma cells in nude mice. *World J. Gastroenterol.* 11: 280–284.

36. Su, J.L. et al., 2005. Resveratrol induces FasL-related apoptosis through Cdc42 activation of ASK1/JNK-dependent signaling pathway in human leukemia HL-60 cells. *Carcinogenesis* 26: 1–10.

37. Chen, Z.H. et al., 2004. Resveratrol inhibits TCDD-induced expression of CYP1A1 and CYP1B1 and catechol estrogen-mediated oxidative DNA damage in cultured human mammary epithelial cells. *Carcinogen.* 25: 2005–2013.

38. Azios, N.G. et al., 2005. Resveratrol and estradiol exert disparate effects on cell migration, cell surface actin structures, and focal adhesion assembly in MDA-MB-231 human breast cancer cells. *Neoplasia* 7: 128–140.

39. Provinciali, M. et al., 2005. Effect of resveratrol on the development of spontaneous mammary tumors in HER-2/neu transgenic mice. *Intl. J. Cancer* 115: 36–45.

40. Woo, J.H. et al., 2004. Resveratrol inhibits phorbol myristate acetate-induced matrix metalloproteinase-9 expression by inhibiting JNK and PKC signal transduction. *Oncogene* 23: 1845–1853.

41. Manna, S.K. et al., 2000. Resveratrol suppresses TNF-induced activation of nuclear transcription factors NF-κB, activator protein-1, and apoptosis: potential role of reactive oxygen intermediates and lipid peroxidation. *J. Immunol.* 164: 6509–-6519.

42. Kundu, J.B. et al., 2004. Resveratrol inhibits phorbol ester-induced cyclooxygenase-2 expression in mouse skin: MAPKs and AP-1 as potential molecular targets. *BioFactors* 21: 33–39.

43. Pozo-Guisado, E. et al., 2005. Resveratrol-induced apoptosis in MCF-7 human breast cancer cells involves a caspase-independent mechanism with downregulation of Bcl-2 and NF-κB. *Intl. J. Cancer* 115: 74–84.

44. Lian, Y.N. et al., 2016. Protective effect of grape seed oligomeric PACs extract against cisplatin-induced nephrotoxicity in HEK293 cell and effect on anticancer activity of cisplatin in human lung cancer cells. *Shipin Kexue* (Beijing, China) 37(7): 182–186.

45. Mao, J.T. et al., 2016. Grape seed procyanidin extract mediates antineoplastic effects against lung cancer via modulations of prostacyclin and 15-HETE eicosanoid pathways. *Cancer Prev. Res.* 9(12): 925–932.

46. Yi, W.G. et al., 2006. Effects of phenolic compounds in blueberries and muscadine grapes on HepG2 cell viability and apoptosis. *Food Res. Int.* 39: 628–638; 2005. Study of anticancer activities of muscadine grape phenolics in vitro. *J. Agricul. Food Chem.* 53: 8804–8812.

47. Lopez de las Hazas, M.-C. et al., 2017. Exploring the colonic metabolism of grape and strawberry anthocyanins and their in vitro apoptotic effects in HT-29 colon cancer cells. *J. Agricul. Food Chem.* 65 (31):6477–87.

48. Kaur, M. et al., 2009. Gallic acid, an active constituent of grape seed extract, exhibits anti-proliferative, pro-apoptotic and anti-tumorigenic effects against prostate carcinoma xenograft growth in nude mice. *Pharm. Res.* 26: 2133–2140.

49. Mertens-Talcott, S.U. et al., 2006. Induction of cell death in Caco-2 human colon carcinoma cells by ellagic acid rich fractions from Muscadine grapes (Vitis rotundifolia). *J. Agricul. Food Chem.* 54: 5336–5343.

50. Nirmala, J.G. et al., 2017. Vitis vinifera peel and seed gold nanoparticles exhibit chemopreventive potential, antioxidant activity and induce apoptosis through mutant p53, Bcl-2 and pan cytokeratin downregulation in experimental animals. *Biomed. Pharmacother.* 89: 902–917.

51. Nirmala, J.G. et al., 2017. Vitis vinifera peel polyphenols stabilized gold nanoparticles induce cytotoxicity and apoptotic cell death in A431 skin cancer cell lines. *Advanced Powder Technol.* 28(4):1170-84.

40. GUAVA

Goyaves   Guave   La guayaba

番石榴   グアバ   구아바

Psidium guajava

Myrtaceae

Guava is a fruit of a Myrtaceae plant *Psidium guajava* that is native to southern Mexico. Now, the tree grows in tropical and subtropical areas of the world. Widely relished in the tropical regions, its fruit has several varieties depending on the fruit shape, size, and color. Guava fruits are usually consumed in fresh and processed forms, including beverage, syrup, ice cream, and jam. The skin of guava fruit is prominently rich in vitamin C, whose content is highest in guava compared to most other fruits; for example, four times more than in orange and 3.7 times more than in papaya. Thus, guava fruit provides remarkable antioxidant capacity. The root, bark, leaf, and immature fruit of *P. guajava* are commonly employed as traditional medicines in many cultures throughout Central America, the Caribbean, Africa, and Southern Asia for treatment of gastroenteritis, diarrhea, dysentery, ulcers, and so on. These herbs derived from guava plants have been validated by pharmacological studies to possess significant bioactivities including cancer inhibition and prevention.

SCIENTIFIC EVIDENCE OF CANCER PREVENTION

Polyphenols are widely distributed in the fruits and usually serve various biological benefits such as antioxidant, anti-inflammatory, and anticarcinogenic activities. The polyphenolic contents were found to be the highest in guava peels (10.36 g/100 g) and the lowest in guava jam (1.47 g/100 g) in dry weight, but the amount in guava jam was twice that in guava peel.[1] HPLC analysis has identified and quantified the polyphenolics in different parts of guava fruit, revealing that the highest level of phenolics was those of galangin (68.2 mg/100 g), homogentisic acid (10.2 mg/100 g), and catechin (29.2 mg/100 g) in guava peel, homogentisic acid (7.5 mg/100 g) and gallic acid (1.7 mg/100 g) in guava flesh, and gallic acid (6.8 mg/100 g), kaempferol (138 mg/100 g), and cyanidin 3-glucoside (2.8 mg/100 g) in guava seed.[2] The HPLC also showed almost exclusively lycopene (45.3 µg/g) and small amounts of lutein (2.1 µg/g), β-carotene (2.0 µg/g), and β-cryptoxanthin in Horana-red variety of Guava in FW.[3] These constituents were demonstrated to play important roles in antioxidative activities that are believed to largely contribute to cancer prevention.

Antioxidative effects of guava fruit: Usually, the potent antioxidant activity may interfere with cancers, which are initiated by oxidative and free radical damage to DNA and cell components. Total soluble phenolics, vitamin C, lycopene, and total carotenoids were found to be correlated with the total antioxidant capacity (TAOC) of hydrophilic and lipophilic extracts from guava fruits, whose TAOC was measured using six different assays: DPPH, *N,N*-dimethyl-*p*-phenylendiamine (DMPD), ferric-ion-reducing antioxidant power (FRAP), trolox equivalent antioxidant capacity (TEAC), oxygen radical absorbance capacity (ORAC), and total oxidant scavenging capacity (TOSC).[4] The phenolic content in guava peel displayed ten times higher antioxidant capacity than that in guava pulp and the hydrophilic extracts of guava exerted the highest antioxidant capacity.[4,5] The results from the six assays also revealed that the contents of vitamin C and total soluble phenols in the hydrophilic extracts of guava fruit were highly correlated with TAOC, whereas the lipophilic extracts, β-carotene, and total carotenoids from guava fruit were only highly active in the DMPD assay.[4] Besides the extractable polyphenols (2.62%–7.79%), the hydrophilic extracts from the pulp and peel of guava also contain high content of dietary fiber (48.55%–49.42%), whose antioxidant activity was confirmed by three assays, DPPH, FRAP, and LDL (copper-catalyzed low-density lipoprotein oxidation).[6] Pink guava puree in other experiments diminished LPO and enhanced the activities of antioxidant enzymes such as catalase, SOD, glutathione peroxidase, and glutathione reductase in spontaneous hypertensive rat's blood.[7] All these antioxidant capacities of guava fruits led to remarkable contribution to the cancer prevention.

Antiproliferative activities of guava fruit: The phenolic extract from whole fruit of guava in *in vitro* models inhibited the proliferation of two human cancer cell lines with IC_{50}s of 20.94 or 33.60 mg/mL in HepG2 hepatoma cells and 15.93 mg/mL in Caco colon cancer cells.[8,9] The antiproliferative capacities of A549 (lung), HepG2 (liver), HT-29 (colon), and MCF-7 (breast) human cancer cell lines were 73.6%, 71%, 83%, and 56.3% for guava peel, 92%, 89%, 91%, and 66% for guava flesh, and 94%, 91%, 95%, and 95% for guava seed, respectively.[2] In the *in vitro* and/or *ex vitro* assays, total acetone extract of guava fruit was effective in eliciting the proliferative suppression and apoptotic death of human NB4 promyelocitic leukemia, AML #106 primary acute myeloid leukemia blasts, and MDA-MB-231 breast cancer cell lines, but not U937 acute myeloid leukemia and U-2 OS osteosarcoma cells.[10] Both crude water-soluble and alcohol-soluble flavone extracts from the fruits exerted the growth inhibition against human Ec109 (esophagus) and HeLa (cervix) cancer cell lines. However, their antigrowth potencies were less than those of the extracts from guava leaves.[11] Moreover, lycopene is a prominent preventive agent against cancer and carcinogenesis (the detail data of lycopene in the cancer inhibition and prevention were summarized in the section on papaya). The investigations characterized the pulp, peel, and seed of guava fruit to be most relevant to cause cell cycle arrest and apoptosis, whereas the peel was also responsible for prompting cell differentiation of certain carcinomas.[7] In addition, the crushed guava fruit has been tested for antimutagenic activity, wherein its aqueous extract diminished the mutagenicity of *Salmonella typhimurium* caused by mutagens such as 4-nitro-*o*-phenylenediamine, sodium azide, and 2-aminofluorene.[12]

Anticancer activity of guava leaves: Owing to marked inhibitory effects against a variety of neoplastic cell lines, the extracts of guava leaves have gained much more interest in the discovery of novel cancer inhibitors and bioactive constituents with antimicrobial, antidiabetic, cardioprotective, neuroprotective, hepatoprotective, and antioxidant activities. All the aqueous, ethanol, chloroform, and hexane extracts and essential oil of guava leaves have demonstrated anticancer and antioxidant potentials on many different tumor cell lines. From these extracts, many phenolics, flavonoids, carotenoids, and terpenes were isolated and showed to be responsible for moderate to weak antiproliferative and antioxidant activities of guava leaves, especially the meroterpenes, for example, guajadial (**1**), psidial-A (**2**), psiguadial-A (**3**), psiguadial-B (**4**), and the sesquiterpenes, for example, β-caryophyllene oxide separated from the hexane extract and essential oil of guava leaves exhibited more potential for further development as cancer chemotherapy and chemoprevention.[13-16] The leaves are inedible, but young leaves of the guava tree can be brewed to make a kind of tea that affords potentially significant health benefits.

CONCLUSION AND SUGGESTION

The dietary guava fruits have gained a lot of attention for their antioxidant and anticarcinogenic potential and health-promoting nutrients and many anticancer constituents and effects have been reported for guava leaves and stems. As a rich source of vitamin C, carotenoids, and polyphenolics, the fruits can make a beneficial contribution to variety of bioactivities in hampering oxidative stress, scavenging free radicals, and eliminating the factors in cancer initiation in humans. The cancer prevention from dietary guava fruits is figured out to be closely correlated with the excellent antioxidant, antiproliferative, and antimutative effects. As an economical fruit, guava fruits are a good choice for potentiating the antioxidant capacity of the human body and lessening the incidence of carcinogenesis and mutagenesis. Moreover, the young leaves of guava may be valuable to be further developed as a tea-like health supplement.

REFERENCES

1. Marquina, V. et al., 2008. Composition and antioxidant capacity of the guava (Psidium guajava) fruit, pulp and jam. *Arch. Latinoam Nutr.* 58: 98–102.
2. Chen, Y.H. et al., 2015. Evaluation of antioxidant and anticancer activities of guava. *Int. J. Food Nutr. Safety* 6: 1–9.
3. Chandrika, U. et al., 2009. Carotenoid content and in vitro bioaccessibility of lycopene from guava (Psidium guajava) and watermelon (Citrullus lanatus) by high-performance liquid chromatography diode array detection. Int. J. Food Sci. Nutr. 60: 558–566.
4. Corral-Aguayo, R.D. et al., 2008. Correlation between some nutritional components and the total antioxidant capacity measured with six different assays in eight horticultural crops. *J. Agric. Food Chem.* 56: 10498–10504.
5. Sato, R. et al., 2009. Anticancer activity of guava (Psidium guajava) extracts anticancer activity of guava (Psidium guajava) extracts. *J. Complement. Integrative Med.* 7: Dec. Article: 43.
6. Antonio, J.E., 2001. Guava fruit (Psidium guajava L.) as a new source of antioxidant dietary fiber. *J. Agric. Food Chem.* 49: 5489–5493.
7. Wang, F. et al., 2014. Chemical components and bioactivities of Psidium guajava. *Int. J. Food Nutr. Safety* 5: 98–114.
8. Li, W. et al., 2013. Antioxidant and antiproliferative activities of polyphenol extract from 12 tropical fruits. *Xiandai Shipin Keji* 29: 2383–2387.
9. Liu, D. et al., 2015. Evaluation of the anti-proliferative activities of major fruits in China on human hepatic carcinoma (HepG2) and colon adenocarcinoma (Caco-2) cells. *Xiandai Shipin Keji* 31: 23–28.
10. Bontempo, P. et al., 2012. Psidium guajava L. anti-neoplastic effects: induction of apoptosis and cell differentiation. *Cell Proliferation* 45: 22–31.
11. Zou, X.H. et al., 2012. Effect of flavone extract from Psidium guajava L. on HeLa and Ec109 cell growth. *Guangdong Yixue* 33: 914–916.
12. Grover, I.S. et al., 1993. Studies on antimutagenic effects of guava (Psidium guajava) in Salmonella typhimurium. *Mutat. Res.* 300: 1–3.
13. Feng, X.H. et al., 2015. Cytotoxic and antioxidant constituents from the leaves of Psidium guajava. *Bioorg. Med. Chem. Lett.* 25(10): 2193–2198.
14. Ashraf, A. et al., 2016. Chemical composition, antioxidant, antitumor, anticancer and cytotoxic effects of Psidium guajava leaf extracts. *Pharm. Biol.* (Abingdon, U.K.) 54(10): 1971–1981.
15. Anand, V. et al., 2016. Phytopharmacological overview of Psidium guajava Linn. *Pharmacog. J.* 8(4): 314–320.
16. Rizzo, L.Y. et al., 2014. In vitro, in vivo and in silico analysis of the anticancer and estrogen-like activity of guava leaf extracts. *Current Med. Chem.* 21(20): 2322–2330.

41. HAWTHORN BERRY

Aubépine   Weißdorn

山楂 サンザシ 호손

Crataegus monogyna, C. laevigata, C. pinnatifida, C. azarolus

Rosaceae

Hawthorn berry is the fruits of five species of Crataegus genus plants, *Crataegus monogyna, C. laevigata, C. pinnatifida, C. azarolus*, and *C. mexicana*. The ripe fruits of these hawthorns have been utilized in a similar manner, that is using as a folk medicine and producing soft drinks, jelly, jam, and candy. The fresh fruit (*C. pinnatifida*) is a very common children's food in northern China, where the fruits on a stick are coated with candy. Hawthorn berry is a good source of vitamins C and B complex, vitexin, rutin, catechins, saponins, tannins, dietary fiber, calcium, potassium, iron, and various anthocyanids that act as antioxidants within the human body. The pharmacological examinations established that the hawthorn fruits possess hypotensive, hypolipidemic, antioxidant, cardiovascular-strengthening, immunopotentiating, antimyocardial ischemia, blood cholesterol-lowering, anti-inflammatory, and antibacterial properties. Therefore, the dried fruits of hawthorn in China are often used as an herb for treating digestion-related disorders, coronary artery disease, tachycardia, palpitations, cardiomyopathy, hypercholesterolemia, hypertension, angina, and varicose veins.[1]

Scientific Evidence of Cancer-Preventive Effect

Nitrosamine is a carcinogen that occurs in many processed foods. The hawthorn berry extracts were reported to be able to obstruct the synthesis of nitrosamine through elimination of its precursor.[2] Experimental murine animal models confirmed that hawthorn extract prominently blocked the synthesis pathway of methylbenzyl nitrosamine.[3] An acetone extract of *C. pinnatifida* showed obvious inhibitory effect against the mutagenesis and carcinogenesis caused by aflatoxin B1.[4] The hawthorn berry extracts were capable of effectively scavenging free radicals. A hot water extract derived from *C. cuneate* fruits at higher concentrations could synergically augment the cytotoxicity of ascorbate on human oral squamous cell cancer and salivary gland tumor cell lines.[5] Thus, the findings designated that the hawthorn berries are a functional food that may be useful for the cancer prevention and health promotion. In addition, the aqueous extract of *C. monogyna* fruits could serve as a protective substance against reproductive toxicity caused by a chemo drug cyclophosphamide in a rat model.[6]

Scientific Evidence of Antitumor Constituents

Bioactive ingredients found in hawthorn plants (fruits, leaves, and stems) include tannins, phenolic acids, flavonoids, C-glycosylated flavones, oligomeric PACs, and triterpene acids. These phytochemicals respond to the health-promoting and body protective advantages of hawthorns, including antioxidation and anticarcinogenesis.

1. Triterpenoids

Bioassay-guided separation of the berry of *C. pinnatifida* gave several cytotoxic triterpenoids with ursane-type and olean-type skeletons, as well as sitosterol. Uvaol (**1**) and ursolic acid (**2**) demonstrated moderate cytotoxicity against murine L1210 leukemia cells, but showed only weak activities against human SKOV-3 (ovary), XF498 (brain), A549 (lung), SK-MEL-2 (skin), and HCT-15 (colon) neoplastic cell lines *in vitro*.[7] Corosolic acid (**3**) acted as an inhibitor of protein kinase-C (PKC) to display the inhibitory effect similar to that of ursolic acid toward several human cancer cell lines *in vitro*.[8] 3β,6β,18β,23-Tetrahydroxy-olean-12-en-28-oic acid (**4**), 2α,3β,6β,18β-tetrahydroxy-olean-12-en-28-oic acid (**5**), and 2α,3β,6β,18β,23-pentahydroxy-olean-12-en-28-oic acid (**6**) exerted highly potent inhibitory activity toward the proliferation of human HepG2 (liver) and MCF-7 (breast) cancer cell lines (EC_{50}s < 5 μM).[9] The antioxidant capacity of 3β,6β,18β-trihydroxy-olean-12-en-28-oic acid and 2α,3β,19α-trihydroxy-olean-12-en-28-oic acid was 70 and 28 times higher than that of ascorbic acid.[9] A triterpenes-enriched fraction from the hexanoic extract of *C. monogyna* demonstrated significant cytotoxic effect against cultured human HEp-2 laryngeal carcinoma cells. After treatment with a dose 6 μg/mL for 72 h, the fraction obstructed the growth of HEp-2 cells by 93%.[10]

Moreover, *N*-(3-acetoxyurs-12-en-28-oyl)-3-morpholin-4-yl-1-propylamine (**7**) was produced by the modification of ursolic acid (**2**) structure. *In vitro* treatment with the derivative (**7**) at a concentration of 10 mol/L for 96 h showed markedly enhanced suppressive effect against the proliferation of human SKOV-3 (ovary), BGC-823 (stomach), and HeLa (cervix) carcinoma cell lines with the inhibitory rates of 62.28%, 85.03%, and 92.97%, respectively. The results revealed that the acetylation at C-3 and coupling with selected amino acid methyl esters at C-28 could augment the antineoplastic potency.[11] In addition, a sitosterol isolated from hawthorn berry also showed marginal antiproliferative effect on three cancer cell lines (HepS, sarcoma 180, and EAC), probably by causing apoptosis.[12]

2. Flavonoids

Total flavonoids isolated from the hawthorn fruits exerted the inhibitory effect against the proliferation of HEp-2 laryngocarcinoma cells obviously in a dose-dependent manner. When treated with the total flavonoids for 48 h, the intracellular calcium concentration was amplified notably and the DNA content was declined remarkably in the HEp-2 cells, suggesting that the antitumor activities might be related to the blocking of signal transduction and DNA synthesis.[13] The total flavonoids also displayed marginal *in vitro* inhibitory effect against the cell growth of human HepG2 liver and Caco colorectal cancer cell lines and exerted antioxidant effect in free radical-scavenging assays.[14] In addition, the hawthorn flavonoids could elicit the apoptotic death of hepatic stellate cells in rats.[15]

Vitexin (**8**), a natural flavonoid, is found in fruits, flowers, and/or leaves of Crataegus genus plants such as *C. pinnatifida* and has been reported to exhibit certain levels of antioxidative, anti-inflammatory, anti-metastatic, and antitumor properties. At a concentration range of 5.0–80.0 μM, vitexin (**8**) impeded the viability and proliferation of EC-109 human esophageal cancer cells in a dose- and time-dependent manner. By the induction of p53-dependent metastatic and apoptotic pathway, including increase in PAI-1 and downexpression MMP-2, vitexin (**8**) hindered the viability and metastasis of OC2 human oral cancer cells in 25–100 μM concentrations; by the inhibition of HIF-1α (hypoxia inducible factor-1α) and decrease in hypoxia-induced genes, vitexin (**8**) exerted the anti-metastatic effect in rat PC12 pheochromocytoma cells at >20 μM and the antimigratory effect in human MCF-7/T47D breast cancer cells at 2 μM. In an earlier study, the proapoptotic effect of vitexin (**8**) was observed in human U937 lymphomic leukemia cells, but its antitumor activity on U937 cells was weak (IC$_{50}$ ~200.34 μM).[16,17]

3. Polyphenols

CF-TP, a polyphenolic fraction, was derived from the hot-water extract of hawthorn fruits, which notably restrained BAP/TPA-induced melanoma formation and decreased the incidence of skin carcinogenesis. This chemopreventive potential of the melanoma might be partially correlated to its significant suppressive effects against the expressions of COX-2, iNOS, NF-κB, and AP-1, the generation of reactive oxygen species (ROS), and the activation of ODC.[18] Several polyphenolic extracts prepared from the fruit peels, leaves, pulp, or syrup of *C. azarolus* and the fruit peels or leaves of *C. monogyna* showed antiproliferation of human Caco-2 colon cancer cells, and only the extracts from the pulp and syrup of *C. azarolus* had the inhibitory effects in B16F10 melanoma cell model.[19] The azarole polyphenolic extracts also exerted protective effect against oxidative damage.[20] Likewise, an extract derived from the flower buds of *C. monogyna* presented moderate to weak antiproliferative effects on human MCF-7 (breast), NCI-H460 (lung), HeLa (cervix), and HepG2 (liver) carcinoma cell lines (GI$_{50}$s of 63.55–88.45 μg/mL) and its activities were much better than those of the extracts obtained from the fruits of *C. monogyna*. According to characterization by HPLC–DAD–ESI/MS methods, the extract was revealed to be rich in phenolic acids such as quinic acid and its derivatives, caffeic acid and its derivatives, and *p*-coumaric acid derivatives.[20]

4. Neolignans

Eighteen 8-O-4′ neolignans were obtained from the isolation of 70% ethanolic extract of hawthorn seeds. In *in vitro* system, pinnatifidanins-BVII (**9**), -BIX (**10**), *erythro*-(7S,8R)-guaiacylglycerol-β-coniferylaldehyde ether (**11**), and *threo*-(7R,8R)-guaiacylglycerol-β-coniferylaldehyde ether (**12**) showed moderate to week inhibitory effect against the cell viability of human neoplastic cells lines (HepG2, A549, HL-60, A375-S2, HCT-116, and HT1080 cells) but were inactive to other four human cancer cells (HeLa, K562, MCF-7, and Mrc5). The presence of an aldehyde group at C-9′ and a double bond at C-7′/C-8′ next to the aromatic ring (π–π conjugation) might augment the cytotoxicity of the neolignans. Pinnatifidanins-BVII (**9**) exerted much stronger inhibitory effect against human U937 leukemic monocyte lymphoma cells compared to an anticancer drug 5-fluorouracil (IC$_{50}$s of 2.71 μM vs. 23.93 μM), but the other three (**10–12**) showed no inhibitory effect against the U937 cells. Consideration of the structure–bioactivity relationships suggested that a methoxy group at C-7 might play an important role in the selectivity of anti-U937 activities.[21] Also, 7R,8S-balanophonin (**13**) exhibited cytotoxicity on human HT-1080 fibrosarcoma cells and its IC$_{50}$ was lower than that of 5-fluorouracil (8.86 μM vs. 35.62 μM), but it displayed moderate to weak inhibitory effect on human HeLa, HepG2, A375-S2, and HL-60 cancer cell lines.[18,22] In addition, many of the isolates from the plant showed marked antioxidant properties.[22]

CONCLUSION AND SUGGESTION

The experimental observations demonstrated that the bioactive components in hawthorn berries were triterpenoids, flavonoids, polyphenolics, and neolignans, which were mostly responsible for the medical functions of hawthorn fruits. These components showed only moderate to weak range of antitumor activities but were safely available for the antioxidative and preventive activities to lessen the risk of certain types of carcinogenesis such as that in liver, stomach, esophagus, larynx, colon, breast, and cervix. There is no question that frequent dietary intake of hawthorn fruit with its biologically active constituents may offer an advantageous protection for the human body to be in a good condition to minimize the threat of cancer in addition to improving cardiovascular function. However, overdose of hawthorn fruits should be avoided, as it may cause cardiac arrhythmia and dangerously low blood pressure.

OTHER BIOACTIVITIES OF THE COMPONENTS

The levels of flavonoid components and proanthocyanins are quite high in hawthorn fruits, matured flower buds, and young leafy spring tips of the plant. The hawthorn flavonoids are also available for treating diabetes and arthritis, as well as for strengthening and repairing connective tissue, and the procyanadins are effective on cardiotonic.[23]

REFERENCES

1. Jurikova, T. et al., 2012. Polyphenolic profile and biological activity of Chinese hawthorn (Crataegus pinnatifida Bunge) fruits. *Mol.* 17: 14490–14509.
2. Gu, F.C. et al., 1989. The hawthorn extract eliminating nitrite. *J. Henan Med. Univ.* 24: 27–31.
3. Liu, Z.P. et al., 1991. The blocking effect of hawthorn extract on the internal synthesis of methylbenzyl-nitrosamine and its carcinogenesis. *J. Henan Med. Univ.* 26: 349–352.
4. Yuan, C.C. et al., 1989. Inhibition of 12 Chinese traditional medicinal herbs on mutagenic effect induced by aflatoxin B1. *Aizheng* 8: 29–31.
5. Satoh, K. et al., 1998. Enhancement of radical intensity and cytotoxic activity of ascorbate by Crataegus cuneata Sieb et. Zucc. Extracts. *Anticancer Res.* 18: 2749–2753.
6. Jalali, A.S. et al., 2012. Crataegus monogyna aqueous extract ameliorates cyclophosphamide-induced toxicity in rat testis: Stereological evidences. *Acta Medica Iranica* 50: 1–8.
7. Min, B.S. et al., 2000. Cytotoxic triterpenes from Crataegus pinnatifida. *Archiv. Pharm. Res.* 23: 155–158.
8. Ahn, K.S. et al., 1998. Corosolic acid isolated from the fruit of Crataegus pinnatifida var. psilosa is a protein kinase C inhibitor as well as a cytotoxic agent. *Planta Med.* 64: 468–470.
9. Qiao, A.M. et al., 2015. Novel triterpenoids isolated from hawthorn berries functioned as antioxidant and antiproliferative activities. *J. Functional Foods* 13: 308–313.
10. Saenz, M.T. et al., 1997. Extracts from Viscum and Crataegus are cytotoxic against larynx cancer cells. *Z Naturforsch C.* 52: 42–44.
11. Meng, Y.Q. et al., 2010. Synthesis and in vitro cytotoxicity of novel ursolic acid derivatives. *Mol.* 15: 4033–4040.
12. Dong, H. et al., 2009. Inhibition of tumour cells with sitosterol from hawthorn fruits. *Zhongguo Shenghua Yaowu Zazhi* 30: 270–272.
13. Zhang, Y. et al., 2004. Isolation and purification of total flavonoids from Crataegus pinnatifida and its antitumor activity. *Zhongcaoyao* 35: 787–789.
14. Liu, J. et al., 2010. Hawthorn flavonoid extract: antioxidant activity and growth inhibition effect on cancer cells. *Shipin Kexue* (Beijing, China) 31: 220–223.
15. Li, Z.G., 2013. Emodin and hawthorn flavonoids induce rat hepatic stellate cell apoptosis. *Zhongguo Yaowu Yu Linchuang* 13: 740–741.
16. Yang, S.H. et al., 2013. The novel p53-dependent metastatic and apoptotic pathway induced by vitexin in human oral cancer OC2 Cells. *Phytother. Res.* 27: 1154–1161.
17. He, M. et al., 2016. A review on the pharmacological effects of vitexin and isovitexin. *Fitoterapia* 115: 74–85.
18. Kao, E. et al., 2007. Effects of polyphenols derived from fruit of Crataegus pinnatifida on cell transformation, dermal edema and skin tumor formation by phorbol ester application. *Food Chem. Toxicol.* 45: 1795–1804.
19. Belkhir, M. et al., 2016. Protective effects of azarole polyphenolic extracts against oxidative damage using in vitro biomolecular and cellular models. *Industrial Crops Prod.* 86: 239–250.
20. Rodrigues, S. et al., 2012. Crataegus monogyna buds and fruits phenolic extracts: Growth inhibitory activity on human tumor cell lines and chemical characterization by HPLC-DAD-ESI/MS. *Food Res. Intl.* 49: 516–523.
21. Huang, X.X. et al., 2013. The cytotoxicity of 8-O-4' neolignans from the seeds of Crataegus pinnatifida. *Bioorg. Med. Chem. Lett.* 23: 5599–5604.
22. Huang, X.X. et al., 2013. Cytotoxic and antioxidant dihydrobenzofuran neolignans from the seeds of Crataegus pinnatifida. *Fitoterapia* 91: 217–223.
23. Yu, B.B. et al., 2015. Research progress in pharmacological activities and mechanism of hawthorn. *Zhongnan Yaoxue* 13: 745–748.

42. JUJUBE

Jujube   Jujube   Pastilla

紅棗 ナツメ 대추

Ziziphus jujuba

Rhamnaceae

2. R$_1$ = –CH$_3$, R$_2$ = –H
3. R$_1$ = –H, R$_2$ = –CH$_3$

Jujube (Chinese date) is the ripe fruit of a Rhamnaceae plant *Ziziphus jujuba*. As the fruits are great source of a nutritional food and a folk medicine, jujube today has been widely consumed in Asian countries. Fresh jujube is a rich source of vitamin C that helps stave off harmful free radicals from the human body, whereas dried jujube is a good source of vitamins B2, B1, and C, manganese, phosphorus, and iron. The dried jujube is traditionally consumed as a Chinese herb for its various physiological functions, such as immunostimulant, antiulcer, antispastic, cardiotonic, sedative, antioxidant, anti-inflammatory, hypotensive, antiobesity, hepato- and gastrointestinal-protective, hypnotic, antinephritic, antiallergic, and wound-healing properties. A controlled clinical trial found the fruits are helpful for chronic constipation. In addition, an extract derived from jujube leaves exhibited antiobese activity in rats.[1]

Scientific Evidence of Antitumor Activity

Jujube possesses multiple health benefits including anticarcinogenetic and immunoenhancing activities. When rats freely drank water added *N*-methyl-*N*′-nitro-*N*-nitrosoguanidine (MNNG, a mutagene) and ate 1 g of jujube daily at the same time for ten successive months, the incidence of gastric adenocarcinogenesis was significantly dropped.[2,3] Its water extract demonstrated marked growth inhibitory and apoptosis-inducing effects in human Jurkat (leukemic), HEp-2 (larynx), and HeLa (cervix) neoplastic cell lines *in vitro*, wherein Jurkat leukemic cells were the most sensitive to the extract with IC$_{50}$ of 0.1 μg/mL.[4] ZE1 (n-hexane extract), ZE2 (chloroform extract), and ZE4 (ethyl acetate partition fraction) were prepared from the jujube, showing obvious antiproliferative effects on both MCF-7 estrogen receptor (ER)α-positive (IC$_{50}$s 14.42, 7.64, and 1.69 μg/mL) and SKBR3 ERα-negative (IC$_{50}$s 14.06, 6.21, and 3.70 μg/mL) human breast cancer cell lines but no influence on viability of both nonmalignant breast epithelial MCF-10A cells and normal human fibroblast BJ1-hTERT cells.[5] The MCF-7 and SKBR3 breast cancer cell lines were elicited to apoptosis after the ZEs treatments and the effective ZE2 and ZE4 were found to share a number of triterpenic acids as anticancer agents.[5] These extracts of jujube were also able to reduce the viability of human HepG2 hepatoma cells. The antihepatoma effect of CHCl$_3$-F (a chloroform fraction) was found to be closely associated with the induction of apoptosis and cell cycle arrest. The cell cycle arrest was mediated by two different mechanisms, that is, CHCl$_3$-F at a low concentration (100 μg/mL) induced G1 cell cycle arrest of HepG2 cells via increase of p27Kip1 activity and Rb hypophosphorylation and decrease of phosphorylated Rb and at a high concentration (200 μg/mL) resulted in G2/M cell cycle arrest of HepG2 cells by decrease in the p27Kip1 levels and increase in p27Kip1 phosphorylation.[6] When combined with green tea extract, the chemotherapeutic activity of CHCl$_3$-F on the hepatoma concomitant could be enhanced, with notable downregulation of APRIL (a proliferation-inducing ligand) expression.[7]

In the long-term administration, jujube, which is rich in betulinic acid, and its derivatives demonstrated suppressive effects against broad spectrum of malignant tumors in stomach, colon, breast, lung, cervix, ovary, prostate, oral cavity, larynx, liver, pancreas, kidney, bladder, and skin, and against glioblastoma, leukemia, and myeloma. The antigrowth effect of jujube was always accompanied by inhibition of PKC activity and elicitation of cell apoptosis in the neoplastic cells.[8,9] In addition, orally given to mice as an extract of Dongzao Jujube (a jujube cultivar), it restrained the growth of sarcoma 180 together with activation of SOD, decline of malondialdehyde (MDA) level in plasma, and lessening of red blood cell hemolytic degree *in vivo*.[10] Interestingly, a recent report revealed that 95% ethanolic extract derived from the fruit seeds of some jujube cultivars markedly suppressed the proliferation of human Jurkat leukemia T cells *in vitro* and induced both extrinsic and intrinsic apoptosis pathways by increasing caspase-8 and caspase-9 activity, respectively.[11]

SCIENTIFIC EVIDENCE OF ANTITUMOR CONSTITUENTS AND ACTIVITIES

1. Triterpenoids

A group of triterpenoid acids including zizyberenalic acid (**1**), oleanonic acid (**2**), ursolonic acid (**3**), and betulonic acid (**4**) were isolated from Jujube. High concentrations of the triterpenoids exhibited moderate to weak antiproliferative effect against a viral produced MS-G2 hepatoma cells *in vitro*. The four major triterpenoids also displayed anti-HBsAg and anti-HBeAg effects in the MS-G2 cells.[12] Other isolated triterpenoic acids, especially 3-O-*trans-p*-coumaroyl-alphitolic acid (**5**), exerted *in vitro* cytotoxicities against a panel of tumor cell lines such as B16-F10, LOX-IMVI, and SK-MEL-2 (skin), PC3 (prostate), K562 (leukemic), and A549 (lung) cells. Comparison of the relationship between their structures and activities suggested that a coumaroyl moiety at C-3 position of the lupane-type triterpenoids might play an important role in enhancing the cytotoxicity.[13] Moreover, the self-assembled betulinic acid, which was prepared by dissolving 10 mg of betulinic acid in a mixture of ethanol:water (16:4), could protect human peripheral blood lymphocytes (PBLs) from a chemo drug doxorubicin (DOX) induced apoptosis via reduction of ROS-TNFα-caspase-3 pathway to lessen DOX-caused side effects and to ameliorate DOX-induced chemotherapeutic toxicity.[14] In addition to the fruits, the roots of the jujube plant also are rich in ceanothane-type and lupane-type triterpenoids, some of the triterpenes showed moderate cytotoxic effect on human HepG2 hepatoma cells with IC$_{50}$ values ranging from 1.9 to 5.9 μM.[15]

2. Saponins

Jujuboside-B is one of the saponins isolated from the seeds of *Z. jujuba* var. *spinosa*, whose antigrowth effects were weak in human AGS (stomach) and HCT-116 (colon) cancer cell lines (IC$_{50}$s 107–114 μM), but it triggered both apoptotic and autophagic death of the two cell lines. Mechanistic explorations revealed that jujuboside-B-induced apoptosis of the AGS cells was mediated by an extrinsic pathway via upregulation of FasL and caspase-8 and activation of p38/JNK. The *in vivo* suppressive effect of jujuboside-B was further observed in a nude mice xenograft model implanted HCT-116 cells.[16]

3. Peptide

An antitumor peptide extract was prepared from jujube by electromagnetic cracking device. Daily administration of the peptide extract for 10 continuous days obviously obstructed the growth of sarcoma 180, Hep, and MFC tumor cells in tumor-bearing mice and prolonged the survival time of the sarcoma 180-bearing mice even at a lower dose. *In vitro* studies further found the peptide extract could augment phagocytic index and thymus co-effecter and potentiate the transformation of lymphocyte function. These evidences indicated that the jujube peptide extract exerted immuno-potentiating anticarcinoma effects.[17]

4. Polysaccharide

Jujube fruit is rich in functional polysaccharides. From the fruits, a deproteinized polysaccharide (DPP) was prepared. DPP was composed of two fractions with average molecular weights of 143,108 Da and 67,633 Da, respectively. The antiproliferative and G2/M cell cycle arrest-inducing effects were observed in melanoma cells in a dose- and time-dependent manner. The IC_{50} of DPP was around 3.99 mg/mL (in 24 h) and 3.36 mg/mL (in 48 h).[1,18] After the DPP treatment, the apoptotic bodies were generated in association with activation of caspases-3 and -9.[18] Likewise, two acidic polysaccharides, HJP1 and HJP3, were isolated from the fruits of Z. jujuba cv. Muzao. Their molecular weights were 6.762×10^4 Da and 2.936×10^4 Da, respectively, composed of mannose, rhamnose, galactose, galacturonic acid, glucose, and arabinose. Both HJP1 and HJP3 could inhibit the growth of human HepG2 hepatoma cells, and HJP3 showed stronger cytotoxicity on the HepG2 cells than HJP1.[19] Therefore, the results suggest that these functional polysaccharides may potentially be used in the prevention and treatment of liver and skin cancers.

CONCLUSION AND SUGGESTION

Extensive investigations over the past 20 years have demonstrated that dietary jujube can provide considerable chemopreventive potential against the carcinogenesis in skin, stomach, colon, liver, breast, prostate, lung, larynx, cervix, and so on, in addition to the immunostimulating and anti-inflammatory activities. The major biologically active phyto components in the jujube fruits are vitamins B and C, polyphenolics, flavonoids, triterpenic acids, peptides, and polysaccharides. Some of the molecules, especially triterpenic acids and polysaccharides, demonstrated anticancer activities by provoking antiproliferative and apoptotic effects in the experimental models. The polyphenolic content in the jujube was positively correlated with antioxidant activities by regulating antioxidant enzyme functions, whose effects may be conducive to lowering the risk of cancer and chemoresistance.[20,21] Considering jujube has a long history of usage as a fruit and remedy, it is recommended for the safe prevention of carcinogenesis and health enhancement by dietary consumption.

REFERENCES

1. Ji, X.L. et al., 2017. Isolation, structures and bioactivities of the polysaccharides from jujube fruit (Ziziphus jujuba Mill.): A review. *Food Chem.* 227: 349–357.
2. Lin, B.S. et al., 1982. *Tianjing Yiyao Zhongliuxue, Supplement* 9: 62; 1999. Chinese Materia Medica, Vol. 5, Published by Shanghai Science Technology Express, 5-4208, pp. 258.
3. Song, W.M. et al., 1991. Anti-mutagenic effect of Chinese date. *Zhongyao Yaoli yu Linchuang* 7: 25.
4. Vahedi, F. et al., 2008. Evaluation of inhibitory effect and apoptosis induction of Zyzyphus jujube on tumor cell lines, an in vitro preliminary study. 2008. *Cytotechnol.* 56: 105–111.
5. Plastina, P. et al., 2012. Identification of bioactive constituents of Ziziphus jujube fruit extracts exerting antiproliferative and apoptotic effects in human breast cancer cells. *J. Ethnopharmacol.* 140: 325–32.
6. Huang, X.D. et al., 2007. Mechanism of the anticancer activity of Zizyphus jujuba in HepG2 cells. *Am. J. Chin. Med.* 35: 517–532.
7. Huang, X.D. et al., 2009. Combination of Zizyphus jujuba and green tea extracts exerts excellent cytotoxic activity in HepG2 cells via reducing the expression of APRIL. *Am. J. Chinese Med.* 37: 169–179.
8. Ramadoss, S. et al., 2000. Use of betulinic acid and its derivatives for inhibiting cancer growth and a method of monitoring this. *US* 6048847 A 20000411.
9. Mukherjee, R. et al., 2004. Method for treating cancer using betulinic acid-rich Ziziphus extract. *US Pat. Appl. Publ.* 20040116394 A1 20040617.
10. Ma, L. et al., 2008. Study on antioxidant activity of DJE on S180 tumor-bearing mice. *Qingdao Daxue Xuebao, Tech. Edition* 23: 30–34.

11. Taechakulwanijya, N. et al., 2016. Apoptosis-inducing effects of jujube (Zao) seed extracts on human Jurkat leukemia T cells. *Chinese Medicine* (London, U.K.) 11: 15/1-15/13.

12. Huang, R.L. et al., 2001. Cytotoxic triterpenes from the fruit of Ziziphus jujuba. *Chin. Pharm. J.* (T.W.) 53: 179–184.

13. Lee, S.M. et al., 2003. Cytotoxic triterpenoids from the fruits of Ziziphus jujuba. *Planta Med.* 69: 1051–1054.

14. Dash, S.K. et al., 2015. Self-assembled betulinic acid protects doxorubicin induced apoptosis followed by reduction of ROS-TNF-α-caspase-3 activity. *Biomed. Pharmacother.* 72: 144–157.

15. Kang, K.B. et al., 2016. Cytotoxic ceanothane- and lupane-type triterpenoids from the roots of Ziziphus jujuba. *J. Nat. Prod.* 79(9): 2364–2375.

16. Xu, M.Y. et al., 2014. Antitumor activity of jujuboside B and the underlying mechanism via induction of apoptosis and autophagy. *J. Nat. Prod.* 77: 370–376.

17. Sun, X. et al., 2008. Experimental study on antitumor effect of jujube peptide prepared with electromagnetic cracking device. *Shipin Kexue* (Beijing, China) 29: 597--600.

18. Hung, C.F. et al., 2012. Antiproliferation of melanoma cells by polysaccharide isolated from Zizyphus jujuba. *Nutr.* (Burbank, Los Angeles County, Calif.) 28: 98–105.

19. Wang, Y.J. et al., 2015. Structural characterization and in vitro antitumor activity of polysaccharides from Zizyphus jujuba cv. Muzao. *RSC Advances* 5: 7860–7867.

20. Siriamornpun, S. et al., 2015. Bioactive compounds and health implications are better for green jujube fruit than for ripe fruit. *J. Functional Foods* 12: 246–255.

21. Tahergorabi, Z. et al., 2015. "Ziziphus jujuba": A red fruit with promising anticancer activities. *Pharmacognosy Reviews* 9: 99–106.

43. KIWI FRUIT

獼猴桃　キウイ　키위

Actinidia chinensis

Actinidiaceae

1. $R_1 = R_2 = -H$
2. $R_1 = -H, R_2 = -CH_3$
3. $R_1 = R_2 = -CH_3$
4. $R_1 = -H, R_2 = -Ac$

6. $R_1 = R_2 = H$, 3beta-OH.
7. $R_1 = -H, R_2 = -OH$, 3alpha-OH.
9. $R_1 = -OH, R_2 = -H$, 3alpha-OH.

Kiwi is the fruit of the Actinidia tree, wherein *A. chinensis* is the most popular kiwi plant that is native to the Yangtze River valley of China and the coast of eastern China. Today, kiwi is a favorite fruit commercialized around the world as it is rich source of vitamin C and good source of vitamins K, E, and dietary fiber. The fruit pulp contains bioactive carotenoids (β-carotene, lutein, and zeaxanthin), and the fruit seed oil contains α-linolenic acid (an omega-3 fatty acid) in average 62%. Kiwi fruit not only acts as nutritional supplement but also plays functional roles in DNA protection, antioxidation, cardiovascular improvement, and macular degeneration protection, hepatoprotection, blood lipid reduction, antianoxemia, and antiasthma.[1] A 70% methanol extract of kiwi fruits was reported to have significant anti-HIV, anti-free radical, and peroxide-eliminating activities. In China, the fresh and dried fruits, roots, and stems (>10 years old) of kiwi plant are used as folk medicines.

Scientific Evidence of Cancer Prevention

Antimutagenic activity: Owing to the heterocyclic amines and the polycyclic aromatic hydrocarbon produced in foods because of high-temperature cooking, this oncogenes-related mutagenesis is relevant to humans. Kiwi fruit juice and its extracts were able to repress the mutagenesis caused by chemical carcinogens (such as heterocyclic amines and imidazoquinolines) in the *in vitro* assays.[1] Kiwi fruits exerted antimutagenic effect against picrolonic acid or BAP-induced mutation.[2] Kiwi fruit juice could inhibit nitrosamine formation and deter mutagenicity of α-*tert*-butane-O-benzoquinone.[3,4] *In vivo* experiments showed that the juice was able to obstruct nitritoproline production in rats, pregnant mice, pregnant women, healthy persons, and patients with chronic atrophic gastritis.[5,6]

Antioxidant and DNA protective activities: Kiwi fruit is a rich source of potential antioxidant polyphenols in addition to its high content of vitamin C. Kiwi fruit juice showed SOD-like activity in the *in vitro* test, and it potently restrained lipid oxidation and eliminated hydrogen peroxide-induced oxidative stress. Seventy percent methanol extract of kiwi fruit exhibited marked superoxide radical-scavenging activity. In DPPH assay, the antioxidant activities of several types of kiwi fruits were confirmed and the fruit extract of *A. kolomikta* showed the highest DPPH scavenging effect, an activity that was attributed to the highest content of vitamin C and total phenolics in kiwi fruit (*A. kolomikta*). However, the total antioxidation capacity of kiwi fruit was lower than that of raspberry, strawberry, plum, and orange but greater than that of grapefruit, apple, and pear.[1] Moreover, in human intervention studies, kiwi fruit intake showed certain defensive potentials against DNA damage, such as reduction of DNA strand breaks, decline of endogenous oxidative levels of pyrimidines and purines, improvement of DNA repair capacity, and amplification of lymphocyte DNA resistance to hydrogen peroxide-induced oxidative damage.[1]

Anticancer activity: The extracts from kiwi fruits or roots in the *in vitro* assays exerted certain cytotoxic effect against human solid tumor cell lines of oral, esophagus, stomach, colon, and lung.[7-11] An extract prepared from hardy kiwi fruit (*A. argute*) in an *in vitro* assay displayed antiproliferative effects to Hep3B (liver) and HeLa (cervix) cancer cells but not to HepG2 (liver), HT-29, and LoVo (colon) cancer cells.[12] The polyphenol-rich crude extracts, which were derived from the fruits of three kiwi cultivars with 60% ethanol, exhibited antiproliferative activity against human A549 (lung) and HeLa (cervix) cancer cell lines *in vitro*, wherein the extract derived from *A. argute* exerted greater inhibition than others.[13]

Kiwi essence, a nutritional supplement sold in Chinese markets, is made of 60% concentration of kiwi fruit seed oil, which contains >50% linolenic acid. The kiwi essence was found to have an ability to sensitize chemotherapeutics (cisplatin and gemcitabine) to hamper the growth of allotransplantation tumors in mice with lung adenocarcinoma, associated with downregulation of excision repair cross-complementation group 1 (ERCC1) and upregulation of ribonucleotide reductase subunit M1 (RRM1).[14] Kiwi essence also obviously reversed the multidrug resistance of lung adenocarcinoma to GP chemotherapy (a combination with gemcitabine and cisplatin) in mice bearing tumor xenografts of Lewis cells via downregulation of *P*-glycoprotein (*P*-gp) and glucose-regulated protein 78 (GRP78).[15] In addition, an ethyl acetate extract from kiwi root (*A. chinensis*) could restrain the proliferation of human A549 lung cancer cells in concentrations of 40–160 µg/mL in association with block of DNA synthesis and reduction of Ki-67 antigen expression.[16] A n-butanol lysate of alcohol extract from *A. rufa* root showed the antitumor effect on SGC-7901 human gastric tumor cells by inducing the injury of DNA and stimulating apoptosis.[17]

Scientific Evidence of Antitumor Constituents and Activities

Phytochemical investigations disclosed that kiwi fruits contain multiple components such as water-soluble vitamins, pigments (including chlorophylls, carotenoids, lutein, and anthocyanins), myosmine, serotonin, alkaloids, saponins, and free galactose. Kiwi fruits are also known to contain appreciable amounts of proteases. The phytochemical and nutritional properties of kiwi fruits may be impacted by various factors such as kiwi fruit species, cultivation, harvesting, storage, and processing. However, compared with kiwi fruits, phytochemists usually prefer to explore the kiwi roots as their projects due to the roots presenting more interesting bioactivities and chemical characteristics.[18]

1. Flavonoids

From the roots of Kiwi (*A. chinensis*), twelve phenolic constituents and four pairs of isomeric flavonoids were isolated. The four phenolic compounds designated as planchols A–D (**1–4**) possess a novel skeleton, demonstrating marked inhibition of murine P388 leukemia cells and human A549 lung adenocarcinoma cells *in vitro*. The IC_{50} values were 2.5–5.05 µM in the P388 cells and 1.44–4.5 µM in the A549 cells. The preliminary SAR analysis showed that the hydroxyl groups in **1–4** are essential for the inhibitory effect because the cytotoxicity was reduced when the hydroxyl group was substituted by methoxylation or acetylation.[19]

2. Triterpenoids

A group of triterpenoids was isolated from the roots of *A. chinensis*. Of them, 2α,3β-dihydroxyolean-12-en-28-oic acid (DHOA, **5**), 2α,3β-dihydroxyurs-12-en-28-oic acid (DHUA, **6**), and 2α,3α,24-trihydroxyurs-12-en-28-oic acid (**7**) showed moderate inhibition of human LoVo colon cancer cells (IC_{50}s 6.0, 2.9, and 13.9 µg/mL, respectively), and DHUA (**6**) restrained the growth of human HepG2 hepatoma cells (IC_{50} 9.2 µg/mL) *in vitro*.[20] 12α-Chloro-2α,3β,13β,

23-tetrahydroxyolean-28-oic acid-13-lactone (**8**), 2α,3α,23-trihydroxyurs-12-en-28-oic acid (**9**), and the above-mentioned three triterpenoids (**5–7**) were also effective in the inhibition of human A549 pulmonic cancer cells with IC_{50}s between 30.4 and 34.6 μg/mL, whereas pseudotaraxasterol and the triterpenoids (**8** and **9**) showed similar levels of suppressive effect on the Lovo cell line (IC_{50}s 31.1–31.6 μg/mL). Except for DHUA (**6**), the above-mentioned triterpenes displayed moderate cytotoxic effect on the HepG2 cells (IC_{50}s 25.5–35.7 μg/mL).[20] 2α,3α,23-Trihydroxy-12-en-28-ursolic acid induced the apoptosis of HeLa cells, associated with the activation of caspases-3 and -7 and inactivation of NF-κB.[21] A HUVEC assay exhibited the antiangiogenic potential of DHUA (**6**), 2α,3α,23-trihydroxyurs-12-en-28-oic acid (**9**), 2α,3α,24-trihydroxyolean-12-en-28-oic acid, and Asiatic acid.[22] These antiangiogenic agents are worthy of further translational research. In addition, corosolic acid isolated from *A. valvata* root effectively enhanced S cell cycle arrest and apoptotic death of human HeLa cervical cancer cells and deterred the viability of HeLa cells (IC_{50} of 28 μM in 72 h), whose proapoptotic effect was mediated by a caspases-dependent mitochondrial pathway.[23] Similarly, 2β,3β,23-trihydroxy-urs-12-ene-28-olic acid isolated from the roots showed antiproliferative effect on human Hela cervical cancer and NCI-H460 NSCLC cells *in vitro*, wherein inhibition in the NCl-H460 cells was found to be mediated by prompting apoptotic death, activating IκBα, and hindering NF-κB (p65).[24] The isolated corosolic acid impeded hepatocellular carcinoma cell migration *in vitro* by targeting VEGFR2/Src/FAK pathway and lessening F-actin formation and deterred the growth of hepatoma cells in a mouse model in a dose of 5 mg/kg/day.[25] All these positive findings suggested that the triterpenoid-rich extract from *A. chinensis* roots can be developed as an adjuvant and supplement to help the prevention of cancers in colon, lung, liver, cervix, and so on.

3. Polysaccharides

The anticancer polysaccharides such as ACPS-R, ACPS, and FP2 were prepared from the kiwi roots and/or fruits of *A. chinensis* by different research groups, displaying potent *in vivo* suppressive effect against the growth carcinoma cells. The i.p. injection of ACPS-R at doses of 75–125 mg/kg to tumor-bearing mice resulted in noticeable inhibitory rates, >88.8% on ascetic hepatoma, and EAC and >49.6% on solid hepatoma. The life spans of mice bearing EAC or P388 were prolonged significantly and the percentage of EAC-free mice was increased by the ACPS-R treatment. ACPS-R was also capable of potentiating the cytotoxicity of an anticancer drug 5-FU in a co-treatment.[26] Also, the growth suppression of ACPS-R was apparent in a clinical cancer trial.[26]

By v.c. injection, ACPS obviously restrained B16 melanoma and promoted the spleen index of tumor-bearing mice, resulting in antitumor rates of 40.90%–48.67% in the middle and high doses. Its therapeutic potencies were correlated with its abilities to distribute cell cycle at G1/S phase and regulate immunization.[27] *A. chinensis* root polysaccharide (ACP) induced the apoptosis of anterior gastric cancer MFC cells and orthotopic transplanted gastric cancer cells *in vitro and in vivo* via downregulation of Mcl-1, Bcl-2, and Bcl-xl expressions and upregulation of Bak and Bax expressions, leading to the antitumor effects.[28] An injection derived from kiwi root polysaccharide obstructed the growth of H22 hepatoma cells by 68.5% in its best dose *in vivo* and also retarded the growth of orthotopic transplanted tumor of gastric cancer and partly improved the immune function in mice, in whom anticancer effect was found to be associated with lessening of PCNA expression and/or p53 activity and inducing a toxic effect on mitochondrial.[29]

FP2 is a kiwi fruit-derived polysaccharide that is principally composed of D-glucose, D-mannose, and D-galactose. In a dosage of 150 mg/kg, FP2 evidently decreased the weight of sarcoma 180 in mice and raised the inhibitory rate to 54.2%.[30]

4. Enzyme

A type of proteolytic enzyme prepared from the kiwi fruits, actinidine was claimed to be an inhibitor of tumor proliferation and metastasis as well as remover of albuminoids (e.g., skin aging spot, wart, etc.). It was considered useful for anticarcinogenic and prevention of Alzheimer's disease as a supplement.[31]

CONCLUSION AND SUGGESTION

The observations and findings from scientific studies provided deeper and wider insight into the medical function of Actinidia plants and demonstrated that kiwi fruits have marked health benefits. A rich source of vitamin C, polyphenolics, and antioxidants, dietary kiwi fruits can diminish the contents of potential mutagens and carcinogens and enhance the antioxidant and anticarcinogenic defenses, leading to the inhibition of the initiation and growth of some human carcinomas. The cancer preventive efficacy of kiwi fruit is also partly dependent on its ability to promote immune function. Moreover, the anticancer constituents (flavonoids, triterpenoids, and polysaccharides) discovered from the kiwi roots showed useful potentials, which can be developed as adjuvants and supplements for treatment of some carcinomas in clinics and improvement of the conventional chemotherapy against cancers.

REFERENCES

1. Singletary, K. et al., 2012. Kiwifruit, overview of potential health benefits. *Nutr. Today* 47: 133–147.
2. Lee, H. et al., 1988. Antimutagenic activity of extracts from anticancer drugs in Chinese medicine. *Mutation Res.* 204: 229–234.
3. Mizuno, M. et al., 1988. Desmutagenic effects of sulfhydryl compounds on a mutagen formed from butylated hydroxyanisole reacted with sodium nitrite. *Agricul. Biol. Chem.* 52: 2843–2849.
4. Song, P.J. et al., 1984. Cancer preventive effect of Actinidia sinensis Planch fruit juice. II. Detection of the blocking of N-nitrosamine formation in simulated human gastric juice in vitro by the Ames test. *Yingyang Xuebao* 6: 241–246.
5. Song, P.J. et al., 1988. The block of N-nitritoproline synthesis in rats and healthy persons. *Yingyang Xuebao* 10: 50; 1984. 6: 109.
6. Xu, Y. et al., 1988. Anticancer effects of Actinidia chinensis. *Yingyang Xuebao* 10: 130; 10: 230.
7. Motohashi, N. et al., 2002. Cancer prevention and therapy with kiwifruit in Chinese folklore medicine: A study of kiwifruit extracts. *J. Ethnopharm.* 81: 357–364.
8. Cao, S.F. et al., 2007. The inhibitory effect of an ethyl acetate extract from Teng-Li roots against the growth of human cells. *J. Shanxi Med. Univ.* 38: 413–416.
9. Wei, P.F. et al., 2005. Studies on the extract of Teng-Li roots induces gastric cancer cell apoptosis. *J. Shaanxi TCM Univ.* 28: 52.
10. Sun, X.F. et al., 2006. Studies on the inhibition of Teng-Li roots extract against human lung adenocarcinoma A539 cells. *Shandong Yiyao* 46: 40–41.
11. Hu, B. et al., 2013. Root of Actinidia chinensis Planch induces anoikis in colon carcinoma RKO cells. *Zhongguo Shiyan Fangjixue Zazhi* 19: 242–245.
12. Lim, S.Y. et al., 2016. Inhibition of hardy kiwifruit (Actinidia aruguta) ripening by 1-methylcyclopropene during cold storage and anticancer properties of the fruit extract. *Food Chem.* 190: 150–157.
13. Zuo, L.L. et al., 2013. Antiproliferative activity of three kiwi polyphenol crude extracts on A549 and Hela cells. *Shipin Gongye Keji* 34: 358–361.
14. Xiao, H. et al., 2016. Effect of Kiwi essence on response of chemotherapy for non-small cell lung cancer in mice. *Zhongguo Shiyan Fangjixue Zazhi* 22: 132–136.
15. He, J.B. 2014. Reversing multidrug resistance of lung adenocarcinoma xenografts to gemcitabine in combination with cisplatin in mice by Kiwi essence and its mechanism. *Zhongliu* 34: 1120–1125.
16. Du, Q.C. et al., 2011. Effects of ethyl acetate extracts of Actinidia chinensis on proliferation of lung cancer A549 cells. *Zhongguo Laonianxue Zazhi* 31: 4180–4183.
17. Lin, G. et al., 2008. Antitumor mechanism of active components from extract of Actinidia rufa root. *Zhongguo Zhong Yao Za Zhi.* 33: 2100–2104.
18. He, J. et al., 2015. Advances on chemical constituents and antitumor effects of root of Actinidia chinensis. *Zhongguo Shiyan Fangjixue Zazhi* 21(4): 213–218.
19. Chang, J. et al., 2005. Cytotoxic phenolic constituents from the root of Actinidia chinensis. *Planta Med.* 71: 955–959.
20. Xu, Y.X. et al., 2010. Two new triterpenoids from the roots of Actinidia chinensis. *Fitoterapia* 81: 920–924.

21. Cheng, Q.L. et al., 2014. Apoptosis of cervical carcinoma HeLa cells induced by ursane triterpene compound A from roots of Actinidia chinensis Planch. and primary research on its action mechanisms. *Shizhen Guoyi Guoyao* 25: 2094–2095.

22. Zhu, W.J. et al., 2013. Antiangiogenic triterpenes isolated from Chinese herbal medicine Actinidia chinensis Planch. *Anti-Cancer Agents in Med. Chem.* 13: 195–198.

23. Xu, Y. et al., 2009. Corosolic acid induces apoptosis through mitochondrial pathway and caspases activation in human cervix adenocarcinoma HeLa cells. *Cancer Lett.* 284: 229–237.

24. Cheng, Q.L. et al., 2015. Effect of ursolic compound A from root of Actinidia chinensis on proliferation of cervical cancer HeLa cells. *Zhongguo Shiyan Fangjixue Zazhi* 21(24): 84–87; 2β,3β,23-trihydroxy-urs-12-ene-28-olic acid (TUA) isolated from Actinidia chinensis Radix inhibits NCI-H460 cell proliferation by decreasing NF-κB expression. *Chemico-Biol. Interact.* 240, 1–11.

25. Ku, C.Y. et al., 2015. Corosolic acid inhibits hepatocellular carcinoma cell migration by targeting the VEGFR2 /Src/FAK pathway. PLoS One 10(5): e0126725.

26. Lin, P.F. et al., 1988. Antitumor effect of Actinidia chinensis polysaccharide on murine tumor. *Zhonghua Zhongliu Zazhi* 10: 441–444.

27. Shi, S.L. et al., 2009. Antitumor effect and its mechanism of Actinidia chinensis polysaccharide on B16-bearing mice. *Zhonghua Zhongyiyao Zazhi* 24: 777–779.

28. Shen, L. et al., 2014. Effect of Actinidia chinensis polysaccharide on apoptosis of MFC and their orthotopic transplanted tumor of gastric cancer. *Zhongcaoyao* 45: 673–678.

29. Zhang, G.J. et al., (a) 2013. Influence of Actinidia chinensis polysaccharide on expression of PCNA and p53 in orthotopic transplanted cancer of gastric tumor in 615 mice. *Zhonghua Zhongyiyao Zazhi* 28: 2538–2541; (b) 2012. Mechanism study of kiwifruit root polysaccharide antitumor injection on tumor in vivo. *Zhonghua Zhongyiyao Zazhi* 27: 2177–2179.

30. Lu, D. et al., 2005. Studies on purification and antitumor activity of fruit polysaccharide isolated from Actinidia chinensis Planch. *Shipin Kexue* (Beijing, China) 26: 213-5.

31. Tanaka, K. 2001. Actinidine as tumor proliferation and metastasis-inhibiting enzyme for removal of albuminoids. *Jpn. Kokai Tokkyo Koho* JP 99-332014 A 20010605.

44. MANGO

Mangue Mango Mango

芒果 マンゴー 망고

Mangifera indica

Anacardiaceae

Mango tree (Mangifera indica) is native to south central areas of Asia. Now, several cultivated varieties of mango have been introduced to other warm regions of the world as far as Africa, Brazil, and Mexico. Mango is one of the most popular tropical fruits in world supermarkets. In recent decades, mango fruit has increased in popularity in Western countries as a source of a variety of nutrients. Vitamin C and folate are found in significant amounts along with vitamin A, vitamin K, vitamin B complex, and minerals (potassium and magnesium). Other parts of the mango tree, such as leaf, stem bark, and fruit peel are reported to have multiple biological properties including antioxidative and radical-scavenging, anti-inflammatory, antidiabetic, and anticancer activities. Particularly, mango leaves can afford ideal antioxidants and mango peels show better values than the fruit flesh in nutrition and bioactivities.[1]

SCIENTIFIC EVIDENCE OF CANCER-PREVENTIVE CONSTITUENTS

In several *in vitro* assays, MJ, a fully ripe mango juice, hindered cell cycle of HL-60 leukemia cells at G0/G1 stage and deterred BAP-induced cancer transformation of BALB/c 3T3 mammalian cells in a dose-dependent manner, besides showing radical-scavenging effect.[2] Methanol extracts from mango peels of three cultivars (Irwin, Nam Doc Mai, and Kensington Pride) restrained the proliferation of human MCF-7 breast cancer cells concomitant with blockage of intracellular calcium signaling, but the corresponding mango flesh extracts showed no inhibition of the MCF-7 cells.[3] Exposure of 80% ethanol extracts of mango peels (either unripened or ripened fruits) exerted greater suppressive effect against the proliferation of human HeLa (cervix), AGS (stomach), and HepG2 (liver) cancer cell lines compared with the extracts from mango flesh in 125–1,000 µg/mL concentrations, but showed almost no effect on normal human lung fibroblast cells (CCD-25Lu).[4] The peel extracts were also able to hamper oxidative stress-triggered DNA damage in HepG2 cells.[4] During the treatments of HeLa cells, these peel extracts induced the cell apoptosis by downregulation of Bcl-2 expression, activation of caspases, and degradation of PARP.[5] However, giving Ataulfo mango (0.02–0.06 g/mL) mixed in drinking to rats resulted in no influence of *N*-methyl-*N*-nitrosourea on breast carcinogenesis. When the dietary intake lasted for a long period, plasma antioxidant capacity was enhanced in a dose-dependent manner.[6] In addition, mango kernel ethanolic extract was effective in suppressing both estrogen-positive (MCF-7) and -negative (MDA-MB-231) breast cancer cell lines and not active in normal breast cells (MCF-10A). The IC_{50}s were 15 and 30 µg/mL in the MCF-7 and MDA-MB-231 cell lines, respectively.[7] The peel extract also exerted protection against oxidative damage to erythrocytes caused by hydrogen peroxide in rats.[8] In addition, under nutrient-deprived condition, a methanol extract of *M. indica* bark could preferentially hamper the survival of PANC-1 human pancreatic cancer cells.[9]

SCIENTIFIC EVIDENCE OF CANCER PREVENTERS

1. Polyphenolics

According to the HPLC-ESI-MS analysis, the peel extract was revealed to be rich in polyphenols and flavonoids, such as gallic acid, gallotannins, galloyl glycosides, quercetin 3-O-galactoside, isomangiferin gallate, mangiferin gallate, mangiferin, and quercetin-3-O-arabinopyranoside, along with unsaturated fatty acids, linoleic acid, ethyl linoleate, and oleic acid, as well as carotenoids, vitamin E, and vitamin C. Mango peel extracts exhibited better free radical scavenging and cancer preventive activities than mango flesh, owing to higher contents of polyphenols and flavonoids.[4] All five polyphenolic extracts from the pulps of five mango varieties (Francis, Ataulfo, Tommy Atkins, Kent, and Haden) showed antiproliferative effect against human SW480 colon cancer cells; the Ataulfo and Haden extracts had superior efficacy to the SW480 cells than the extracts of Kent, Francis, and Tommy Atkins, with IC_{50}s of 1.6, 2.3, 5.0, 8.2, and 27.3 mg GAE (gallic acid equivalent)/L, respectively. The Ataulfo and Haden polyphenolics were also effective in inhibiting the proliferation of human Molt-4 (leukemic), MDA-MB-231 (breast), A549 (lung), and LNCap (prostate) neoplastic cell lines but not active to noncancer CCD-18Co colon cells.[10] The mango pulp polyphenolics extracted as a mixture of ethanol–methanol–acetone (1:1:1) deterred the proliferation and growth of human BT474 breast cancer cells *in vitro* and *in vivo* along with modulation of miRNAs and downregulation of NF-κB (p65), pAkt, pPI3K, HIF-1α, and VEGF protein expressions.[11]

Gallotannins: The gallotannin-rich 80% acetone extracts were isolated from kernel and peel of three Chinese mango cultivars (Maqiesu, Tainong-1, and Zihuamang), with the kernel containing much richer gallotannins than its peel. These extracts in the *in vitro* model showed antiproliferative effects against human MDA-MB-231 (breast), HepG2 (liver), and HL-60 (leukemic) carcinoma cell lines. The IC_{50}s were 8.31–11.02 μg/mL for the kernel extracts (KE) and 12.27–15.84 μg/mL for the peel extracts (PE) in MDA-MB-231 cells, 14.68–28.72 μg/mL for KE and 11.46–38.37 μg/mL for PE in HL-60 cells, and 33.91–41.50 μg/mL for KE and 43.01–53.33 μg/mL for PE in HepG2 cells, implying that the sensitivities of cancer cell lines to these extracts were of the order MDA-MB-231 > HL-60 >> HepG2. Likewise, the peel extracts from Zihuamang and Tainong-1 cultivars were more effective to HL-60 cells (IC_{50} of 11.46–12.04 μg/mL) than other extracts. Five gallotannins, that is, penta-, hexa-, hepta-, octa-, and nona-O-galloyl-glucoside were isolated from the peel extracts; penta-O-galloyl-glucoside was revealed to have higher antioxidant and antiproliferative activities.[12] These data showed that the gallotannins from mango peels and kernels have moderate to weak levels of antiproliferative activities on the three types of carcinomas in leukemia, breast, and liver.

Mangiferin: Mangiferin (**1**) is a special polyphenol with xanthone skeleton and C-glucosyl linkage in *Mangifera indica*. It can be extracted from pulp, peel, seed, leaf, and bark of mango plant, and its content varies from pulp (34 g/kg), peel (87 g/kg), kernel (66 g/kg), bark (107 g/kg), and leaf (172 g/kg), though the data depend on the factors such as variety, soil, and origin of mango cultivations.[13] Due to nutraceutical and medicinal significances, mangiferin (**1**) has gained much attention in recent years for its potential in hindering mutagenesis, carcinogenesis, oxidation, inflammation, and some degenerative diseases. A 0.1% mangiferin in a diet significantly limited the development of ACF in bowel caused by AOM in rats in a short-term assay, and significantly lowered the incidence and multiplicity of AOM-induced intestinal neoplasms in a long-term assay.[14] Administration of mangiferin orally in a dose 100 mg/kg/d for 18 weeks markedly restrained BAP-induced lung carcinogenesis in experimental animals by decreasing the ROS levels and enhancing antioxidant status, together with markedly lowering the levels of glycoproteins, membrane ATPases and membrane lipid peroxidation to near-normal lines, and recovering the activities of electron transport chain complexes and TCA cycle key enzymes such as isocitrate dehydrogenase (ICDH), succinate dehydrogenase (SDH), α-ketoglutarate dehydrogenase (α-KGDH), and malate dehydrogenase (MDH).[15] The *in vivo* models disclosed that mangiferin (1) exerted the antigrowth activity against A549 lung adenocarcinoma xenograft and MCF-7 and MDA-MB-231 breast carcinoma xenografts to reduce the tumor volume and weight and to prolong the life span of xenograft mice.[13,16,17]

In other cases, mangiferin (1) treatment was able to elicit the cell apoptosis and/or cell cycle blockage of human carcinoma cell lines such as K562 and HL-60 (leukemic), MCF-7 and MDA-MB-231 (breast), A549 (lung), U87 (brain), CNE2 and CNE3 (nasopharynx) cells, and IM9, RPMI8226, ARH-77, and RPMI1788 (multiple myeloma) cells, leading to the inhibitory effect against the proliferation of these cancer cells.[18-29] After mangiferin (1) treatment at 200 μmol/L concentration for 24–96 h, the proliferation of K562 chronic myeloid leukemia cells was markedly inhibited in a dose- and time-dependent manner, and the inhibitory rates were 48.19–83.50%.[30] The proapoptotic mechanisms were revealed to be associated with (i) enlarging Bax gene expression, lessening the mRNA expressions of Bcl-2, survivin, and BCR/ABL protein P210, lowering bcr/abl gene expression, upregulating Fas protein expression, and impeding telomerase activity (such as in K562 cells); (ii) decreasing Bcl-2 and survivin expressions and reducing NF-κB, Bcl-xL, and XIAP expressions (such as in HL-60 cells); (iii) blocking β-catenin pathway, upregulating E-cadherin expression and downregulating MMPs-7 and -9 expressions and vimentin (such as in MDA-MD-231 cells); (iv) blocking PKC/NF-κB pathway (such as in A549 and MCF-7 cells); (v) inducting miR-15b and obstructing MMP-9 expression (such as in U87 cells); and (vi) hampering XIAP, survivin, and Bcl-xL proteins and inactivating NF-κB-inducing kinase (NIK) (such as in multiple myeloma cells).[18-26] The G2/M phase cell cycle was blocked in the mangiferin-treated HL-60, A549, and MCF-7 cell lines via downregulation of cdc2-cyclin B1 signaling pathway[16,17,31] and the G2/M and S phases cell cycle blockage in NCE2 and NCE3 nasopharyngeal cancer cells was triggered in a time- and dose-dependent manner.[27-29]

Mangiferin (1) also could obviously hinder the invasive abilities of cancer cells such as in HL-60 acute myeloid leukemia cells through lessening the cell adhesion capability and FAK mRNA expression in Raji lymphoma cells by downregulating Tiam1 mRNA and U87MG glioma cells via specifically impeding MMP-9 expression and secreting and blocking DNA binding and transcriptional activities of NF-κB and AP-1.[32-34] A test of Matrigel invasion exhibited that mangiferin (1) markedly deterred TNFα-induced invasion of LNCaP prostate neoplastic cells via downregulation of MMP-9.[13] At 12.5–25 μg/mL concentrations, mangiferin (1) restrained endothelial cell proliferation along with inhibition of both basic fibroblast growth factor and VEGF in human dermal microvasculature cells.[13] Subcutaneous injection of mangiferin (0.5–4 mg/kg) in mice suppressed the metastasis of lung cancer cells and the proliferation of B16 melanoma cells. These findings showed that antiangiogenic activity of mangiferin (1) might be correlated with the retardation of tumor metastasis.[13]

Furthermore, the synergistic capacity of mangiferin (1) was explored in combination treatments with some chemotherapeutic agents. Addition of 10 μg/mL mangiferin obviously amplified the proapoptotic and antiproliferative efficacies of oxaliplatin on HT-29 colon cancer cells by 3.4-fold and on HeLa cervical cancer cells by 1.7-fold, together with downregulation of NF-κB, activation of caspase-3, and counteraction of drug resistance in the cancer cells.[35] Mangiferin (1) was able to enhance the antiproliferative effects of cisplatin on A549 lung cancer cells.[23] In a S180 tumor model, mangiferin (1) antagonized the toxicity of cyclophosphamide (CP) on the body and maintained the immunity at normal level by promoting IL-2 content, stabilizing TNF-α level, and reducing cAMP content in spleen T-lymphocytes, thereby enhancing the antitumor effect of CP.[36] In addition, mangiferin (1) is a Nrf2 activator that exerts multipotent anti-inflammatory and cytoprotective potentials via activation of Nrf2-ARE pathway, significantly increases NQO1 expression, and reduces intracellular ROS level, thereby leading to lowering of oxidative stress and reduction of drugs (such as etoposide) and toxics (such as galactosamine and rotenone)-induced DNA damage to protect normal cells.[37–42] Also, in a rat model, the cardiotoxicity caused by doxorubicin (a chemo drug) could also be reversed by the treatment with mangiferin (1) in oral doses of 50 and 100 mg/kg for five weeks.[43]

Overall, these scientific observations substantiated the remarkable anticancer, anticarcinogenic, and detoxication activities of mangiferin (1) in mango, besides its antioxidant and anti-inflammatory properties, and suggested that it may be a potential chemotherapy adjuvant and a chemopreventive agent, especially for protection of lung, prostate, brain, breast, cervix, and hematopoietic system from carcinogenesis.

2. Triterpenes

Lupeol (2) is a major triterpene constituent found in mango and other common fruits as well as some vegetables and herbs. It has been reported to possess a wide range of health benefits including marked antioxidant, antimutagenic, anti-inflammatory, and antiarthritic effects. In the assays, either lupeol (2) or mango pulp extract (MPE) treatment prominently induced the apoptosis of human LNCaP prostate cancer cells *in vitro* by a ROS-triggered mitochondrial pathway.[44] Daily dose of lupeol (2) of 25 mg/kg or 1 mL of 20% aqueous MPE to mice by oral intubation for a week effectively lessened DMBA-elicited oxidative stress and LPO, enhanced the antioxidant enzyme activities and mitochondrial transmembrane potential, and diminished the DMBA-caused DNA fragmentation, leading to protection of hepatocytes from DMBA, a carcinogen.[45] Similarly, pretreatment with lupeol (1 mg/animal) or MPE (1 mL, 20%) orally for 7 days prior to BAP inoculation obviously amplified mitotic index and decreased the incidence of aberrant cells and micronuclei in the tested mouse bone marrow tissues, achieving an *in vivo* protective effect against the BAP-caused clastogenicity.[46] By modulating NF-κB and PI3K/Akt pathways, lupeol (1–2 mg/mouse), when applied topically onto the skin of CD-1 mice prior to giving TPA (3.2 nmol/mouse), notably obstructed the TPA-promoted skin inflammation and skin carcinogenesis in a time- and dose-dependent manner, an effect that was evidenced by the reduction of skin edema and hyperplasia, inhibition of epidermal ODC activity, and diminution of protein expression of ODC, COX-2, and NO synthase.[47] Significantly, the lupeol and MPE at the effective therapeutic doses showed safe and no toxicity to normal cells and tissues.[48] These results from the preclinical investigations showed the benefit of dietary mango fruits for chemoprevention of some carcinogenesis and inflammation.

In addition, mangiferolate-B and isoambolic acid were the bioactive triterpenoids present in the methanol extract of the *M. indica* bark; under the nutrition-deprived condition, both compounds showed potent preferential cytotoxic effect against human PANC-1 pancreatic cancer cells.[9]

NANOFORMULATION

Currently, the biosynthesis of nanoparticles is a growing research field for promoting the drug delivery efficacy and the drug bioavailability. An aqueous extract of mango seeds was used for the formulation of barium carbonate nanoparticles (BaCO$_3$-NPs). The BaCO$_3$-NPs (average size: 18.3 nm) showed significant suppressive effect against cervical cancer cells concomitant with activation of caspase-3.[49]

CONCLUSION AND SUGGESTION

All these scientific investigations have truly approved the benefits of mango fruits, especially mango peel and kernel (the major byproduct in the food industry), for their certain cancer chemoprevention and antioxidant benefits. The prominent bioactive constituents such as polyphenolics (gallic acid derivatives, gallotannins, and mangoferin) and triterpene (lupeol), especially mangoferin (1), are primarily responsible for the bioactivities and health functions of mango fruits, which have marked potentials in natural chemoprevention and health improvement. The total polyphenolic extract of mango showed better efficacy in the antioxidant and anticarcinogenesis than vitamin C, vitamin F, mangiferin, and β-carolence. Consequently, its dietary intake of the favorable mango fruits should be encouraged because they are helpful in gaining a natural power and nutrition for safe prevention of carcinogenesis and effective invigoration of health. In addition, considering the facts, that is, the byproducts (mango peel and kernel) and mango leaves are a rich and higher source of biologically active polyphenolic compounds, mango leaves, peels, and kernels should be used in the food industry for the production of nutritional and functional supplements.

REFERENCES

1. Khurana, R.K. et al., 2016. Mangiferin: A promising anticancer bioactive. *Pharm. Patent Analyst* 5: 169–81.
2. Percival, S.S. et al., 2006. Neoplastic transformation of BALB/3T3 cells and cell cycle of HL-60 cells are inhibited by mango (mangifera indica L.) juice and mango juice extracts. *J. Nutr.* 136: 1300–1304.
3. Taing, M.W. et al., 2015. Mango fruit extracts differentially affect proliferation and intracellular calcium signalling in MCF-7 human breast cancer cells. *J. Chem.* 613268.
4. Kim, H. et al., 2010. Antioxidant and antiproliferative activities of mango (Mangifera indica L.) flesh and peel. *Food Chem.* 121: 429–436.
5. Kim, H.J. et al., 2012. Induction of apoptosis by ethanolic extract of mango peel and comparative analysis of the chemical constituents of mango peel and flesh. *Food Chem.* 133: 416–422.
6. Garcia-Solis, P. et al., 2008. Study of the effect of 'Ataulfo' mango (Mangifera indica L.) intake on mammary carcinogenesis and antioxidant capacity in plasma of N-methyl-N-nitrosourea (MNU)-treated rats. *Food Chem.* 111: 309–315.
7. Abdullah, A.S.H. et al., 2014. Cytotoxic effects of Mangifera indica L. kernel extract on human breast cancer (MCF-7 and MDA-MB-231 cell lines) and bioactive constituents in the crude extract. *BMC Complem. Altern. Med.* 14: 199/1–199/10; 2015. Oxidative stress-mediated apoptosis induced by ethanolic mango seed extract in cultured estrogen receptor positive breast cancer MCF-7 cells. *Int. J. Mol. Sci.* 16: 3528–3536.
8. Ajila, C.M. et al., 2008. Protection against hydrogen peroxide induced oxidative damage in rat erythrocytes by Mangifera indica peel extract. *Food Chem. Toxicol.* 46: 303–309.
9. Nguyen, H.X. et al., 2016. Chemical constituents of Mangifera indica and their antiausterity activity against the PANC-1 human pancreatic cancer cell line. *J. Nat. Prod* 79(8): 2053–2059.
10. Noratto, G.D. et al., 2010. Anticarcinogenic effects of polyphenolics from mango (Mangifera indica) varieties. *J. Agricul. Food Chem.* 58: 4104–4112.
11. Banerjee, N. et al., 2015. Mango polyphenolics suppressed tumor growth in breast cancer xenografts in mice: role of the PI3K/AKT pathway and associated microRNAs. *Nutr. Res.* (NY, NY, US) 35: 744–751.
12. Luo, F.L. et al., 2014. Identification and quantification of gallotannins in mango (Mangifera indica L.) kernel and peel and their antiproliferative activities. *J. Functional Foods* 8: 282–291.
13. Selles, A.J.N. et al., 2016. The potential role of mangiferin in cancer treatment through its immuno-modulatory, anti-angiogenic, apoptopic, and gene regulatory effects. *BioFactors* Ahead of Print.
14. Yoshimi, N. et al., 2001. The inhibitory effects of mangiferin, a naturally occurring glucosylxanthone, in bowel carcinogenesis of male F344 rats. *Cancer Lett.* (Shannon, Ireland) 163: 163–170.
15. Rajendran, P., 2008. Chemopreventive efficacy of mangiferin against benzo(a)pyrene induced lung carcinogenesis in experimental animals. *Envir. Toxicol. Pharmacol.* 26: 278–282; *Basic Clin. Pharmacol. Toxicol.* 103; 137–142; *Nat. Prod. Res.* 22: 672–680.
16. Shi, W. et al., 2016. Molecular mechanisms underlying mangiferin-induced apoptosis and cell cycle arrest in A549 human lung carcinoma cells. *Mol. Med. Reports* 13: 3423–3432.
17. Lv, J.Z. et al., 2013. Mangiferin induces apoptosis and cell cycle arrest in MCF-7 cells both in vitro and in vivo. *J. Animal Veterinary Advances* 12: 352–359.
18. Peng, Z.G. et al., 2004. CML cell line K562 cell apoptosis induced by mangiferin. *Zhongguo Shiyan Xueyexue Zazhi* 12: 590–594; 2007. Apoptotic mechanism of leukemic K562 cells induced by mangiferin. *Zhongcaoyao* 38: 715–719.

19. Cheng, P. et al., 2007. Effect of mangiferin on telomerase activity and apoptosis in leukemic K562 cells. *Zhongyaocai* 30: 306–309.
20. Peng, Z. G. et al., 2010. Effect of mangiferin on proliferation and apoptosis of leukemia cell line HL-60. *Shizhen Guoyi Guoyao* 21: 2462–2465.
21. Shoji, K. et al., 2011. Mangiferin induces apoptosis by suppressing Bcl-xL and XIAP expressions and nuclear entry of NF-κB in HL-60 cells. *Archiv. Pharmacol Res.* 34: 469–475.
22. Lu, J.Z. et al., 2013. Anti-proliferation effect and mechanism of mangiferin on human lung cancer cell line A549. *Sichuan Daxue Xuebao, Ziran Kexueban* 50: 611–614.
23. Liu, J.H., 2012. Effects of mangiferin on proliferation and apoptosis of lung cancer A549 cells. *Xinxiang Yixueyuan Xuebao* 29: 900–903.
24. Li, H.Z. et al., 2013. Mangiferin exerts antitumor activity in breast cancer cells by regulating matrix metalloproteinases, epithelial to mesenchymal transition, and β-catenin signaling pathway. *Toxicol. AppliedPharmacol.* 272: 180–190.
25. Xiao, J.S. et al., 2015. Mangiferin regulates proliferation and apoptosis in glioma cells by induction of microRNA-15b and inhibition of MMP-9 expression. *Oncol. Report* 33: 2815–2820.
26. Takeda, T. et al., 2016. Mangiferin induces apoptosis in multiple myeloma cell lines by suppressing the activation of nuclear factor-kB-inducing kinase. *Chemico-Biol. Interactions* 251: 26–33.
27. Yang, X.L. et al., 2009. Effects of mangiferin on proliferation, apoptosis and cycle of nasopharyngeal carcinoma CNE2 cells. *Shandong Yiyao* 49(39): 23–24.
28. Liu, X.C. et al., 2009. Study on mangiferin to proliferation inhibition and cell cycle blockage of naso-pharyngeal carcinoma CNE3 cells. *Xiandai Jianyan Yixue Zazhi* 24: 10-2.
29. Pan, L.L. et al., 2014. Mangiferin induces apoptosis by regulating Bcl-2 and Bax expression in the CNE2 nasopharyngeal carcinoma cell line. *Asian Pac J Cancer Prev.* 15: 7065–7068.
30. Peng, Z.G. et al., 2004. Inhibitory effect of mangiferin on the proliferation of K562 leukemia cells. *Guangxi Yike Daxue Xuebao* 21: 168–170.
31. Yao, Y.B. et al., 2010. Effects of mangiferin on cell cycle status and CDC2/CyclinB1 expression of HL-60 cells. *Zhongyaocai* 33: 81–85.
32. Tang, Y.L. et al., 2010. Effect of mangiferin on the invasive ability of leukemia HL-60 cells. *Zhongyao Yaoli Yu Linchuang* 26: 15–18.
33. Ding, D. et al., 2010. Effect of mangiferin on proliferation and invasion of lymphoma Raji cells and Tiam1 gene. *Guangxi Yike Daxue Xuebao* 27: 852–855.
34. Jung, J. S. et al., 2012. Selective inhibition of MMP-9 gene expression by mangiferin in PMA-stimulated human astroglioma cells: Involvement of PI3K/Akt and MAPK signaling pathways. *Pharmacol. Res.* 66: 95–103.
35. du Plessis-Stoman, D. et al., 2011. Combination treatment with oxaliplatin and mangiferin causes increased and downregulation of NF-kB in cancer cell lines. *Afr. J. Tradit. Complem. Alternative Med.* 8: 177–184.
36. Yun, C.X. et al., 2010. Effects of mangiferin on levels of cytokines and second messenger in carcinoma-tous mice after chemotherapy. *Guangxi Yike Daxue Xuebao* 27: 829–832.
37. Saha, S. et al., 2016. Mangiferin: A xanthonoid with multipotent anti-inflammatory potential. *BioFactors* (2016), Ahead of Print.
38. Zhang, B.P. et al., 2014. Mangiferin activates Nrf2-antioxidant response element signaling without reducing the sensitivity to etoposide of human myeloid leukemia cells in vitro: a novel Nrf2 activator without a "dark side" *Acta Pharmacologica Sinica* 35: 257–266.
39. Zhang, B.P. 2015. Mangiferin activates the Nrf2-ARE pathway and reduces etoposide-induced DNA damage in human umbilical cord mononuclear blood cells. *Pharm. Biol.* (London, UK) 53: 503–511.
40. Das, J. et al., 2012. Mangiferin exerts hepatoprotective activity against D-galactosamine induced acute toxicity and oxidative/nitrosative stress via Nrf2-NFκB pathways. *Toxicol. Applied Pharmacol.* 260: 35–47.
41. Zhao, J. et al., 2014. Mangiferin increases Nrf2 protein stability by inhibiting its ubiquitination and degradation in human HL60 myeloid leukemia cells. *Int. J. Mol. Med.* 33: 1348–1354.
42. Kavitha, M. et al., 2014. Mangiferin antagonizes rotenone: Induced apoptosis apoptosis through attenu-ating mitochondrial dysfunction and oxidative stress in SK-N-SH neuroblastoma cells. *Neurochem. Res.* 39: 668–676.
43. Arozal, W. et al., 2015. The effects of mangiferin (Mangifera indica L) in doxorubicin-induced cardio-toxicity in rats. *Drug Res.* (Stuttgart, Germany) 65: 574–580.

44. Prasad, S. et al., 2008. Induction of apoptosis by lupeol and mango extract in mouse prostate and LNCaP cells. *Nutr. Cancer* 60: 120–130.
45. Prasad, S. et al., 2007. Hepatoprotective effects of lupeol and mango pulp extract of carcinogen induced alteration in Swiss albino mice. *Mol. Nutr. Food Res.* 51: 352–359.
46. Prasad, S. et al., 2008. Protective effects of lupeol against benzo[a]pyrene induced clastogenicity in mouse bone marrow cells. *Molecular Nutr. Food Res.* 52: 1117–1120.
47. Saleem, M. et al., 2004. Lupeol modulates NF-κB and PI3K/Akt pathways and inhibits skin cancer in CD-1 mice. *Oncogene* 23: 5203–5214.
48. Saleem, M. et al., 2009. Lupeol, a novel anti-inflammatory and anticancer dietary triterpene. *Cancer Lett.* 285: 109–115.
49. Nagajyothi, P. C. et al., 2016. In vitro anticancer potential of BaCO3 nanoparticles synthesized via green route. *J. Photochem. Photobiol. B: Biol.* 156: 29–34.

45. PAPAYA

番木瓜　パパイヤ　파파야

Carica papaya

Caricaceae

Papaya (*Carica papaya*, Caricaceae) is a popular fruit crop in tropical and subtropical regions, where it is widely cultivated. Nutritionally, papaya fruit is a significant source of vitamin C and a source of folate. Besides the favorable papaya fruits, papaya leaves, barks, latex, flowers, and seeds are broadly used as folk medicines, with great reputation as a remedy for various diseases. Pharmacological approaches have established the fact that the papaya plant possesses multiple properties, such as anti-inflammatory, antihypertensive, hypoglycemic, hypolipidemic, neuroprotective, free radical scavenging, wound healing, diuretic, anthelmintic, antiprotozoan, antifungal, antiviral, antibacterial, antisickling, antifertility, and abortifacient effects.

Scientific Evidence of Cancer Prevention

A variety of phytochemicals have been discovered in papaya peels, pulp, and seeds, wherein the constituents such as carotenoids, polyphenols, and isothiocyanates have been revealed to be responsible for the bioactive activities including antioxidant and anticarcinogenic effects. 0.5% and 1% aqueous extract of papaya fruit showed modest suppressive effect on the proliferation of MCF-7 human breast cancer cells after 72 h of treatment.[1] RS4 is a lipophilic extract rich in carotenoid and prepared from fully ripe papaya fruit pulp (*C. papaya* cv *Maradol*). It exerts antiproliferative effect on estrogen receptor positive MCF-7 breast cancer cells (IC_{50} of 20 mg/mL) but not on estrogen receptor negative MDA-MB-231 breast cancer cells and MCF-12F nontumoral mammary epithelial cells.[2] Compared with RS4, other extracts prepared from not fully ripe papaya fruit pulps had no such inhibition on the MCF-7 cells.[2]

Although other portions of papaya plant are inedible, the antioxidant and anticancer-related properties have been also found in the extracts of papaya fruit peels, seeds, and leaves. A papaya peel extract exerted inhibitory effect against AOM-induced oxidative stress and colon carcinogenesis after eight weeks of oral treatment in a rat model.[3] In the *in vitro* models, the peel extract showed marked abilities in scavenging free radicals, enhancing antioxidant enzymes (e.g., SOD, CAT, GPx, GR), inhibiting COX-2 activity, and inducing the apoptosis of cancer cells (such as HepG2 hepatoma).[4] The n-hexane extract from papaya seeds was effective in inducing cell apoptosis and viability inhibition (IC_{50} of 20 μg/mL) and repressing the superoxide generation in human HL-60 acute promyelocytic leukemia cells, while the extract from papaya pulp showed no effect on HL-60 cells even at 100 μg/mL concentration.[5] The *in vitro* cytotoxicities of aqueous and ethanolic extracts of papaya leaves, which were found to contain high levels of phenolic and flavonoid components, have been shown in human SCC25 oral squamous cell carcinoma cells.[6] These approvals disclosed that not only papaya fruit is a functional food for the cancer prevention and antioxidation but also papaya leaves and discarded fruit seeds and peels are potential sources for the development of health-promoting adjuvant.

1. Carotenoids

The most abundant carotenoids in red-fleshed papaya were in order lycopene (**1**), β-criptoxanthin, ζ-carotene, and β-carotene (**2**), but those in yellow-fleshed papaya were β-cryptoxanthin, ζ-carotene, and β-carotene with no lycopene. The amounts of the carotenoids and vitamin C would be amplified in the red-fleshed fruits as they ripen.[7-9] Per 100 g (dried weight) of papaya fruit contains lycopene from 0.36 to 3.40 mg, β-criptoxanthin from 0.28 to 1.06 mg, β-carotene from 0.23 to 0.50 mg, and vitamin C from 25.07 to 58.59 mg. Besides papaya, lycopene is also extracted from tomato, Gac, watermelon, pink grapefruit, pink guava, and red carrot. Lycopene (**1**), an acyclic isomer of β-carotene, has been shown to be effective in diminishing the oxidation and reducing the risk of carcinogenesis in many organs and retarding the growth of cancer.[7,8] Especially, lycopene (**1**) can reach much higher concentration in prostate tissue than in other tissues, leading to the stronger suppression and prevention of prostate carcinoma.[10] The modulation of PI3K/Akt pathway is one of major mechanisms for the anticancer activity of lycopene.[11] Moreover, combinational treatment with other bioactive agents and lycopene (**1**) may have a promising potential for cancer therapy and prevention. Oral administration of lycopene (20 mg/kg) and genistein (2 mg/kg) alone or in combination for 20 weeks (3 times/week) suppressed the incidences of breast cancer developed by DMBA in rat, where reduction in tumor weight by 48%, 61%, and 67% and reduction in mean tumor volume by 18%, 35%, and 65%, respectively, indicated that the combination of genistein and lycopene was more effective in hindering DMBA-induced breast cancer and inducing apoptosis.[12] No single treatment reduced PC-346C prostate tumor volume, but the lycopene (**1**) treatment combined with vitamin E at 5 mg/kg dose suppressed orthotopic growth of PC-346C cancer cells *in vivo* by 73% at day 42 and amplified the survival by 40%.[13] More detailed anticancer properties of lycopene (**1**) are summarized in the section on tomato.

Moreover, a synergistic anticancer effect was observed in human HepG2 hepatoma cells after dietary intake of ascorbic acid and β-carotene (**2**) together, a treatment that elicited oxidative, genotoxic, and cytotoxic damage of HepG2 cells and enhanced the cell apoptosis and necrosis.[14] Giving β-carotene (**2**) in a dose of 250 mg/kg every other day to mice by o.s. obstructed the growth of mouse mammary cancer by 49.1% and prolonged survival of the tested animals. The inhibitory rate was augmented to 60.5% when combination of β-carotene (**2**) with a chemotherapeutic protocol, which result was slightly better than that of the chemotherapy alone. β-carotene (**2**) also could alleviate toxic side-effects caused by the chemotherapeutic drugs.[15] Accordingly, dietary supplementation with lycopene- and β-carotene-rich ripened papaya fruit can provide a wide range of chemopreventive effects against cancer, carcinogenesis, and damages from radiation and radiotherapy.[7,8,16]

2. Benzyl isothiocyanate

Organosulfur compounds such as isothiocyanates are a group of promising chemopreventive agents largely found in cruciferous vegetables (such as broccoli, watercress, Brussels sprouts, cabbage,

Japanese radish, and cauliflower). Benzyl isothiocyanate (BITC, **3**) and benzylglucosinolate (BG, **4**), two of the major isothiocyanate compounds, were also discovered from the pulp and seed of papaya fruit. As a precursor of BITC, BG (**4**) can be hydrolyzed into BITC (**3**) in the catalysis of myrosinase. They, especially BITC (**3**), displayed inhibitory effect against tumor cell growth and proliferation specifically and showed antioxidant effect in an electrophilic reaction-dependent manner. At 80 µmol concentration for 24 h, BITC (**3**) suppressed the proliferation of HLE and Bel-7402 hepatoma cells by 67.19% and 46.94%, respectively, accompanied by the induction of apoptosis and cell cycle arrest via activation of a caspase signal pathway and arrest of cell cycle progression.[17] At higher concentration, BITC (**3**) exerted better inhibition rate on cell proliferation on human H69 lung cancer cells *in vitro*, and its IC_{50} value was 6.5 µmol/L.[18] Exposure of human Jurkat T-cell leukemia, HL-60 promyelocytic leukemia, and HeLa cervical cancer cell lines to BITC (**3**) resulted in cell cycle G2/M arrest that coincided with proapoptosis through activation of JNK/p38 MAPK pathway.[19] The growth of HeLa cells was hindered by 41%–79% after treatment with 2.5 µM BITC (**3**).[21] α-Tocopherol could sensitize the HL-60 cells to apoptosis elicited by BITC (**3**).[20] Co-treatment of HL-60 cells with BITC (**3**) followed by cisplatin elicited a significant decrease in the cell viability and a notable increase in apoptotic cell death, which synergic inhibition was mediated by the generation of ROS, depletion of GSH, and ERK signaling in HL-60 cells. However, BITC did not enhance the cytotoxicity of cisplatin in normal human lymphocytes.[22]

Moreover, the broad anticancer spectrum of BITC (**3**) was demonstrated by the use of diverse neoplastic cell lines. BITC (**3**) at 30 µM was effective in killing all five tested HNSCC cell lines (1483, UM-22B, UPCI:SCC103, PCI-37A, and PCI-15B). The inhibitory rates were 71.69%–74.19% in the first four cell lines and 65.03% in PCI-15B cells, and the IC_{50} (24 h) values were 22 and 17 µM for 1483 and UM-22B cell lines, respectively. The studies further found that both p38 MAPK and p44/42 MAPK pathways were triggered by BITC in 1483 cells, and both p38 MAPK and MEK/MAPK pathways are activated in UM-22B cells.[23] BITC (**3**) treatment also could induce the apoptotic death and/or cell cycle arrest in human CFPAC-1 and Hs 766T pancreatic carcinoma cells, androgen-independent human PC3 prostate cancer cells, and human 697 pre-B leukemic cells.[24] The proapoptosis of another androgen-independent human DU-145 prostate cancer cell was mediated by ROS and Ca^{2+} increases-promoted mitochondrial signaling pathway, followed by decrease in mitochondrial membrane potential, release of AIF and Endo G from mitochondria, and activation of caspases-3, -8, and -9.[25] Similarly, through ROS-triggered both mitochondria-dependent and death receptor-mediated multiple signaling pathways, BITC (**3**) elicited cell cycle arrest and apoptosis in human A375.S2 melanoma cells and U-2 OS osteogenic sarcoma cells.[26,27] BITC treatment caused cell survival inhibition and cell apoptosis in human pancreatic cancer BxPC-3, AsPC-1, Capan-2, and MiaPaCa-2 cell lines in vitro and restrained the growth of BxPC-3 pancreatic tumor xenografts *in vivo*, associated with inhibiting STAT3 signaling pathway.[28] Similarly, by blocking a PI3K/Akt/FOXO pathway, BITC (**3**) hindered the proliferation of BxPC-3 and PanC-1 pancreatic cancer cell lines.[29] Also, BITC (**3**) was able to sensitize human PANC-1 and MIAPaCa-2 cell to radiation by inducing apoptosis.[30] The inhibition of human breast cancer cells by BITC was observed in MCF-7 and MDA-MB-231 cell lines associated with upregulation of p53-induced modulator of apoptosis (PUMA) protein. The enhanced PUMA was relatively more pronounced in MCF-7 cells with wild-type p53 than in MDA-MB-231 cells with mutant p53. The antigrowth effect of BITC was further proved in MDA-MB-231 breast cancer xenograft *in vivo*.[31]

The anti-metastatic and anti-invasive potentials of BITC were proved in human neoplastic cell lines such as SK-Hep1 (liver), AGS (stomach), HT-29 (colon), MDA-MB-231 (breast), BxPC-3 and PanC-1 (pancreas), and murine 4T1 breast cancer cells through mechanism that was mainly connected with inhibition of MMPs-2 and -9 by impeding the mitogen-activated protein kinase, blocking ERK signal pathways, repressing uPA via PKC and MAPK signaling pathway, and/or deterring HIF-α/VEGF/Rho-GTPases.[32–36] The antiangiogenic effect of BITC (**3**) was markedly propitious to hindering the invasion and metastasis of human pancreatic cancer cells and murine 4T1 breast cancer cells *in vivo*.[36,37] Moreover, the anticarcinogenic properties of

BITC (**3**) were demonstrated in more *in vivo* murine models. It obstructed diethylnitrosamine-caused hepatocarcinogenesis and methylazoxymethanol acetate-caused intestinal carcinogenesis in rats, suppressed polycyclic aromatic hydrocarbon-caused or BAP and 4-(methylnitrosamino)-1-(3-pyridyl)-1-butanone-caused lung tumorigenesis in mice, prevented breast carcinogenesis in female MMTV-neu mice, repressed *N*-butyl-*N*-(4-hydroxybutyl)nitrosamine-induced urinary bladder carcinogenesis in rat, and inhibited *N*-nitrosobis (2-oxopropyl)amine-elicited pancreatic carcinogenesis in hamster.[7] Exposure of mouse skin to BITC (**3**) attenuated TPA-induced oxidative damage via inhibition of NAD(P)H oxidase system and leukocyte clearance at the inflamed region. Topically, application of BITC (**3**) suppressed DMBA-initiated and TPA-promoted papilloma formation in ICR mouse skin in a dose-dependent manner.[37–39] The studies also found that BITC (**3**) is not only a potent inhibitor of leukocytic NAD(P)H oxidase but also an inducer of phase II xenobiotic metabolizing enzymes.

Because of the specific content of BITC (**3**), papaya fruits are paid much more attention as a functional food for lowering the risk of cancer and scavenging free radicals. The quantities of BITC (**3**) and BG (**4**) in different stages of papaya fruits have been analyzed. The data showed that the amount of BITC (**3**) in pulp was maximum during 90–120 days after anthesis, while that of BG (**4**) in pulp and peel decreased during this period. The BITC levels were 0.0038 μmol/kg in the pulp on 6th day and 1.3 μmol/kg in the peel on 10th day after harvest, whereas the BG levels were around 0.05 μmol/kg in the pulp on 8th and 9th days and around 2.2 μmol/kg in the peel on 9th and 10th days after harvest. Along with the fruit maturation, both levels continued to decline. Compared to that in the pulp and peel, the content levels of BITC and BG were higher in the seeds.[42] However, the antiproliferative and proapoptotic effects were also observed in the BITC-treated normal human colon CCD-18Co cells and normal rat liver epithelial RL34 cells *in vitro*.[40,41] Therefore, it should be suggested that dietary papaya fruit is best when fully mature, and it is best to avoid its over intake.

3. Cysteine proteases

In an *in vitro* test, papain, a cysteine protease prepared from papaya fruit, diminished the proliferation, invasion, and migration of cholangiocarcinoma (CC) cells in association with inhibition of NF-κB/AMPK signaling as well as the downstream signaling proteins such as p-Akt, p-ERK, p-Stat3, and partial downregulation of MMP-9 and other epithelial–mesenchymal transition markers. Bromelain (a cysteine protease from pineapple fruit) showed a similar type of inhibition of the CC cells, but was better than papain in impairing tumor growth by NF-κB/AMPK signaling.[43]

CONCLUSION AND SUGGESTION

According to the findings described earlier, it is clear that papaya is not only a nutritional supplement but also a functional food due to two major cancer preventive compounds discovered from papaya fruit. The chemical biology studies demonstrated that lycopene (**1**) and benzyl isothiocyanate (**3**) are the most important contributors for the antioxidant and cancer inhibitory properties of papaya fruits. However, the two constituents, lycopene (**1**) and benzyl isothiocyanate (**3**), exist in the fruit in two reverse directions, namely, the level of lycopene (**1**) is maximum in the fully ripened red-flesh fruit, while the level of BITC (**3**) is minimum at the same time. The two compounds may provide their advantages in the cancer prevention individually or collectively. The studies also showed that a large consumption of fully ripened papaya fruit is recommendable, but excessive dietary papaya should be avoided. In addition to the major compounds, the peel and pulp of papaya are also rich in polyphenols, which usually exert prominent antioxidative effects, closely contributing to the anticarcinogenic function. Likewise, the leaves of papaya plant also demonstrated to have more potent efficacies in the cancer prevention and inhibition.[44] Therefore, papaya leaves may have a potential for development of a chemotherapeutic adjuvant used in medicinal practice.

ATTENTION

A latex fluid released from unripened papaya fruit may cause irritation and an allergic reaction in some people. Papaya seeds also contain a cyanogenic glycoside termed prunasin, which can be hydrolyzed to produce hydrogen cyanide, and, therefore, be toxic.

REFERENCES

1. García-Solís, P. et al., 2009. Screening of antiproliferative effect of aqueous extracts of plant foods consumed in México on the breast cancer cell line MCF-7. *Int. J. Food Sci. Nutr.* 60, Suppl 6: 32–46.
2. Sancho, L.E. et al., 2014. Inhibition of proliferation of breast cancer cells MCF-7 and MDA-MB-231 by lipophilic extracts of papaya (Carica papaya L. var. Maradol) fruit. *Food Nutr.* Sci. 5: 2097–2103.
3. Waly, M.I. et al., 2014. Amelioration of azoxymethane induced-carcinogenesis by reducing oxidative stress in rat colon by natural extracts. *BMC Complem. Alternat. Med.* 14, 60/1–60/10.
4. Salla, S. et al., 2016. Antioxidant and apoptotic activity of papaya peel extracts in HepG2 cells. *Food Nutr. Sci.* 7(6): 485–494.
5. Nakamura Y. et al., 2007. Papaya seed represents a rich source of biologically active isothiocyanate. *J. Agric. Food Chem.* 55: 4407–4413.
6. Nguyen, T.T. et al., 2016. Chemical characterization and in vitro cytotoxicity on squamous cell carcinoma cells of Carica papaya leaf extracts. *Toxins* 8(1): 7/1–7/11.
7. Nguyen, T.T., 2013. Anticancer activity of Carica papaya: a review. *Mol. Nutr. Food Res.* 57: 153–164.
8. Johary, A. et al., 2012. Role of lycopene in the prevention of cancer. *Int. J. Nutr. Pharmacol. Neurol. Diseases* 2: 167–170.
9. Chandrika, U. et al., 2003. Gamage carotenoids in yellow- and red-fleshed papaya (Carica papaya L). *J. Sci. Food Agric.* 83: 1279–1282.
10. Pisipati, S.V.V. et al., 2012. Lycopene: redress for prostate cancer. *J. Basic and Clinical Pharmacy* 3: 261–264.
11. Chen, J.Z. et al., 2014. The effect of lycopene on the PI3K/Akt signalling pathway in prostate cancer. *Anti-Cancer Agents in Med. Chem.* 14: 800–805.
12. Sahin, K. et al., 2011. Inhibitory effects of combination of lycopene and genistein on 7,12-dimethyl benz(a)anthracene-induced breast cancer in rats. *Nutr. Cancer-an Int. J.* 63: 1279–1286.
13. Limpens, J. et al., 2006. Combined lycopene and vitamin E treatment suppresses the growth of PC-346C human prostate cancer cells in nude mice. *J. Nutr.* 136, 1287–1293.
14. Yurtcu, E. et al., 2011. Effects of ascorbic acid and β-carotene on HepG2 human hepatocellular carcinoma cell line. *Mol. Biol. Rep.* 38: 4265–4272.
15. Zhu, Y. et al., 1991. Effect of beta-carotene on mouse transplantable mammary cancer MA737. *Zhonghua Zhongliu Zazhi* 21: 262–264.
16. Gajowik, A. et al., 2014. Lycopene - antioxidant with radioprotective and anticancer properties. A review. *Roczniki Panstwowego Zakladu Higieny* 65: 263–271.
17. Zhu, M.Y. et al., 2014. Benzyl isothiocyanate induces apoptosis of hepatocarcinoma cells. *Shijie Huaren Xiaohua Zazhi* 22: 2277–2284.
18. Li, Z. Y. et al., 2012. Content determination of benzyl glucosinolate and anticancer activity of its hydrolysis product in Carica papaya L. *Asian Pacific J. Tropical Med.* 5: 231–233.
19. (a) Miyoshi, N. et al., 2004. A link between benzyl isothiocyanate-induced cell cycle arrest and apoptosis: Involvement of mitogen-activated protein kinases in the Bcl-2 phosphorylation. *Cancer Res.* 64: 2134–42; (b) 2004. Benzyl isothiocyanate modifies expression of the G2/M arrest-related genes. *Bio Factors* 21: 23–26.
20. Abe, N. et al., 2012. Alpha-tocopherol sensitizes human leukemia HL-60 cells to apoptosis induced by benzyl isothiocyanate. *Biosci. Biotechnol. Biochem.* 76: 381–383.
21. Hasegawa, T. et al., 1993. Isothiocyanates inhibit cell cycle progression of HeLa cells at G2/M phase, *Anti-Cancer Drugs* 4: 273–279.
22. Lee, Y.H. et al., 2012. Enhancement of cisplatin cytotoxicity by benzyl isothiocyanate in HL-60 cells. *Food Chem. Toxicol.* 50: 2397–2406.
23. Lui, V.W.Y. et al., 2003. Requirement of a carbon spacer in benzyl isothiocyanate-mediated cytotoxicity and MAPK activation in head and neck squamous cell carcinoma. *Carcinogenesis* 24: 1705–1712.
24. Bsu, A. et al., 2008. Dietary isothiocyanate mediated apoptosis of human cancer cells is associated with Bcl-xL phosphorylation. *Intl. J. Oncol.* 33: 657–663.

25. Liu, K.C. et al., 2011. The roles of AIF and Endo G in the apoptotic effects of benzyl isothiocyanate on DU 145 human prostate cancer cells via the mitochondrial signaling pathway. *Int. J. Oncol.* 38: 787–796.

26. Huang, S.H. et al., 2012. Benzyl isothiocyanate (BITC) induces G2/M phase arrest and apoptosis in human melanoma A375.S2 cells through reactive oxygen species (ROS) and both mitochondria-dependent and death receptor-mediated multiple signaling pathways. *J. Agric. Food Chem.* 60: 665–675.

27. Wu, C.L. et al., 2011. Benzyl isothiocyanate (BITC) and phenethyl isothiocyanate (PEITC)-mediated generation of reactive oxygen species causes cell cycle arrest and induces apoptosis via activation of caspase-3, mitochondria dysfunction and nitric oxide (NO) in human osteogenic sarcoma U-2 OS cells. *J. Orthop. Res.* 29: 1199–209.

28. Sahu, R.P. et al., 2009. The role of STAT-3 in the induction of apoptosis in pancreatic cancer cells by benzyl isothiocyanate. *J. Natl. Cancer Inst.* 101: 176–193.

29. Boreddy, S.R. et al., 2011. Pancreatic tumor suppression by benzyl isothiocyanate is associated with inhibition of PI3K/AKT/FOXO pathway. *Clin. Cancer Res.* 17: 1784–1795.

30. Ohara, M. et al., Benzyl isothiocyanate sensitizes human pancreatic cancer cells to radiation by inducing apoptosis. *Int. J. Mol. Med.* 28: 1043–1047.

31. Antony, M. L. et al., 2012. Critical role of p53 upregulated modulator of apoptosis in benzyl isothiocyanate-induced apoptotic cell death. *PLoS One* 7: e32267.

32. Hwang, E.S. et al., 2008. Benzyl isothiocyanate inhibits metalloproteinase-2/-9 expression by suppressing the mitogen-activated protein kinase in SK-Hep1 human hepatoma cells. *Food Chem. Toxicol.* 46: 2358–2364.

33. Kim, E.J. et al., 2012. Benzyl isothiocyanate inhibits basal and hepatocyte growth factor-stimulated migration of breast cancer cells. *Mol. Cell. Biochem.* 359: 431–440.

34. Ho, C.C. et al., 2011. Benzyl isothiocyanate (BITC) inhibits migration and invasion of human gastric cancer AGS cells via suppressing ERK signal pathways. *Hum. Exp. Toxicol.* 30: 296–306.

35. Lai, K.C. et al., 2010. Benzyl isothiocyanate (BITC) inhibits migration and invasion of human colon cancer HT29 cells by inhibiting matrix metallo-proteinase-2/-9 and urokinase plasminogen (uPA) through PKC and MAPK signaling pathway. *J. Agric. Food Chem.* 58: 2935–2942.

36. Boreddy, S.R. et al., 2011. Benzyl isothiocyanate suppresses pancreatic tumor angiogenesis and invasion by inhibiting HIF-α/VEGF/Rho-GTPases: pivotal role of STAT-3. *PLoS One* 6: e25799.

37. Kim, E. J. et al., Oral administration of benzyl-isothiocyanate inhibits solid tumor growth and lung metastasis of 4T1 murine mammary carcinoma cells in BALB/c mice. *Breast Cancer Res. Treat.* 2011, 130, 61–71.

38. Miyoshi, N. et al., 2004. Benzyl isothiocyanate inhibits excessive superoxide generation in inflammatory leukocytes: implication for prevention against inflammation-related carcinogenesis, *Carcinogenesis* 25: 567–575.

39. Nakamura, Y. et al., 2004. Benzyl isothiocyanate inhibits oxidative stress in mouse skin: Involvement of attenuation of leukocyte infiltration, *Bio Factors* 21: 255–257.

40. Nakamura, Y. et al., 2002. Involvement of the mitochondrial death pathway in chemopreventive benzyl isothiocyanate-induced apoptosis, *J. Biol. Chem.* 277: 8492–8499.

41. Miyoshi, N. et al., 2007. Selective cytotoxicity of benzyl isothiocyanate in the proliferating fibroblastoid cells. *Int. J. Cancer*, 120: 484–492.

42. Rossetto, M.R. et al., 2008. Benzylglucosinolate, benzylisothiocyanate, and myrosinase activity in papaya fruit during development and ripening. *J. Agric. Food Chem.* 56: 9592–9599.

43. Muller, A. et al., 2016. Comparative study of antitumor effects of bromelain and papain in human cholangiocarcinoma cell lines. *Int. J. Oncol.* 48: 2025–2034.

44. Nguyen, T.T. et al., 2016. Traditional aboriginal preparation alters the chemical profile of Carica papaya leaves and impacts on cytotoxicity towards human squamous cell carcinoma. *PLoS One* 11: e0147956.

46. PERSIMMON

Kaki   Persimmon   Caqui

柿子 柿 감

Diospyros kaki

Ebenaceae

Persimmon is the edible fruits of a number of *Diospyros* trees (Ebenaceae), which is one of the favorable fruits in East Asia. *Diospyros kaki* is the most broadly cultivated *Diospyros* tree and is usually called oriental persimmon. The fully ripened persimmon has high sweet taste and delicate flavor, but unripened persimmon is rich in soluble tannins, which brings astringency. Although the oriental persimmon has no significant nutrients, it contains higher contents of dietary fibers, carotenoids (such as β-cryptoxanthin, β-carotene, and zeaxanthin), and manganese. The ripened persimmon fruits can afford multiple advantages on health, including improvement in eye health and skin care, boosting of digestion, upgrading of immune system and cognitive function, lowering of cholesterol and blood pressure, increase in blood circulation, anti-inflammation, and cancer prevention. In Eastern Asia, especially in China, many parts of *D. kaki* plant, such as its fresh and dried fruits, fruit stalk, peel, leaf, root, wood bark, flower, and lacquer, have been traditionally used as folk medicine. However, compared to the oriental persimmon, fresh ripened American persimmon fruit (*D. virginiana*) is an excellent source of vitamin C and iron.

Scientific Evidence of Cancer Prevention and Constituents

The ripened persimmon fruits possess high nutraceutical value and contain many biologically active substances including antioxidants, dietary fiber, and triterpenoids. The health and medicinal benefits of persimmon are considered to relate to the hydrophilic and lipophilic antioxidants largely in the fruit, including PACs, polyphenols, flavonoids, vitamin C, and carotenoids. In comparison, the leaves of *Diospyros* plants comprise of more kinds of constituents such as flavonoids, terpenes, naphthoquinones, naphthols, coumarins, sterols, organic acids, volatiles, and other ingredients to exert diverse biological activities.

1. Anticancer activity of persimmon fruits

The fruit extract strongly inhibited the growth of human Molt-4B lymphoid leukemia cells and induced the cell apoptosis *in vitro* in a concentration-dependent manner. The anticancer constituents in the fruits were identified to be polyphenol-type principles such as catechin, epicatechin,

epicatechin gallate, epigallocatechin, and epigallocatechin gallate. Treatment with these polyphenols individually for 3 days *in vitro* not only caused the irregular shape of Molt 4B cell leading to apoptotic death but also restrained the activity of ODC (a rate-limiting enzyme of polyamine biosynthesis).[1] The condensed tannins contained in the fruits are useful for prevention of UV-induced skin cancer and skin aging.[2] β-Cryptoxanthin (**1**), a natural carotenoid pigment, was separated from the fruits, showing abilities to prevent free radical damage to DNA and to exert its antioxidant activity to repair DNA oxidative damage. The investigations further revealed that the β-cryptoxanthin (**1**) has anticancer potential for the prevention of lung carcinogenesis.[3–5]

Two acetone fractions (A4 and A5) derived from the fruit peel were found to have moderate cytotoxic activity against human HSC-2 oral squamous cell carcinoma cells and HSG submandibular gland tumor cells, with IC_{50}s ranging from 21 to 59 μg/mL. Other four fractions, H3 and H4 (derived from n-hexane extract of the peel) and M2 and M3 (prepared from 70% methanolic extract of the peel), demonstrated a remarkable reversal activity on multidrug resistance (MDR).[6] The fractions M2–M4 displayed marked O^{2-} radical-scavenging function.[6] All the evidences support the use of persimmon fruits as a potential functional food for cancer chemoprevention and antioxidation.

Moreover, the *in vitro* experimental results revealed that the hydroalcoholic extracts of persimmon peel and fruit pulp (*D. kaki*) could protect PC12 rat pheochromocytoma cells from glucose-oxygen-serum deprivation (GOSD)-caused oxidative injury via antioxidant mechanisms. The finding suggested a possibility to translate the persimmon fruit extracts to a therapeutic application for treatment of cerebral ischemic and other neurodegenerative disorders and prevention of brain tumorigenesis.[7]

2. Anticancer activity of persimmon leaves

A water extract of persimmon leaves was dose-dependently effective in the tumor inhibition and the life prolongation of mice implanted H22 hepatoma or sarcoma 180.[8] In the *in vitro* assay, the extracts of unsaponifiable matter, ethyl acetate, and ethanol from the leaves showed the suppressive activities against MCF-7 breast cancer cells (respective IC_{50}s 25.4, 19.8, and 50 μg/mL) and HeLa cervical cancer cells (respective IC_{50}s 7.8, 16.7, and 46.2 μg/mL).[9] From the ethyl acetate extract, four growth inhibitors such as 24-hydroxyursolic acid (**2**), kakisaponin-A (**3**), 4,4′-dihydroxy-α-truxillic acid (**4**), and tatarine-C (**5**) were isolated, and the late three (**3–5**) were shown to have cytotoxicities against human A549 (lung), HepG2 (liver), and HT-29 (colon) neoplastic cell lines, with IC_{50}s in a range of 9.3–21.1 μM.[10,11] The proapoptotic effect of 24-hydroxyursolic acid (**2**) in HT-29 cells was found to closely correlate with the inhibition of COX-2 and the activation of PARP, AMP (ataxia telangiectasia-mutated)-activated protein kinase, caspase-3, and p53 phosphorylation.[11] An isolated triterpenoid termed lupeol (**6**) moderately deterred the MCF-7 and HeLa cell lines (respective IC_{50}s 20.7 and 23.7 μg/mL).[9] Betulinic acid (**7**) was isolated from many *Diospyros* tree leaves, which attracted more attention due to its apparent inhibitory activity against the viability and proliferation of various cancer cell lines including neuroblastoma, multiple myeloma, glioma, rhabdomyosarcoma-medulloblastoma, leukemia, and the carcinomas of thyroid, breast, lung, colon, cervix, ovary, and prostate. These antitumor activities ranged from moderate to weak but it also exhibited apoptosis-inducing, antiangiogenic, anti-inflammatory and immuno-modulatory properties. The *in vivo* anticancer effects of betulinic acid (**7**) against the growth of breast, pancreatic, cervical, ovarian, colon, prostate, and skin carcinomas have been observed in several mouse models.[12,13]

An acetone extract of the leaves was able to promote the differentiation of human HL-60 acute promyelocytic leukemia cells. Especially, it synergistically enhanced the HL-60 cell differentiation to monocytes or granulocytes when the treatment was combined with 1,25-dihydroxyvitamin D3 or all-*trans* retinoic acid.[14] In addition, persimmon leaf flavonols (PLF) could significantly augment cytotoxicity of heavy ion irradiation on the A549 cells *in vitro* and *in vivo* and obstruct the tumor growth through modulation of DNA damage response,[15] implying that PLF is an useful adjuvant for clinical application in combination with heavy ion radiotherapy.

3. Anticancer activity of persimmon

An extract derived from the calyx of *D. kaki* cv. *Hachiya* in 500 µg/mL concentration exhibited extensive cell death against human HT-29 colon cancer cells,[16] and both methanolic extracts of the calyx and the seeds of persimmon serve the antioxidant activity.[17]

CONCLUSION AND SUGGESTION

The significance of persimmon fruits and leaves for cancer prevention has been demonstrated by the extensive chemical biology studies as shown in the earlier summary. These anticancer molecules discovered from the fruits and leaves of persimmon showed only moderate to weak activities against the cancer cell viability and proliferation, but persimmon fruits comprise a complete antioxidant composition including carotenoid, PACs, flavonoids, phenols, and vitamins C, A, and K. These antioxidants synergistically exert prominent effects on scavenging free radicals and protecting from the damage of free radicals. These interactions would be helpful for improving overall body defense ability and eliminating health risks of developing tumors. Other biologically active constituents (such as triterpenoids and dietary fiber) and the antioxidants are also directly linked to preventing various types of carcinogenesis. Consequently, dietary intake of persimmon fruits should be a wise choice for gaining a functional benefit of lowering the cancer threat. The persimmon leaves can provide additional anticancer and antioxidant responses when utilized in combination with the cancer chemotherapy and chemoprevention.

REFERENCES

1. Achiwa, Y. et al., 1997. Inhibitory effects of persimmon (Diospyros kaki) extract and related polyphenol compounds on growth of human lymphoid leukemia cells. *Biosci. Biotech. Biochem.* 61: 1099–1101.
2. Tsukumo, K. et al., 1997. Mutation inhibitors containing persimmon condensed tannin for UV-induced mutation. *Jpn. Kokai Tokkyo Koho* JP 09315992 A 19971209.
3. Lorenzo, Y. et al., 2008. The carotenoid β-cryptoxanthin stimulates the repair of DNA oxidation damage in addition to acting as an antioxidant in human cells. *Carcinogenesis* 30: 308.
4. Lian, F.Z. et al., 2006. β-Cryptoxanthin suppresses the growth of immortalized human bronchial epithelial cells and non-small-cell lung cancer cells and up-regulates retinoic acid receptor b expression. *Int. J. Cancer* 119: 2084–2089.
5. Takahashi, E. et al., 2004. Manufacture of β-cryptoxanthin-containing extracts from persimmon (Diospyros kaki). *Jpn. Kokai Tokkyo Koho* JP 2004331528 A 20041125.
6. Kawase, M. et al., 2003. Biological activity of persimmon (Diospyros kaki) peel extracts. *Phytotherapy Res.* 17: 495–500.
7. Forouzanfar, F. et al., 2016. Protective effect of diospyros kaki against glucose-oxygen-serum deprivation-induced PC12 cells injury. *Adv. Pharmacol. Sci.* 2016: 3073078.
8. Tang, X.N. et al., 2009. Experimental study on antitumor effect of water extract of persimmon leaves. *Zhongguo Yaoshi* (Wuhan, China) 12: 31–33.
9. Abozaid, H. et al., 2014. Phytochemical and biological study of Diospyros kaki L. growing in Egypt. *World J. Pharm. Res.* 3: 1786–1795.
10. Chen, G. et al., 2007. Chemical constituents of the leaves of Diospyros kaki and their cytotoxic effects. *J. Asian Nat. Prods. Res.* 9: 347–353.
11. Khanal, P. et al., 2010. 24-hydroxyursolic acid from the leaves of the Diospyros kaki (persimmon) induces apoptosis by activation of AMP-activated protein kinase. *Planta Med.* 76: 689–693.
12. Gheorgheosu, D. et al., 2014. Betulinic acid as a potent and complex antitumor phytochemical: A inmi review. *Anti-Cancer Agents in Med. Chem.* 14: 936–945.
13. Zhang, D.M. et al., 2015. Betulinic acid and its derivatives as potential antitumor agents. *Med. Res. Reviews* 35: 1127–1155.
14. Kim, S.H. et al., 2010. Effects and action mechanism of Diospyros kaki on the differentiation of human leukemia HL-60 cells. *Oncol. Reports* 23: 89–95.

15. Kawakami, K. et al., 2013. Persimmon leaf flavonols enhance the anti-cancer effect of heavy ion radiotherapy on murine xenograft tumors. *J. Cancer Ther.* 4: 1150–1157.

16. Jo, Y.H. et al., 2010. Antioxidant and anticancer activities of methanol extracts prepared from different parts of Jangseong daebong persimmon (Diospyros kaki cv. Hachiya). *Han'guk Sikp'um Yongyang Kwahak Hoechi* 39: 500–505.

17. Jo, Y.H. et al., 2010. Antioxidant and anticancer activities of methanol extracts prepared from different parts of Jangseong Daebong Persimmon (Diospyros kaki cv. Hachiya). *Han'guk Sikp'um Yongyang Kwahak Hoechi* 39: 500–505.

47. POMEGRANATE

Grenade   Granatapfel   Granada

石榴   ザクロ   석류나무

Punica granatum

Punicaceae

Pomegranate is now known to be an extremely healthy fruit, whose fruit-bearing deciduous shrub is called *Punica granatum*. Several anatomical component of pomegranate, especially its fruits/ intact ariles, have been used in cooking, baking, meal garnishes, juice blends, and alcoholic beverages for many years, whereas its peels, seeds, leaves, and roots of the plant are used in folk medicines in the plant distribution areas. The fruits are a source of vitamins K, C, and folate and the seeds are an excellent source of dietary fiber. Polyphenols, including hydrolyzable tannins, are the most abundant phytochemicals in pomegranate fruit juice and are responsible for many biological benefits of the fruits, whereas punicic acid, a polyunsaturated fatty acid (18:3), is the major constituent (65.3%) of the seed oil. Pharmacological researches have established pomegranate fruits as possessing potent antioxidant, anti-inflammatory, antidiabetes, antihypertensive, antidiarrhea, antihelminth, and antipathogenic microbe properties besides anticancer-related potentials.[1]

Scientific Evidence of Antitumor Activities

Pomegranate fruit including peel, intact arile, juice, and seed is gaining tremendous attention for its wide spectrum of health benefits. In the past decade, plenteous studies have reported the suppressive effect of pomegranate extracts on human breast, prostate, lung, and colon cancer cell lines *in vitro* as well as the prevention and treatment of breast, colon, skin, lung, and prostate tumors in preclinical animal models.

1. Anticancer activities of its fruits

An acetone extract of pomegranate fruits (PFE) displayed anticancer, anticarcinogenic, and antitumor-promoting effects in the *in vitro* and *in vivo* approaches. Oral administration of PFE in drinking water to A/J mice for 140 days markedly reduced the incidence of lung cancer induced by BAP or *N*-nitrosotrischloroethylurea (NTCU) by 61.6% and 65.9%, respectively. The treatments elicited multiple inhibitions toward the proliferation, angiogenesis, and inflammation in the BAP- and NTCU-elicited lung carcinogenesis *in vivo*.[2] Similarly, by modulation of MAPK and NF-κB pathways and prominent inhibitions of ODC and COX-2, PFE significantly diminished TPA-elicited melanoma promotion in CD-1 mice.[3] A combined treatment with PFE and diallyl sulfide (DAS) exerted synergistic suppression against two-stage mouse skin tumorigenesis via inhibition of the activated MAPKs/NF-κB.[4] In addition, treatment of normal human epidermal keratinocytes with PFE in 20 μg/mL concentration inhibited UVB-mediated nuclear translocation and NF-κB/p65 phosphorylation in dose- and time-dependent manner via modulation of NF-κB and MAPK pathways, resulting in photochemopreventive effects against the skin carcinogenesis from UVB radiation.[5]

The antiproliferative and proapoptotic properties of PFE were further demonstrated in both *in vitro* and *in vivo* models with human prostate and lung carcinoma cell lines. PFE (10–100 μg/mL; 48 h) treatment of PC3 highly aggressive prostate cancer cells led to dose-dependent suppression of cell growth/viability and promotion of cell apoptosis. Oral administration of PFE (0.1% and 0.2%, wt/vol) to athymic nude mice implanted with androgen-sensitive CWR22Rv1 prostate tumor cells resulted in a marked suppression of the tumor growth concomitant with a significant decrease in the PSA levels in serum.[6,7] Likewise, *in vitro* treatment of A549 lung carcinoma cells with PFE (50–150 μg/mL) for 72 h elicited a suppression of the cell viability and induced dose-dependent cell cycle arrest at G0/G1 phase, while it had only minimal effects on normal human bronchial epithelial cells *in vitro*. The chemotherapeutic potential of PFE has also been proven in nude mice implanted with A549 cells given oral doses of 0.1% and 0.2% (wt/vol).[8] All these evidences provide a suggestion that the pomegranate fruit can be a chemopreventive/chemotherapeutic agent/adjuvant against the carcinomas in lung, prostate, and skin. According to analysis by matrix-assisted laser desorption/ionization time-of-flight mass spectrometry, PFE was found to be rich in anthocyanins, ellagitannins, and hydrolyzable tannins.[3]

2. Anticancer activity of its fruit/intact arile juice

Pomegranate fruits are widely consumed as juice (PJ), which was actually derived from its pulps and intact ariles. PJ is rich in polyphenols with potent antioxidant activity and capable of hampering the proliferation, invasion, and promoting apoptosis in various neoplastic cells. In PJ, the most abundant antioxidant punicalagin and the enrichment of ellagitannins, anthocyanins, hydroxycinnamic acids, and ellagic acid may provide the majority of the bioactivities of PJ. Consumption of PJ, in a rat model, diminished AOM-induced colorectal ACF and dysplastic ACF by 29% and 53.5%, respectively, and lowered the proliferation of mucosa cells notably, associated with down-regulation of NF-κB and VCAM-1 expressions and significant repression of proinflammatory enzymes (NOS and COX-2). PJ's therapeutic potentials in the colon tumorigenesis were mediated in part by targeting miR-126-regulated pathways.[9] The chemopreventive efficacy of PJ on DMBA-caused carcinogenesis was mediated by significant diminishing of chronic unpredictable stress and its overall antioxidant potential via reducing the antioxidant enzymes activities and altering the levels of glutathione, malondialdehyde, glutamate oxaloacetate transaminase, and glutamate pyruvate transaminase.[10] In the *in vitro* assays, PJ exerted the greatest antiproliferative effect against all tested human oral, colon, and prostate tumor cell lines, with inhibitory rates ranging from 30% to 100%. At 100 μg/mL, PJ induced the apoptosis in HT-29 colon cancer cells but not in HCT-116 colon cells. Other experiments revealed that PJ treatment also restrained the inflammatory cell signaling proteins (such as COX-2, NF-κB, and p65 subunit phosphorylation) in HT-29 cells and repressed the phenol sulfotransferase activity and 1-naphthol sulfoconjugation in Caco-2 colon cancer cells.[11,12] After treatment of an ethanol extract with PJ, the proliferation of T24 urinary bladder urothelial cancer cells was hindered through restriction of PTEN/Akt/mTORC1 pathway and upregulation of profiling-1, and the cell apoptosis was evoked via overexpression of Diablo.[13]

Furthermore, a PJ concentrated extract (2.5–50 μg/mL) deterred the growth of human BT-474 and MDA-MB-231 breast cancer cells but not non-cancer MCF-10F and MCF-12F breast cells, effects that were further proved in nude mice bearing BT474 tumor as xenografts.[14] By induction of mitochondrial damage and death receptor signaling pathways, PJ treatment triggered the apoptosis of DU-145 prostate cancer cells and effectively hindered the growth of DU-145 cells.[15] The antiproliferative and proapoptotic effects of PJ were also observed in LNCaP prostate cancer cells *in vitro* and in human LAPC-4 prostate cancer xenograft *in vivo*.[16,17] The PJ treatment in several phase II trials obviously prolonged prostate-specific antigen (PSA) doubling time in prostate cancer patients, with a rising PSA and displayed antiproliferation and proapoptotic effects on the prostate cancer cells with no serious adverse effects.[16,17] Besides, PJ also was able to enhance the cell adhesion and reduce the cell migration by upregulation of cell adhesion-related genes (such as E-cadherin and ICAM-1) and anti-invasive microRNAs and down-regulation of cell migration-related genes and proinvasive microRNA. Concurrently, PJ declined secretion levels of proinflammatory cytokines/chemokines (such as IL-6, IL-12p40, IL-1β, and RANTES) and retarded the ability of chemokine SDF1α to chemoattract the prostate cancer cells, implying that PJ has abilities for lessening of cancer cell metastasis to the bone.[18]

Five series of fractions were derived from PJ by solid-phase extraction, and its acetonitrile fractions contained higher polyphenol content than other fractions. The acetonitrile fractions were rich in ellagitannins, ellagic acid, and hydroxycinnamic acid derivatives but depleted in anthocyanins. In the *in vitro* experiments, only the acetonitrile fraction promoted the cell apoptosis and S-phase cell cycle arrest and declined adenosine triphosphate (ATP) levels in all four tested leukemia cell lines (CCRF-CEM, HL-60, Molt-3, and THP-1), wherein CCRF-CEM were the most sensitive cells and THP-1 cells were the least affected.[19]

3. Anticancer activity of POMx

POMx is a highly concentrated blend of natural polyphenol antioxidants from pomegranate fruits that contains punicalagins (37%–40%), free ellagic acid (3.4%), and no anthocyanin as determined by HPLC. POMx is prepared by the means of POM Wonderful for use as a dietary ingredient from its skin and arils minus seeds after squeezing out the juice. On the basis of the positive data, dietary POMx have received increasing attention for preventing many types of malignancies. Treatment with 10 μg/mL POMx exerted antigrowth and proapoptotic effects in human LAPC4 androgen-independent prostate cancer cells via a NF-κB-dependent mechanism.[16,20] When co-treated with POMx and IGFBP-3, a synergistic stimulation was observed in the proapoptosis and suppression against the growth of prostate cancer cells. However, treatment with IGF-1 (100 ng/mL) completely blocked the POMx-triggered apoptosis of 22RV-1 prostate carcinoma cells. The findings implied that the IGF/IGFBP system was involved in the POMx-induced apoptosis in human prostate cancer cells.[20,21]

More *in vitro* and *in vivo* results pointed toward the antiangiogenic and anti-metastatic functions of POMx. POMx significantly inhibited the proliferation of HUVEC cells *in vitro* and decreased prostate cancer xenograft size, tumor vessel density, VEGF peptide levels, and HIF-1α expression *in vivo* in SCID mice.[22] POMx treatment effectively obstructed survivin, induced apoptosis, retarded C4-2 metastatic castration-resistant prostate cancer cell growth, and pointedly enhanced the efficacy of docetaxel in athymic nude mice.[23] These evidences proved that the ellagitannin-rich POMx is capable of impeding tumor-related angiogenesis and metastasis for slowing the growth of prostate cancer cells.[23] Moreover, POMx as well as pomegranate juice and seed oil are able to reduce UVB-induced MMPs-2 and -9 activities and to diminish UVB-induced c-Fos protein expression and c-Jun phosphorylation, thereby protecting human reconstituted skin from UVB-caused damage and carcinogenesis.[24]

In addition, PE is a standardized whole-fruit extract of pomegranate, which is similar to POMx but produced by different manufacturers. *In vitro* treatment with PE elicited cell cycle arrest and inhibited the proliferation of human PANC-1 and AsPC-1 pancreatic cancer cell lines. PE was more effective in deterring PANC-1 cell proliferation than paclitaxel, a chemo drug.[25] According to these evidences, POMx and PE may be candidates for further preclinical testing for chemotherapy and chemoprevention of prostate cancer, pancreatic cancer, and melanoma.

4. Anticancer activity of its peels, rinds, husks, and pericarps

Pomegranate peels, rinds, husks, and pericarps have also attracted much attention as the valuable byproducts in the food industry due to their extensive range of bioactivities. Their extracts contain significant amounts of polyphenolic compounds such as ellagic acid (10%–25%), gallic acid (0.80%–1.2%), and punicalagin (35%–53%), and possess marked antioxidant and anticarcinogenic properties.[26] Compared to the fruit pulps, the fruit peels showed more potent suppressive effects toward the oxidative stress and carcinogenesis. The extracts from pomegranate rinds demonstrated suppressive and proapoptotic effect against the growth of human A549 NSCLC cells.[27,28] The methanolic extracts from pomegranate pericarps/peels could hinder estradiol binding to estrogen receptor (ER) and selectively change estrogen receptor modulator profile, thereby restraining the proliferation of ER+-breast cancer cells.[29] The apoptosis of MCF-7 and MDA-MB-231 breast cancer cells and the G2/M cell cycle arrest of MDA-MB-231 cells were prominently promoted by the peel extract, leading to the antigrowth and antiproliferative effects.[30,31] An aqueous ethanol extract of the fruit peel hindered the growth of K562 chronic myeloid leukemia cells mainly via G2/M cell cycle arrest,[32] and it potently inhibited the proliferation in two thyroid cancer cell lines (BCPAP and TPC-1) in vitro and in a mouse model implanted with BCPAP cells, together with apoptosis induction via a mitochondria-mediated apoptotic pathway.[33] The peel extract could markedly impede the migration and invasion of thyroid cancer cells as well inhibiting MMP-9 expression.[33] Oral administration of the 95% ethanol peel extract in a dose of 50 mg/kg for 10 days resulted in 93.9% inhibition against the tumor growth and 64.7% life elongation of mice in an *in vivo* model bearing Ehrlich ascites carcinoma (EAC) cells. In parallel, the antiangiogenic potential of the peel extract was observed clearly.[34]

In addition, the hexane, chloroform, and ethyl acetate extracts from *P. granatum* fruit peels exhibited marked inhibition on cathepsin-D activity, implying the chemopreventive potential of these extracts on the breast carcinoma. A bioactivity-guided isolation of hexane- and chloroform-soluble fractions yielded piperine and ursolic acid, which were identified as the bioactive constituents for the inhibition of cathepsin-D protease activity.[35] Also, the methanol, ethanol, and water extracts of pomegranate peels displayed significant anticarcinogenesis-related antioxidant and free radical scavenging activities.[36]

5. Anticancer activity of its pomegranate emulsion

P-emulsion is a product of Rimonest Ltd., Haifa, Israel and is composed of pomegranate aqueous phase extract and pomegranate seed oil. The aqueous phase of pomegranate juice, peels, leaves, and flowers was fermented with *Saccharomyces cerevisiae*, whereas the seed oil was extracted from dried seeds with cold press. Chemical analyses of the P-emulsion showed the presence of mixed octadecatrienoic acids, sterols and steroids, γ-tocopherol, tocol in the lipid phase and caffeic acid, corilagin, ellagic acid, ferulic acid, gallic acid, protocatechuic acid, 5-hydroxymethyl-furfural, punicalagins, and *trans-p*-coumaric acid in the aqueous phase. In the *in vivo* experiments, the P-emulsion restrained diethylnitrosamine (DENA)-induced rat hepatocarcinogenesis via blockage of Nrf2-mediated redox signaling and NF-κB-regulated inflammatory pathway, and also substantially induced the tumor cell apoptosis and inhibited the cell proliferation by enhancing Bax expression, deterring Bcl-2, and modulating Wnt/β-catenin signaling pathway.[37-39] Oral administration of pomegranate emulsion (PE) to rats hampered DMBA-inflicted mammary carcinogenesis, a chemopreventive effect that was accompanied by antiproliferative and proapoptotic activities of PE. The antiproliferative effect of PE was mediated by disruption of estrogen receptor (ER) and Wnt/β-catenin signaling pathways and inhibition of cyclin-D1, and the proapoptotic effect was triggered by upregulation of Bax and downregulation of Bcl-2 in concert with caspase cascades.[40,41]

6. Anticancer activity of its seeds and seed oil

Pomegranate seed ethanolic extract showed a promising antiproliferative effect against human breast cancer cells (IC_{50} of 9.6 μg/mL) and against hormone-dependent human LNCaP prostate carcinoma cells with three times lower IC_{50} value than that of vinblastine. Phytochemical analysis revealed that the seed extract contained bioactive lipid compounds, such as neutral lipids, glycolipids, and phospholipids.[42] The seed oil obtained by cold-press acutely restrained the proliferation of LNCaP, PC3, and DU-145 human prostate carcinoma cells *in vitro*. The oil in a concentration of 35 μg/mL induced the apoptosis of androgen-independent DU-145 cells and accumulated G2/M cells after 4 h treatment, and also potently hampered the PC3 cell invasion through Matrigel.[43] Administration of 5% pomegranate seed oil notably reduced the incidence and multiplicity of skin tumor caused by DMBA and lowered TPA-induced ODC activity.[44] Giving the seed oil (0.01%–1%) in the diet notably declined the incidence of AOM-induced colonic adenocarcinogenesis. According to the essential oil analysis, the pomegranate seed oil was known to contain more than 70% *cis*-9, *trans*-11, *cis*-13-punicic acid (18:3, n-5) as a conjugated linolenic acid (CLN).[45,46]

Furthermore, the seed oil was able to hinder the oxidation and prostaglandin synthesis and to suppress the proliferation and invasion of breast cancer cells. It also showed antiangiogenic potentials based on the evidences from the inhibition of human umbilical vein endothelial cells *in vitro* and blockage of new blood vessel formation *in vivo* in a chicken chorio-allantoic membrane model.[45] Moreover, the seed oil extracted by supercritical CO_2 exerted potent antigrowth effect against PC3 prostate cancer xenograft in athymic mice.[43]

SCIENTIFIC EVIDENCE OF ANTITUMOR CONSTITUENTS AND ACTIVITY

More detail bioactivity-integrated phytochemical investigations disclosed that the most therapeutically beneficial constituents in pomegranate fruit are polyphenols, phenolic acids, and flavonoids, which are receiving substantial importance due to their exceptional properties, that is, anticarcinogenesis, antioxidation, and anti-inflammation.[40,41] Furthermore, some polyunsaturated fatty acids and polysaccharides isolated from pomegranate were found to have the potential effects in the cancer prevention.

1. Polyphenols

Granatum polyphenols (GP), the peel polyphenols (PP), and fermented juice polyphenols (FJP) in the *in vitro* assays moderately inhibited the proliferation of LNCaP, PC3, and DU-145 prostate cancer cell lines and potently repressed the invasion of PC3 cells and HeLa cells through Matrigel, whereas normal prostate epithelial cells were significantly less affected. The *in vivo* antigrowth effect on the PC3 xenograft was further proved in athymic mice. The ED_{50}s of GP were 70 and 78.13 µg/mL in LNCaP (prostate) and HeLa (cervix) cancer cells, respectively.[43,47-50] These results showed a capability of pomegranate polyphenols to arrest proliferation and stimulate apoptosis in human androgen-dependent and androgen-independent prostate cancer cells, effects that were accompanied by downregulation of androgen-synthesizing genes, such as SRD5A1 in LNCaP, LNCaP-AR, and DU-145 cells, HSD3B2 in LNCaP and LNCaP-AR cells, and AKR1C3 in DU-145 cells.[51] The tumor inhibitory potencies of FJP and GP were according to estrogen-dependent MCF-7 cells > estrogen-independent MB-MDA-231 cells >> normal human breast epithelial cells (MCF-10A).[52] Furthermore, by treatment with the pomegranate polyphenols, HUVEC proliferation and tubule formation were repressed, VEGF expression in MCF-7 estrogen-dependent breast cancer cells and MCF-10A immortalized normal breast epithelial cells were hindered, and migration inhibitory factor activity in MDA-MB-231 estrogen-resistant breast carcinoma cells was enhanced. These data demonstrated the significant potential of pomegranate polyphenols for antiangiogenic effect in human breast carcinoma cells.[53]

By phytochemical analysis, the major polyphenolic components in pomegranate were identified to be phenolic acids (e.g., ellagic acid), anthocyanins/anthocyanidins, condensed tannins (PACs), hydrolysable tannins (e.g., ellagitannins and gallotannins), as well as flavonoids.

Phenolic derivatives: Ellagic acid (**1**) is an important bioactive compound in pomegranate, which exhibited both antimutagenic and anticarcinogenic activities against a wide range of carcinogens in several tissues *in vitro* and/or *in vivo*. For instance, ellagic acid (**1**) obstructed DNA adduction induced by a carcinogen dibenzo[a,l]pyrene in MCF-7 human breast cancer cells,[54] deterred a 2-amino-fluorene-DNA adduct formation and NAT activity in human bladder tumor cell lines (T24 and TSGH 8301),[55] and hindered a tobacco-specific carcinogen 4-(methylnitrosamino)-1-(3-pyridyl)-1-butanone causing lung tumorigenesis in A/J mice.[56] It also showed a direct suppression against the mutagenicity of aflatoxin B1 in *Salmonella* microsuspension assay.[57]

In the studies with rat and mouse models, ellagic acid (**1**) exerted significant inhibition on the cancers of colon, esophagus, tongue, liver, lung, and skin and caused the cell apoptosis of some carcinomas. At doses between 12.5 and 100 µg/mL, ellagic acid (**1**) restrained the proliferation of all tested neoplastic cell lines in a dose-dependent manner. The inhibitory rates were from 45% to 88% in KB oral cancer cells, from 26% to 69% in CAL27 oral cancer cells, from 49% to 76% in SW480 colon carcinoma cells, from 14% to 35% in SW620 metastatic colon cancer cells, from 53% to 87% in HCT-116 colon cancer cells, from 0% to 21% in HT-29 colon cancer cells, from 43% to 94% in 22Rv1 metastatic prostate carcinoma cells, and from 78% to 92% in RWPE-1 immortalized prostate epithelial cells.[58] Compared to LNCaP-AR cell line, ellagic acid (**1**) treatment resulted in a relatively higher apoptotic response in LNCaP and DU-145 prostate cancer cells. Both *in vitro* and *in vivo* data showed that the LNCaP (androgen-dependent) cells were more sensitive to ellagic acid (**1**) in the apoptosis induction than PC3 and DU-145 (androgen-independent) cells.[59]

Besides inducing apoptosis, ellagic acid (**1**) arrested the cell cycle of SW480 (colon) and CaSki (cervix) cancer cell lines at G1/S phase and G1 phase, respectively.[60,61] Likewise, ellagic acid (**1**) obstructed the proliferation and induced apoptosis of human 4T1 breast cancer cells *in vitro* and *in vivo*, and simultaneously increased spleen lymphocyte, NK, LAK, and CTL activities and serum TNF levels to significantly improve specific antitumor immune response in tumor-bearing mice.[62] The proliferation and viability of mouse WA4 breast cancer cells could be obstructed by ellagic acid (**1**) and luteolin (**2**) *in vitro* in a dose- and time-dependent manner.[63] Moreover, ellagic acid (**1**), luteolin (**2**), and caffeic acid were potential inhibitors against the invasion of PC3 human prostate cancer cells across Matrigel. Combination of caffeic acid or luteolin with punicic acid could synergistically achieve the anti-invasive effect on the PC3 cells.[64]

Ellagitannins: Ellagitannins are the most abundant polyphenols present in pomegranate, and puni-calagin (3) is the most important ingredient in the pomegranate ellagitannins that exhibits various bioactivities. In the *in vitro* assays, punicalagin (3) markedly reduced ATP levels lines and promoted the apoptosis in four leukemia cell lines. The IC_{50}s were 5 μmol/L in CCRF cells, 17 μmol/L in HL-60 cells, 18 μmol/L in Molt-3 cells, and 69 μmol/L in THP-1 cells.[19] The apoptosis of HT-29 and HCT-116 human colon cancer cell lines was also stimulated by punicalagin (3) when administered at a dose of 100 μg/mL. Treatment with pinicalagin (3) in the same dose hindered the proliferation of KB and CAL27 oral cancer cells by 42% and 96%, SW480, SW620, HT-29, and HCT-116 colon cancer cells by 65%, 57%, 55%, and 72%, respectively, and RWPE-1 and 22Rv1 prostate cancer cells by 94% and 90%, respectively.[58] The antiproliferative ability of punicalagin was proved in human MCF-7 (breast) and LNCaP (prostate) cancer cells as well.[65] Punicalagin (3) at 1–30 μg/mL concentrations obstructed the viability of U87MG human glioma cells in a dose-dependent manner and enhanced both apoptotic and autophagic pathways in U87MG cells.[66] Further, punicalagin (3) was capable of promoting the process of autophagic cell death of human BCPAP papillary thyroid carcinoma markedly, then leading to the antigrowth effect. The autophagy-inducing effect in the BCPAP cells was associated with (i) activating MAPK and deterring mTOR signaling pathways and (ii) increasing LC3-II conversion and beclin-1 expression and promoting p62 degradation.[67]

In addition, the ellagitannins including punicalagin can be converted to urolithins during the human intestinal metabolism by bacteria. Urolithin-A (4) and urolithin-C (5) suppressed the pro-liferation and clonogenic efficiency of HT-29 colon cancer cells concomitant with cell cycle arrest at G0/G1 and G2/M stages followed by apoptosis induction.[68] These findings highlight that the pome-granate fruit ellagitannins in considerable amounts can potentially curtail the risk of many types of cancer development, and the anticarcinoma effect of punicalagin (3) is substantially linked to its abilities to induce autophagic and apoptotic cell death.

Flavonoids: Both *in vitro* and *in vivo* assays demonstrated that flavonoid-rich fractions from the pomegranate fruit exert antiproliferative, anti-invasive, and proapoptotic activities in breast and prostate cancer cell lines and antiangiogenic activity. The flavonoid-rich fractions from fresh (J) and fermented (W) pomegranate juice and from an aqueous extract (P) of pomegranate pericarps not only displayed proportional inhibitory effect on the proliferation of human HL-60 promyelocytic leukemia cells but also showed differentiation-promoting effect in the HL-60 cells.[69] The results highlighted the cancer preventive potential of pomegranate juice, its fermented juice and pericarp extracts.

Anthocyanins were water-soluble vacuolar pigments belonging to one kind of flavonoid groups and having an array of health-promoting benefits, including antioxidant and anticarcinogenic activ-ities. Two anthocyanins separated from pomegranate fruits were elucidated as delphinidin-3-O-glucoside (6) and cyanidin-3-O-glucoside (7), both of which significantly inhibited ATP levels in four tested leukemia cell lines (CCRF, HL-60, Molt-3, and THP-1). Delphinidin-3-glucoside (6) was moderately toxic to HL-60, CCRF, and Molt-3cells with IC_{50}s of 19, 35, and 35 μmol/L, respec-tively, whereas cyanidin-3-glucoside (7) required high concentrations to inhibit 50% of these leu-kemia cells (IC_{50}s: 89–91 μmol/L). The THP-1 leukemia cell line was the least sensitive to the anthocyanins.[19]

2. Polysaccharides

The polysaccharide components prepared from pomegranate peels/rinds were reported to have potential anticancer property. PPP, a polysaccharide from the peels, in an *in vitro* model, promoted G2/M cell arrest and apoptosis of human U-2 osteosarcoma cancer cells by the means of obstruct-ing the proliferation of U-2 cells. The apoptosis of U-2 cells triggered by PPP was mediated by an intrinsic mitochondrial pathway.[70] PSP001 is a galactomannan-type polysaccharide isolated from the fruit rinds. Besides excellent antioxidant, radical-scavenging, and immunomodulatory properties, PSP001 also exerted antiproliferative effect against human MCF-7 (breast), KB (naso-pharyngy), HCT-116 (colon), K562 (leukemic), A375 (skin), and HepG2 (liver) cancer cell lines as well as murine cancer cell lines (DLA and EAC), together with the proapoptosis. The IC_{50}s (in 72 h) were 52.8 and 97.21 μg/mL, respectively, in K562 and MCF-7 cells. The *in vivo* antitumor efficacy of PSP001 was tested in DLA and EAC murine ascites and EAC solid tumor mouse models. Either treatment with PSP001 alone or in combination with doxorubicin resulted in an obvious decrease in the tumor burden and an increase of life span of tested mice.[71,72] The evidences provided the scientific support for using the pomegranate polysaccharides as an adjuvant in the cancer prevention.

3. Fatty acids

Two linolenic acid isomers, punicic acid (**8**) and α-eleostearic acid (**9**), in the seed oil of pome-granate are selective modulators of estrogen receptor (ER). Both isomers hindered ERα at con-centrations of 7.2 and 6.5 μM and ERβ at 8.8 and 7.8 μM, respectively, and induced ERα and ERβ mRNA expressions in MCF-7 breast cancer cells but not in MDA-MB-231 breast cancer cells.[73] Punicic acid (**8**), a ω-5 long-chain polyunsaturated fatty acid (18:3), at 40 μM concentra-tion, hampered the proliferation of estrogen-insensitive MDA-MB-231 breast cancer cells and estrogen-sensitive MDA-ERα7 breast cancer cells by 92 and 96%, respectively, *in vitro*, together with elicitation of 86% MDA-MB-231 cells and 91% MDA-ERα7 cells to apoptosis via disruption of cellular mitochondrial membrane potential. The antiproliferative effect of punicic acid (**8**) in the breast cancer cell lines was further revealed to be dependent on its abilities to suppress LPO and PKC pathway.[74]

OTHER MEDICINAL USES

Today, pomegranate fruits have been clinically tested for the treatment of cardiovascular disease, neurodegenerative diseases, diabetes, bacterial infections, and UV radiation-induced skin dam-age, showing therapeutic potential in the trials for the treatment of infant brain ischemia, male infertility, Alzheimer's disease, arthritis, and obesity.[75]

NANOFORMULATION

For improving the efficacy of drug delivery, the pomegranate fruit extract was combined with gold nanoparticles (AuNPs) by the green synthesis. The formulated PF-AuNPs (size: 5–20 nm) showed an excellent cytotoxic effect against HeLa cervical cancer cells *in vitro* and the similar AuNPs of the fruit extract exerted a synergistical effect to enhance the therapeutic efficacy of 5-FU (a chemo-therapeutic drug) on MCF-7 breast cancer cells and to attenuate the side effects.[76,77] Likewise, pome-granate seed oil nanoemulsions (PSO-NEs) reduced C6 glioma cell viability to 47% and promoted the radical-scavenging capacity.[78]

Pomegranate polyphenols are the important antioxidant and chemopreventive component, and punicalagin (PU) is a major polyphenol in pomegranates. The pomegranate fruit extract (PE) and punicalagin (PU) were encapsulated by poly(d,l-lactic-co-glycolic acid)-poly(ethylene glycol) nanoparticles, respectively. The synthesized PE-NPs and PU-NPs exerted 2.3- and 5.5-fold enhanced inhibitory effect on MCF-7 breast cancer cells and 2.1- and 11.8-fold effect on Hs578-T breast cancer cells *in vitro*. The PU-NPs were obviously more potent than the PE-NPs, with IC_{50} values of 8.13 and 4.45 μg/mL on the MCF-7 and Fs578-T cells, respectively.[79] Accordingly, these approaches highlighted that the nanoencapsulation is a prospective formulation in the functional food and clinical fields for the cancer chemoprevention.

CONCLUSION AND SUGGESTION

In recent years, multiple pharmacological and physiological functions have been demonstrated, especially antioxidant, anticarcinogenic, anticancer, and heart blood-vessel protective activities, for pomegranate fruit. The importance of gaining health benefits from dietary pomegranate fruits have drawn more and more attention, especially for the cancer prevention and heart protection. The polyphenols including the hydrolyzable tannins (ellagitannins) and phenolic acids are the most abundant phytochemicals in pomegranate fruits, wherein ellagic acid (1) and punicalagin (3) are the major constituents, all of which have been scientifically corroborated in *in vitro* and/or *in vitro* explorations to be potent antioxidants and cancer inhibitors. Their antiproliferative, anti-invasive, and antiagiogenic activities are in moderate to weak levels, but the polyphenols can play a helpful role in cancer prevention; their anticarcinogenic profits have been reported to be associated largely with their remarkable antioxidative and radical-scavenging properties. On the basis of the experimental data, the pomegranate polyphenols may be good for protection of human leukocyte/blood, breast, prostate, colon, esophagus, liver, lung, bladder, and skin from cancer threat.

In addition to the rich polyphenols, other anticarcinogenic substances such as punicic acid (a polyunsaturated 18:3 fatty acid) in the seed oil exerted more potent suppressive effects against the prostate and breast cancer cells than the polyphenols in the *in vitro* models. Polysaccharides in the peel/rind and anthocyanins in the red color juice also contributed to the anticarcinogenic property. Compared with the pulps, the inedible pomegranate peels and seeds contain three times more total amount of polyphenols. Therefore, besides pomegranate fruits that are consumed as functional supplement for cancer prevention, dietary intake of the fruit seeds is encouraged for obtaining more nutritional and anticancer benefits. The pomegranate peels/rinds normally are waste after the production of juice, but the peels/rinds still contain higher polyphenol components, which may be used as byproduct for producing dietary supplements and food preservatives.

REFERENCES

1. Wang, R.F. et al., 2010. Pomegranate: Constituents, bioactivities and pharmacokinetics fruit, vegetable and cereal science and biotechnology, *Global Sci. Books*, 77–87.
2. Khan, N. et al., 2007. Oral consumption of pomegranate fruit extract inhibits growth and progression of primary lung tumors in mice. *Cancer Res.* 67: 3475–3482.
3. Afaq, F. et al., 2005. Anthocyanin- and hydrolyzable tannin-rich pomegranate fruit extract modulates MAPK and NF-κB pathways and inhibits skin tumorigenesis in CD-1 mice. *Intl. J. Cancer* 113: 423–433.
4. George, J. et al., 2011. Synergistic growth inhibition of mouse skin tumors by pomegranate fruit extract and diallyl sulfide: Evidence for inhibition of activated MAPKs/NF-κB and reduced cell proliferation. *Food Chem. Toxicol.* 49: 1511–1520.
5. Afaq, F. et al., 2005. Pomegranate fruit extract modulates UV-B-mediated phosphorylation of mitogen-activated protein kinases and activation of nuclear factor kappa B in normal human epidermal keratinocytes. *Photochem. Photobiol.* 81(Jan./Feb.): 38–45.
6. Malik, A. et al., 2005. Pomegranate fruit juice for chemo-prevention and chemotherapy of prostate cancer. *Proc. Nat. Acad. Sci. U.S.A.* 102: 14813–14818.
7. Malik, A. et al., 2006. Prostate cancer prevention through pomegranate fruit. *Cell Cycle* 5: 371–373.
8. Khan, N. et al., 2007. Pomegranate fruit extract inhibits prosurvival pathways in human A549 lung carcinoma cells and tumor growth in athymic nude mice. *Carcinogenesis* 28: 163–173.
9. Banerjee, N. et al., 2013. Pomegranate polyphenolics suppressed azoxymethane-induced colorectal aberrant crypt foci and inflammation: Possible role of miR-126/VCAM-1 and miR-126/PI3K/AKT/mTOR. *Carcinogenesis* 34: 2814–2822.
10. Hasan, S. et al., 2016. Chronic unpredictable stress deteriorates the chemopreventive efficacy of pomegranate through oxidative stress pathway. *Tumor Biol.* 37: 5999–6006.
11. Adams, L.S. et al., 2006. Pomegranate juice, total pomegranate ellagitannins and punicalagin suppress inflammatory cell signaling in colon cancer cells. *J. Agricul. Food Chem.* 54: 980–985.

12. Saruwatari, A. et al., 2008. Pomegranate juice inhibits sulfoconjugation in Caco-2 human colon carcinoma cells. *J. Med. Food* 11: 623–628.

13. Wu, T.F. et al., 2016. Clarification of the molecular pathway of Taiwan local pomegranate fruit juice underlying the inhibition of urinary bladder urothelial carcinoma cell by proteomics strategy. *BMC Complem. Alternat. Med.* 16: 96/1–96/10.

14. Banerjee, N. et al., 2012. Cytotoxicity of pomegranate polyphenolics in breast cancer cells in vitro and vivo: Potential role of miRNA-27a and miRNA-155 in cell survival and inflammation. *Breast Cancer Res. Treatment* 136: 21–34.

15. Lee, S. et al., 2012. Proteomic exploration of the impacts of pomegranate fruit juice on the global gene expression of prostate cancer cells. *Proteomics* 12: 3251–3262.

16. Pantuck, A.J. et al., 2006. Phase II study of pomegranate juice for men with rising prostate-specific antigen following surgery or radiation for prostate cancer. *Clin. Cancer Res.* 12: 4018–4026.

17. Seeram, N.P. et al., 2007. Pomegranate ellagitannin-derived metabolites inhibit prostate cancer growth and localize to the mouse prostate gland. *J. Agricul. Food Chem.* 55: 7732–7737.

18. Wang, L. et al., 2011. Cellular and molecular mechanisms of pomegranate juice-induced anti-metastatic effect on prostate cancer cells. *Integr. Biol.* 3: 742–754.

19. Dahlawi, H. et al., 2013. Polyphenols are responsible for the proapoptotic properties of pomegranate juice on leukemia cell lines. *Food Sci. Nutrition* 1: 196–208.

20. Rettig, M.B. et al., 2008. Pomegranate extract inhibits androgen-independent prostate cancer growth through a nuclear factor-κB-dependent mechanism. *Mol. Cancer Therap.* 7: 2662–2671; 7: 3654.

21. Koyama, S. et al., 2010. Pomegranate extract induces apoptosis in human prostate cancer cells by modulation of the IGF-IGFBP axis. *Growth Hormone & IGF Res.* 20: 55–62.

22. Sartippour, M.R. et al., 2008. Ellagitannin-rich pomegranate extract inhibits angiogenesis in prostate cancer in vitro and in vivo. *Intl. J. Oncol.* 32: 475–480.

23. Wang, Y.R. et al., 2014. Pomegranate extract inhibits the bone metastatic growth of human prostate cancer cells and enhances the in vivo efficacy of docetaxel chemotherapy. *Prostate* (Hoboken, NJ, USA) 74: 497–508.

24. Afaq, F. et al., 2009. Protective effect of pomegranate-derived products on UVB-mediated damage in human reconstituted skin. *Experim. Dermatol.* 18: 553–561.

25. Nair, V. et al., 2011. Pomegranate extract induces cell cycle arrest and alters cellular phenotype of human pancreatic cancer cells. *Anticancer Res.* 31: 2699–2704.

26. Gao, X.L. et al., 2014. Antitumor polyphenol active part extracted from punica granatum peel, manufacture method thereof and application. *Faming Zhuanli Shenqing* CN 103505480 A 20140115.

27. Jayakumar, S. et al., 2012. Anticancer activity of Punica granatum rind extracts against human lung cancer cell line. *Asian J. Pharm. Clin. Res.* 5(2): Supplement, p204.

28. Sangeetha, J. et al., 2015. Apoptosis induction of Punica granatum extract on human lung cancer cells. *Am. J. Pharm Tech Res.* 5: 478–485.

29. Sreeja, S. et al., 2012. Pomegranate extract demonstrate a selective estrogen receptor modulator profile in human tumor cell lines and in vivo models of estrogen deprivation. *J. Nutr. Biochem.* 23: 725–32.

30. Dikmen, M. et al., 2011. The antioxidant potency of Punica granatum L. fruit peel reduces cell proliferation and induces apoptosis on breast cancer. *J. Med. Food* 14: 1638–1646.

31. Zhang X. et al., 2012. Effects of extract of pomegranate peel on proliferation and apoptosis of breast cancer cell line mda-mb-231. *Tianjin Zhongyiyao Daxue Xuebao* 31: 214–217.

32. Asmaa, M.J.S. et al., 2015. Growth inhibitory effects of crude pomegranate peel extract on chronic myeloid leukemia, K562 cells. *Int. J. Applied & Basic Med. Res.* 5: 100–105.

33. Li, Y.J. et al., 2016. Punica granatum (pomegranate) peel extract exerts potent antitumor and antimetastasis activity in thyroid cancer. *RSC Advances* 6(87): 84523–84535.

34. Oliveira, L.P. et al., 2010. Cytotoxic and antiangiogenic activities of Punica granatum, Punicaceae. *Revista Brasileira de Farmacognosia* 20: 201–207.

35. Chaturvedi, A.K. et al., 2013. Inhibition of Cathepsin D protease activity by Punica granatum fruit peel extracts, isolates, and semisynthetic analogs. *Med. Chem. Res.* 22: 3953–3958.

36. Mahmoud, S. et al., 2014. Antioxidant and antitumor activities of Pomegranate (*Punica granatum*) peel extracts. *World J. Pharm. Sci.* 2: 1441–1445.

37. Bishayee, A. et al., 2013. Pomegranate phytoconstituents blunt the inflammatory cascade in a chemically induced rodent model of hepatocellular carcinogenesis. *J. Nutr. Biochem.* 24: 178–187.

38. Bhatia, D. et al., 2013. Pomegranate bioactive constituents suppress cell Proliferation and induce apoptosis in an experimental model of hepatocellular carcinoma: Role of Wnt/β-Catenin Signaling Pathway. *Evidence-Based Complem. Altern. Med.* (2013): Article ID 371813.

39. Bishayee, A. et al., 2011. Pomegranate-mediated chemoprevention of experimental hepatocarcinogenesis involves Nrf2-regulated antioxidant mechanisms. *Carcinogenesis* 32: 888–896.

40. Bishayee, A. et al., 2016. Pomegranate exerts chemoprevention of experimentally induced mammary tumorigenesis by suppression of cell proliferation and induction of apoptosis. *Nutr. Cancer* 68: 120–130.

41. Mandal, A. et al., 2015. Mechanism of breast cancer preventive action of pomegranate: disruption of estrogen receptor and Wnt/β-catenin signaling pathways. *Mol.* 20: 22315–22328.

42. Lucci, P. et al., 2015. Punica granatum cv. Dente di Cavallo seed ethanolic extract: Antioxidant and antiproliferative activities. *Food Chem.* 167: 475–483.

43. Albrecht, M. et al., 2004. Pomegranate extracts potently suppress proliferation, xenograft growth, and invasion of human prostate cancer cells. *J. Med. Food* 7: 274–283.

44. Hora, J.J. et al., 2006. Chemopreventive effects of pomegranate seed oil on skin tumor development in CD1 mice. *J. Med. Food* 6: 157–161.

45. Kohno, H. et al., 2004. Pomegranate seed oil rich in conjugated linolenic acid suppresses chemically induced colon carcinogenesis in rats. *Cancer Sci.* 95: 481–486.

46. Aruna, P. et al., 2016. Health benefits of punicic acid: A review. *Compr. Rev. Food Sci. Food Saf.* 15: 16–27.

47. Cavalcanti, R.N. et al., 2012. Supercritical carbon dioxide extraction of polyphenols is from pomegranate (Punica granatum L.) leaves: chemical composition, economic evaluation and chemometric approach. *J. Food Res.* 1: 282–294.

48. Hussein, S.A. 2014. Punica granatum as antioxidants, anticancers, antiestrogens, ethnomedical, and isolated of phenolic components, Abstracts of Papers, *248th ACS National Meeting & Exposition*, San Francisco, CA, United States, August 10-14, (2014), BIOL-62.

49. Yang, B. et al., 2010. Extraction of granatum polyphenols and its effect on human cervical cancer HeLa cells. *Shandong Yiyao* 50: 50–51.

50. Ma, G.Z. et al., 2015. Effect of pomegranate peel polyphenols on human prostate cancer PC3 cells in vivo. *Food Sci. Biotechnol.* 24: 1887–1892.

51. Hong, M.Y. et al., 2008. Pomegranate polyphenols down-regulate expression of androgen-synthesizing genes in human prostate cancer cells overexpressing the androgen receptor. *J. Nutr. Biochem.* 19: 848–855.

52. Kim, N.D. et al., 2002. Chemopreventive and adjuvant therapeutic potential of pomegranate (Punica granatum) for human breast cancer. *Breast Cancer Res. Treatment* 71: 203–217.

53. Toi, M. et al., 2003. Preliminary studies on the anti-angiogenic potential of pomegranate fractions in vitro and in vivo. *Angiogenesis* 6: 121–128.

54. Smith, W.A. et al., 2001. Effect of chemopreventive agents on DNA adduction induced by the potent mammary carcinogen dibenzo[a, l]pyrene in the human breast cells MCF-7. *Mutat. Res.* 480-1, 97–108.

55. Lin, S.S. et al., 2001. Ellagic acid inhibits arylamine N-acetyltransferase activity and DNA adduct formation in human bladder tumor cell lines (T24 and TSGH 8301). *Urol. Res.* 29: 371–376.

56. Castonguay, A. et al., 1997. Antitumorigenic and antipromoting activities of ellagic acid, ellagitannins and oligomeric anthocyanin and procyanidin. *Intl. J. Oncol.* 10: 367–373.

57. Loarca-Pina, G. et al., 1998. Inhibitory effects of ellagic acid on the direct-acting mutagenicity of aflatoxin B1 in the Salmonella microsuspension assay. *Mutat. Res.* 398: 183–187.

58. Seeram, N.P. et al., 2005. In vitro antiproliferative, apoptotic and antioxidant activities of punicalagin, ellagic acid and a total pomegranate tannin extract are enhanced in combination with other polyphenols as found in pomegranate juice. *J. Nutr. Biochem.* 16: 360–367.

59. Naiki-Ito, A. et al., 2015. Ellagic acid, a component of pomegranate fruit juice, suppresses androgen-dependent prostate carcinogenesis via induction of apoptosis. *Prostate* (Hoboken, NJ, US) 75: 151–160.

60. Narayanan, B.A. et al., 2001. IGF-II down regulation associated cell cycle arrest in colon cancer cells exposed to phenolic antioxidant ellagic acid. *Anticancer Res.* 21(1A): 359–364.

61. Narayanan, B.A. et al., 1999. p53/p21(WAF1/CIP1) expression and its possible role in G1 arrest and apoptosis in ellagic acid treated cancer cells. *Cancer Lett.* (Ireland) 136: 215–221.

64. Lansky, E. et al., 2005. Pomegranate (Punica granatum) pure chemicals show possible synergistic inhibition of human PC3 prostate cancer cell invasion across Matrigel. *Investig. New Drugs* 23: 121–122.

62. Zhang, Y.M. et al., 2014. Influence of pomegranate peel ellagic acid on the immune function of mice with 4T1 breast cancer. Xiandai *Zhongxiyi Jiehe Zazhi* 23: 1597–1599, 1602.

63. Dai, Z.L. et al., 2010. Pomegranate extract inhibits the proliferation and viability of MMTV-Wnt-1 mouse mammary cancer stem cells in vitro. *Oncol. Reports* 24: 1087–1091.

65. Orgil, O. et al., 2014. The antioxidative and anti-proliferative potential of non-edible organs of the pomegranate fruit and tree. *LWT-Food Sci. Technol.* 58: 571–577.

66. Wang, S.G. et al., 2013. Punicalagin induces apoptotic and autophagic cell death in human U87MG glioma cells. *Acta Pharmacol. Sinica* 34: 1411–1419.

67. Cheng, X. et al., 2016. Punicalagin induces apoptosis-independent autophagic cell death in human papillary thyroid carcinoma BCPAP cells. *RSC Advances* 6: 68485–68493.

68. Kasimsetty, S.G. et al., 2010. Colon cancer chemopreventive activities of pomegranate ellagitannins and urolithins. *J. Agricul. Food Chem.* 58: 2180–2187.

69. Kawaii, S. et al., 2004. Differentiation-promoting activity of pomegranate (Punica granatum) fruit extracts in HL-60 human promyelocytic leukemia cells. *J. Med. Food* 7: 13–18.

70. Li, J. et al., 2014. A polysaccharide from pomegranate peels induces the apoptosis of human osteosarcoma cells via the mitochondrial apoptotic pathway. *Tumor Biol.* 35: 7475–7482.

71. Joseph, M.M. et al., 2012. Evaluation of antioxidant, antitumor and immuno-modulatory properties of polysaccharide isolated from fruit rind of Punica granatum. *Mol. Med. Reports* 5: 489–496.

72. Joseph, M.M. et al., 2013. A galactomannan polysaccharide from Punica granatum imparts in vitro and in vivo anticancer activity. *Carbohydrate Polymers* 98: 1466–1475.

73. Tran, H.N.A. et al., 2010. Pomegranate (Punica granatum) seed linolenic acid isomers: Concentration-dependent modulation of estrogen receptor activity. *Endocrine Res.* 35: 1–16.

74. Grossmann, M.E. et al., 2010. Punicic acid is a ω-5 fatty acid capable of inhibiting breast cancer proliferation. *Intl. J. Oncol.* 36: 421–426.

75. NIH-listed human clinical trials on pomegranate. *Clinicaltrials.gov. Retrieved* 2013-11-19.

76. Lokina, S. et al., 2014. Spectroscopic investigations, antimicrobial, and cytotoxic activity of green synthesized gold nanoparticles. *Spectrochimica Acta, Part A: Mol. Biomol. Spectros.* 129: 484–490.

77. Ganeshkumar, M. et al., 2013. Spontaneous ultra fast synthesis of gold nanoparticles using Punica granatum for cancer targeted drug delivery. *Coll. Surf., B: Biointerfaces* 106: 208–216.

78. Mota Ferreira, L. et al., 2016. Pomegranate seed oil nanoemulsions with selective antiglioma activity: Optimization and evaluation of cytotoxicity, genotoxicity and oxidative effects on mononuclear cells. *Pharm. Biol.* (Abingdon, U.K.) 54(12): 2968–2977.

79. Shirode, A.B. et al., 2015. Nanoencapsulation of pomegranate bioactive compounds for breast cancer chemoprevention. *Int. J. Nanomed.* 10: 475–484/1-475-484/10.

48. UME, CHINESE PLUM, OR JAPANESE APRICOT

Prune   Pflaume   Ciruela

烏梅   ウメ   오매

Prunus mume

Rosaceae

Ume is the dried fruit of *Prunus mume*, a tree commonly grown in South China, Japan, Korea, Vietnam, and Taiwan island. The deciduous plant has been cultivated for over 2,000 years as a highly valued ornamental in Eastern Asia with numerous members of cultivars. Besides being used in oriental medicine, the ume fruits are often used in the Eastern Asian region as sauces for oriental cooking, sousing pickle, preparing juice and sauce, and flavoring for alcohol brewage. Pharmacological studies revealed that the ume extract possesses antioxidant, hepatoprotective, immunoenhancing, gastroprotective, and antimicrobial properties. Owing to resistance to *Helicobacter pylori*, the ume extract can be used to remedy gastritis and gastric ulcers. Ume is able to retard oral microbial diseases and prevent dental diseases caused by several oral pathogenic bacteria.

Scientific Evidence of Antitumor Activity

In early investigation, ume showed the inhibitory effect against human megakaryoblastic leukemia and promyelocytic leukemia cells *in vitro*.[1] The extracts of hot water, water, acetone, ethanol, ethyl acetate, chloroform, and hexane from *P. mume* fruits and leaves have been screened *in vitro*. Some of the extracts from the fruits and all extracts from the leaves showed DPPH and ABTS radical-scavenging activities and the protective effects against oxidative stress in L-132 cells. Probably due to higher total polyphenol contents (523 mg vs. 336.41 mg GAE/100 g), the extract of leaves showed better antioxidant activities than the extracts of fruits.[2] The extracts of ethyl acetate, chloroform, hexane, and ethanol from the fruits and leaves exerted anticancer activities against human A549 (lung), HeLa (cervix), and U87 (brain) cancer cell lines, and the two ethanol extracts showed no toxicity in normal cells (BNLCL2).[2] The ethanol extracts were also able to induce the apoptotic death of human U937 leukemia cells.[3] These examinations revealed that the antioxidant and anticancer activities of *P. mume* fruits and leaves were attributed to the contents of polyphenolics.

MK615: MK615 is an extract prepared from ume fruits and it contains hydrophobic substances. In the recent seven years, MK615 showed a broad anti-neoplastic spectrum.[4,5] It suppressed the cell growth and induced the death of a variety of neoplastic cells, including promyelocytic leukemia (HL-60), breast (MDA-MB-468, MCF-7, FM3A), pancreatic (Mia PaCa-2, PANC-1, PK-1, PK45H), liver (HuH7, HepG2, Hep3B), gastric (Kato-III), esophageal (YES-2), colon (SW480, Colo, and

WiDr), skin (A375, SK-MEL-28), and lung (H1299, H157) cancer cell lines *in vitro*.[4,5] At a dosage of 300 µg/mL, MK615 could inhibit the growth of MDA-MB-468 and MCF-7 cells by 52.4%–52.7%. When the dose rose to 600 µg/mL, the inhibitory percentage of MK615 reached 83.5% for the MCF-7 cells.[6] *In vitro* treatment of human pancreatic cancer cell lines with MK615 at a concentration of 600 µg/mL resulted in the antigrowth effects for 67.1% in PANC-1 cells, 45.7% in PK-1 cells, and 52.1% in PK45H cells.[7] *In vivo* assay further approved the anticarcinoma activity of MK615 in a nude mouse model inoculated human MiaPaCa pancreatic cancer cells. Daily treatment with 0.2 mL of 25% MK615 in phosphate-buffered saline solution (2.5 mL/kg/day) by oral administration markedly inhibited the growth of pancreatic cancer cells without apparent adverse effects. When combined with gemcitabine by an i.p. dose of 20 mg/kg, 3 times per week for two weeks, MK615 synergistically enhanced the chemotherapeutic effect of gemcitabine against the pancreatic cancer.[8]

The anticancer effect of MK615 was found to correlate with its multiabilities in the inhibition of cell proliferation, induction of cell cycle arrest, and increase in apoptosis and autophagy. MK615 acted as an inducer of arrest of the cell cycle at G0/G1 stage in NSCLC cells (H1299, H157)[9] and at sub-G1 phase in SK-MEL-28 melanoma cells in a dose-dependent manner, thereby eliciting the cells to apoptotic death.[10] In breast carcinoma cells (MDA-MB-468 and MCF-7) and pancreatic neoplastic cells (PANC-1, PK-1, and PK45H), MK615 treatment augmented the cell proportion at G2/M phase together with the inhibition of Aurora-A and/or Aurora-B kinases.[8,11] The proapoptotic mechanisms of MK615 were characterized to be associated with (i) reduction of Id-1 expression level and blockage of ERK1/2-Id-1 pathway (such as in A375 cells);[12] and (ii) increase in reactive oxygen species (such as in MiaPaCa-2 cells).[8] MK615 also exerted the anticancer effects through induction of autophagy-related and caspase-independent cell death. The induction of massive cytoplasmic vacuoles (i.e., autophagosomes) including mitochondria and Golgi apparatus was found to be involved in the mechanism of autophagic death in the colon cancer cell lines (SW480, Colo, and WiDr cells).[13] The H1299 and H157 human nonsmall-cell cancer cells were highly sensitive to MK615. The growth inhibitory effect of MK615 on these cell lines was found to correlate with the induction of autophagy and G0/G1 cell cycle arrest and the downregulation of IL-8 expression.[9] Moreover, Glycer-AGE was known to exert a potent proliferative effect on hepatoma HuH7 cells, which expressed a high level of RAGE (receptor of advanced glycation end-products) on the cell surface, but MK615 demonstrated the suppressive effect against the proliferative effect of Glycer-AGE in the HuH7 cells by decreasing RAGE expression.[14] MK615 was also demonstrated to strongly suppress cutaneous in-transit metastasis in a patient with malignant melanoma accompanied by the suppression of RAGE expression.[10] *In vitro* studies also showed that MK615 had no inhibitory effect on human A549 alveolar basal epithelial carcinoma cells, mouse EL4 lymphoma cells, and mouse FM3A mammary carcinoma cells with or without irradiation. But, with irradiation *in vivo*, treatment with MK615 (660 µg/day) led to diminished volume in mouse FM3A mammary carcinoma and prolonged the life duration of tumor-bearing mice together with normalization of cellular-mediated immunity level such as enhancing CD4+/CD8+ ratio.[15] In addition, MK615 deterred the release of lipopolysaccharide-induced proinflammatory cytokine via inactivation of MAPK pathway in murine macrophage-like RAW264.7 cells.[16] Hence, these findings approved the functions of MK615 and ume extracts as a potential therapeutic and preventive agent for hampering a variety of malignant tumors, carcinogenesis, as well as some inflammatory diseases.[18]

Fermented Maesil: The fermented Maesil (*P. mume*) with probiotics demonstrated noticeable suppressive effect against mouse skin carcinogenesis caused by DMBA plus TPA, as evidenced by marked decreases in papilloma numbers and epidermal hyperplasia as well as decline in the cellular proliferation and the percentage of proliferating cell nuclear antigen positive cells. During the treatment, the fermented Maesil, in parallel, augmented the TAOC and phase II detoxifying enzymes and lessened the activity level of LPO, indicating these antioxidant effects are responsible for the anticarcinogenesis.[17]

SCIENTIFIC EVIDENCE OF ANTITUMOR CONSTITUENTS

1. Triterpenoids

JAE was a Japanese apricot (ume) extract containing triterpenoids, which include ursolic acid (106 μg/g of JAE), oleanolic acid (41 μg/g of JAE), lupeol, α-amyrin, cycloartenol, 24-methylencycloartanol, and so on. *In vitro* and *in vivo* tests showed that JAE and the triterpenoid compounds (ursolic acid, oleanolic acid, and betulinic acid) exerted synergistic cytotoxic effects against YES-2 esophageal squamous cell carcinoma cells, respectively, in combination with 5-FU, irinotecan, and cisplatin (chemotherapeutic drugs). The JAE and 5-FU combination amplified the suppressive effect against experimental metastasis to peritoneum in mice as well. However, the synergistic effect of JAE was greater than that of ursolic acid (**1**), oleanolic acid, and betulinic acid.[19] Ursolic acid (**1**), a major triterpene constituent in ume, also exhibited certain inhibitory effect on the proliferation of human primary megakaryocytic and myeloblastic leukemia cell lines (HIMeg and HL-60).[20]

2. Coumarins

Four fractions (n-hexane, chloroform, ethyl acetate, and water) prepared from a methanol extract of *P. mume* fruits displayed the suppressive effect on the proliferation of human SKOV-3 (ovary) and HEp-2 (larynx) neoplastic cell lines *in vitro*, wherein the n-hexane fraction exerted greater inhibitory effect. From the n-hexane fraction, a bioactive coumarin compound assigned as pronate (**2**) was isolated. According to HPLC analysis, the quantity of pronate in ume was approximately 1.47–1.70 g/kg. In *in vitro* assays, pronate (**2**) moderately restrained the growth of a panel of human cancer cell lines and its IC_{50}s were in a range of 39–58 μg/mL. The sensitivity of the cancer cell lines to pronate (**2**) was HEp-2 (larynx carcinoma) > SW156 (kidney hypernephroma) > HEC-1-B (uterus adenocarcinoma) > SKOV-3 (ovary neoplasm). At a concentration of 100 μg/mL, pronate (**2**) deterred the proliferation of all tested cancer cells by 81%–96%, but it also had little effect against normal WRL-68 human liver cells and NIH/3T3 mouse embryo cells.[21]

3. Quinic acid analogues

Three acylated quinic acid analogues, 5-O-(E)-p-coumaroylquinic acid ethyl ester, mumeic acid-A, and its methyl ester, were isolated from a methanolic extract of the flower buds of *P. mume*. The acylated quinic acid analogues substantially hindered melanogenesis in theophylline-stimulated B16 melanoma 4A5 cells, but showed no cytotoxicity. The potent inhibitory effect of 5-O-(E)-feruloylquinic acid methyl ester (**3**) on the melanogenesis was much stronger than that of arbutin (a reference compound).[22] The results showed that the acylated quinic acid analogues in ume may be potential therapeutic supplement for the treatment of skin disorders and skin carcinogenesis through the blockage of melanogenesis; also, dietary ume may be good for skin whitening.

CLINIC PRACTICE

MK615 has been used to treat a patient with advanced hepatocellular carcinoma (HCC). The patient was a 60-year-old female who had undergone surgical resection and had moderately differentiated HCC with vascular invasion. MK615 was selected to challenge the recurrence and metastasis of hepatoma. After MK615 treatment for 3 months, α-fetoprotein level declined and both pulmonary metastases and lymph node reduced in size. Then, the patient survived for more than 17 months and was in good condition without serious adverse effects.[23] More clinic trials have approved that MK615 may be a promising hepatoprotective agent for patients with liver disorders.[24]

CONCLUSION AND SUGGESTION

Numerous scientific studies have been performed to investigate the anticarcinogenic and anticancer potential of ume. The results demonstrated that ume is naturally bestowed with two kinds of major bioactive molecules such as triterpenoids and coumarins in the fruits and leaves and quinic acid analogues in the flower buds of *P. mume*; all these molecules were found to be responsible for the antioxidant and cancer preventive properties of ume. These active chemicals together with other types of ume components such as PACs, flavonoids, phenolics/tannins, carotenoids, and dietary fiber are also significant for coronary health because ume has hypocholesterolemia, antidiabetic, antiatherosclerosis, and antioxidant properties. Particularly, MK615, a bioactive extract of ume, displayed remarkable potential as a health-improving agent for preventing and synergistically treating not only a variety of carcinomas in liver, lung, breast, colon, pancreas, and skin but also ailments in oral, digestive tract, liver, and so on, owing to its antiproliferative, proapoptotic, antioxidant, anti-inflammatory, and antimicrobial activities. On the basis of the observations from scientific investigations, ume has been recommended as a dietary supplement for safely hindering the percentages of certain carcinogenesis and development of some diseases. MK615 may be a promising product that can be used to formulate health supplement for increasing cancer prevention and other body defenses.

OTHER BIOACTIVITIES

Experiments in a rat model revealed that the *P. mume* extract could enlarge the oxidative capacity of exercising skeletal muscle and induce the muscle to prefer fatty acids for its fuel use, thus assisting endurance.[25] MK615 is reported to be useful for treating periodontitis.[26]

REFERENCES

1. Shen, H.M. et al., 1995. In vitro antitumor activity and immunomodulatory effects of Wumei. *China J, Chinese Materia Medica* 20: 365–368.
2. Rho, K.A. et al., 2015. Antitumor and free radical—scavenging activities of various extract fractions of fruits and leaves from Prunus mume. *Han'guk Sikp'um Yongyang Kwahak Hoechi (J. Kor. Soc. Food Sci. Nutr.)* 44: 1137–1143.
3. Park, C. et al., 2011. Induction of apoptosis by ethanol extract of Prunus mume in U937 human leukemia cells through activation of caspases. *Oncol Rep.* 26: 987–993.
4. Adachi, M. et al., 2007. The "Prunus mume Sieb. et Zucc" (Ume) is a rich natural source of novel anticancer substance. *Int. J. Food Properties* 10: 375–384.
5. Sawada, T. et al., 2011. MK615, an extract of the Japanese apricot (ume) a promising anticancer and anti-inflammatory compound. Watson, R.R. and Preedy, V.R. (Eds.), *Bioactive Foods and Extracts*, pp. 31–35.
6. Nakagawa, A. et al., 2007. New antineoplastic agent, MK615, from UME (a variety of) Japanese apricot inhibits growth of breast cancer cells in vitro. *Breast J.* 13: 44–49.
7. Toshie, O. et al., 2008. MK615 inhibits pancreatic cancer cell growth by dual inhibition of Aurora A and B kinases. *World J. Gastroenterol* 14: 1378–1382.
8. Hattori, M. et al., 2013. Antitumor effect of Japanese apricot extract (MK615) on human cancer cells in vitro and in vivo through a reactive oxygen species-dependent mechanism. *Tumori.* 99: 239–248.
9. Sunaga, N. et al., 2010. MK615, A compound extract from the Japanese apricot "Prunus mume" inhibits in vitro cell growth and interleukin-8 expression in non-small cell lung cancer cells. *J. Cancer Sci. Therapy* 16: 5334–5341.
10. Shigeto, M. et al., 2010. Advanced malignant melanoma responds to Prunus mume Sieb. et Zucc (Ume) extract: Case report and in vitro study. *Experimental and Therapeutic Med.* (1): 569–574.
11. Okada, T. et al., 2007. A novel anti-cancer substance, MK615, from ume, a variety of Japanese apricot, inhibits growth of hepatocellular carcinoma cells by suppressing Aurora A kinase activity. *Hepato-Gastroenterol.* 54: 1770–1774.
12. Tada, K.-I. et al., 2012. MK615, a Prunus mume Steb. et Zucc (Ume) extract, attenuates the growth of A375 melanoma cells by inhibiting the ERK1/2-Id-1 pathway. *Phytotherapy Res.* 26: 833–838.
13. Mori, S. et al., 2007. New anti-proliferative agent, MK615, from Japanese apricot "Prunus mume" induces striking autophagy in colon cancer cells in vitro. *World J. Gastroenterol.* 13: 6512–6517.
14. Yuhki, S. et al., 2010. MK615 decreases RAGE expression and inhibits TAGE-induced proliferation in hepatocellular carcinoma cells. *World J. Gastroenterol.* 16: 5334–5341.

15. Wael, S. et al., 2011. MK615, a prospective anti-proliferative agent, enhances CD4/CD8 ratio after exposure to irradiation. *Int. J. Radiation Biol.* 87: 81–90.

16. Morimoto, Y. et al., 2009. MK615 attenuates Porphyromonas gingivalis lipopolysaccharide-induced pro-inflammatory cytokine release via MAPK inactivation in murine macrophage-like RAW264.7 cells. *Biochem. Biophys. Res. Commun.* 389: 90–94.

17. Lee, J.A. et al., 2013. Fermented Prunus mume with probiotics inhibits 7,12-dimethylbenz[a]anthracene and 12-O-tetradecanoyl phorbol-13-acetate induced skin carcinogenesis through alleviation of oxidative stress. *Asian Pacific J. Cancer Prevention* 14: 2973–2978.

18. (a) Tokihiko, S. et al., 2010. MK615, an Extract of the Japanese Apricot (ume), A Promising Anticancer and Anti-Inflammatory Compound. In: R. R. Watson and Victor R. Preedy (Eds.), *Bioactive Foods and Extracts, Cancer Treatment and Prevention*, pp. 31–35. CRC Press. (b) Li, Y.Z. et al., 2015. Dietary Chinese Herbs, p. 488. Springer Verlary Wien.

19. Yamai, H. et al. 2009. Triterpenes augment the inhibitory effects of anticancer drugs on growth of human esophageal carcinoma cells in vitro and suppress experimental metastasis in vivo. *Int. J. Cancer* 125: 952–960.

20. Shen, H.M. et al., 1995. Preliminary investigation of immune modulation effect and in vitro antineoplastic activity of Fructus mume. *Zhongguo Zhongyao Zazhi* 20: 365–368.

21. Jeong, J. et al., 2006. Isolation and characterization of a new compound from Prunus mume fruit that inhibits cancer cells. *J. Agricul. Food Chem.* 54: 2123–2128.

22. Nakamura, S. et al., 2013. Acylated sucroses and acylated quinic acids analogs from the flower buds of Prunus mume and their inhibitory effect on melanogenesis. *Phytochem.* 92: 128–136.

23. Hoshino, T. et al., 2013. Advanced hepatocellular carcinoma responds to MK615, a compound extract from the Japanese apricot "Prunus mume" *World J. Hepatol.* 5: 596–600.

24. Hokari, A. et al., 2012. Efficacy of MK615 for the treatment of patients with liver disorders. *World J. Gastroenterol.* 18: 4118–4126.

25. Kim, S. et al., 2008. Prunus mume extract ameliorates exercise-induced fatigue in trained rats. *J Med Food* 11: 460–468.

26. Morimoto-Yamashita, Y. et al., 2015. A natural therapeutic approach for the treatment of periodontitis by MK615. *Medical Hypotheses* 85(5), 618–621.

6 Cancer-Preventive Substances in Flavorings

---

49. Chili Pepper/*Capsicum* Fruits

50. Chinese Pepper/*Zanthoxylum bungeanum, Z. schinifolium*

51. Lemongrass/*Cymbopogon citratus*

52. Fennel/*Foeniculum vulgare*

53. Ginger/*Zingiber officinale*

54. Rosemary/*Rosmarinus officinalis*

55. Star Anise/*Illicium verum*

56. Thyme/*Thymus vulgaris, T. mongolicus, T. quinquecostatus*

In this chapter, eight flavorings, all natural herbs, are selected to discuss the possibility of lessening the incidence of cancer. Most types of flavorings are food additives with long history, and are used in cuisines for the purpose of both augmenting the taste and flavor of food and amplifying the appetite. Owing primarily to containing good amounts of phenolics and terpenes, natural flavorings usually exert marked antioxidant activity. Furthermore, these eight flavorings show certain properties in the anticancer, anticarcinogenesis, and health promotion in the biological assays, and revealed the types of cancer inhibitory constituents by the bioactivity-related phytochemical studies. Even if the anticancer potencies of the ingredients in flavorings are weak, the added phytochemicals influence the food nutrition and function by interaction with the food chemical components through many pathways when flavoring and/or coloring the food. The additive process would improve the absorption of food nutrition and/or enhance the food preservation, and may also be expected to enhance the bioactivities in cancer prevention synergistically when used with the right culinary techniques. For this reason, it is recommended that the addition of flavorings in cooking not only provide food with pleasant taste, but also increase the likelihood of cancer prevention.

Spicy food is highly popular in many areas of the world. The pungent additives in a safe dietary amount play a role in promoting the body's protection against cancer, but it should be advised that intake in excess may have link with the cancer risk. This interesting topic is discussed in the "chili pepper" section of this chapter. In addition, cinnamon and turmeric are two other important and common herbs and flavorings, and they show significant potential in the cancer therapy and prevention as well. Particularly, curcumin, which is a major constituent in turmeric, showed broad anticancer spectrum. The two flavorings are not discussed in this chapter because both have been described in a book titled *Cancer Inhibitors from Chinese Medicines* (published by CRC Press in the end of 2016). On account of high use of cinnamon and turmeric in cooking, reading the related two sections in that book is suggested for gaining more information about the flavorings.

49. CHILI PEPPER

Piment   Chili-Pfeffer   Pimienta de chile

红辣椒   唐辛子   칠레고추

Capsicum Fruits

Solanaceae

Chili peppers are the fruits of *Capsicum* genus, which is one of the Native American native vegetables to global humanity. After the Columbian Exchange, various cultivars of chili pepper were started to spread worldwide and be consumed in both cuisine and medicine. Nowadays, chili peppers have already been an integral part of the human diet in a variety of countries and regions. Compared to green and yellow chilies, red chilies contain richer vitamin C, higher content of vitamin B6, and carotene (provitamin A), and have higher contents of dietary minerals (such as potassium, magnesium, and iron). Due to the composition of its major constituents termed capsaicinoids, chili pepper gives not only spicy hot flavors but also some medicinal benefits, such as lessening of high blood pressure and cholesterol level, decline of levels of triglycerides and platelet aggregation to help protection of heart, increase in fat burn and loss of body weight, remission of several types of pains and intestinal problems, and so on. In addition to the culinary uses, chili pepper has also been utilized in medicinal practices, exerting its functions, such as anticancer, anti-inflammatory, antidiabetic, anticholesteremic, anticlotting, analgesic, and antimicrobial effects.[1]

SCIENTIFIC EVIDENCE OF CANCER PREVENTION

Anticancer activities of chili: An *in vitro* study showed that the ethyl acetate extract of chili at a concentration of 10 μg/mL showed 22.2% suppressive rate against human SNU-1 gastric cancer cells but its water extract had no such effect. The antiproliferative activity of chili was less than hexane and ethyl acetate extracts of onion, though these extracts exhibited strong telomerase-inhibiting activity at a concentration of 10 μg/mL.[2] Chili pepper (*C. annum*), a commonly used spice and food flavor in India, has been screened with five different kinds of neoplastic cell lines at a concentration of 300 μg/mL for 24 h. Its aqueous extract prompted maximal death of TE-13 esophageal cancer cells (65%), HeLa cervical cancer cells (55%), MDA-MB-231 (ER$^-$) breast cancer cells (51%), MCF-7 (ER$^+$) breast cancer cells (50%), and DU-145 prostate cancer cells (29%), whereas its ethanolic extract showed maximal cell death in case of HeLa cells (50%).[3] The anti-growth and anti-survival activities were revealed to be mediated by cell-cycle disruption with subsequent membrane rupture, breakage of DNA, downregulation of Bcl-2 and obviously upregulation of p53 and Bax in the chili-treated cancer cells, but no remarkable cell death or DNA damage presented in the same treated normal human peripheral lymphocytes.[3] In addition, the extract of *C. chinense* fruit was effective in suppressing the proliferation of HepG2 hepatocellular carcinoma cells.[4]

Antioxidant activities of chili: Chili pepper fruits comprised several kinds of antioxidative phytochemicals such as phenolic compounds, anthocyanins, vitamins C and E, which deterred the oxidation to counteract the effects of ROS. Thus, dietary chili peppers in both dried and fresh forms would influence the levels of radical scavenging and antioxidants. Among the commonly consumed fruits and vegetables, the antioxidant capacity of chili pepper was listed only behind spinach, and among the diverse *Capsicum* species and cultivars, Turkish cultivars of chili showed the most potent antioxidant activity. The majority antioxidant potencies from the chili pepper were tightly correlated with the content of phenolics.[4] As substantiated by numerous studies, it is well known that the antioxidants are usually one of the important contributors for the anticarcinogenic potential.

SCIENTIFIC EVIDENCE OF CANCER-PREVENTIVE SUBSTANCES AND ACTIVITIES

In addition to flavonoids, β-catenin, carotenoids (capsanthin, capsorubin, and cryptocapsin), vitamins, glycolipids, and glycerolipids, capsaicinoids are the major components in the chili pepper fruits, which are mainly responsible for the pungent taste. Normally, the acetone and hexane extracts of chili fruits comprise 58.8%–84.5% contents of total capsaicinoids. The major capsaicinoids in chili peppers are capsaicin (37%), dihydrocapsaicin (29%), homocapsaicin, homodihydrocapsaicin, and nordihydrocapsaicin, and minor capsaicinoids are nonvamide and *n*-vanillyl decanamide. The capsaicinoids are oil-soluble, lipophilic, odorless, colorless, and crystalline alkaloids, which demonstrated various biological and physiological properties, such as anti-inflammatory, cardiovascular-improving, and anti-obesity effects beside antitumor potential.[1,4] Capsaicin (**1**) is the main pungent principal of hot pepper and its content would be higher in some chili varieties.

Anticancer and proapoptotic activities of capsaicin: *In vitro* experiments revealed the broad anti-growth spectrum of capsaicin (**1**) against a variety of cancer cell lines, such as leukemia (HPB-ATL-T, HB4-PL, Kasumi-1), myeloma (U266, MM.1S), glioma (A172, FLS, FCI), colon carcinoma (HT-29, Colo 205), tongue cancer (SCC-4), gastric cancer (SNU-1, NIH/3T3), nasopharyngeal cancer (NPC-TW039), esophageal cancer (CE 81T/VGH), lung cancer (NCI-H69, NIC-H82), hepatoma (SK-Hep-1, HepG2), pancreatic cancer (AsPC-1, BxPC-3), breast cancer (MCF-7, SKBR-3, T47D, BT-474, MDA-MB-231), prostate cancer (PC3, DU145, LNCaP), cutaneous cell carcinoma (SRB-12, Colo16), bladder cancer (MBT-2), and oral cancer (KB).[4,5] The treatment concurrently elicited cell-cycle arrest at G1 stage in the lung cancer and cutaneous cell cancer cell lines, at G0/G1 phase in the esophageal cancer cells, and at G2/M phase in the KB cancer cells. The capsaicin (**1**) exposure also caused apoptotic death of the treated neoplastic cell lines through multiple pathways and different mechanisms independent of neoplastic types: (1) increase in oxidative stress and ROS generation, leading to mitochondrial damage in glioma, leukemia, hepatoma, esophageal, pancreatic, and prostate cancers cell lines; (2) block of STAT3 signaling pathway and link to transient receptor potential vanilloid-type-I (TRPV-I) in multiple myeloma cells; (3) loss of mitochondria membrane potential, and subsequently activation caspase signaling pathway; (4) degradation of TAX protein (a human T-cell leukemia virus type-1 transcriptional activator) and increase of NF-κB inhibitor-α (IκBα) in T-cell leukemia cells; (5) upregulation of a tumor suppressor gene p53 and proto-oncogenes (c-myc and c-Ha-ras) in gastric carcinoma cells; (6) induction of endoplasmic reticulum stress, mitochondrial depolarization, and caspase-3 activation in nasopharyngeal cancer cells; (7) obstruction of EGFR/HER-2 pathway, activation of p27, and a caspase-independent pathway in breast cancer cells; (8) repression of plasma membrane NADH oxidoreductase enzyme in mitochondria; (9) stimulation of peroxisome proliferator-activated receptor-γ and/or caspase-8 dependent pathway in colon cancer cells; (10) activation of AMPK pathway in osteo-sarcoma cells; (11) ROS generation and mitochondrial death pathway in pancreatic cancer cells; (12) increase of p-STAT3-dependent autophagy through ROS generation signaling pathways in hepatoma cells, inhibition of autophagy, then enhancing the cell apoptosis; and (13) modulation of epidermal growth factor receptor (EGFR) and decrease of Bcl-2 expression in melanoma cells.[5–11] Furthermore, several characteristic mechanisms were also found to involve in the suppressive effects of capsaicin (**1**) against the cell proliferation; for instance, (1) inhibition of β-catenin-dependent signaling pathway and downregulation of transcription factor 4 (TCF-4) in colorectal carcinoma cells, (2) restriction of E2F (a family of transcription factor genes in higher eukaryotes) responses and proliferative gene expression in small cell lung cancer cells, and (3) downregulation of prostate specific antigen (PSA) and downmodulation of androgen receptor activity at both mRNA and protein levels by restoring miR-449a profiling in prostate cancer cells.[5–12] Both capsaicin (1) and dihydrocapsaicin (2) were effective suppressors of survival of human U251 glioma cells together with stimulation of the apoptosis by Ca^{2+} and ROS-mediated mitochondrial pathway *in vitro* and *in vivo*.[13] In addition, capsaicin (1) was able to prompt the death of breast cancer stem cells via deterring NOTCH signaling pathway, and then impacted the viability of cancer stem cells.[12]

Anti-angiogenic and antimetastatic potentials of capsaicin: Both *in vitro* and *in vivo* investigations established that capsaicin (1) has anti-angiogenic and antimetastatic properties against the malignant tumors. In *in vivo* models, capsaicin (1) treatment inhibited vascular endothelial growth factor (VEGF)-triggered proliferation, migration, and tube formation in endothelial cells and hampered VEGF-induced vessel sprouting and formation in mouse Matrigel. By promoting hypoxia inducible factor-1α (HIF-1α) and impeding VEGF transcription, capsaicin (1) obstructed angiogenic signaling pathways in lung cancer and myeloma tissues.[7] The anti-invasive and anti-migratory activities of capsaicin (1) were further observed in the treated metastatic cancer cells of colon, bladder, breast, prostate, and skin and invasive fibrosarcoma models, effects of which were mediated by hindering the diverse signaling pathways involved in the cell invasion and migration; for instance, (1) downregulating signaling pathways of Akt/FAK, extracellular signal-regulated kinases and p38-MAPK, and then inhibiting MMP-9 in invasive fibrosarcoma cells, (2) notably reducing metastatic burden in mouse prostate adenocarcinoma cells, and (3) blocking PI3K signaling cascade and reduction of RAC1 in skin cancer cells.[7]

Synergistic anticancer effects of capsaicin: When combined with active agents, the activities of capsaicinoids were amplified for the cancer chemotherapy and chemoprevention. The synergistic anti-cancer effects of capsaicin (1) were observed in cotreatments with active natural products, such as with resveratrol (rich in grapes) deterred colon cancer cells via elevation of NO in a p53-dependent manner; with genistein (rich in soybeans)-impeded breast carcinoma cells via modulation of AMPK and COX-2; with pirarubicin (an anthracycline drug) restrained bladder carcinoma cells by TRPV1 activation; with 3,3'-diindolylmethane (an *in vivo* metabolite from cruciferous vegetables) hindered colorectal cancer cells by modulation of NF-κB, p53 and apoptosis-related genes; and with brasinin (a type of indole derived from cruciferous vegetables) hampered prostate cancer cell invasion via inhibition of MMPs-2 and 9.[7,12] Capsaicin (1) also promoted camptothecin (a chemo drug) elicited apoptotic death of human small lung cancer cell by a calpain pathway and elevation of intracellular calcium.[10] In addition, the capsaicin (1) combination would help to reverse the drug resistance of cholangiocarcinoma cells to 5-fluorouracil (an anticancer drug) and then to promote 5-fluorouracil-triggered autophagy.[14] Considering many bioactive agents (such as resveratrol and genistein) that are abundant in common comestibles, it is possible that the intake together with chili pepper would be beneficial to exert the synergistic and additive activities for the cancer prevention. Chili pepper is a great food supplement as well in the diet for cancer patients.

Anticarcinogenic potentials in animal models: In the *in vivo* experiments, the anticarcinogenic effects of capsaicin (1) and chili pepper occurred corresponding to the results from *in vitro* assays. For instance, (1) intake of a solid diet with 0.01% capsaicin for 16 weeks markedly reduced the incidence of lung adenoma (from 56% to 13%) in mice and inhibited the induction of GST-P+ hepatic foci in rats, that tumors were induced by a mixture of carcinogens (DEN+ MNU+DBN); (2) fed with a 0.25% capsaicinoid mixture (64% capsaicin and 32.6% dihydrocapsaicin) in the diet to mice for 79 weeks showed no evidence of carcinogenicity; (3) intraperitoneal (i.p.) administration of capsaicin to adult male mice over an 8-week period failed to cause mutagenic progression; (4) dermal application of capsaicin did not increase the incidence of preneoplastic or neoplastic skin lesions in male or female mice; (5) topical application of capsaicin caused no marked increases in incidence and multiplicity of skin tumors in female mice injected TPA; (6) capsaicin effectively inhibited tumor growth and induced the cell apoptosis in nonobese diabetic severe combined nude mice; and (7) topical applications of capsaicin repeatedly resulted in no promotion on 7,12-dimethylbenz[a] anthracene (DMBA)-initiated mouse skin tumorigenesis, but if capsaicin (1) is given prior to each topical dose of phorbol ester, it moderately inhibited the papilloma formation.[15] These observations exhibited that capsaicin (1), a major active constituent in chili pepper, has the potential to prevent cancer generation.

CONFLICTING OBSERVATIONS FROM ANIMAL ASSAYS AND HUMAN STUDIES

Despite capsaicin (1) showing the direct inhibitory effect and broad anticancer spectrum in the *in vitro* models and exerting the anticarcinogenic effects in the *in vivo* models, the role of capsaicin (1) in a series of *in vivo* and population-based case-control studies is quite controversial, to be carcinogenesis inhibition or to be carcinogenesis induction.

Carcinogenic potentials in animal models: Despite the above-mentioned *in vitro* and *in vivo* assays proving that the anticancer potential for capsaicin in a variety of cancer cells included LNCaP cell line, the viability and proliferation of androgen-responsive prostate carcinoma LNCaP cells was also reported to be enhanced concomitant with the upregulation of androgen receptor after the capsaicin treatment. Similar contradictory results also occurred in animal models exhibiting carcinogenic effects. For example, (1) if fed with a semisynthetic diet mixing 10% chilies to rats resulted in ~60% of them developing live carcinogenesis; (2) given drinking water containing 0.002% capsaicin for 6 weeks stimulated the development of hepatic foci, which was initiated by diethylnitrosamine (DEN) and altered by enzyme in male rats; (3) chili extract promoted the hexachlorocyclohexan (BHC)-induced hepatocarcinogenesis in mice; (4) 0.03% capsaicin in a semisynthetic diet to mice for lifetime generated benign polypoid adenomas in cecum; (5) intake of solid diets with 0.01% capsaicin for 16 weeks enhanced the papillary of nodular hyperplasia in urinary bladder (from 13% to 53%) caused by carcinogens (DEN+MNU+DBN) in mice; (6) treatment with capsaicin (125 mg/kg) resulted in significantly more lung and cardiac metastases in adult mice injected orthotopically with syngeneic 4T1 mammary carcinoma cells; (7) dietary chili extract showed a promoting effect on the development of gastric cancer initiated by methylacetoxy methylnitrosamine and hepatoma elicited by benzene hexachloride in mouse models; (8) capsaicin (1) exerted no preventive effect on lung tumor development induced by nicotine-derived nitrosamine ketone (NNK); (9) injection of capsaicin at 1.46 and 1.94 mg/kg by IP to mice, respectively. At 16th day and 32nd day, a genotoxic response was detected only in the mice that received high dose of capsaicin; (10) capsaicin showed a cocarcinogenic effect in TPA-promoted skin carcinogenesis *in vivo*, the effect of which was mediated by overexpression of TRPV1 and EGFR and activation of EGFR and COX-2; and (11) topical application of capsaicin (1) on the skin of mice augmented the skin carcinogenesis and development, which was initiated by DMBA and promoted by TPA.[12–15]

Case-controlled cohorts in human studies: Several population-based case-controlled surveys and studies have been conducted in some countries and regions with the consumption of chili pepper, resulting in diametrically opposing opinions. In fact, the consumption of chili pepper in various populations obviously ought to differ in the dietary patterns, intensity, the chili varieties, and qualities. These factors might influence the case-controlled cohorts to result in the incompatible views. Therefore, these factors need to be taken into account when reviewing these cohort results.

Two large cohort statistics conducted in the United States and China disclosed an inverse association between chili pepper consumption and mortality from all causes, including cancerous, respiratory, and cardiovascular diseases or diabetes, independent of other risk factors of death. Consumption of spicy foods for 6–7 days per week showed 14% less risk in total mortality compared to <1 day/time a week.[16,17] The researchers advocated that, frequently, dietary spicy foods, especially fresh chili peppers, relatively minimize the total mortality, including delaying the death from cancer. A same suggestion was concluded from a discussion of the molecular targets in 41 common Indian dietary spices with more than 182 spice-derived nutraceuticals for their effects against different stages of tumorigenesis. The data evidenced that spice-derived nutraceuticals can restrain the viability, proliferation, invasion, and angiogenesis of cancer cells and imped inflammatory pathways, as well as lowering the risk of most chronic diseases.[18] An epidemiologic study in Italy revealed that moderate chili consumption was protective against gastric cancer.[19] Nevertheless, two population-based case-control studies, which were conducted in Mexico, presented the evidences for the consumption of chili and capsaicin leading to an obvious trend of increasing risk of gastric carcinogenesis in the people with high intake of chili spices and capsaicinoids compared with non-consumers, the effect of which was independent of *Helicobacter pylori* status,[20] but was ascribed to the gastric mucosa injury and mutation caused by the strong pungent irritation from high intake of chili peppers.

Similarly, high consumption of chili pepper has been shown to elicit gallbladder cancer (GBC) in women based on three case-control studies performed in Chile and Hungary. By multivariate logistic regression analysis, the chili pepper consumption was assigned as a risk factor for GBC in both Chilean and Hungarian women and the populations in Chile and India.[21–24] In many cases, constipation and long-standing gallstone also occurred in the dietary chili pepper.[23–25] However, aflatoxins-contaminated red chili peppers have been found from Chile, Bolivia, and Peru. A high level of consumption of the contaminated red chili peppers was confirmed to associate with a high GBC incidence rate. Thus, it is clear now that the high risk factor for the development of GBC should be largely attributed to the aflatoxins contamination.[26] Another examination also showed none of the abnormal bladder cells and solid invasive cancer cells observed in the patients who received capsaicin treatment over a 5-year period, indicating a lack of bladder carcinogenic property for the capsaicin.[15]

CONCLUSION AND SUGGESTION

All these extensive investigations have provided the solid foundations for scientifically discussing the safety of chili pepper consumption. The conflicting research findings and epidemiologic data exposed two faces of chili pepper, that is, the major components capsaicinoids in chili pepper play roles both in carcinogenesis and cancer prevention. The totally opposing activities should be primarily dependent on the dietary amount and intensity of chili pepper. Long-term and heavy intake of chili pepper/capsaicin would establish the linkage with carcinogenesis, cocarcinogenesis, or tumor promotion, especially in stomach and gallbladder. The frequently topical use of chili cream on human skin would increase the risk of melanoma, especially under UV/sunlight irritation. Contrarily, in moderate and low doses, the chili and capsaicin consumption is able to exert obvious antioxidant and anticancer activity via targeting multiple signaling pathways and downregulating the gene expressions related to different stages of tumor in its initiation, progression, metastasis, apoptosis, and angiogenesis. On the basis of these characteristics, chili pepper at its safe intake range may serve as a healthy food in diet to ward off carcinogenesis and other chronic diseases. In addition, by the cointake of moderate and low amounts of chili/capsaicinoids with other chemopreventive foods or chemotherapeutic agents, their interaction may effectively stimulate the antitumorigenic/anticancer signaling pathways, leading to the helpful effects of lessening the cancer risk. However, although people differ in their sensitivity and tolerance to spicy food, the intensity and frequency need would decline with aging. Thus, intake of chili pepper is better to be limited between moderate to low levels by self. Consequently, it is concluded that chili pepper can be advised as both nutritional and functional food to be used in the prevention of cancer and some other diseases as long as in a safe range.

REFERENCES

1. Rains, C. et al., 1995. Topical capsaicin. A review of its pharmacological properties and therapeutic potential in post-herpetic neuralgia, diabetic neuropathy and osteoarthritis. *Drugs Aging* 7(4): 317–328; Robbins, W., 2000. Clinical applications of capsaicinoids. *Clin. J. Pain* 16(2 Suppl.): S86–S89.
2. Xu, B.J. et al., 2015. Telomerase inhibitory effects and anti-proliferative properties of onion and other natural spices against cancer cells. *Food Biosci.* 10: 80–85.
3. Vinay, D. et al., 2012. In vitro evaluation of the anticancer potential of chili pepper (Capsicum annum): An Indian spice. *Conference: Carcinogenesis-2012*, Delhi, India, November 19–21.
4. Mori, A. et al., 2006. Capsaicin, a component of red peppers, inhibits the growth of androgen-independent, p53 mutant prostate cancer cells. *Cancer Res.* 66(6): 3222–3229.
5. Chamikara, M.D.M. et al., 2016. Dietary, anticancer and medicinal properties of the phytochemicals in chili pepper (Capsicum spp.). *Ceylon J. Sci.* 45(3): 5–20.
6. Cao, S.W. et al., 2015. Anticancer effects and mechanisms of capsaicin in chili peppers. *Am. J. Plant Sci.* 6: 3075–3081.
7. Clark, R. et al., 2016. Anticancer properties of capsaicin against human cancer. *Anticancer Res.* 36: 837–843.
8. Chen, X. et al., 2016. Inhibiting ROS-STAT3-dependent autophagy enhanced capsaicin-induced apoptosis in human hepatocellular carcinoma cells. *Free Radical Res.* 50(7): 744–755.
9. Zhang, R.F. et al., 2008. In vitro and in vivo induction of apoptosis by capsaicin in pancreatic cancer cells is mediated through ROS generation and mitochondrial death pathway. *Apoptosis* 13(12): 1465–1478.
10. Friedman, J.R. et al., 2017. Capsaicin synergizes with camptothecin to induce increased apoptosis in human small cell lung cancers via the calpain pathway. *Biochem. Pharmacol.* (Amsterdam, the Netherlands) 129: 54–56.
11. Zheng, L. et al., 2015. Capsaicin causes inactivation and degradation of the androgen receptor by inducing the restoration of miR-449a in prostate cancer. *Oncol. Rep.* 34(2): 1027–1034.
12. Shim, Y. et al., 2015. Quantum dot nanoprobe-based high content monitoring of notch pathway inhibition of breast cancer stem cell by capsaicin. *Mol. Cell. Probes* 29: 376–381.
13. Xie, L. et al., 2016. Capsaicin and dihydrocapsaicin induce apoptosis in human glioma cells via ROS and Ca2+ mediated mitochondrial pathway. *Mol. Med. Rep.* 14(5): 4198–4208.
14. Hong, Z.F. et al., 2015. Capsaicin enhances the drug sensitivity of cholangiocarcinoma through the Inhibition of chemotherapeutic induced autophagy. *Plos One* 10: e0121538.
15. Bode, A.M. et al., 2011. The two faces of capsaicin. *Cancer Res.* 71(8): 2809–2814.
16. Chopan, M. et al., 2017. The association of hot red chili pepper consumption and mortality: A large population-based cohort study. *Plos One* 12: e0169876.
17. Lv, J. et al., 2015. Consumption of spicy foods and total and cause specific mortality: Population based cohort study. *BMJ* (Clinical researched) 351: h3942.
18. Aggarwal, B.B. et al., 2009. Molecular targets of nutraceuticals derived from dietary spices: Potential role in suppression of inflammation and tumorigenesis. *Exp. Biol. Med.* (Maywood, NJ) 234(8): 825–849.
19. Buiatti, E. et al., 1989. A case-control study of gastric cancer and diet in Italy. *Int. J. Cancer* 44: 611–616; Buiatti, E. et al., 1991. A case-control study of gastric cancer and diet in Italy. III. Risk patterns by histologic type. *Int. J. Cancer* 48(3): 369–374.
20. Lopez-Carrillo, L. et al., 1994. Chili pepper consumption and gastric cancer in Mexico: A case-control study. *Am. J. Epidemiol.* 139(3): 263–271; Lopez-Carrillo, L. et al., 2003. Capsaicin consumption, Helicobacter pylori positivity and gastric cancer in Mexico. *Int. J. Cancer* 106(2): 277–282.
21. Tsuchiya, Y. et al., 2010. Evidence that genetic variants of metabolic detoxification and cell cycle control are not related to gallbladder cancer risk in Chilean women. *Int. J. Biol. Markers* 25(2): 75–78.
22. Nakadaira, H. et al., 2009. A case-control study of gallbladder cancer in Hungary. *Asian Pac. J. Cancer Prev.* 10(5): 833–836.
23. Endoh K. et al., 1997. Risk factors for gallbladder cancer in Chilean females. *Jpn J. Public Health* 44: 113–122.
24. Pandey, M. et al., 2002. Diet and gallbladder cancer: A case-control study. *Eur. J. Cancer Prev.* 11(4): 365–368.
25. Serra, I. et al., 2002. Association of chili pepper consumption, low socioeconomic status and longstanding gallstones with gallbladder cancer in a Chilean population. *Int. J. Cancer* 102(4): 407–411.
26. Asai, T. et al., 2012. Aflatoxin contamination of red chili pepper from Bolivia and Peru, countries with high gallbladder cancer incidence rates. *Asian Pac. J. Cancer Prev.* 13(10): 5167–5170.

50. CHINESE PEPPER

Pfeffer   Poivre   Pimienta

花椒　ハジカミ（山椒）　산초(학명)

Zanthoxylum bungeanum, Z. schinifolium

Rutaceae

1. R = –H, **2.** R = –OH, **3.** R = –OAc

5

6. R = –OCH$_3$
7. R = –H

4

8

Chinese pepper originates from two aromatic Rutaceae shrubs: (1) *Zanthoxylum bungeanum* (Sichuan pepper) and (2) *Z. schinifolium* (Green pepper). The pericarps and leaves of the two trees are widely used as culinary applications and traditional medicines in East Asian countries and the seeds, leaves, stems, and roots are also utilized as folk herbs. The herbs have long been used for treating the common cold, diarrhea, stomach ache, and jaundice. Chinese pepper has been reported to have pharmacological effects such as antiplatelet aggregation, inhibitory activity against mono-amine oxidase, lipid peroxidation inhibition, antioxidant, anti-diabetes, anti-HBV DNA replication, and anti-inflammatory activities. As a condiment, Chinese pepper not only gives a simple pungent taste but also generates a tingly numbness in the mouth; it is heavily used in Szechuan cuisine. The leaves of the Chinese pepper trees can also be used in cooking as a condiment and the leaves collected in spring and summer are sometimes used for preparation of a unique salad in some areas. The related species are also utilized in the cuisines of Tibet, Bhutan, Nepal, Thailand, and some Indian and Indonesian areas.

Scientific Evidence of Cancer-Inhibitory and Cancer-Preventive Constituents

The essential oil (EO) was reported as a major anticancer component extracted from Sichuan pepper (*Z. bungeanum* fruits). A Sichuan pepper extract which was obtained by supercritical fluid extraction in an *in vitro* assay exhibited marked proliferative inhibitory and apoptosis-inducing effects against human SGC-7901 gastric carcinoma cells.[1] Other types of chemical constituents isolated from the green pepper plant (*Z. schinifolium*) were responsible for the cancer suppression as well. The following summarized research results provide scientific supports for use of Chinese pepper for the cancer chemoprevention.

1. Essential oil

The EO extracted from the seeds of Sichuan pepper demonstrated weak antiproliferative activity against human HeLa (cervix), A549 (lung), and K562 (leukemic) cancer cell lines *in vitro*,[2] but at lower concentrations (0.25–1 mg/mL) elicited the apoptosis of human A549 lung carcinoma cells. Its inhibitory rates in the A549 cells would be 40.12% at its 1 mg/mL concentration and 87.19% at its 4–16 mg/mL concentrations.[3] Treatment with the Sichuan pepper EO (1 mg/mL) for 72 h disturbed the cell cycle progression with G2/M arrest and promoted the apoptosis of mouse H22 hepatoma cells and human Caski cervical cancer cells. When the concentration rose to 4 mg/mL, the EO remarkably restrained the proliferation and growth of H22 and Caski tumors by 45% and 46% at 48 h and by 76% and 78% at 72 h, respectively.[4,5] IP injection of the EO in doses of 25, 50, and 100 mg/mL to mice every 2 days for 7 times resulted in the *in vivo* inhibitory rates of 40.03%, 60.25%, and 62.58%, respectively, against H22 hepatoma.[5] During the *in vivo* test, the EO showed no reinforcement of immunity.[5]

A volatile extract obtained from dried pericarps of green pepper consisted of 29.9% geranyl acetate, 15.8% citronella, 15.4% sabinene, and its minor volatile components included β-myrcene, linalool, (-)-isopulegol, citronellyl acetate, 1,4-dimethylpyrazole, α-terpinene, and 3-methyl-6-(1-methylethyl)-2-cyclohexene-1-ol and *trans*-geraniol.[5] The extract restrained the cell viability and elicited apoptosis of human HepG2 hepatoma cells *in vitro* in a concentration- and time-dependent manner and obviously inhibited the development of human Huh-7 hepatoma cells *in vivo*. During the treatments, the volatile extract notably augmented the ROS production with no influence on caspase-3 activity, implying that the ROS was a key signaling molecule for the induction of HepG2 cell apoptosis.[6] Moreover, oral administration of a seed oil of *Z. schinifolium* in a dose of 200 mg/kg per day for 13 weeks amplified the populations of total T-cells, B-cells, cytotoxic T-cells, monocytes, macrophages, and NK cells and enhanced T-cell function but not B-cell function. The treatment did not change the indexes of biological safety such as hematologic enzymes, CBC, and histopathologic morphologies.[7] Therefore, the findings validated that green pepper seed oil is a safe agent for the antitumor and immunomodulating activities.

2. Coumarins

Several coumarins isolated from methylene chloride fraction of green pepper leaves (*Z. schinifolium*) demonstrated moderate-to-weak anticancer property. Among them, the inhibitory coumarins against human HL-60 leukemia cells were identified as collinin (**1**), 8-methoxyanisocoumarin (**2**), acetoxyschinifolin (**3**), phytodor, puberulin, and lacinartin with IC_{50}s of 4.62, 5.02, 5.12, 19.80, 21.77, and 28.18 μM, respectively, the data of which evidenced that the longer side chain in these molecules is important to the anticancer activity on the HL-60 cells. In association with downregulation of p-ERK1/2 MAPK, p-Akt, and c-myc, these coumarins (**1–3**) exerted the apoptosis-inducing effects in the HL-60 cells.[8] In addition, collinin (**1**) exhibited greatest antiproliferative activity against PC3 human prostate cancer cells and SNU-C5 human colorectal cancer cells with IC_{50}s of 4.39 and 6.26 μM, respectively, and the second active coumarin on the PC3 cells was 8-methoxyanisocoumarin (**2**, IC_{50} of 12.22 μM). The IC_{50}s were 33–35 μM for 8-methoxy-anisocoumarin (**2**) and acetoxyschinifolin (**3**) on the SNU-C5 cells.[8] The *in vitro* assay discovered that the auraptene (**4**) and 7-[(E)-3′,7′-dimethyl-6′-oxo-2′,7′-octadienyl]oxy coumarin (**5**) were the most potent to human acute Jurkat T leukemia cells (IC_{50}s of 16.5 and 8.10 μM, respectively), whereas schinilenol (**6**) and 7-[(E)-7′-hydroxy-3′,7′-dimethyl-octa-2′,5′-dienyl-oxy]-coumarin (**7**) were weak to Jurkat cells (IC_{50}s of 60–72 μM).[9,10] In addition, collinin (**1**) exerted weak cytotoxicity on other human cancer cell lines (IC_{50}s of 38.1–111.6 μM) and on human normal breast epithelial MCF-10A cells (IC_{50} 124.4 μM).[11]

The proapoptotic activity of collinin (**1**) in Jurkat T cells was mediated by an intrinsic mitochondrial apoptotic pathway, which was preceded by the activation of Bak and Bax, mitochondrial damage, DNA fragmentation, and resultant activation of caspase cascades, leading to Bcl-2-regulated degradation of poly(ADP-ribose) polymerase (PARP).[11] However, auraptene (**4**), which is just one methoxyl group less in its structure as compared to collinin (**1**), showed a different mechanism in the promotion of Jurkat T-cell apoptosis, that is, endoplasmic reticulum stress-mediated activation of caspase-8, and subsequent JNK activation, cleavage of FLICE inhibitory protein and Bid, release of mitochondrial cytochrome c, activation of caspases 9 and 3, degradation of PARP, and induction of apoptotic DNA fragmentation.[12]

3. Phenyl propanoid

A phenyl propanoid designated as cuspidiol (**8**), which was isolated from the leaves of *Z. schinifolium* exhibited a marked cytotoxicity in the assay against Jurkat T-cell clone E6.1 and its IC_{50} was calculated to be 7.3 μg/mL.[10]

4. Lignans

A group of lignans were separated from a methanol extract of *Z. schinifolium* stems as the major components and were evaluated in the *in vitro* model with human HL-60 (leukemic), PC3 (prostate), and SNU-C5 (colorectal) cancer cell lines. All the 13 lignans obtained showed only modest-to-none inhibitory effect on the tested cell lines. Relatively, the higher effect on the HL-60 cells was exerted by schinifolisatin-A, simplexoside, and (+)-9′-O-*trans*-feruloyl-5,5′-dimethoxyl-ariciresinol with IC_{50}s in a range of 25–29 µM. The IC_{50}s were 58.87 and 74.43 µM for epipinoresinol in PC3 and HL-60 cells and 42.60 and 82.50 µM for schinifolisatin-A in PC3 and SNU-C5 cells, respectively.[8]

Conclusion and Suggestion

The antitumor potential of Chinese pepper has been demonstrated by the scientific approaches with a combination of bioactivities and phytochemistry. The anticancer activity was found to be predominantly attributed to monoterpene-rich EO and volatile extract from the pericarps and seeds of Chinese pepper and to coumarins in the leaves. Their suppressive potencies are only in levels of moderate-to-weak, but consumption of Chinese pepper (pericarps and leaves) may help protect human blood, liver, lung, colon, and/or prostate from the cancer threat. As a condiment, Chinese pepper usually should not be used too much in each cuisine; however, these bioactive components may synergistically integrate with the cancer inhibitors in other materials of cookery to work for the cancer prevention. Interestingly, the spring and summer leaves of Chinese pepper trees are reported to be edible as a wild vegetable for preparation of salad; thus, it is recommended for cancer prevention.

REFERENCES

1. Li, P.A. et al., 2011. Study on the effect of *Pericarpium zanthoxyli* extracts on proliferation and apoptosis of SGC-7901 cells. *J. Anhui Agric. Sci.* 39: 12091–12092.
2. Han, S.N. et al., 2014. Extraction optimization and antitumor activity of Zanthoxylum bungeanum essential oil. *Shipin Kexue(Food Sci.)* 35(18): 13–16.
3. Zang, L.Q. et al., 2006. The antitumor effect of Zanthoxylum Maxim and its mechanism of essential oil of Zanthoxylum Maxim. *J. Snake* 18: 183–186.
4. Yuan, T.N. et al., 2009. Primary study of the inhibitory effect of Zanthoxylum on Caski cervical cancer and its mechanism. *Shizhen Guoyi Guoyao* 20: 1119–1120.
5. Yuan, T.N. et al., 2008. Primary study of the antitumor effect and its mechanism of Zanthoxylum in vivo and in vitro. *Shizhen Guoyi Guoyao* 19: 2915–2916.
6. Paik, S.Y. et al., 2005. The essential oils from *Zanthoxylum schinifolium* pericarp induce apoptosis of HepG2 human hepatoma cells through increased production of reactive oxygen species. *Biol. Pharm. Bull.* 28: 802–807.
7. Seo, J.W. et al., 2012. The *Zanthoxylum schinifolium* seed oil modulates immune function under the biological safety level. *Mol. Cell. Toxicol.* 8: 179–185.
8. Li, W. et al., 2013. Coumarins and lignans from *Zanthoxylum schinifolium* and their anticancer activities. *J. Agric. Food Chem.* 61: 10730–10740.
9. Min, B.Y. et al., 2011. A new cytotoxic coumarin, 7-[(E)-3′,7′-dimethyl-6′-oxo-2′,7′-octadienyl] oxy coumarin, from the leaves of *Zanthoxylum schinifolium. Arch. Pharm. Res.* 34: 723–726.
10. Fang, Z. et al., 2010. Cytotoxic constituents from the leaves of *Zanthoxylum schinifolium. Bull. Korean Chem. Soc.* 31: 1081–1084.
11. Kim, J.S. et al., 2013. Induction of apoptosis by collinin from *Zanthoxylum schinifolium* is mediated via mitochondrial pathway in human Jurkat T cells. *Process Biochem.* (Oxford, UK) 48: 945–954.
12. Jun, D.Y. et al., 2007. Apoptogenic activity of auraptene of *Zanthoxylum schinifolium* toward human acute leukemia Jurkat T cells is associated with ER stress-mediated caspase-8 activation that stimulates mitochondria-dependent or -independent caspase cascade. *Carcinogenesis* 28: 1303–1313.

51. LEMONGRASS

Citronnelle   Zitronengras   La hierba de limón

香茅 レモングラス 레몬 그라스

Cymbopogon citratus

Poaceae

Lemongrass, or *Cymbopogon citratus*, is a perennial Poaceae plant native to India, Southeast Asia, and Oceania. In the regions where the plant grows, its leaves and stems are commonly used in teas, soups, and curries as a condiment. Its stalks are often sold in Asian food markets. It is also a folk medicine in India and Southern China for treating digestive tract spasms, stomachache, high blood pressure, convulsions, vomiting, cough, pain, achy joints, fever, and exhaustion and its EO is often applied directly on local skin for release of headache, stomach ache, muscle pain, and abdominal pain. Pharmacological approaches have proven the multiple health benefits of lemongrass, such as anti-inflammatory, antioxidant, antidiarrheal, hypoglycemic, hypolipidemic, hypocholesterolemic, cardiovascular, neurobehavioral, antimutagenicity, antinociceptive, antifungicidal, and antimycobacterial activities as well as antifilarial, antimalarial, antiamoebic, antiprotozoan ascaricidal, and larvicidal insecticide and pesticide properties.[1] In addition, same other genus plants *C. nardus* (Citronella) and *C. flexuosus* (Cochin grass) are also used as the similar purposes in their growing areas.

SCIENTIFIC EVIDENCE OF CANCER-INHIBITORY AND CANCER-PREVENTIVE CONSTITUENTS

The 50% and 90% ethanolic extracts of lemongrass leaves were assayed in *in vitro* model with four human tumor cell lines such as HCT-116 (colon), MCF-7 and MDA-MB 231 (breast), and SKOV3 and COAV (ovary) cells. The 50% ethanolic extract showed moderate inhibition on MCF-7 cells (IC$_{50}$ of 68 µg/mL) and weak on MDA-MB 231 cells (IC$_{50}$ of ≥200 µg/mL), whereas the 90% ethanolic extract exerted weak suppression on COAV and MCF-7 cells (IC$_{50}$s of 104.6 µg/mL). The antiproliferative effect of the 50% ethanolic extract in MCF-7 cells were correlated to the upregulation of p21 expression in the presence of high level of p27 and p53, leading to elicitation of cell cycle arrest and apoptosis.[2] Dietary 80% ethanolic extract of lemongrass at 0.6% or 1.8% concentrations for 10 weeks exerted an inhibitory activity in male Fischer 344 rats against the early phase of hepatocarcinogenesis caused by diethylnitrosamine (DEN). Together, the extract reduced the numbers of putatively preneoplastic, glutathione *S*-transferase (GST) and placental form-positive lesions and lessened the level of oxidative hepatocyte and nuclear DNA injury.[3] These data designated the anticarcinogenic potentials of lemongrass, especially for prevention of cancers in colon, liver, breast, and ovary. The most important constituents responsible for its anticancer effects were demonstrated to be mono- and sesquiterpenes (citral, β-myrcene, limonene, nerol acetate, neryl acetate, linalool, geranyl acetate, terpinen-4-ol, β-caryophyllene, and geraniol), saponins, flavonoids, tannins, and phenolic molecules. Generally, lemongrass extract and its components showed no toxicity to human, but at high doses the toxicities of the extract, citral, β-myrcene and limonene would be observed.[1]

1. Essential oil

The lemongrass (*C. citratus*) EO (LGEO) was extracted by steam distillation and then subjected to *in vitro* assay using human HCT-116 (colon) and MCF-7 (breast) cancer cell lines. The moderate inhibitory effect of LGEO was observed against the proliferation of HCT-116 and MCF-7 cell lines (respective IC_{50}s of 27.41 and 41.90 µg/mL), whereas citronella (*C. nardus*) EO (CNEO) had no activity on HCT-116 cells.[4,5] However, LGEO and CNEO showed the inhibition in a nontumorigenic cell line (Vero).[6] The anticarcinogenic activity of LGEO was proved *in vivo* against chemical oncogens-induced neoplastic formation. Oral administration of 500 mg/kg LGEO (5 times per week for 5 weeks) markedly reduced the leukocyte DNA damage caused by *N*-methyl-*N*-nitrosurea (MNU). In a medium-term study, LGEO in oral doses of 125 or 500 mg/kg for 6 weeks resulted in an anticarcinogenic activity against DDB-initiated breast carcinogenesis in female mice.[7,8] At 100 µg/mL concentration, LGEO obstructed the angiogenesis in tumor by 99% in a rat aortic ring model.[5] In addition, the free radical scavenging activity of LGEO was also established *in vitro* but not strongly, whose potency was greater than that of CNEO.[4] The lemongrass oil could also offer a protection against benzo[a]pyrene-induced oxidative stress and DNA damage in human embryonic lung fibroblast cells by lessening 8-hydroxydeoxyguanosine level.[9]

C. *flexuosus* EO (CFEO) demonstrated the anticancer potential in both *in vivo* and *in vitro* models. I.p. administration of CFEO significantly inhibited both ascitic and solid forms of Ehrlich tumor and sarcoma-180 in a dose-dependent manner, in which inhibitory rates at 200 mg/kg (i.p.) of CFEO were 97.34% and 57.83% in ascitic and solid forms of Ehrlich carcinoma, and 94.07% and 36.97% in ascitic and solid forms of sarcoma-180, respectively.[10] The *in vitro* studies showed the dose-dependent cytotoxicity against 12 human cancer cell lines and the IC_{50}s were ranged from 4.2 to 79 µg/mL, wherein the highest cytotoxicity was observed in 502713 colon cancer and IMR-32 neuroblastoma cells with IC_{50}s of 4.2 and 4.7 µg/mL, respectively. CFEO moderately promoted the apoptosis and growth inhibition in HL-60 human leukemia cells (IC_{50} of ~30 µg/mL at 48 h).[10,11]

2. Terpenes

Citral (**1**) is a natural mixture of two isomeric acyclic monoterpene aldehydes geranial (*trans*-citral/citral-A, **1a**) and neral (*cis*-citral/citral-B, **1b**) in a proportion of 6:4. Citral (**1**) is a key constituent in the EOs of lemongrass (*C. citratus*) and several aromatic plants.[12] The anti-leukemia activity of citral (**1**) was reported against different types of cell lines such as human B-lymphoma cells, human U937 and HL-60 leukemia cells, human NB4 acute promyelocytic leukemia cells, mouse RL12 and BS-24-1 leukemia cells, and mouse P388 lymphocytic leukemia cells *in vitro*. The IC_{50}s were 4.0 µg/mL in NB4 cells, 47 µg/mL in HL-60 cells, and 77.19 µM in B-lymphoma cells.[13,14] Treatment of the U937, HL60 and RL12 and BS-24-1 leukemic cell lines with citral (45 µg/mL) for 4–24 h resulted in 58%–90% death of cells and activation of caspase-3, which is a parameter of apoptosis.[13] The suppressive effect of citral (**1**) on the NB4 cells was accompanied with proapoptosis in a dose- and time-dependent manner, mechanism of which was involved in a mitochondrial pathway, including upregulation of Bax and downregulation of Bcl-2 mRNA and NF-κB protein.[14] The proapoptotic ability of citral (**1**) is mostly contributed by its core pharmacophore of α,β-unsaturated aldehyde conjunction.[13] Meanwhile, the citral (**1**) had no caspase-3 induction in human MCF-7 and 293T carcinoma cells, normal mouse thymocytes and splenocytes, and no cytotoxic effect to normal spleen cells, but it had only 29% cell death in normal thymocytes.[13] When combined with doxorubicin, citral (**1**) at concentrations of 20 and 40 µM could additively enhance the cytotoxic and proapoptotic effects of this chemo drug on the B-leukemia cells in association with the augmentation of

BAK expression and lessening of Bcl-xL expression to 5.26-fold. In the cotreatment, the enhanced cytotoxicity was not observed in normal human peripheral blood mononuclear cells (PBMCs).[15] Thus, the results evidenced that citral (1) can be beneficial to chemotherapy and chemoprevention of leukemic diseases as an adjuvant.

Besides the anti-leukemia activity, citral (1) treatment was able to cause weak growth inhibition against MCF-7 breast cancer cells (IC$_{50}$ of 18×10^5 M at 48 h) together with a cell cycle arrest in G2/M phase, apoptosis induction, and a decrease in prostaglandin E2 synthesis.[16] An emulsion formulation of citral or lemongrass oil could improve the anticancer potency. In an *in vitro* assay, the two produced emulsions retarded the proliferation of HeLa and ME180 human cervical neoplastic cell lines and induced the cell apoptosis via escalation of intracellular ROS and alteration of mitochondrial membrane potential.[17]

Several other monoterpenes isolated from the EO showed the antitumor activity. Citronellal (2) from the lemongrass oil could selectively suppress the proliferation of MCF-7 breast cancer cell line (IC$_{50}$ of 91 μM).[6] d-Limonene (3) and geraniol (4) from the lemongrass oil were able to stimulate the activity of a detoxifying enzyme, GST, in several tissues of female A/J mice, exerting the anticarcinogenic and chemopreventive potentials.[18] Isointermedeol (ISO, 5), a sesquiterpene, is a constituent of *C. flexuosus* EO, which displayed antiproliferative and proapoptotic effect in human promyelocytic leukemia HL-60 cell line *in vitro*, resulting in its IC$_{50}$ of 20 μg/mL (48 h). During the induction of HL-60 cell apoptosis, ISO (5) amplified ROS formation with concurrent loss of mitochondrial membrane potential, activated apical death receptors TNFR1, DR4 and caspase-8, increased Bax translocation and release of cytochrome c, activated caspase-9, and lessened nuclear NF-κB expression, which in all events implied that both intrinsic and extrinsic pathways involved in the ISO (5) induced HL-60 cell apoptosis.[10]

By gas chromatography–mass spectrometry (GC-MS) examination of LFEO (from *C. flexuosus* collected in Malaysia), 41 compounds, representing 88.5% of LFEO, were identified and the main components were geranial (1a, 44.6%) and neral (1b, 29.8%).[5] The Togo collections showed that the major constituents were geranial (1a, 45.2%), neral (1b, 32.4%), and myrcene (10.2%) for LFEO, and were citronellal (2, 35.5%), geraniol (4, 27.9%), and citronellol (10.7%) for CNEO.[11] Moreover, after the removal of the dominant components (geranial and geraniol), the remaining CNEO was distilled again to collect an oil fraction of 104°C–106°C/7 mm Hg or 103°C–107°C/7–8 mm Hg, oil fraction of which contains terpenes such as elemenes (85%–95%), germacrenes (1%–3%), and bourbonene (3%–10%). An emulsion which was formulated with this redistilled fraction and soybean lecithin milk demonstrated marked anti-growth effect against sarcoma 180, MKN-45 gastric cancer, H22 hepatoma, QGY hepatoma, and G422 brain cancer in animal models, and showed the enhancement of NK activity and lymphocyte production in mice bearing Lewis lung cancer.[19,20] This development provided a novel application of the remained EO for the cancer prevention after the industrial isolation of flavor.

3. Polysaccharides

The antitumor activity of polysaccharides (CCPS) from *C. citratus* was shown in a mouse model inoculated sarcoma 180. IP administration of CCPS (30–200 mg/kg per day) for seven consecutive days restrained the growth of S180 cells with inhibition rates ranging from 14.8% to 37.8%. Simultaneously, CCPS dose-dependent improved immune functions of the tumor-bearing mice, including enlargement of thymus and spleen indexes and splenocyte production and stimulation of the secretions of IL-2, IL-6, IL-12, and TNF-α. The data suggested that *in vivo* anticancer effect of CCPS might also be achieved by immunoenhancement.[21] F1 and F2, two polysaccharide fractions were isolated from the CCPS, both of which were composed of (1-4)-linked β-D-xylofuranose moiety. Both F1 and F2 displayed cytotoxic and proapoptotic effects in human Siha (cervix) and LNCaP (prostate) cancer cell lines *in vitro*. The proapoptotic mechanism was found to relate with the activation of an intrinsic apoptotic signaling pathway, that is, downregulation of Bcl-2 family genes, release of cytochrome c, and activation of caspase-3.[22]

CONCLUSION AND SUGGESTION

Overall, these research data provided encouraging scientific support for the application of lemongrass and lemongrass oil as potentially useful supplements for cancer chemopreventive purpose. The anticancer components with small molecules in the lemongrass were designated as a group of monoterpenoids and/or some sesquiterpenes, which are mostly in lemongrass EO. The major cancer inhibitory monoterpenoids were citral (**1**), geranial (**1a**), and neral (**1b**) in *Cymbopogon citratus* and *C. flexuosus*, which were markedly effective in suppressing various leukemia cell lines and weakly effective in inhibiting breast and cervical cancer cells. Other anticancer compounds in the two plants were citronellal (**2**), *d*-limonene (**3**), geraniol (**4**), and isointermedeol (**5**). Probably owing to the synergistic effect from these bioactive terpenoids, the lemongrass oil exerted greater suppressive effect in the *in vitro* and *in vivo* assays against various cancer cell lines such as breast, colon, and brain and against some chemicals that caused carcinogenesis. These anticancer activities were normally associated with the induction of the cell apoptosis and cell cycle arrest and/or repression of angiogenesis in tumor tissues. Similarly, the preliminary *in vitro* assays revealed that polysaccharides were another important component being responsible for the anticancer property of lemongrass. Accordingly, several Cymbopogon plants such as lemongrass and Cochin grass as well as their EOs are believed to be beneficial to lessening the risk of some malignant neoplastic diseases, if frequently added in the cookeries and food preparation.

REFERENCES

1. Gagan, S. et al., 2011. Scientific basis for the therapeutic use of *Cymbopogon citratus*, stapf (Lemon grass). *J. Adv. Pharm. Technol. Res.* 2: 3–8; Kouame, N.M. et al., 2016. *Cymbopogon citratus* (DC.) ethnopharmacology, phytochemical, pharmacological activities and toxicology. *Phytotherapie* 14(6): 384–392.
2. Mohammed, F. et al., 2014. Anti-proliferative effect and phytochemical analysis of *Cymbopogon citratus* extract. *BioMed Res. Int.* 2014: 8.
3. Puatanachokchai, R. et al., 2002. Inhibitory effects of lemon grass (*Cymbopogon citratus*, Stapf) extract on the early phase of hepato-carcinogenesis after initiation with diethylnitrosamine in male rats. *Cancer Lett.* 183: 9–15.
4. Mitoshi, M. et al., 2012. Effects of essential oils from herbal plants and Citrus fruits on DNA polymerase inhibitory, cancer cell growth inhibitory, antiallergic, and antioxidant activities. *J. Agric. Food Chem.* 60: 11343–11350.
5. Piaru, S.P. et al., 2012. Chemical composition, anti-angiogenic and cytotoxicity activities of the essential oils of *Cymbopogan citrates* (lemon grass) against colorectal and breast carcinoma cell lines. *J. Essent. Oil Res.* 24: 453–459.
6. Stone, S.C. et al., 2013. Evaluation of potential use of Cymbopogon sp. essential oils, (R)-citronellal and N-citronellylamine in cancer chemotherapy. *Int. J. Appl. Res. Nat. Prod.* 6: 11–15.
7. Bidinotto, L.T. et al., 2011. Protective effects of lemongrass (*Cymbopogon citratus* STAPF) essential oil on DNA damage and carcinogenesis in female Balb/C mice. *J. Appl. Toxicol.* 31: 536–544.
8. DDB: 7,12-dimethylbenz(a)antracene, 1,2-dimethylhydrazine and N-butyl-N-(4-hydroxibuthyl) nitrosamine.
9. Jiang, J. et al., 2017. Protective effects of lemongrass essential oil against benzo(a)pyrene-induced oxidative stress and DNA damage in human embryonic lung fibroblast calls. *Toxicol. Mech. Methods* 27(2): 121–127.
10. Sharma, P.R. et al., 2009. Anticancer activity of an essential oil from *Cymbopogon flexuosus*. *Chem. Biol. Interact.* 179: 160–168.
11. Kumar, A. et al., 2008. An essential oil and its major constituent isointermedeol induce apoptosis by increased expression of mitochondrial cytochrome c and apical death receptors in human leukaemia HL-60 cells. *Chem. Biol. Interact.* 171: 332–347.
12. Dudai, N. et al., 2005. Citral is a new inducer of caspase-3 in tumor cell lines. *Planta Med.* 71: 484–488.
13. Dubey, N.K. et al., 1997. Citral: A cytotoxic principle isolated from the essential oil of *Cymbopogon citratus* against P388 leukemia cells. *Curr. Sci.* 73: 22–24.
14. Xia, H.L. et al., 2013. The in vitro study of apoptosis in NB4 cell induced by citral. *Cytotechnology* 65: 49–57.

15. Dangkong, D. et al., 2014. Effect of citral on the cytotoxicity of doxorubicin in human B-lymphoma cells. *Pharm. Biol.* 53: 262–268.
16. Chaouki, W. et al., 2009. Citral inhibits cell proliferation and induces apoptosis and cell cycle arrest in MCF-7 cells. *Fundam. Clin. Pharmacol.* 23: 549–556.
17. Ghosh, K. et al., 2013. Anticancer effect of lemongrass oil and citral on cervical cancer cell lines. *Pharmacogn. Commun.* 3: 41–48.
18. Zheng, G.Q. et al., 1993. Potential anticarcinogenic natural products isolated from lemongrass oil and galanga root oil. *J. Agric. Food Chem.* 41: 153–156.
19. Dou, Y.Q. et al., 2005. Non-dominant components of citronella oil and their tumorostatic activity. *Shanxi Med. J.* 34: 375–376.
20. Li, D.S. et al., 2010. The extraction of an antitumor fraction from citronella oil and its emulsion formulation. Chinese Patent CN 1970054 B, CN 200610129740; May 12.
21. Bao, X.L. et al., 2015. Polysaccharides from *Cymbopogon citratus* with antitumor and immunomodulatory activity. *Pharm. Biol.* (London, UK) 53: 117–124.
22. Thangam, R. et al., 2014. Activation of intrinsic apoptotic signaling pathway in cancer cells by *Cymbopogon citratus* polysaccharide fractions. *Carbohydr. Polym.* 107: 138–150.

52. FENNEL

Fenouil   Fenchel   Hinojo

茴香 ウイキョウ 회향

Foeniculum vulgare

Umbellifereae

1. R = –H
2. R = –OH

R = -β-D-glucopyranose

Fennel is the dried fruit and seeds of an Umbellifereae plant *Foeniculum vulgare*. Today, fennel is broadly used in culinary art as an anise-flavored spice. Nutritionally, it is a good source of vitamin B complex, vitamin C, dietary fiber, and several dietary minerals, especially manganese, magnesium, calcium, iron, phosphorus, and potassium. Fennel is also a highly aromatic herb in folk medicine for the treatment of ailments related to digestive, endocrine, reproductive, and respiratory systems, and it is helpful for some women to improve the flow of breast milk to promote menstruation and to ease the birthing process. The compiled experimental evidences indicated the efficacy of fennel in pharmacological properties such as anti-inflammatory, antimutagenic, antipyretic, hypoglycemic, antinociceptive, antispasmodic, antilipid peroxidant, hypolipidemic, cardiovascular-improving, hepatoprotective, memory-enhancing, antithrombotic, antiviral, and antimicrobial effects, besides its anticarcinogenic potential.[1] In addition, the bulbs, stalks, and leaves of fennel plant are all edible.

SCIENTIFIC EVIDENCE OF CANCER-INHIBITORY AND CANCER-PREVENTIVE ACTIVITIES

In *in vitro* models, the aqueous extracts of fennel seeds, which were prepared with different pH conditions, displayed high radical-scavenging activity and moderate antitumor activity against Ehrlich ascites carcinoma (EAC) cells in a high concentration of 900 μg/mL.[1] IP injection of its methanol extract of fennel seeds (FSME) in a dose of 100 mg/kg into mice for 30 days with or without exposure to radiation prolonged the life span of EAC-bearing hosts, the effect of which was mediated by augmenting antioxidant defense system and deterring lipid peroxidation.[2] The moderate inhibitory effect of FSME was also confirmed *in vitro* against the proliferation of human carcinoma cell lines and the IC_{50}s were 50 μg/mL in MCF-7 breast cancer cells and 48 μg/mL in HepG2 hepatoma cells.[2] Fennel ethanolic extract induced the cell apoptosis and inhibited the cell proliferation of mouse breast cancer 4T1 cell line (very closely mimic human breast cancer) *in vitro*.[3] Due to 100% strong free-radical scavenging activity, FSME reduced the oxidative stress and protected the cells from the damage caused by ROS.[2]

Similarly, fennel volatile oil exerted the anticarcinogenic and cytotoxic activities against human tumor cell lines *in vitro* and against murine EAC cells *in vivo*.[4] A diet with fennel seeds significantly diminished the incidences of BAP-induced forestomach papillomagenesis and DMBA-induced skin carcinogenesis in murine model systems. During the treatment, the activities of antioxidant enzymes were significantly enhanced and the activities of defensive enzymes were augmented, especially in 4% or 6% test diets. Simultaneously, the activity of glyoxalase-I and the content of glutathione (GSH) were markedly elevated, and the levels of peroxidative damage and the activity of lactate dehydrogenase were significantly reduced at all test diets.[5] Hence, these findings were clearly indicative of the safe and effective chemoprevention and antioxidation of fennel against the carcinogenesis.

Scientific Evidence of Cancer-Inhibitory and Cancer-Preventive Constituents

The phytochemical examination revealed the presence of different types of components in the FSME such as flavonoids, terpenoids, alkaloids, polyphenols, and sterols. The predominant constituents in the FSME (the herb of which was collected in north Egypt) were identified as estragole (71.10%), gallic acid (18.90%), and L-limonene (11.97%), whereas the major constituents of volatile oil (which were extracted from fennel seeds produced in China) were trans-anethole (63.4%), limonene (13.1%), fenchenone (12.1%), estragole (4.7%), γ-terpinene (2.7%), and α-pinene (1.9%).[6,7] Despite estragole (a major compound in Egypt FSME) exhibited no cytotoxic and proapoptotic activities,[5] but anethole (1, a major compound in Chinese FSME) was found to be an important anticancer agent in fennel oil.[8,9]

1. Anethole

The anticarcinogenic potential of anethole (1) was first demonstrated in the paw of Swiss albino mice-transplanted EAC, where it expanded the survival time and diminished the tumor weight and volume of EAC-bearing mice accompanied with decline of nucleic acids and malondialdehyde (MDA) levels and increase of glutathione (NP-SH) concentrations.[9] Its estrogen receptor independently suppressed the survival and proliferation of human MCF-7 and MDA-MB-231 breast cancer cell lines in parallel with the promotion of apoptosis via activation of caspase-9 and PARP1/2 cleavage, increase of c-FLIP and p53 expressions, and decrease of NF-κB transcriptional activity, in which optimal concentration of anethole (1) for the suppression was 1×10^{-3} M in the breast cancer cells.[8] More evidences showed that the block of NF-κB, AP-1, JNK, and MAPK-kinase pathways by anethole (1) also closely correlated to its role in the anticarcinogenesis and anti-inflammation.[10]

Despite only weak cytotoxicity to highly metastatic HT-1080 human fibrosarcoma cell line, the anethole treatment dose-dependently restrained the adhesion to Matrigel and the invasion of HT-1080 cells, and exerted antimetastatic effect against the HT-1080 cells via the inhibition of MMPs-2, 9, and Akt/mitogen-activated kinase/NF-κB signaling pathways.[11] Anethole (1) also had no cytotoxicity on human DU-145 prostate cancer cells but it similarly exerted preventive effect against the metastatic progression of DU-145 cells.[12,13] In addition, binary combination of anethole (1) and curcumin with platinum drugs cisplatin and oxaliplatin to treat three epithelial ovarian cancer cell lines, (1) A2780 (parent), (2) A2780cisR (cisplatin-resistant), and (3) A2780ZD0473R (ZD0473-resistant), resulted in synergistic effects in the growth inhibition of these ovarian cancer cells and the reversal of drug resistance.[14]

2. 4-methoxycinnamyl alcohol and syringin

4-methoxycinnamyl alcohol (2) and syringin (3) were also found from F. vulgare as bioactive constituents. Both were toxic to human HeLa (cervix), MCF-7 (breast), and DU145 (prostate) cancer cell lines in an in vitro assay. The IC_{50} values of 4-methoxycinnamyl alcohol (2) in all these tested cancer cell lines were 7.82, 14.24, and 22.10 μg/mL, respectively. 4-Methoxycinnamyl alcohol (2) at a concentration of 10 μg/mL did not elicit the apoptosis of cancer cells after 48 h exposure, but it caused the cell necrosis.[15,16]

3. Polysaccharides

From the dried fennel seeds, bioactive polysaccharides were isolated, which could restrain the growth of sarcoma 180 cells by 55.1% and extend the survival time by 1.2% in a mouse model with a dose of 10 mg/kg/day (i.p.).[17]

Conclusion and Suggestion

The scientific observations presented the anticancer potential of fennel seeds against the carcinomas of breast, liver, and skin in a moderate level concomitant with noticeable antioxidant activity.

Anethole (**1**) as the major constituent in fennel is markedly responsible for the anticarcinogenic, anti-cancer, and antimetastatic potentials of fennel and other bioactive constituents such as 4-methoxy-cinnamyl alcohol (**2**), syringin (**3**), gallic acid, and polysaccharides are also found to be in charge of the cancer inhibitory effect *in vitro* or *in vivo*. Consequently, the studies with phytochemistry-related chemical biology substantiated that consumption of fennel in the cuisine can afford some level of cancer preventive function to protect breast, liver, skin, prostate, and cervix, in addition to a pleasing and rich flavor and taste. The evidences clearly suggested that the frequency of fennel application in cooking should be amplified for effectively augmenting the body's capability to prevent cancer.

REFERENCES

1. Badgujar, S.B. et al., 2014. Foeniculum vulgare Mill: A review of its botany, phytochemistry, pharmacology, contemporary application, and toxicology. *BioMed Res. Int.* 2014: 842674.
2. Taie, H.A.A. et al., 2013. Chemical composition and biological potentials of aqueous extracts of fennel (Foeniculum vulgare L). *J. Appl. Sci. Res.* 9: 1759–1767.
3. Mohamad, R. et al., 2011. Antioxidant and anticarcinogenic effects of methanolic extract and volatile oil of fennel seeds (Foeniculum vulgare). *J. Med. Food* 14: 986–1001.
4. Mansourabadi, A.H. et al., 2015. Effects of fennel, asafetida and ginseng ethanolic extracts on growth and proliferation of mouse breast cancer 4T1 cell lines. *Adv. Herb. Med.* 1: 34–39.
5. El-Bastawesy, A.M. et al., 2008. Fennel seeds (Foeniculum vulgare) methanolic extract and volatile oil as antioxidant and anti-carcinogenic agents. *Egypt. J. Food Sci.* 36: 61–80.
6. Singh, B. et al., 2008. Chemomodulatory action of Foeniculum vulgare (fennel) on skin and forestomach papillomagenesis, enzymes associated with xenobiotic metabolism and antioxidant status in murine model system. *Food Chem. Toxicol.* 46: 3842–3850.
7. Villarini, M. et al., 2014. Investigation of the cytotoxic, genotoxic, and apoptosis-inducing effects of estragole isolated from fennel (Foeniculum vulgare). *J. Nat. Prod.* 77: 773–778.
8. Zhao, S.P. et al., 1991. Chemical studies on the essential oils of Foeniculum vulgare. *Acta Bot. Sin.* 33: 763–765; Wu, M.B. et al., 2001. Study on chemical components of essential oil in fructus Foeniculi from ten different areas by GC-MS. *Chin. J. Pharm. Anal.* 21: 415–418.
9. Chen, C.H. et al., 2012. Anethole suppressed cell survival and induced apoptosis in human breast cancer cells independent of estrogen receptor status. *Phytomedicine* 19: 763–767.
10. Chainy, G.B.N. et al., 2000. Anethole blocks both early and late cellular responses transduced by tumor necrosis factor: Effect on NF-κB, AP-1, JNK, MAPKK and apoptosis. *Oncogene* 19: 2943–2950.
11. Al-Harbi, M.M. et al., 1995. Influence of anethole treatment on the tumour induced by Ehrlich ascites carcinoma cells in paw of Swiss albino mice. *Eur. J. Cancer Prevent.* 4: 307–318.
12. Choo, E.J. et al., 2011. Anethole exerts antimetastatic activity via inhibition of matrix metalloproteinase 2/9 and AKT/mitogen-activated kinase/nuclear factor-κB signaling pathways. *Biol. Pharm. Bull.* 34: 41–46.
13. Rhee, Y.H. et al., 2014. CXCR4 and PTEN are involved in the anti-metastatic regulation of anethole in DU145 prostate cancer cells. *Biochem. Biophys. Res. Commun.* 447: 557–562.
14. Ha, B.C. et al., 2014. Regulation of crosstalk between epithelial to mesenchymal transition molecules and MMP-9 mediates the antimetastatic activity of anethole in DU145 prostate cancer cells. *J. Nat. Prod.* 77: 63–69.
15. Nessa, M.U. et al., 2012. Studies on combination of platinum drugs cisplatin and oxaliplatin with phytochemicals anethole and curcumin in ovarian tumor models. *Anticancer Res.* 32: 4843–4850.
16. Lall, N. et al., 2015. Cytotoxicity of syringin and 4-methoxycinnamyl alcohol isolated from Foeniculum vulgare on selected human cell lines. *Nat. Prod. Res.* 29: 1752–1756.
17. Moon, C.K. et al., 1985. Antitumor activities of several phytopolysaccharides. *Arch. Pharm. Res.* 8: 42–44.

53. GINGER

Gingembre   Ingwer   Ingwer

薑 姜 생강

Zingiber officinale

Zingiberaceae

Ginger, the rhizomes of the Zingiberaceae plant *Zingiber officinale*, is the most commonly used natural spice and condiment for various cuisines and beverages worldwide. It contains good contents of vitamin B6 and B complex, magnesium, manganese, and potassium, though it shows low nutritional value. Due to rich aromatic ingredients, ginger has a long history of medicinal application for treatment of varied human ailments, such as nausea, dysentery, heartburn, flatulence, diarrhea, loss of appetite, infections, cough, and bronchitis in different parts of the globe. Pharmacological approaches have proven ginger to possess antioxidant, anti-inflammatory, antihepatotoxic, cardiotonic, antimutagenic, antimycobacterial, and antifungal properties.

SCIENTIFIC EVIDENCE OF ANTICARCINOGENIC ACTIVITIES

Anticarcinogenic activities of ginger: Oral supplementation of ginger in a dose of 50 mg/kg/day to rats for 30 weeks significantly lessened the incidence of colon carcinogenesis caused by 1,2-dimethylhydrazine (DMH) and repressed the proliferation of colon cancer cells. Ginger also optimized tissue lipid peroxidation and antioxidant status in DMH-treated rats.[1] When the experimental rats were treated with ginger, the ethionine-induced hepatocarcinogenesis, SOD activity, and malondialdehyde level were markedly diminished and the catalase activity was amplified *in vivo* due to the abilities of ginger in repressing circulating lipid peroxidation, deterring the activities of mucinase and β-glucuronidase and potentiating the activities of glutathione peroxidase, GST, glutathione reductase, superoxide dismutase, and catalase.[2] The evidences indicated that the anticarcinogenic activity of ginger in the liver and colon was largely achieved by scavenging free-radical formation and reducing lipid peroxidation and SOD activity.[1–6] In addition, if treated with 1% ginger diet, lack of carcinogenic activity of ginger was reported.[2]

Anticancer activities of ginger: By interacting directly with cellular microtubules and disrupting tubulin structure, the aqueous ethanolic extract of ginger (GAE) suppressed the cell viability and promote the cell apoptosis of human A549 nonsmall lung cancer and HeLa cervical cancer cells *in vitro* and *in vivo*.[7] The mechanism in A549 cells was found to be also mediated by impeding two prominent targets, (1) human telomerase reverse transcriptase (hTERT) and c-myc, and (2) upregulating p53 and Bax expressions.[8] Treatment with GAE hampered the cell cycle progression, and consequently elicited human pancreatic cancer cell lines to apoptosis *in vitro* and repressed the growth of pancreatic cancer *in vivo* by inducing ROS-mediated autotic cell death without serious adverse effects.[9] GAE at 50 μg/mL concentration exerted modest inhibitory and proapoptotic effects against human HepG2 (liver), HEp-2 (larynx), and CL-6 (cholangiole) cancer cell lines, wherein the lowest IC_{50} was 9.67 μg/mL observed in HepG2 cells.[10] By an increase in superoxide production and reactive oxygen species, a saline extract prepared from ginger at a dose of 250 mg/mL markedly triggered the apoptosis of HEp-2 laryngeal cancer cells.[11] Administration of ginger ethanolic extract by lavage to mice in 40 mg/kg dose per day for 20 days promoted human HepA hepatoma cell apoptosis and the cell proliferative inhibition by 32.4%, thereby notably prolonging the survival of tumor-bearing mice.[12] More comprehensive studies have revealed that its aqueous methanolic extract disturbed the cell-cycle progression, induced a caspase-driven and mitochondrial-mediated apoptosis, then impaired the viability of human PC3 prostate cancer cells. Oral feeding of the extract (100 mg/kg per day) inhibited the growth of PC3 cell xenografts in nude mice by approximately 56% with the lack of toxicity.[13] A dietary of ginger inhibited the growth of epithelial ovarian cancer cells and modulated the secretion of angiogenic factors simultaneously.[14,15] In an *in vitro* assay, ginger EO exerted cytoxic effect against Dalton's lymphoma ascites and EAC cell lines with IC_{50}s of 18 and 11 μg/mL and against L929 mouse fibroblasts and Vero Monkey kidney epithelial cells with IC_{50}s of 41 and >100 μg/mL, respectively. The antitumor activity of ginger oil was further obseved *in vivo* against both solid and ascites types of Dalton tumors.[16] However, ginger extract did not decrease the development of mouse bladder carcinoma induced by *N*-butyl-*N*-(4-hydroxybutyl) nitrosamine (BBN).[17] If the ginger plant grew under elevated CO_2 concentration since its young age, the produced ginger demonstrated enriched antioxidant activity and moderate suppressive effect obviously in two human breast cancer cells (MCF-7 and MDA-MB-231) *in vitro*.[14]

Protective activities of ginger: P.O. giving GAE (200 and 400 mg/kg) to rat demonstrated nephroprotective effect on doxorubicin (DXN)-induced acute renal damage by preventing renal antioxidant status and increasing the activity of GST.[18] The protective effect of ginger was also observed against cisplatin-induced renal damage in rats.[19] Treatment of albino rats with ginger water extract for 4 or 6 weeks could reverse adriamycin (ADR) caused histological harm and lessened alanine aminotransferase and aspartate aminotransferase in serum together with reduced malondialdehyde (a lipid peroxidation marker) level and activated superoxide dismutase, leading to excellent antioxidant and protective effects against hepatotoxicity induced by ADR.[20]

On the basis of these findings, ginger and its extracts were known to be beneficial as a supplement agent in the cancer prevention and therapy and the decrease of toxicity caused by chemotherapeutic agents.

SCIENTIFIC EVIDENCE OF CANCER-INHIBITORY AND CANCER-PREVENTIVE CONSTITUENTS

Ginger rhizome is an excellent source of bioactive phenolics. In fresh ginger, the gingerols were identified as the major components that showed the great bioactivities in the treatment of various diseases. The anticarcinogenic property of ginger was primarily attributed to the presence of nonvolatile pungent phenolics such as gingerols (1), shogaols (2), paradols (3), as well as other curcumin-like constituents.[21–23] These representative ginger phenolic compounds showed marked antioxidant activity and remarkable potentials in anticarcinogenesis and anticancer.

1. Gingerols

6-Gingerol (1) has demonstrated proapoptotic effect in human HL-60 promyelocytic leukemia cells and human A431 epidermoid cancer cells, the effect of which was triggered by the generation of ROS. The increase of ROS level led to decrease of mitochondrial membrane potential and subsequent release of cytochrome c, activation of Apaf-1 and caspase cascade, leading the carcinoma cells to apoptotic death.[24,25] By treatment with 6-gingerol (1), the benzo[a]pyrene-induced mouse skin tumorigenesis was suppressed and the apoptosis of melanoma cells was promoted via elevating the levels of p53 and Apaf-1 and lessening the expressions of Bcl-2 and survivin.[26] 6-gingerol (1) inhibited the cell proliferation and induced apoptosis of human SW-480 colon cancer cells in association with activation of caspases and cleavage of poly(ADP-ribose) polymerase (PARP). By inhibition of ERK1/2/JNK/AP-1 pathway and activation of AP-1 (a transcription factor), 6-gingerol (1) deterred phorbol myristate acetate (PMA)-triggered proliferation of SW-480 cells.[27] Similarly, 6-gingerol (1) weakly hindered the growth of HeLa cervical cancer cells with IC_{50} of 96.32 μM concomitant with the induction of G0/G1 cell-cycle arrest and apoptosis via downregulating cyclins (A, D1, E1), activating PI3K/Akt phosphorylation with reduced P70S6K expression, and suppressing mTOR phosphorylation. Though its anti-growth rate was only 10.75%, it could sensitize the HeLa cells to chemotherapeutic drugs (e.g., 5-FU) to result in the stimulation of cell proapoptosis and the obstruction of cell growth.[28]

Moreover, the proliferation of human endothelial cells induced by both vascular endothelial growth factor (VEGF) and basic fibroblast growth factor (bFGF) was inhibited and the cell cycle was arrested in G1 phase by the 6-gingerol treatment, indicating the anti-angiogenic potential. The capillary-like tube formation in endothelial cells was blocked and the endothelial cell sprouting in rat aorta and the formation of new vessels in mouse cornea were strongly deterred in response to the anti-VEGF effect of 6-gingerol (1).[28] Therefore, due to the obvious anti-angiogenic effect, i.p. injection of 6-gingerol (1) markedly reduced the lung metastasis in mice transplanted B16F10 melanoma.[29] In addition, the migratory and invasive abilities of human HepG2 and Hep3B hepatoma cells and human MDA-MB-231 breast cancer cells were attenuated dose-dependently by 6-gingerol (1) in association with blockage of MMPs-2 and 9 activities.[30,31]

In addition, 6-gingerol (1) was capable of decreasing the TNF-α expression and inducible nitric oxide synthase (iNOS) and hindering NF-κB nuclear translocation and IκBα phosphorylation to exert chemopreventive and anti-inflammatory effects.[20] By extensive metabolism, (3R,5S)-6-gingerdiol and (3S,5S)-6-gingerdiol were formed by 6-gingerol (1) as two major metabolites in H-1299 human lung carcinoma cells. Both the metabolites were cytotoxic to the H-1299 cells after 24 h exposure. The inhibitory potency of (3R,5S)-6-gingerdiol were comparable to that of 6-gingerol (1) in the H-1299 cells.[32]

2. Shogaols

Shogaols (2) are the dehydration products of corresponding gingerols during thermal processing and storage. 6-, 8-, and 10-Shogaols, especially, 6-shogaol demonstrated stronger growth inhibitory effects ($IC_{50} \sim 8$ μM) than 6-, 8-, and 10-gingerols against human H-1299 (lung) and HCT-116 (colon) neoplastic cell lines.[33] Similar to 6-gingerol (1), 6-shogaol (2) obstructed the proliferation of human Colo205 colon cancer cells and promoted the apoptosis through modulation of ROS-involved mitochondrial functions, release of cytochrome c, and activation of caspase in Colo 205 cells, the effect of which on the Colo205 cells was much greater than 6-gingerol (1).[34] 6-Shogaol (2) effectively hampered the survival of human LNCaP, DU145, and PC3 and mouse HMVP2 prostate cancer cell lines in vitro and the growth of HMVP2 prostate cancer in vivo via blockage of STAT3 and NF-κB signaling, and induced the apoptosis of these prostate cancer cells by modulation mRNA levels of chemokine, cytokine, cell cycle, and apoptosis regulatory genes (IL-7, CCCL5, Bax, Bcl-2, p21, and p27).[35] Through a process involving caspase-mediated cleavage of eIF2α, 6-shogaol (2) markedly deterred the cell growth and elicited the apoptosis of human leukemia cell lines (U937 and Jurkat).[36] 6-shogaol (2) also displayed potent cytotoxic effect against human A549 (lung), SK-MEL-2 (skin), H-1299 (lung), HCT15 and HCT116 (colon), SKOV3 (ovary), KB (oral), and HL-60 (leukemic) cancer cell lines.[37,38] The markedly antiviability effect of 6-shogaol (2) in human oral carcinoma OC2 cells was found to be accompanied with a significant rise in $[Ca^{2+}]i$ and induction of Ca^{2+} influx via a phospholipase A^{2-} and La^{3+}-sensitive pathway.[39] The proliferation of transgenic mouse ovarian cancer cell lines such as C1 genotype (p53-/-, c-myc, K-ras) and C2 genotype (p53-/-, c-myc, Akt) could be obviously restrained by 6-shogaol (2) with $ED_{50}s$ of 0.58 and 10.7 μM, respectively.[40] In addition, 8-shogaol exerted the suppressive effect against human HL-60 promyelocytic leukemia cells *in vitro* in a concentration- and time-dependent manner, anti-leukemia activity of which was in parallel with induction of apoptosis via generation of ROS and depletion of GSH.[41] Because of some similarity in the structures, both 6-shogaol (2) as well as turmeric's curcumin influenced mPGES-1, GSK3β, and β-catenin pathway, thereby exerting the anticancer effect against A549 lung cancer cells.[42,43]

Moreover, a combined treatment with 6-shogaol (2) and TRAIL markedly induced apoptosis in various cancer cell lines (such as Caki renal cancer, MDA-MB-231 breast cancer, and U118MG glioma), but not in normal mesangial cells and normal mouse kidney cells. The 6-shogaol enhanced TRAIL-mediated apoptosis in Caki cells in association with ROS-mediated cytochrome c release and downregulation of c-FLIP(L) expression, whereas 6-gingerol (1) had no such ability.[44,45] 6-Shogaol (2), 4-shogaol as well as 8- and 10- shogaols were potent inhibitors on the invasion and migration of human MDA-MB-231 breast cancer cells and/or human HepG2 and Hep3B hepatoma cells, anti-invasive mechanisms of which were correlated with the reduction of MMP-9 (and/or MMP-2) transcription and the inhibition of NF-κB activation cascade in the breast cancer and hepatoma cells. The regulation of urokinase-type plasminogen activity was also found to be involved in the inhibition of hepatoma cell invasion by these shogaols.[30,33,44–46]

3. Paradols

Similar to 6-gingerol (1), 6-paradol (3) and its synthetic 6-dehydroparadol possess significant antitumor-promoting property with evidences in the inhibition of skin papillomagenesis and the decrease of incidence and multiplicity of melanoma initiated by 7,12-dimethylbenz[a]anthracene (DMBA) and promoted by TPA in mice. The TPA-stimulated inflammation, TNF-α production, epidermal ornithine decarboxylase activity, and the H_2O_2/UV-induced formation of oxidized DNA could be attenuated by 6-paradol (3) and 6-dehydroparadol, then resulting in the inhibitory effect on the carcinogenesis.[47–49] 6-Paradol (3) and its analogs (10-paradol, 3-dehydroparadol, 6-dehydroparadol, and 10-dehydro-paradol) displayed a marked ability to promote the apoptotic death of KB oral squamous cancer cells, where 6-dehydroparadol and 3-dehydroparadol appeared to be more potent.[50] *In vitro* experiments also proved that 6-paradol (3) and 6-gingerol (1) could promote the apoptosis of HL-60 leukemia cells and suppress the superoxide production stimulated by TPA in the differentiated HL-60 cells.[47–49] Moreover, oral administration of 6-paradol (3) in a dose of 30 mg/kg to DMBA-treated hamsters every 2 days for 14 weeks showed potent chemopreventive, antioxidant, and antilipid peroxidative activities against DMBA-induced hamster buccal pouch carcinogenesis, together with the reduction of GSH and the modulation of phase-II detoxification enzyme.[51]

4. Gingerdione

6-dehydrogingerdione (6-DG, 4) as an active constituent in ginger was effective in the inhibition of human MDA-MB-231 and MCF-7 breast cancer cells and human HepG2 hepatoma cells *in vitro*. The anti-growth effect was closely correlated to its ability to induce the cancer cells undergoing cell-cycle arrest and apoptosis via ROS generation and c-Jun *N*-terminal kinase (JNK) activation in the breast cancer cells, and via mitochondrial and Fas receptor-mediated pathways in the hepatoma cells.[52,53] 6-DG (4) was also able to sensitize HepG2 hepatoma cells synergistically to TRAIL-induced apoptotic death in association with ROS-mediated increase of DR5 expression.[53]

5. Diarylheptanoids

Some of the diarylheptanoids isolated from ginger demonstrated moderate-to-weak cyto-toxic effect and proapoptotic activity in HL-60 leukemia cells. A diarylheptanoid identified as 3,5-diacetyl-1-(3-methoxyl-4,5-di-hydroxyphenyl)-7-(4-hydroxy-3-methoxyphenyl)-heptane (5) was able to impede the proliferation of human K562 chronic myelogenous leukemia cells and adriamycin-resistant K562/ADR cells. (5) showed antioxidative (such as scavenging radicals and inhibiting lipid peroxidation) and neuroprotective activities as well.[54,55] Hexahydrocurcumin (6), a constituent present in ginger, was cytotoxic to human SW480 colorectal cancer cells followed by G1/G0 cell-cycle arrest.[56] Moreover, other diarylheptanoids isolated from ginger, such as gin-gerenone-A (7), curcumin, (E)-1,7-bis(4-hydroxy-3-methoxy-phenyl)-hept-1-ene-3,5-dione, and (E)-7-(4-hydroxy-3-methoxyphenyl)-1-(4-hydroxyphenyl)-hept-1-ene-3,5-dione were active in the inhibition of HeLa cervical cancer and MNK-45 gastric cancer cells, but 7-(3,4-dihydroxyphenyl)-5-hydroxy-1-(4-hydroxy-3-methoxyphenyl)-heptan-3-one was only active to HeLa cells. The IC_{50}s were 6.4 µmol/L in the HeLa cells, and 7.8 µmol/L in the MNK-45 cells after treatment with gingerenone-A (7).[57]

6. Zingerone

Zingerone (8), one of the active phenolics isolated from *Z. officinale*, has both antioxidant and anticar-cinogenic properties. Administration of zingerone (8) for 16 weeks suppressed 1,2-dimethylhydrazine (DMH)-induced colon carcinogenesis effectively in male Wistar rats together with modulation of tissue lipid peroxidation level and antioxidant status.[58] When cotreated with zingerone (8) and its derivative ZD-2, the metastasis (included migration and invasion) of SNU182 hepatocellular carci-noma cells synergistically deterred via blocking TGF-β1–induced epithelial–mesenchymal transi-tion, obviously hindering TGF-β1–regulated MMPs-2, -9 and Smad-2/3 activation, and restraining NF-κB nuclear translocation.[59]

7. Terpenoids

Terpenoids presented in the steam distilled extract of ginger (SDGE) are potent inhibitors on the proliferation of endometrial cancer cell lines, Ishikawa and ECC-1, at IC_{50} of 1.25 µg/mL. SDGE was also effective in eliciting cancer cell apoptosis via a rapid and strong increase of intracellular calcium, activation of p53 protein, and decrease in the mitochondrial membrane potential. Besides, SDGE could potentiate the cytotoxic effect of radiation and cisplatin.[60]

CONCLUSION AND SUGGESTION

The broad *in vitro* and *in vivo* evidences demonstrated the chemopreventive and chemothera-peutic potentials of ginger and its active components. From the proven scientific information, it is clear that ginger is a health-helpful condiment and herb being able to exert a pleiotropy of antioxidant, anti-inflammatory, antiemetic, anticancer, anticarcinogenic, and antimutagenic effects. The experimental studies have established that phenolic components of ginger, particu-larly 6-gingerol (1) and 6-shogaol (2) as the major aromatic constituents provoking the apoptotic death and inhibited the cell proliferation, viability, invasion, and metastasis against various types of neoplasm with moderate-to-weak degree. Compared to 6-gingerol (1), 6-shogaol (2) also has much stronger inhibitory effects on arachidonic acid release and nitric oxide (NO) synthe-sis to play positive roles in cancer chemopreventive, chemotherapeutic, and anti-inflammatory activities.[32] On the basis of these findings, ginger and its bioactive components have been demon-strated to be a safe, cheap, and effective complementary agent and functional condiment, being beneficial for humans in cancer prevention and treatment. Especially, it may provide certain levels of protection to stomach, colon, prostate, breast, liver, larynx, skin, and blood away from the cancer threats.

REFERENCES

1. Manju, V. et al., 2010. Effect of ginger on lipid peroxidation and antioxidant status in 1,2-dimethyl hydrazine induced experimental colon carcinogenesis. *J. Biochem. Technol.* 2: 161–167.
2. Dias, M.C. et al., 2006. Lack of chemopreventive effects of ginger on colon carcinogenesis induced by 1,2-dimethyl-hydrazine in rats. *Food Chem. Toxicol.* 44: 877–884.
3. Yusof, Y.A.M. et al., 2008. Chemopreventive efficacy of ginger (Zingiber officinale) in ethionine induced rat hepatocarcino-genesis. *Afr. J. Tradit. Complement. Altern. Med.* 6: 87–93.
4. Ahmad, N. et al., 2006. Effects of ginger extract (Zingiber officinale Roscoe) on antioxidant status of hepato-carcinoma induced rats. *Malays. J. Biochem. Mol. Biol.* 14: 7–12.
5. Manju, V. et al., 2006. Effect of ginger on bacterial enzymes in 1,2-dimethylhydrazine induced experimental colon carcinogenesis. *Eur. J. Cancer Prev.* 15: 377–383.
6. Manju, V. et al., 2005. Chemopreventive efficacy of ginger, a naturally occurring anticarcinogen during the initiation, post-initiation stages of 1,2 dimethyl-hydrazine-induced colon cancer. *Clin. Chim. Acta* 358: 60–67.
7. Choudhury, D. et al., 2010. Aqueous extract of ginger shows antiproliferative activity through disruption of microtubule network of cancer cells. *Food Chem. Toxicol.* 48: 2872–2880.
8. Tuntiwechapikul, W. et al., 2010. Ginger extract inhibits human telomerase reverse transcriptase and c-Myc expression in A549 lung cancer cells. *J. Med. Food* 13: 1347–1354.
9. Akimoto, M. et al., 2015. Anticancer effect of ginger extract against pancreatic cancer cells mainly through reactive oxygen species-mediated autotic cell death. *Plos/One* 10(5): e0126605.
10. Mahavorasirikul, W. et al., 2010. Cytotoxic activity of Thai medicinal plants against human cholangiocarcinoma, laryngeal and hepatocarcinoma cells in vitro. *BMC Complement. Alternat. Med.* 10: 55.
11. Padma, V.V. et al., 2007. Induction of apoptosis by ginger in HEp-2 cell line is mediated by reactive oxygen species. *Basic Clin. Pharmacol. Toxicol.* 100: 302–307.
12. Liu, H. et al., 2011. Ethanol extract of Zingiber officinale Rosc induces cell apoptosis and inhibits cell proliferation in mice with HepA liver cancer. *Guangdong Yixue* 32: 969–970.
13. Karna, P. et al., 2012. Benefits of whole ginger extract in prostate cancer. *Br. J. Nutr.* 107: 473–484.
14. Rahman, S. et al., 2011. In vitro antioxidant and anticancer activity of young Zingiber officinale against human breast carcinoma cell lines. *BMC Complement. Altern. Med.* 11: 76.
15. Rhode, J. et al., 2007. Ginger inhibits cell growth and modulates angiogenic factors in ovarian cancer cells. *BMC Complement. Altern. Med.* 7: 44.
16. Jeena, K. et al., 2015. Antitumor and cytotoxic activity of ginger essential oil (Zingiber officinale roscoe). *Int. J. Pharm. Pharm. Sci.* 7: 341–344.
17. Bidinotto, L.T. et al., 2006. Effects of ginger on DNA damage and development of urothelial tumors in a mouse bladder carcinogenesis model. *Environ. Mol. Mutagen.* 47: 624–630.
18. Ajith, T.A. et al., 2008. Protective effect of Zingiber officinale roscoe against anticancer drug doxorubicin-induced acute nephrotoxicity. *Food Chem. Toxicol.* 46: 3178–3181.
19. Ali, D.A. et al., 2015. Histological, ultrastructural and immunohistochemical studies on the protective effect of ginger extract against cisplatin-induced nephrotoxicity in male rats. *Toxicol. Ind. Health* 31: 869–880.
20. Sakr, S.A. et al., 2011. Protective effect of ginger (Zingiber officinale) on adriamycin-induced hepatotoxicity in albino rats. *J. Med. Plants Res.* 5: 133–140.
21. Shukla, Y. et al., 2007. Cancer preventive properties of ginger: A brief review. *Food Chem. Toxicol.* 45: 683–690.
22. Oyagbemi, A.A. et al., 2010. Molecular targets of 6-gingerol: Its potential roles in cancer chemoprevention. *BioFactors* 36: 169–178.
23. Ghosh, A.K. et al., 2011. Gingerol might be a sword to defeat colon cancer. *Int. J. Pharm. Bio. Sci.* 2: 816–827.
24. Wang, C.C. et al., 2003. Effects of [6]-gingerol, an antioxidant from ginger, on inducing apoptosis in human leukemic HL-60 cells. *In Vivo* 17: 641–645.
25. Nigam, N. et al., 2009. [6]-Gingerol induces reactive oxygen species regulated mitochondrial cell death pathway in human epidermoid carcinoma A431 cells. *Chem. Biol. Interact.* 181: 77–84.
26. Nigam, N. et al., 2010. Induction of apoptosis by [6]-gingerol associated with the modulation of p53 and involvement of mitochondrial signaling pathway in B[a]P-induced mouse skin tumorigenesis. *Cancer Chemother. Pharmacol.* 65: 687–696.
27. Radhakrishnan, E.K. et al., 2014. 6-gingerol induces caspase-dependent apoptosis and prevents PMA-induced proliferation in colon cancer cells by inhibiting MAPK/AP-1 signaling. *PLoS One* 9: e104401/1–e104401/13.

28. Zhang, F. et al., 2017. Assessment of anti-cancerous potential of 6-gingerol (Tongling White Ginger) and its synergy with drugs on human cervical adenocarcinoma cells. *Food Chem. Toxicol.* 109(Pt 2): 910–922.
29. Kim, E.C. et al., 2005. [6]-Gingerol, a pungent ingredient of ginger, inhibits angiogenesis in vitro and in vivo. *Biochem. Biophys. Res. Commun.* 335: 300–308.
30. Weng, C.J. et al., 2010. Anti-invasion effects of 6-shogaol and [6]-gingerol, two active components in ginger, on human hepatocarcinoma cells. *Mol. Nutr. Food Res.* 54: 1618–1627.
31. Lee, H.S. et al., 2008. [6]-Gingerol inhibits metastasis of MDA-MB-231 human breast cancer cells. *J. Nutr. Biochem.* 19: 313–319.
32. Lv, L.S. et al., 2012. 6-gingerdiols as the major metabolites of 6-gingerol in cancer cells and in mice and their cytotoxic effects on human cancer cells. *J. Agric. Food Chem.* 60: 11372–11377.
33. Sang, S.M. et al., 2009. Increased growth inhibitory effects on human cancer cells and anti-inflammatory potency of shogaols from Zingiber officinale relative to gingerols. *J. Agric. Food Chem.* 57: 10645–10650.
34. Pan, M.H. et al., 2008. [6]-Shogaol induces apoptosis in human colorectal carcinoma cells via ROS production, caspase activation, and GADD 153 expression. *Mol. Nutr. Food Res.* 52: 527–537.
35. Saha, A. et al., 2014. 6-Shogaol from dried ginger inhibits growth of prostate cancer cells both in vitro and in vivo through inhibition of STAT3 and NF-κB signaling. *Cancer Prev. Res.* 7: 627–638.
36. Liu, Q. et al., 2013. 6-Shogaol induces apoptosis in human leukemia cells through a process involving caspase-mediated cleavage of eIF2α. *Mol. Cancer* 12: 135/1–135/12.
37. Zhu, Y.D. et al., 2013. Metabolites of ginger component [6]-shogaol remain bioactive in cancer cells and have low toxicity in normal cells: Chemical synthesis and biological evaluation. *PLoS One* 8: e54677.
38. Peng, F. et al., 2012. Cytotoxic, cytoprotective and antioxidant effects of isolated phenolic compounds from fresh ginger. *Fitoterapia* 83: 568–585.
39. Kim, J.S. et al., 2008. Cytotoxic components from the dried rhizomes of Zingiber officinale Roscoe. *Arch. Pharm. Res.* 31: 415–418.
40. Chen, C.Y. et al., 2010. Effect of 6-shogaol on cytosolic Ca^{2+} levels and proliferation in human oral cancer cells (OC2). *J. Nat. Prod.* 73: 1370–1374.
41. Han, M.A. et al., 2015. 6-Shogaol enhances renal carcinoma Caki cells to TRAIL-induced apoptosis through reactive oxygen species-mediated cytochrome c release and down-regulation of c-FLIP(L) expression. *Chem. Biol. Interact.* 228: 69–78; Shieh, P.C. et al., 2010. Induction of apoptosis by [8]-shogaol via reactive oxygen species generation, glutathione depletion, and caspase activation in human leukemia cells. *J. Agric. Food Chem.* 58: 3847–3854.
42. Eren, D. et al., 2016. Revealing the effect of 6-gingerol, 6-shogaol and curcumin on mPGES-1, GSK-3β and β-catenin pathway in A549 cell line. *Chem. Biol. Interact.* 258: 257–265.
43. Xu, J.P., 2016. *Cancer Inhibitors from Chinese Natural Medicines*. Boca Raton, FL: CRC Press.
44. Ling, H. et al., 2010. 6-shogaol, an active constituent of ginger, inhibits breast cancer cell invasion by reducing matrix metalloproteinase-9 expression via blockade of nuclear factor-κB activation. *Br. J. Pharmacol.* 161: 1763–1777.
45. Hsu, Y.L. et al., 2012. 4-Shogaol, an active constituent of dietary ginger, inhibits metastasis of MDA-MB-231 human breast adenocarcinoma cells by decreasing the repression of NF-κB/Snail on RKIP. *J. Agric. Food Chem.* 60: 852–861.
46. Chung, W.Y. et al., 2001. Antioxidative and antitumor promoting effects of [6]-paradol and its homologs. *Mutat. Res.* 496: 199–206.
47. Lee, E. et al., 1998. Induction of apoptosis in HL-60 cells by pungent vanilloids, [6]-gingerol and [6]-paradol. *Cancer Lett.* 134: 163–168.
48. Surh, Y.J. et al., 1999. Anti-tumor-promoting activities of selected pungent phenolic substances present in ginger. *J. Environ. Pathol. Toxicol. Oncol.* 18: 131–139.
49. Han, M.A. et al., 2015. 6-Shogaol enhances renal carcinoma Caki cells to TRAIL-induced apoptosis through reactive oxygen species-mediated cytochrome c release and down-regulation of c-FLIP(L) expression. *Chem. Biol. Interact.* 228: 69–78.
50. Keun, Y.S. et al., 2002. Induction of apoptosis and caspase-3 activation by chemo-preventive [6]-paradol and structurally related compounds in KB cells. *Cancer Lett.* 177: 41–47.
51. Suresh, K. et al., 2010. Chemopreventive and antioxidant efficacy of [6]-paradol in 7,12-dimethylbenz(a)anthracene induced hamster buccal pouch carcinogenesis. *Pharmacol. Rep.* 62: 1178–1185.
52. Hsu, Y.L. et al., 2010. 6-Dehydrogingerdione, an active constituent of dietary ginger, induces cell cycle arrest and apoptosis through reactive oxygen species/c-Jun N-terminal kinase pathways in human breast cancer cells. *Mol. Nutr. Food Res.* 54: 1307–1317.

53. Chen, C.Y. et al., 2010. 6-Dehydrogingerdione sensitizes human hepatoblastoma HepG2 cells to TRAIL-induced apoptosis via reactive oxygen species-mediated increase of DR5. *J. Agric. Food Chem.* 58: 5604–5611.

54. Wei, Q.Y. et al., 2005. Cytotoxic and apoptotic activities of diarylheptanoids and gingerol-related compounds from the rhizome of Chinese ginger. *J. Ethnopharmacol.* 102: 17784.

55. Yang, L.X. et al., 2009. Antioxidative and cytotoxic properties of diarylheptanoids isolated from zingiber officinale. *Zhongguo Zhongyao Zazhi* 34: 319–323.

56. Chen, C.Y. et al., 2011. Cytotoxic activity and cell cycle analysis of hexahydrocurcumin on SW480 human colorectal cancer cells. *Nat. Prod. Commun.* 6: 1671–1672.

57. Li, N. et al., 2012. Antioxidant and cytotoxic diaryl-heptanoids isolated from Zingiber officinale rhizomes. *Chin. J. Chem.* 30: 1351–1355.

58. Vinothkumar, R. et al., 2014. Chemopreventive effect of zingerone against colon carcinogenesis induced by 1,2-dimethylhydrazine in rats. *Eur. J. CancerPrev.* 23: 361–371.

59. Kim, Y.J. et al., 2017. Combined treatment with zingerone and its novel derivative synergistically inhibits TGF-β1 induced epithelial-mesenchymal transition, migration and invasion of human hepatocellular carcinoma cells. *Bioorg. Med. Chem. Lett.* 27(4): 1081–1088.

60. Liu, Y. et al., 2012. Terpenoids from Zingiber officinale (ginger) induce apoptosis in endometrial cancer cells through the activation of p53. *PLoS One* 7: e53178.

54. ROSEMARY

Romarin   Rosmarin   Romero

迷迭香 ローズマリー 로즈메리

Rosmarinus officinalis

Lamiaceae

Rosemary, or *Rosmarinus officinalis* (Lamiaceae), originates from the needle-like leaves of an aromatic evergreen shrub. The plant has been recognized as both healthy spice and herb for culinary use and as a remedy by the European Food Safety Authority (EFSA). Rosemary carries very good amounts of vitamins A, C, and B complex and provides a good source of dietary minerals such as potassium, calcium, iron, manganese, copper, and magnesium. It is frequently consumed in Italian and Mediterranean cuisines. Besides the culinary uses, rosemary tea is a traditionally natural remedy for nervous headache, colds, and depression, and its EO is a rubefacient used to soothe the pains caused by rheumatism, gout, and neuralgia. When often daubing over the scalp, rosemary extract would help to stimulate the hair bulbs and prevent premature baldness.

SCIENTIFIC EVIDENCE OF CANCER-INHIBITORY AND CANCER-PREVENTIVE ACTIVITIES

Not only having antioxidant and anti-inflammatory activities, rosemary extract, which has antioxidant and anti-inflammatory properties, has received greater attention recently due to its reputation for anticarcinogenic benefits. At 20–80 μg/mL concentrations, the extract was able to significantly diminish the growth of both M14 and A375 human melanoma cell lines and to induce cell apoptotic demise.[1] The methanolic extract of rosemary and its *n*-hexane and chloroform fractions exerted a dose-dependent cytotoxic effect on human HeLa (cervix), HepG2 (liver), A549 (lung), HT-29 (colon), and AGS (stomach) cancer cell lines. Associating with increases of caspase-3 level and cleaved PARP, treatment with the two fractions elicited the apoptosis of HeLa and AGS cells.[2] In association with inactivation of Akt and downstream mTOR and p70S6K, the proliferation and clonogenic survival of human A549 nonsmall cell lung cancer cells was deterred together with proapoptosis after treatment with rosemary extract.[3] The extract was also effective in obviously deterring human A2780 ovarian cancer cells and CDDP-resistant A2780CP70 daughter cells together with stimulation of cell-cycle arrest and apoptosis.[4] Similarly, by directly hindering the activity of P-glycoprotein (P-gp, a transmembrane transport pump) and blocking the binding to P-gp, rosemary extract impeded the efflux of doxorubicin and vinblastine and amplified the intracellular accumulation of chemotherapeutic drugs in multidrug-resistant MCF-7 breast cancer cells.[5]

Compared to its normal extracts, supercritical fluid CO_2 rosemary extract (SFRE) displayed superior anticancer effect against various human cancer cell lines, including NCI-H82 (small cell lung carcinoma), Hep3B (hepatoma), K562 (chronic myeloid leukemia), MCF-7 and MDA-MB-231 (breast adenocarcinoma), DU-145 (prostate cancer), and prostate adenocarcinoma (PC3), though both the extracts exhibited moderate effects. The IC_{50}s attained between 12.50 and 25.98 µg/mL by SFRE but between 17.63 and 47.55 µg/mL by the normal extracts. Comparatively, K562 leukemia cells were mostly sensitive to the rosemary extracts.[6] In association with downregulation of ER-α and Her2 receptors, SFRE treatment repressed the proliferation of breast cancer cell sublines with estrogen-dependent and Her2 overexpressions. Moreover, the SFRE was also able to largely enhance the effect of anticancer drugs (tamoxifen, trastuzumab, and paclitaxel) in the chemotherapy of breast cancer.[7] The SFRE augmented the suppressive effect in both 5-FU-sensitive and 5-FU-resistant colon cancer cells in 5-FU-chemotherapy through downregulation of TYMS and TK1 enzymes, which were related to 5-FU resistance.[8]

The anticarcinogenic activity of rosemary extract was further demonstrated by *in vivo* investigations. A diet with 1.0% extract to mice significantly lessened 7,12-dimethylbenz[a]anthracene (DMBA)-induced mammary cancer formation by 47%, and markedly inhibited DMBA binding to DNA in the breast epithelial cells by ≈42%, resulting in remarkable suppressive effect against the breast gland tumorigenesis.[9] Similarly, feeding a diet with rosemary restrained benzo[a]pyrene (BAP)-induced forestomach and lung tumorigenesis.[10] The *in vivo* treatment with rosemary extract also obstructed azoxymethane (AOM)-induced colon tumorigenesis and reduced DMBA-initiated and TPA-promoted skin carcinogenesis and the melanoma size.[11,12] In addition, rosemary extract potently obstructed the DNA adduct formation induced by BAP or aflatoxin B1, together with lessening the metabolic activation of procarcinogens catalyzed by phase-I cytochrome P450 enzymes and amplification of the detoxification pathway induced by phase-II enzymes such as GST, leading to the chemopreventive action in human liver and bronchial cell models.[13] Overall, the bioactivity combined phytochemistry explorations revealed the capability of rosemary in the anticancer, anticarcinogenesis, reversal of drug resistance, and apoptosis induction but the potencies are in the ranges of moderate-to-weak.

SCIENTIFIC EVIDENCE OF CANCER-INHIBITORY AND CANCER-PREVENTIVE CONSTITUENTS

The dried powder extract of rosemary normally comprises about 16.5% ursolic acid, 3.8%–4.6% carnosol, 0.1%–0.5% carnosic acid, and several flavonoid and phenolic glycosides. The major components were assigned to be diterpenes and triterpenes in the herb. Bioactivity related chemical investigations have demonstrated that the anticancer and antioxidant properties of rosemary were principally attributed to its polyphenols and diterpenoids. Carnosol and carnosic acid were found to contribute approximately 90% of rosemary antioxidant activity.[9] The rosemary EO also exhibited the potential in the anticarcinogenesis.

1. Essential oil

By GC–MS analysis, 18 compounds were detected from the EO, which was isolated from rosemary collected in Guangzhou, China, whereas 37 compounds were identified from the EO, which was derived from rosemary collected in south France during the flower season. In the EOs, oxygenated monoterpenes constituted the main chemical class, wherein 1,8-cineole (24.10%–27.23%), α-pinene (19.43%), camphene (11.52%), camphor (14.26%), and β-pinene (6.71%).[14–16] After treatment with the EO in different concentrations, the antiproliferative effect was observed in the tested human

HeLa (cervix) and A549 (lung) tumor cell lines with IC_{50}s of 73.6 µg/mL (48h) and 8.50 µg/mL (72h), respectively.[14,15] The EOs also showed the remarkable cytotoxicity toward three other human tumor cell lines *in vitro* and its IC_{50}s were 0.025%, 0.076%, and 0.13% (v/v), respectively, in SKOV3 and HO-8910 ovarian cancer cell lines and Bel-7402 hepatoma cells. α-Pinene, β-pinene, and 1,8-cineole were effective in the *in vitro* assay against the three cancer cell lines. The IC_{50}s were 0.052%, 0.11%, and 0.32% for α-pinene, 0.12%, 0.16%, and 0.43% for β-pinene, and 1.10%, 2.90%, and 3.47% for 1,8-cineole, respectively. However, the results indicated that the major components showed lower inhibitory activity than rosemary EO in the anticancer test system and the SKOV3 cells were more sensitive to all the tested samples compared to HO-8910 and Bel-7402 cells.[16] The EOs were also able to promote the apoptosis of human HepG2 hepatoma cells in a dose- and time-dependent manner.[17] In addition, the rosemary EOs exhibited effective radical-scavenging capacity in a DPPH assay.[16] These findings disclosed that the rosemary EO provides a safe chemopreventive and adjuvant therapeutic benefits probably on hepatoma, ovarian cancer, and lung cancer.

2. Polyphenols

Rosmarinic acid (**1**, RA) is a major antioxidative polyphenol isolated from rosemary, which also exists in many kinds of plants. Pharmacological tests have proven that RA (**1**) possesses a number of biological activities, such as antifibrotic, hepatoprotective, antineurodegenerative, and anti-inflammatory properties in addition to the anticancer and anticarcinogenic potentials.

Anticarcinogenic activities of rosmarinic acid: The rosemary polyphenols were tested in chemical-elicited murine animal models for the anticarcinogenic activity. Oral RA supplementation (5 mg/kg body weight, every day for a total period of 30 weeks) to rats significantly diminished 1,2-DMH-induced colon polyps and inhibited the proliferation of colon tumor cell associated with marked protection from DMH-caused DNA damage and amplification of antioxidant status.[18–20] Similarly, oral administration of RA (**1**) completely prevented *in vivo* carcinoma formation against 7,12-dimethylbenz[a]anthracene (DMBA)-prompted skin carcinogenesis in mice and DMBA-caused oral carcinogenesis in hamsters. The anticarcinogenic effect was found to be correlated with the activation of apoptotic markers (p53, Bcl-2, caspases-3, and -9), suppression of lipid peroxidant, and stimulation of detoxification enzyme activities.[21,22] More findings revealed that RA (**1**) is an effective inhibitor against AP-1-dependant COX-2 activation and ERK1/2 activation in both HT-29 colon cancer and MCF-7 breast cancer cell lines.[23] When combined with doxorubicin (15 mg/kg), treatment with different concentrations of RA (50–200 mg/kg) noticeably diminished the frequency of micronuclei *in vivo*, presenting the antimutagenicity and cancer-preventive activity.[24]

Anticancer activities of rosmarinic acid: In an *in vitro* model, RA (**1**) exerted some suppressive effect against APC10.1 cells derived from ApcMin mouse colorectal adenoma (IC_{50} of 43 µM). *In vivo* experiment further confirmed that the chronic consumption of RA (**1**) could keep the quantifiable levels in the plasma and intestinal tract of ApcMin mice to slow the adenoma development.[25] By blockage of a MAPK/ERK pathway partly, RA (**1**) induced apoptosis of human colon carcinoma cell lines (HCT15 and CO115).[26] Treatment with RA (**1**) hampered TNFα-induced ROS generation and NF-κB activity and enhanced TNFα-induced apoptosis of human U937 leukemia cells, anti-leukemia effect of which was associated with downregulation of NF-κB-dependent antiapoptotic proteins (IAP-1, IAP-2, and XIAP), nuclear translocation of p50 and p65, and collapse of mitochondrial potential.[27] In HL-60 promyelocytic leukemia cells, RA (**1**) dose-dependently induced the cell growth inhibition and apoptosis, along with exerting radical scavenging potential and lessening nuclear deoxyribonucleoside triphosphate (dNTP) levels.[28] Similarly, RA (**1**) dose-dependently impeded parental CCRF–CEM acute lymphoblastic leukemia cells and multidrug-resistant cells (CEM/ADR5000), but had less effect on normal lymphocytes. During the anti-leukemia effect, RA (**1**) enhanced the cell apoptosis and necrosis via loss of mitochondrial membrane potential and induction of PARP-cleavage and ROS-independent DNA damage in a caspase-independent manner.[29] In addition, in a cotreatment, RA (**1**) augmented all-*trans* retinoic acid (ATRA)-induced macrophage differentiation in NB4 acute promyelocytic leukemia (APL) cells, indicating that combination of RA and ATRA has potential in the APL leukemic therapy.[30]

Antimetastatic activities of rosmarinic acid: RA (**1**) is capable of deterring the invasion and metastasis of cancer cells. The antiinvasive and antiadhesion effects of RA (**1**) were observed on human Ls174-T colon cancer cells *in vitro* and *in vivo* together with decreasing ROS level by enhancing the reduced glutathione hormone level and repressing MMPs-2 and 9 activities. Thus, i.p. administration of 2 mg of RA (**1**) lessened the Ls174-T tumor weight and the numbers of lung nodules significantly in an animal experiment.[31] Through a pathway of the receptor activator of NF-κB ligand/RANK/osteoprotegerin and blocking of IL-8 expression, RA (**1**) dose-dependently inhibited the migration of MDA-MB-231BO human bone homing breast cancer cells and repressed the bone metastasis from the breast cancer cells.[32]

Anti-angiogenic activities of rosmarinic acid: In human umbilical vein endothelial cells, RA (**1**) showed a series of important inhibitory effects against the cell angiogenesis, proliferation, migration, adhesion, and tube formation in a dose-dependent manner, showing a potential to choke blood streaming and new vessel formation in the tumor tissue. The anti-angiogenic effect of RA (**1**) was accompanied with lessening of ROS-associated VEGF expression, release of IL-8 as well as its antioxidative activity.[33] In H22 hepatoma-bearing mice, the inflammation and angiogenesis of hepatocellular carcinoma could be hindered by intragastric administration of RA (**1**) in daily oral doses of 75–300 mg/kg for 10 consecutive days, associated with block of NF-κB signaling.[34]

Radiation-protective activity of rosmarinic acid: RA (**1**) and other natural antioxidants (such as caffeic acid and *trans*-cinnamic acid) have been assayed for the abilities of radiation protection. The results displayed that the three antioxidants in nontoxic concentrations were capable of protécting human HaCaT keratinocytes from γ-radiation by 20%, 40%, and 15%, respectively, through scavenging γ-radiation-provoked intracellular ROS and declining numbers of post irradiation 53bp1 foci.[35] These findings suggest that these polyphenolics may have a potential to safeguard multiple targets in the chemo radiotherapy.

3. Diterpenoids

Carnosic acid (**2**), carnosol (**3**), rosmanol (**4**), and sageone (**5**) are the four benzenediol abietane diterpenes found from rosemary being responsible for anticarcinogenic, antioxidant, and anti-inflammatory activities. Particularly, carnosic acid (**2**) and carnosol (**3**) are the two major bioactive constituents present in the herb. They both exerted marked antiproliferative activity against a variety of cancer cells.

Anti-leukemia activities of the diterpenes: Both carnosic acid (**2**) and caronsol (**3**) were effective in the inhibition of human HL-60 promyelocytic leukemia cells *in vitro* and the IC_{50}s were 1.7 μM for carnosic acid (**2**) and 5.5 μM for carnosol (**3**).[36] During the suppression, both stimulated the apoptotic death of HL-60 cells via induction of intracellular ROS generation and mitochondrial membrane depolarization, release of cytochrome c from mitochondria, and activation of caspases cascade.[37] Carnosol (**3**) was also reported to restrain the synthesis of DNA and RNA in HL-60 cells dose-dependently.[38] The growth arrest of U937 human myeloid leukemia cells occurring by carnosic acid (**2**) at 2.5–10 μM concentration (IC_{50}s ~7 μM) was concomitant with a G1 cell-cycle arrest but no apoptosis or necrosisinduction.[39] Interestingly, carnosic acid (**2**) at low concentrations substantially augmented (100- to 1000-fold) the leukemia cell differentiation caused by all-*trans* retinoic acid- or 1,25-dihydroxyvitamin-D_3. When combined with any of these differentiation inducers, carnosic acid (**2**) synergistically obstructed the proliferation and cell-cycle progression of the leukemia cells.[39] Moreover, treatment with carnosol (**3**) promoted the apoptotic death of B-lineage leukemia cells (BLL) and adult T-cell leukemia/lymphoma (ATL).[40,41] From the findings, it is recognized that there is only one difference between carnosic acid (**2**) and carnosol (**3**) without or with lactone in their structures but largely influenced their anti-leukemia mechanisms. A methyl esteration of the carboxylic acid group in carnosic acid (**2**) would enhance the cytotoxicity against leukemia cells; however, the synthesis of carnosic acid fatty ester derivatives would reduce the anticancer and antioxidant activities.[42]

Anti-colon cancer activities of the diterpenes: *In vitro* assays showed that carnosic acid (**2**) exerted moderate-to-weak inhibitory effect against the viability of human colon cancer cell lines (HCT116, SW480, HT-29, Caco-2, and LoVo) (IC$_{50}$s 24–96 μM).[43,44] The proapoptotic effect of carnosic acid (**2**) in HCT116, SW480, and HT-29 colon cancer cells was mediated by the generation of ROS, activation of p53 and caspases, and inhibition of STAT3 signaling pathway.[45] Carnosic acid (**2**) also notably upregulated nuclear factor erythroid 2-related factor 2 (Nrf2) expression in the colon cells and deterred HCT116 xenograft tumor formation in mice.[45] In the Caco-2 cells, carnosic acid (**2**) not only promoted the cell death by apoptosis after 24 h treatment but also inhibited the cell adhesion and migration by blocking COX-2 pathway and declining the activity of secreted proteases such as uPA and MMPs.[44,47]

By augmenting ROS production and p53 function, inhibiting STAT3 signaling pathway and activating caspases, carnosol (**3**) elicited the apoptotic death and viability arrest in human HCT116 colon cancer cells in a dose- and time-dependent manner.[48] The IC$_{50}$s in human Colo205 colorectal adenocarcinoma cells were ~42 μM for rosmanol (**4**) and 29.9 μM for carnosol (**3**). When treated with 50 μM of rosmanol (**4**) for 24 h, the Colo205 cells presented a strong proapoptotic response contaminant with the regulation of both mitochondrial pathway and death receptor pathway.[49] Other diterpenes, 12-methoxycarnosic acid, taxodione, hinokione, and betulinic acid, were also found to contribute to the antiproliferative activity of rosemary in human colon cancer cells.[50]

Anti-breast and ovarian cancer activities of the diterpenes: When i.p. injection of 200 mg/kg of carnosol (**3**) or rosemary extract for 5 days, the mammary DMBA–DNA adduct formation was markedly restrained by 40% and 44% in female rats, and the DMBA-triggered breast adenocarcinoma was diminished by 65% and 74% in rats, respectively.[51] Treatment with carnosic acid (**2**) potently inhibited the proliferation of ER-human MCF-7 breast cancer cells and induced G1 cell-cycle arrest, especially for the cells transfected by Her2. However, the mechanisms were different in the ER$^-$-MCF-7 cells when treated with higher or lower doses of carnosic acid (**2**). The anti-growth effect on the ER$^-$-human breast cancer cells could be synergized with turmeric/curcumin through inhibition of Na$^+$/K$^+$-ATPase activity.[52] Similarly, carnosol (**3**) and rosmanol (**4**) also impeded the proliferation of MCF-7 breast cancer cells and metastatic F3II breast cancer cells but caused little inhibition of normal mammary cells. Under the same tested conditions, carnosic acid (**2**) and rosemary extract had only weak inhibitory effects and rosmarinic acid (**1**) had no such effect on F3II breast cancer cells.[53] The presence of carnosic acid (**2**) could counteract aflatoxin B1-induced oxidative stress and toxicity on the breast cells to achieve the anticarcinogenic activity by its remarkable free-radical scavenging capacity.[52] In addition, both carnosol (**3**) and carnosic acid (**2**) could augment the cytotoxicity of cisplatin against human A2780 ovarian tumor cells and drug-resistant A2780CP70 cells, where the A2780 cells were more sensitive to the two agents than A2780CP70 cells. At the same range of concentrations (2.5 and 20 μg/mL), carnosol (**3**) exhibited greater synergistic anticancer effect with cisplatin on the A2780 cells than carnosic acid (**2**).[4] Dietary of carnosol (**3**) also obstructed the cell adhesion on fibronectin and suppressed EGF-induced epithelial–mesenchymal transition in the ovarian cancer cell line besides suppression of the cell viability and growth in human breast, ovarian, and intestinal carcinoma cell lines.[54] If combined with curcumin, the anticancer potencies of carnosol (**3**) could be boosted synergistically against the viability of SKOV3 ovarian cancer and MDA-231 breast cancer cells and against the viability of primary cancer cells, which were derived from pleural fluid or ascites of patients with metastatic cancers.[54]

Other anticancer activities of the diterpenes: More data showed that carnosic acid (**2**) was able to elicit the apoptosis of human MDA-MB-361 (breast), SK-HEP1 (liver), and Caki (kidney) carcinoma cells and IMR-32 neuroblastoma cells, thereby hindering the cell proliferation and viability, but no effects in normal human skin fibroblast cells and normal mouse kidney epithelial TMCK-1 cells.[43,44,55] The studies revealed that the proapoptotic mechanisms of carnosic acid (**2**) were mediated by multiple pathways in different types of cancer cell lines. For instance, ROS-mediated p38 MAPK activation played a critical role in carnosic acid-induced apoptosis of IMR-32 neuroblastoma cells, and functional reactivation of p53 pathway, particularly involved in carnosol (**3**)-elicited U87MG glioblastoma cells, leading to decreasing the proliferation of brain tumor cells and sensitizing the tumor cells to chemotherapy.[55] The apoptosis of Caki renal cancer cells elicited by carnosic acid (**2**) was primarily mediated by induction of ROS-mediated endoplasmic reticulum stress, activation of p53 and endoplasmic reticulum stress marker proteins (ATF4 and CHOP), and inactivation of Src/STAT3 signaling pathway.[43] Oral administration of carnosic acid (**2**) at a dose of 10 mg/kg to hamsters completely repressed the tumor formation caused by DMBA, inhibition of hamster buccal pouch carcinogenesis which was attributed to the activities of antiproliferation, anti-inflammation, anti-angiogenesis, and apoptotic promotion.[56] Sageone (**5**) displayed cytotoxic effect against SNU-1 human gastric cancer cells with an IC$_{50}$ of 9.45 μM. In a cotreatment, sageone (**5**) elicited the SNU-1 cell apoptosis via dramatic upexpression of Akt, and then synergistically amplified the cytotoxicity of cisplatin in SNU-1 cells. The observation implied that sageone (**5**) has a great developing potential for chemotherapy of gastric cancer.[57]

Moreover, the anticarcinogenic activities of carnosol (**3**) were demonstrated in murine animal models. Dietary administration of 0.1% carnosol (**3**) lessened the intestinal tumor multiplicity by 46% and prevented colon adenoma formation *in vivo*.[58] Topical application of 10 μmol carnosol (**3**) together with 5 nmol TPA twice weekly for 20 weeks to the backs of mice previously initiated with DMBA inhibited the number of skin tumors in mouse by 78%.[59] In addition, carnosol (**3**) was able to restrain nitric oxide production and iNOS expression by blocking NF-κB activation, inhibit BAP-increased cytochrome P4501A1 activity, and strengthen the detoxifying functions of NAD(P)H quinone oxidoreductase and GST, leading to the cancer chemopreventive and anti-inflammatory effects.[38,60]

Anti-invasive and anti-angiogenic effects of the diterpenes: Anti-invasive and antimigratory effects of carnosic acid (**2**) and carnosol (**3**) were confirmed in highly metastatic mouse B16/F10 melanoma cells. In an *in vitro* Transwell system, carnosic acid (**2**) suppressed the migration and adhesion of B16F10 cells in association with an important inhibition on the epithelial–mesenchymal transitions, that is, (1) diminishment of the secretion of MMP-9, TIMP-1, uPA, and VCAM-1; (2) suppression of the mesenchymal markers snail, slug, vimentin, and *N*-cadherin, induction of epithelial marker E-cadherin; and (3) blocking of phosphorylation of Src, FAK, and Akt.[47] The anti-invasive activity of carnosol (**3**) in B16/F10 cells was also reported to primarily correlate with the inhibition of MMP-9 activity through lessening ERK1/2, Akt, p38, and JNK signaling pathway and declining NF-κB and AP-1 binding activity and c-Jun activation.[61] In addition, the anti-angiogenic activities of carnosic acid (**2**) and carnosol (**3**) were evidenced by the assays *in vitro* with endothelial cells and *in vivo* with chick chorioallantoic membrane, the anti-angiogenic property of which was believed to contribute to the inhibitory activities of rosemary extract against the proliferation and metastasis of cancer cells.[62]

4. Triterpenoids

A mixture of oleanolic acid and ursolic acid (1:1) extracted from rosemary exhibited cytotoxicity in colon cancer cells with IC$_{50}$ of 2.8 μg/mL, whereas ursolic acid showed the cytotoxicity in the same tumor cells at IC$_{50}$ value of 6.8 μg/mL, suggesting the synergistic effect of the mixture to the colon neoplastic cells.[63] Topical application of 0.1–2 μmol ursolic acid together with 5 nmol TPA twice weekly for 20 weeks to mice diminished the incidence of DMBA-initiated skin tumorigenesis by 45%–61%,[59] though ursolic acid had no inhibition in rat mammary tumorigenesis.[51] Treatment with ursolic acid could induce the apoptosis of human HL-60 leukemia cells via increasing intracellular ROS generation and mitochondrial membrane depolarization, release of cytochrome c to cytosol, and activation of caspases-3 and 9.[37] In addition, the anti-inflammatory effect of ursolic acid was found to be correlated with the inhibition of NF-κB, AP-1, and NF-AT, interactions of which might partially contribute to cancer prevention.[64]

5. Flavonoids

Several flavonoids were isolated from rosemary and some of them were found to have certain anti-tumor and antimutagenic activities. Luteolin and kaempferol were effective as the antiproliferative agents against HL-60 leukemia cells (respective IC_{50}s of 39.6 and 82.0 μM).[31] Salvigenin and cirsimaritin exhibited potent 82.0%–94.9% mutagenicity inhibition.[65]

OTHER BIOACTIVITIES

Rosemary and its bioactive constituents, especially caffeic acid derivatives, including rosmarinic acid, have multiple therapeutic potentials in treatment or prevention of bronchial asthma, spasmogenic disorders, inflammatory diseases, hepatotoxicity, peptic ulcer, atherosclerosis, ischemic heart disease, cataract, and poor sperm. Pharmacological tests have proven that rosmarinic acid possesses a number of interesting biological activities, such as antioxidative, antifibrotic, hepatoprotective, antineurodegenerative, neuroprotective,[66] and anti-inflammatory properties. Monoterpenes (such as cineol, camphene, borneol, bornyl acetate, and α-pinene) in rosemary EOs showed rubefacient, anti-inflammatory, antiallergic, antifungal, and antiseptic activities.

CONCLUSION AND SUGGESTION

As a source of both condiment and herb, the phytochemistry and chemical biology of rosemary leaves have been extensively investigated. The research results clearly disclosed that a variety of biological activities of rosemary are mostly contributed by its major constituents, that is, three diterpenes (carnosic acid, carnosol, and rosmanol) and one polyphenol (rosmarinic acid). These important constituents, in particular, have received the most attention in the exploration of their anticancer spectrum and mechanisms. The observed data provided evidences of these bioactive molecules to modulate multiple signaling pathways in different solid and blood cancers, which exerted the moderate-to-weak inhibitory effects against the carcinoma cell initiation, proliferation, invasion, and metastasis. The anticancer and anticarcinogenic activities of rosemary and these constituents should be closely associated with its antioxidant, anti-inflammatory, proapoptotic, anti-angiogenic, and radioprotective properties. Overall, these findings suggested the potential utility of rosemary as a complementary herb in the chemotherapy and chemoprevention of various types of cancers. In consideration of its other bioactivities, it is sure that incorporation of rosemary into our food system and dietary intake would show positive impact on human health promotion and cancer prevention.

REFERENCES

1. Russo, A. et al., 2009. Rosmarinus officinalis extract inhibits human melanoma cell growth. *Nat. Prod. Commun.* 4: 1707–1710; Cattaneo, L. et al., 2015. Anti-proliferative effect of Rosmarinus officinalis L. extract on human melanoma A375 cells. *PLoS One* 10: e0132439/1–e0132439/18.
2. Choi, J.H. et al., 2009. Effect of Rosmarinus officinalis L. on growth inhibition and apoptosis induction in cancer cells. *Han'guk Sikp'um Yongyang Kwahak Hoechi* 38: 1008–1015.
3. Moore, J. et al., 2016. Rosemary extract reduces Akt/mTOR/p70S6K activation and inhibits proliferation and survival of A549 human lung cancer cells. *Biomed. Pharmacother.* 83: 725–732.
4. Tai, J. et al., 2012. Antiproliferation effect of rosemary (Rosmarinus officinalis) on human ovarian cancer cells in vitro. *Phytomedicine* 19: 436–443.
5. Plouzek, C.A. et al., 1999. Inhibition of P-glycoprotein activity and reversal of multidrug resistance in vitro by rosemary extract. *Eur. J. Cancer* 35: 1541–1545.
6. Yesil-Celiktas, O. et al., 2010. Inhibitory effects of Rosemary extracts, carnosic acid and rosmarinic acid on the growth of various human cancer cell lines. *Plant Foods Hum. Nutr.* (NY, NY, USA) 65: 158–163.
7. Gonzalez-Vallinas, M. et al., 2014. Modulation of estrogen and epidermal growth factor receptors by rosemary extract in breast cancer cells. *Electrophoresis* 35: 1719–17127.

8. Gonzalez-Vallinas, M. et al., 2013. Antitumor effect of 5-fluorouracil is enhanced by rosemary extract in both drug sensitive and resistant colon cancer cells. *Pharmacol. Res.* 72: 61–68.

9. Singletary, K.W. et al., 1991. Inhibition of 7,12-dimethylbenz[a]anthracene (DMBA)-induced mammary tumorigenesis and of in vivo formation of mammary DMBA-DNA adducts by rosemary extract. *Cancer Lett.* 60: 169–175.

10. Huang, M.T. et al., 1997. Antitumorigenic activity of rosemary. In: Ohigashi H., Osawa T., Terao J., Watanabe S., and Yoshikawa T. (Eds.), *Food Factors for Cancer Prevention*, pp. 253–256. Tokyo, Japan: Springer.

11. Shao, Y. et al., 1997. Antioxidative and antitumorigenic properties of rosemary. *Book of Abstracts, 213th ACS National Meeting*, San Francisco, CA, April 13–17, AGFD-174.

12. El-Rahman, S.S.A., 2010. West-Libyan propolis and rosemary have synergistic antitumor effect against 12-O-tetradecanoylphorbol 13-acetate-induced skin tumor in BULB/C mice previously initiated with 7,12-dimethylbenz[a]anthracene. *Basic Appl. Pathol.* 3: 46–51.

13. Offord, E.A. et al., 1997. Mechanisms involved in the chemoprotective effects of rosemary extract studied in human liver and bronchial cells. *Cancer Lett.* 114: 275–281.

14. Wei, F.X. et al., 2008. Apoptosis of cervical carcinoma HeLa cells induced by essential oils from *Rosmarinus officinalis* L. *Zhongshan Daxue Xuebao, Yixue Kexueban* 29(3S): 23–25.

15. Miladi, H. et al., 2013. Essential oil of *Thymus vulgaris* L. and *Rosmarinus officinalis* L. gas chromatography-mass spectrometry analysis, cytotoxicity and antioxidant properties and antibacterial activities against foodborne pathogens. *Nat. Sci.* (Irvine, CA, USA) 5: 729–739.

16. Wang, W. et al., 2012. Antibacterial activity and anticancer activity of *Rosmarinus officinalis* L. essential oil compared to that of its main components. *Molecules* 17: 2704–2713.

17. Wei, F.X. et al., 2008. Expressions of bcl-2 and bax genes in the liver cancer cell line HepG2 after apoptosis induced by essential oils from Rosmarinus officinalis. *Zhongyaocai* 31: 877–879.

18. Karthikkumar, V. et al., 2015. Rosmarinic acid inhibits DMH-induced cell proliferation in experimental rats. *J. Basic Clin. Physiol. Pharmacol.* 26: 185–200.

19. Venkatachalam, K. et al., 2013. The effect of rosmarinic acid on 1,2-dimethylhydrazine induced colon carcinogenesis. *Exp. Toxicol. Pathol.* 65: 409–418; Venkatachalam, K. et al., 2016. Biochemical and molecular mechanisms underlying the chemopreventive efficacy of rosmarinic acid in a rat colon cancer. *Eur. J. Pharmacol.* 791: 37–50.

20. Furtado, R.A. et al., 2015. Chemopreventive effects of rosmarinic acid on rat colon carcinogenesis. *Eur. J. Cancer Prev.* 24: 106–112.

21. Sharmila, R. et al., 2012. Antitumor activity of rosmarinic acid in 7,12-dimethylbenz(a)anthracene (DMBA) induced skin carcinogenesis in Swiss albino mice. *Ind. J. Exp. Biol.* 50: 187–194.

22. Anusuya, C. et al., 2011. Antitumor initiating potential of rosmarinic acid in 7,12-dimethylbenz(a) anthracene-induced hamster buccal pouch carcinogenesis. *J. Envir. Pathol. Toxicol. Oncol.* 30: 199–211.

23. Scheckel, K.A. et al., 2008. Rosmarinic acid antagonizes activator protein-1-dependent activation of cyclooxygenase-2 expression in human cancer and nonmalignant cell lines. *J. Nutr.* 138: 2098–2105.

24. Furtado, M.A. et al., 2008. Antimutagenicity of rosmarinic acid in Swiss mice evaluated by the micronucleus assay. *Mutat. Res.* 657: 150–154.

25. Karmokar, A. et al., 2012. Dietary intake of rosmarinic acid by ApcMin mice, a model of colorectal carcinogenesis: Levels of parent agent in the target tissue and effect on adenoma development. *Mol. Nutr. Food Res.* 56: 775–783.

26. Xavier, C.P.R. et al., 2009. Salvia fruticosa, Salvia officinalis, and rosmarinic acid induce apoptosis and inhibit proliferation of human colorectal cell lines: The role in MAPK/ERK pathway. *Nutr. Cancer* 61: 564–571.

27. Moon, D.O. et al., 2010. Rosmarinic acid sensitizes cell death through suppression of TNF-α-induced NF-kB activation and ROS generation in human leukemia U937 cells. *Cancer Lett.* 288: 183–191.

28. Saiko, P. et al., 2015. Epigallocatechin gallate, ellagic acid, and rosmarinic acid perturb dNTP pools and inhibit de novo DNA synthesis and proliferation of human HL-60 promyelocytic leukemia cells: Synergism with arabinofuranosylcytosine. *Phytomedicine* 22: 213–222.

29. Wu, C.F. et al., 2015. Molecular mechanisms of rosmarinic acid from Salvia miltiorrhiza in acute lymphoblastic leukemia cells. *J. Ethnopharmacol.* 176: 55–68.

30. Heo, S.K. et al., 2015. Rosmarinic acid potentiates ATRA-induced macrophage differentiation in acute promyelocytic leukemia NB4 cells. *Eur. J. Pharmacol.* 747: 36–44.

31. Xu, Y.C. et al., 2010. Anti-invasion effect of rosmarinic acid via the extracellular signal-regulated kinase and oxidation-reduction pathway in Ls174-T cells. *J. Cell. Biochem.* 111: 370–379.

32. Xu, Y.C. et al., 2010. Inhibition of bone metastasis from breast carcinoma by rosmarinic acid. *Planta Med.* 76: 956–962.

33. Huang, S.S. et al., 2006. Rosmarinic acid inhibits angiogenesis and its mechanism of action in vitro. *Cancer Lett.* 239: 271–280.

34. Cao, W. et al., 2016. Rosmarinic acid inhibits inflammation and angiogenesis of hepatocellular carcinoma by suppression of NF-κB signaling in H22 tumor-bearing mice. *J. Pharmacol. Sci.* (Amsterdam, Netherlands) 132: 131–137.

35. Hakkim, F.L. et al., 2014. An in vitro evidence for caffeic acid, rosmarinic acid and trans-cinnamic acid as a skin protectant against γ-radiation. *Int. J. Low Radiation* 9: 305–116.

36. Bai, N.S. et al., 2010. Flavonoids and phenolic compounds from *Rosmarinus officinalis*. *J. Agric. Food Chem.* 58: 5363–5367.

37. Lin-shiau, S. et al., 2003. Induction of apoptosis by rosemary polyphenols in HL-60 cells. *ACS Symposium Series*, 859(Oriental Foods and Herbs), pp. 121–141. Washington, DC: American Chemical Society.

38. Ho, C.T. et al., 1998. Antioxidative and antitumorigenic properties of rosemary. *ACS Symposium Series*, 702(Functional Foods for Disease Prevention II: Medicinal Plants and Other Foods), pp. 153–161. Washington, DC: American Chemical Society.

39. Steiner, M. et al., 2001. Carnosic acid inhibits proliferation and augments differentiation of human leukemic cells induced by 1,25-dihydroxyvitamin D3 and retinoic acid. *Nutr. Cancer* 41: 135–144.

40. Ishida, Y.I. et al., 2014. Carnosol, rosemary ingredient, induces apoptosis in adult T-cell leukemia/lymphoma cells via GSH depletion: Proteomic approach using fluorescent two-dimensional differential gel electrophoresis. *Hum. Cell* 27: 68–77.

41. Dorrie, J. et al., 2001. Carnosol-induced apoptosis and down-regulation of Bcl-2 in B-lineage leukemia cells. *Cancer Lett.* 170: 33–39.

42. Prasad, A. et al., 2011. Anticancer and antioxidant activities of fatty ester derivatives of carnosic acid. *Abstracts of Papers, 241st ACS National Meeting & Exposition*, Anaheim, CA, March 27–31, AGFD-123.

43. Min, K.J. et al., 2014. Carnosic acid induces apoptosis through reactive oxygen species-mediated endoplasmic reticulum stress induction in human renal carcinoma Caki cells. *J. Cancer Prev.* 19: 170–178; Park, J.E. et al., 2016. Carnosic acid induces apoptosis through inactivation of Src/STAT3 signaling pathway in human renal carcinoma Caki cells. *Oncol. Rep.* 35(5): 2723–2732.

44. Barni, M.V. et al., 2012. Carnosic acid inhibits the proliferation and migration capacity of human colorectal cancer cells. *Oncol. Rep.* 27: 1041–1048.

45. Kim, D.H. et al., 2016. Carnosic acid inhibits STAT3 signaling and induces apoptosis through generation of ROS in human colon cancer HCT116 cells. *Mol. Carcinog.* 55: 1096–1110.

46. Yan, M. et al., 2015. Standardized rosemary (Rosmarinus officinalis) extract induces Nrf2/sestrin-2 pathway in colon cancer cells. *J. Funct. Foods* 13: 137–147.

47. Park, S.Y. et al., 2014. Carnosic acid inhibits the epithelial-mesenchymal transition in B16F10 melanoma cells: A possible mechanism for the inhibition of cell migration. *Int. J. Mol. Sci.* 15: 12698–12713.

48. Park, K.W. et al., 2014. Carnosol induces apoptosis through generation of ROS and inactivation of STAT3 signaling in human colon cancer HCT116 cells. *Int. J. Oncol.* 44: 1309–1315.

49. Cheng, A.C. et al., 2011. Rosmanol potently induces apoptosis through both the mitochondrial apoptotic pathway and death receptor pathway in human colon adenocarcinoma COLO 205 cells. *Food Chem. Toxicol.* 49: 485–493.

50. Borras-Linares, I. et al., 2015. A bioguided identification of the active compounds that contribute to the antiproliferative/cytotoxic effects of rosemary extract on colon cancer cells. *Food Chem. Toxicol.* 80: 215–222.

51. Singletary, K. et al., 1996. Inhibition by rosemary and carnosol of 7,12-dimethylbenz[a]anthracene-induced rat mammary tumorigenesis and in vivo DMBA-DNA adduct formation. *Cancer Lett.* (Shannon, Ireland) 104: 43–48.

52. Einbond, L.S. et al., 2012. Carnosic acid inhibits the growth of ER-negative human breast cancer cells and synergizes with curcumin. *Fitoterapia* 83: 1160–1168; Costa, S. et al., 2007. Carnosic acid from rosemary extracts: A potential chemoprotective agent against aflatoxin B1. *J. Appl. Toxicol.* 27: 152–159.

53. Cao, S.W. et al., 2001. Study on anti-mammary cancer activity of rosemary extract and its anti-oxidative constituent. *Yingyang Xuebao* 23: 225–229.

54. Vergara, D. et al., 2014. Antitumor activity of the dietary diterpene carnosol against a panel of human cancer cell lines. *Food Funct.* 5: 1261–1269.

55. Tsai, C.W. et al., 2011. Carnosic Acid, a rosemary phenolic compound, induces apoptosis through reactive oxygen species-mediated p38 activation in human neuroblastoma IMR-32 cells. *Neurochem. Res.* 36: 2442–2451; Giacomelli, C. et al., 2016. New insights into the anticancer activity of carnosol: p53 reactivation in the U87MG human glioblastoma cell line. *Int. J. Biochem. Cell Biol.* 74: 95–108.

56. Rajasekaran, D. et al., 2013. Proapoptotic, anti-cell proliferative, anti-inflammatory and anti-angiogenic potential of carnosic acid during 7,12 dimethylbenz[a]anthracene-induced hamster buccal pouch carcinogenesis. *Afr. J. Tradit. Complement. Altern. Med.* 10: 102–112.

57. Shrestha, S. et al., 2016. Sageone, a diterpene from Rosmarinus officinalis, synergizes with cisplatin cytotoxicity in SNU-1 human gastric cancer cells. *Phytomedicine* 23: 1671–1679.

58. Moran, A.E. et al., 2005. Carnosol inhibits β-catenin tyrosine phosphorylation and prevents adenoma formation in the C57BL/6J/Min/+(Min/+) mouse. *Cancer Res.* 65: 1097–1104.

59. Huang, M.T. et al., 1994. Inhibition of skin tumorigenesis by rosemary and its constituents carnosol and ursolic acid. *Cancer Res.* 54: 701–708.

60. Lin, J.K. et al., 2003. Carnosol from rosemary suppresses inducible nitric oxide synthase through down-regulating NF-κB in murine macrophages. *ACS Symposium Series*, 859(Oriental Foods and Herbs), pp. 66–86. Washington, DC: American Chemical Society; Lo, A.H. et al., 2002. Carnosol, an antioxidant in rosemary, suppresses inducible nitric oxide synthase through down-regulating NF-κB in mouse macrophages. *Carcinogenesis* 23: 983–991.

61. Huang, S.C. et al., 2005. Carnosol inhibits the invasion of B16/F10 mouse melanoma cells by suppressing metalloproteinase-9 through down-regulating NF-kB and c-Jun. *Biochem. Pharmacol.* 69: 221–232.

62. Lopez-Jimenez, A. et al., 2013. Anti-angiogenic properties of carnosol and carnosic acid, two major dietary compounds from rosemary. *Eur. J. Nutr.* 52: 85–95.

63. Barcia, R.N. et al., 2014. Antitumor triterpenoid acids extracted from *Thymus mastichina*. Portuguese Patent Application PT 106536 A 20140313.

64. Checker, R. et al., 2012. Potent anti-inflammatory activity of ursolic acid, a triterpenoid antioxidant, is mediated through suppression of NF-κB, AP-1 and NF-AT. *PLoS One* 7: e31318.

65. Nakasugi, T. et al., 1997. Antimutagenic and anticancer salvigenin and cirsimaritin from Rosmarinus officinalis. Jpn. Kokai Tokkyo Koho JP 09176009 A 19970708.

66. Roberto de Oliveira, M., 2016. Carnosic acid affords mitochondrial protection in chlorpyrifos-treated Sh-Sy5y cells. *Neurotoxic. Res.* 30: 367–379; Roberto de Oliveira, M., 2016. Protective effect of carnosic acid against paraquat-induced redox impairment and mitochondrial dysfunction in SH-SY5Y cells: Role for PI3K/Akt/Nrf2 pathway. *Toxicol. In Vitro* 32: 41–54.

55. STAR ANISE

Anis étoilé   Sternanis   Anís estrellado

八角茴香 スターアニス 팔각회향

Illicium verum

Winteraceae

Star anise, or *Illicium verum*, is a dried fruit with eight-pointed star from a Winteraceae plant native to southern China and southern Asia. This is an EO-rich tree widely grown in most Asian countries. Star anise is not only commonly used as a condiment in culinary art, but also prescribed as an herb for promotion of appetite and digestion and treatment of abdominal pain and digestive disturbances. Star anise also provides a relief from rheumatism and escalates mother breast-milk secretion. Pharmacological inspections ascertained that star anise has carminative, stomachic, stimulant, estrogen-like, leukocyte-increasing, antioxidant, diuretic, antifungal, and antibacterial properties. However, other similar *Illicium* trees and their fruits look similar to those of star anise but the fruits with six- or seven-pointed star are inedible due to high toxicity; for instance, Japanese star anise (*I. anisatum*) causes severe inflammation of kidneys, urinary tract, and digestive organs by its toxicins anisatin, shikimin, and sikimitoxin.

SCIENTIFIC EVIDENCE OF CANCER-INHIBITORY AND CANCER-PREVENTIVE CONSTITUENTS

The chemopreventive potential of star anise was evaluated in an *in vivo* model with *N*-nitrosodiethylamine (NDEA) initiated and phenobarbital (PB) promoted hepatocarcinogenesis. Treatment with ethanol–water (1:1) soluble extract of star anise for 20 weeks could reduce nodule incidence and nodule size/volume significantly in rats and lowered the lipid peroxidation in liver and erythrocytes. Simultaneously, the decreased oxidative stress and the increased phase-II enzymes were accompanied by the anticarcinogenic effect, that is, GST level notably declined in the erythrocyte and liver; CAT activity was augmented in the erythrocyte, and GSH level in the liver and superoxide dismutase activity in the erythrocyte and liver were restored to normal levels, then leading to the contribution for anti-hepatocarcinogenic effect.[1] Star anise EO showed prominent antioxidant and radical scavenging effects in DPPH and FRAP models and exerted moderate suppressive effect against the proliferation, migration, invasion, and colony formation of human HCT-116 colon cancer cells in an *in vitro* model together with inducing cell apoptotic death. The IC_{50} value was 50.34 μg/mL and one of the major compounds was identified as *trans*-anethole in the EO by GC–MS inspection.[2]

1. Phenolics

Shikimic acid (1) is a key aromatic compound isolated from star anise seeds, the time- and dose-dependently of which suppressed the proliferation of HepG2 hepatoma cells in an *in vitro* assay and elicited the cell apoptosis and G1 cell-cycle arrest, proapoptotic effect of which was mediated by downregulation of Bcl-2 and NF-κB (p65) expressions and upregulation of Bax expression.[3,4] In addition, anethole (2) demonstrated the inhibitory effects against the growth of human MCF-7 and MDA-MB-231 breast neoplastic cell lines regardless of estrogen receptor statuses.[5] The antiinvasive and antimetastatic effect of anethole (2) was showed in human HT-1080 highly metastatic fibrosarcoma cells and human DU-145 prostate cancer cells despite its weak cytotoxicity.[6–8] Its *in vivo* anticarcinoma activity was established in the paw of Swiss albino mice implanted EAC.[9] Other two phenolics, illiciumflavane acid (3) and (E)-1,2-bis(4-methoxyphenyl)ethene (4) were also separated from the fruits of *I. verum*, two of which obviously deterred the proliferation of human A549 lung adenocarcinoma cells with IC_{50}s of 4.63 and 9.17 μM, respectively.[10]

2. Structural modification

Anethole dithiolethione (= anethole trithione, 5), a substituted dithiolthione of anethole, was produced by structural modification, which displayed a more chemopreventive potential in both *in vivo* and *in vivo* models. Dietary anethole trithione (5) at 40% and 80% maximum tolerated doses to the tested animals obstructed azoxymethane (AOM)-induced colon carcinogenesis significantly.[11] In a protocol, the animals were exposed to nontoxic doses of anethole trithione (5) in the diet markedly inhibiting the multiplicity of DMBA-caused mammary cancer cells but not effecting cancer incidences.[12] A randomized phase-IIb trial further confirmed the chemopreventive activity of the anethole derivative. Thrice-daily oral administration of 25 mg anethole dithiolethione (5) to smokers with bronchial dysplasia for 6 months infectiously declined the lung carcinogenic rates. The chemopreventive and chemotherapeutic effect was found to be mainly contributed by its radical scavenging and GSH-inducing properties.[13,14]

3. Polysaccharides

Crude polysaccharides were extracted from star anise fruits with 10.50% yield, which consisted of xylose, arabinose, and glucose in molar ratios of 1:4.8:18.3. In an *in vivo* test, the star anise polysaccharides suppressed the growth of sarcoma 180 cells by 30.92% at a dose of 720 mg/kg without obvious influences on the indexes of spleen and thymus as compared with a control model.[15]

CONCLUSION AND SUGGESTION

The present reported research results demonstrated that the anticarcinogenic and anticancer potentials and remarked antioxidant, radical scavenging, and hepatoprotective properties of star anise fruits. Due to these biological activities, star anise and its EO effectively hampered the liver cancer initiation and the proliferation and invasion of colon cancer cells. The isolated polyphenolics such as shikimic acid (1), anethole (2), illiciumflavane acid (3), and (E)-1,2-*bis*(4-methoxyphenyl)ethene (4) were designated to be molecules being responsible for the cancer suppressive effect against several human hepatoma, breast cancer, and lung cancer cell lines *in vitro*. Most important, anethole (2) showed obvious antimetastatic potential in prostate cancer and fibrosarcoma cell lines. In addition, the polysaccharides from star anise fruits were also found to possess certain antitumor activity in an *in vivo* model. According to these scientific observations, star anise can be considered as a cancer preventive flavoring, which not only gives us delighted taste but also enhances some possibilities to lessen cancer risk, as well as other health benefits, including stomachic, antioxidant, stimulant, diuretic, and leukocyte-increasing effects.

REFERENCES

1. Yadav, A.S. et al., 2007. Chemopreventive effect of star anise in N-nitrosodiethylamine initiated and phenobarbital promoted hepatocarcinogenesis. *Chem. Biol. Interact.* 169: 207–214.
2. Asif, M. et al., 2016. Anticancer attributes of Illicium verum essential oils against colon cancer. *South Afr. J. Bot.* 103: 156–161.
3. Zhu, K.M. et al., 2014. Influence of shikimic acid on proliferation and expression of nuclear factor-κB in human hepatoma HepG2 cells. *Zhongguo Shiyan Fangjixue Zazhi* 20: 126–129.
4. Zhu, K.M. et al., 2014. Shikimic acid inducing apoptosis on hepatocellular carcinoma HepG2 cells through decreasing the ratio of Bcl-2/Bax. *Zhongguo Shiyan Fangjixue Zazhi* 20: 154–158.
5. Chen, C.H. et al., 2012. Anethole suppressed cell survival and induced apoptosis in human breast cancer cells independent of estrogen receptor status. *Phytomedicine* 19: 763–767.
6. Choo, E. et al., 2011. Anethole exerts antimetastatic activity via inhibition of matrix metalloproteinase 2/9 and AKT/mitogen-activated kinase/nuclear factor-κB signaling pathways. *Biol. Pharm. Bull.* 34: 41–46.
7. Rhee, Y.H. et al., 2014. CXCR4 and PTEN are involved in the anti-metastatic regulation of anethole in DU145 prostate cancer cells. *Biochem. Biophys. Res. Commun.* 447: 557–562.
8. Ha, B.C. et al., 2014. Regulation of crosstalk between epithelial to mesenchymal transition molecules and MMP-9 mediates the antimetastatic activity of anethole in DU145 prostate cancer cells. *J. Nat. Prod.* 77: 63–69.
9. Chainy, G.B.N. et al., 2000. Anethole blocks both early and late cellular responses transduced by tumor necrosis factor: Effect on NF-κB, AP-1, JNK, MAPKK and apoptosis. *Oncogene* 19: 2943–2950.
10. Wu, L.D. et al., 2016. A new flavane acid from the fruits of Illicium verum. *Nat. Prod. Res.* 30: 1585–1590.
11. Reddy, B.S. et al., 1994. Chemoprevention of colon cancer by thiol and other organosulfur compounds. *ACS Symposium Series*, 546(Food Phytochemicals for Cancer Prevention I), pp. 164–172. Washington, DC: American Chemical Society.
12. Lubet, R.A. et al., 1997. Chemopreventive efficacy of anethole trithione, N-acetyl-L-cysteine, miconazole and phenethylisothiocyanate in the dmba-induced rat mammary cancer model. *Int. J. Cancer* 72: 95–101.
13. Lam, S. et al., 2002. A randomized phase IIb trial of anethole dithiolethione in smokers with bronchial dysplasia. *J. Nat. Cancer Inst.* 94: 1001–1009.
14. Christen, M.O. et al., 2002. Anethole dithiolethione: A radical scavenger beneficial in bronchial dysplasia in smokers. In: Pasquier, C. (Ed.), *Proceedings of Biennial Meeting of the Society for Free Radical Research International, 11th*, Paris, France, July 16–20, pp. 433–438.
15. Shu, X. et al., 2010. Extraction, characterization and antitumor effect of the polysaccharides from star anise (Illicium verum Hook.f.). *J. Med. Plants Res.* 4: 2666–2673.

56. THYME

Thym   Thymian   Tomillo

百里香 タイム 백리향

Thymus vulgaris, T. mongolicus, T. quinquecostatus

Lamiaceae

Thyme is the dried leaves of several *Thymus* genus plants. *Thymus vulgaris* is the most common variety, the evergreen subshrub of which is useful in the garden as a groundcover and in cooking and natural remedy since the ancient era in the regions of Egypt, Greece, and southern Italy. Nutritionally, thyme is an excellent source of vitamin C and a good source of vitamin A, iron, manganese, copper, and fiber. It acts as a health beneficial herb and affords noteworthy biological properties. Especially, thyme oils demonstrated a wide range of chemotherapeutic effects such as anti-inflammatory, antirheumatic, antispasmodic, carminative, cardiac, diuretic, expectorant, and antimicrobial activities. The EOs are very helpful for the treatment of cystitis and urethritis.

SCIENTIFIC EVIDENCE OF CANCER-INHIBITORY AND CANCER-PREVENTIVE ACTIVITIES

In an *in vitro* assay, an ethyl acetate fraction, which was fractionated from the ethanolic extract of *T. quinquecostatus*, markedly suppressed the proliferations of human K562 and HL-60 leukemia cell lines in a concentration-dependent manner, together with the induction of the leukemia cells to apoptosis.[1] Daily intragastric administration of ethanolic extract of *T. quinquecostatus* to mice in doses of 40 g (crude drug)/kg and 20 g (crude drug)/kg for 9 days resulted in the inhibitory effect against the growth of sarcoma 180 cells *in vivo* by 51.5% and 36.4%, respectively. However, the extract at its higher dose simultaneously caused abnormal immunological reactions, that is, decrease of spleen index and thymus index, and then inclination of the spleen index to normal level.[2] A methanolic extract of *T. serpyllum* (wild thyme) prompted significant cytotoxicity in human MCF-7 and MDA-MB-231 breast cancer cell lines *in vitro* but not in normal cells. The extract also elicited the apoptosis of MDA-MB-231 cells together with inhibiting the activities of DNA methyltransferase (DNMT) and histone deacetylase (HDAC).[3] Consequently, the bioactivity related phytochemical approaches provided a comprehensive insight into the anticarcinogenic, anticancer, and antioxidant properties of thyme. Despite the fact that the cancer inhibition observed in the investigations was low, the application of thyme (a natural food flavor additive) can be encouraged as a valuable supplementation for the prevention and therapy of malignant tumors.

Scientific Evidence of Cancer-Inhibitory and Cancer-Preventive Constituents

1. Essential oils

The aromatic EO derived from three thyme plants (*T. vulgaris*, *T. serpyllum*, and *T. algeriensis*) showed obvious inhibitory effect on the cancers in the *in vitro* assays. The EO from *T. vulgaris* (TVEO) was effective in the growth suppression of various human neoplastic cell lines, such as A549 lung adenocarcinoma, head and neck squamous cell carcinoma (HNSCC), MCF-7 breast adenocarcinoma, MDA-MB-435 breast cancer, NCI-H460 nonsmall cell lung carcinoma, U937 lymphoma, THP-1 monocytic leukemia, AGS gastric cancer, HCT-115 and HCT-116 colon cancer and HepG2 hepatoma, and murine P815 mastocytoma, with moderate-to-weak active degrees.[1–11] The IC_{50} values of TVEO were 10 µg/mL in U937 cells and MDA-MB-435 cells,[8] 10.50 µg/mL (72 h) in A549 cells,[5] 41 µg/mL (48 h) in HepG2 cells, 60 µg/mL (48 h) in MCF-7 cells, and 75 µg/mL (48 h) in A549 cells.[6] The cell apoptotic promotion and cell-cycle arrest elicited by TVEO in the HNSCC cells were mediated by the regulation of interferon signaling, *N*-glycan biosynthesis and ERK5 signaling pathways.[4] The suppression of TVEO in the HCT-116 colon cancer cells was correlated with apoptotic promotion as evidenced by activation of caspases-3 and 7. The TVEO also exerted antimigratory and anti-invasive activities on the HCT-116 cells through blocking the adhesion to fibronectin in a dose-dependent manner.[10] The TVEO showed no efficacy against PLP2 nontumor cells and less sensitivity to lymphocytes and nonmalignant cells.[6,8]

Similarly, the EOs extracted from *T. algeriensis* (TAEO) and *T. serpyllum* (TSEO) showed the levels of inhibitory effects in four human neoplastic cell lines (NCI-H460, MCF-7, HCT-15, and AGS), but the activities of TSEO were better due to the GI_{50} of 7.02–52.69 µg/mL for TSEO, 62.12–64.79 µg/mL for TAEO, and 76.02–180.40 µg/mL for TVEO. The MCF-7 breast carcinoma cells were the most resistant to these EOs among the tested tumor cell lines and the TSEO was the most potent on all the tested cells.[8] The EO extracted from Moroccan endemic thyme (*T. broussonettii*), which contains carvacrol as a major component, showed interesting cytotoxic effect against several drug-resistant human ovarian adenocarcinoma cell lines *in vitro*, and exerted a significant anti-growth effect on murine P815 mastocytoma *in vivo* by intratumoral injection.[12] The EO of *T. citriodorus* having borneol and thymol as the major components exerted potent cytotoxic effect in human HepG2 hepatoma cells and stimulated the cell apoptosis.[13]

Furthermore, the EO and the extracts derived from thyme displayed potent free-radical scavenging and lipid peroxidation-inhibiting activities in the antioxidant assays, the capacities of which importantly contributed to the anticarcinogenetic and anticancer potentials of thyme.[5,9] Nevertheless, the thyme EOs, especially thymol (its major component), also possess immunosuppressive function. Other *in vitro* tests showed that the EOs dose-dependently restrained the inducible lymphocytes and human peripheral blood mononuclear cells.[14,15] Daily intragastric administration of the thyme oil to mice-implanted sarcoma 180 in two doses (40 g or 20 g crude drug/kg) for 9 days elicited abnormal interactions on immune, that is, augmentation of spleen index but declination of thymus index.[2]

2. Monoterpenes

The hydrodistilled EOs obtained from several thyme species were analyzed by GC–MS. TVEO (endemic to France) were revealed to contain 31 different compounds, which represented 99.64% the thyme oil, wherein thymol (41.33%) was identified as a major constituent.[5] In addition, a range of other monoterpenes, such as *p*-cymene, myrcene, borneol, and linalool, were detected from the thyme oil.[5] The chemical composition of Moroccan thyme populations showed that the major constituents were thymol, borneol, *p*-cymene, and carvacrol.[14] From the TVEO, of which *T. vulgaris* was purchased from local markets in Jazan, Saudi Arabia, 42 compounds in total were examined to represent more than 97.6% of the oil composition, wherein the major components were thymol (54.26%), γ-terpinene (9.50%), *p*-cymene (7.61%), carvacrol (4.42%), terpinolene (3.27%), α-terpinene (2.36%), α-terpineol (1.63%), and α-tujene (1.52%).[6] In addition, the GC–MS examination of three thyme oils revealed thymol (**1**) being 48.9%, 56.0%, and 38.5%, respectively, in *T. vulgaris*, *T. algeriensis*, and *T. serpyllum*, plants of which were collected from other different places.[16]

In various *in vitro* models, thymol (**1**) and carvacrol (**2**) displayed an important dose-dependent inhibitory effect against the proliferation of human HepG2 and/or Bel-7402 hepatoma and Caco-2 colon cancer cell lines, murine P815 mastocytoma, and hamster V79 lung tumor cell lines and showed a potent antioxidant effect against H_2O_2-elicited DNA strand breaks in HepG2 and Caco-2 cells,[14–18] wherein carvacrol (**2**) was mildly more active than thymol (**1**) and Caco-2 cells were more resistant to the both monoterpenes than V79 and HepG2 cells.[17] The anti-growth activity of carvacrol (**2**) in HepG2 cells was found to be associated with the promotion of the cell apoptosis. The results also implied that a mitogen-activated protein kinase pathway played an important role in the antihepatoma effect of carvacrol (**2**).[19] Interestingly, thymol (**1**) showed higher cytotoxicity in drug-resistant H1299 human lung cancer cells, although both thymol (**1**) and carvacrol (**2**) were weakly cytotoxic to its parental H1299 cells.[20] More *in vitro* antiproliferative effects of carvacrol (**2**) were observed in the treatment of human tumor cell lines such as A549 (nonsmall cell lung), DU-145 (prostate), HeLa and SiHa (cervix), MDA-MB-231 and MCF-7 (breast) cancer cells, and rat leiomyosarcoma cells, showing moderate-to-weak degree of anticancer activities.[21–26] The inhibitory effect on the DU-145, HeLa, SiHa, MDA-MB-231, and MCF-7 tumor cell lines were closely correlated with the proapoptosis.[22–25] Carvacrol (**2**) also significantly deterred the invasion capability of DU-145 prostate cancer cells via suppression of MMP-2 activity.[22] At 200–600 μM, carvacrol (**2**) accelerated the cell apoptosis and at ~800 μM killed human glioblastoma cells. The cell apoptosis induction might be mediated by a ROS-increase and $[Ca^{2+}]$i-rise mechanism.[27]

Besides, the anticarcinogenic activity of carvacrol (**2**) was observed in several *in vivo* models. I.p. injection of 0.1 mg/kg carvacrol (**2**) to rats resulted in potent inhibitory effect against 7,12-dimethylbenz[a]anthracene-triggered lung tumor.[28] The incidences of benzo[a]pyrene-caused leimyosarcoma and fibrosarcoma in rats were also lessened by 30% and the survival rates of the rats were extended after the administration of carvacrol (**2**).[26] In diethylnitrosamine (DEN)-induced hepatocellular carcinogenesis in rats, the inhibitory effect of carvacrol (**2**) was accompanied with markedly diminishment of lipid peroxidation and hepatic cell damage and improvement of antioxidant system *in vivo*.[29] The antiproliferative and antimetastatic effects of carvacrol (**2**) were also observed in male rat model with DEN-induced hepatocellular carcinoma.[30]

Terpinolene (**3**) is another monoterpene present in the EOs of many aromatic plant species, including thyme. Through diminution of Akt1 expression, the proliferation of human K562 erythroleukemic cells was restrained by terpinolene (**3**) *in vitro*.[31] *In vivo* treatment with terpinolene (**3**) at various doses obviously hindered the proliferation of rat N2a neuroblastoma cells. However, if in the doses of ≥100 mg/L, terpinolene (**3**) elicited the inhibition on primary rat neurons.[32] Similarly, carvacrol (**2**) at 200 and 400 mg/L was able to minimize the proliferation rates markedly in both K562 and N2a cell lines.[33] These findings suggested that terpinolene (**3**) and carvacrol (**2**) in the suitable dose range may be safe antiproliferative and antioxidative agents in some types of carcinoma cells, including erythroleukemia and brain cancer cells.

3. Phenols and flavonoids

Four acetophenone glycosides were isolated from a butanol-soluble extract of thyme. Among them, 4-hydroxyaceto-phenone 4-O-[5-O-(3,5-dimethoxy-4-hydroxybenzoyl)-β-D-apiofuranosyl]-(1-2)-β-D-glucopyranoside (**4**) showed some cytotoxic and DNA synthesis-inhibiting activities in human HL-60 leukemia cells *in vitro* with IC_{50}s of 40 μM.[34] Naringenin (**5**), a natural flavanone separated from *T. vulgaris*, demonstrated anti-growth effect against human breast (HTB26 and HTB132) and colorectal (SW1116 and SW837) cancer cell lines (IC_{50}s of 4.0 mM) in a dose- and time-dependent manner together with the induction of S and G2/M cell-cycle arrest and apoptotic cell death, where the proapoptotic effects were mediated by upregulation of proapoptotic genes (p18, p19, p21, caspases, Bak, AIF, and Bax), downregulation of antiapoptotic genes (Cdk4, Cdk6, Cdk7, Bcl-2, x-IAP, and c-IAP-2), and suppression of cell-survival factors (PI3K, pAkt, pIκBα, and NF-κBp65).[35] In addition, a rosmarinic acid and methoxylated flavones-rich polyphenol extract, which was derived from *T. vulgaris* plant cultivated in the Campania region (Italy), repressed the cell viability and induced the apoptosis of SH-SY5Y and SK-N-BE$_2$-C neuroblastoma cell lines at 62.5–125 µg/mL concentrations, antibrain cancer effects of which were found to be associated with the inhibition of mitochondrial redox activity, increase of intracellular ROS levels, activation of caspases-8 and 3, and significant decrease of nucleic acid/amide-II ratio.[36]

OTHER BIOACTIVITIES

By pharmacological investigations, the therapeutic significance of carvacrol (**2**) has also been revealed to have antioxidant, antihelmintic, antiplatelet aggregation, analgesic, antifungal, antibacterial, and insecticidal properties.

CONCLUSION AND SUGGESTION

A wide range of chemical biology investigations have been carried out on the cancer-inhibitory and preventive effects of thyme leaves. The thyme extracts from *T. quinquecostatus* and *T. serpyllum* showed the antiproliferative and antiviability effects against human leukemia cells and human breast carcinoma cells, respectively. The cancer inhibitors in the thymes (*T. vulgaris*, *T. algeriensis*, and *T. serpyllum*) were revealed to be in the monoterpenes-rich EOs, monoterpenes, flavonoids, and polyphenols. The EOs in the *in vitro* assays displayed broad anticancer spectrum with moderate-to-weak active degrees, and showed the *in vivo* anti-growth activity on mouse sarcoma 180 and P815 mastocytoma. Two major monoterpenes assigned as thymol (**1**) and carvacrol (**2**) in the EOs, especially carvacrol (**2**), were mostly in charge of the anticancer and anticarcinogenic activities of EOs, but thymol (**1**) was the major constituent in thyme EOs. Terpinolene (**3**) is another monoterpene from thyme EOs, which exerted the inhibitory effect against human leukemia and brain cancer cell lines *in vitro*. In addition of the EOs and monoterpenes, polyphenols and flavonoids are also the different types of cancer inhibitors isolated from thyme against several human leukemic, colon, breast, and brain cancer cell lines but showing weak activities. Most of the anticancer and anticarcinogenic effects were confirmed to closely correlate with their abilities of antioxidant and apoptosis induction. Despite the fact that the anticancer potencies of all these bioactive molecules are far from meeting the chemotherapeutic requirement, thymes containing these anticancer constituents can be useful for cancer chemoprevention and may be considered as one kind of food supplement and a potential therapy adjuvant.

REFERENCES

1. Sun, Z.X. et al., 2005. Antitumor effect of ethanol extracts from *Thymus quinquecostatus* Celak on human leukemia cell line. *Zhongxiyi Jiehe Xuebao* 3: 382–385.
2. Sun, Z.X. et al., 2003. Original studies on antitumor and immunological effect of extracts from *Thymus quinquecostatus* Celak in mice. *Zhongxiyi Jiehe Xuebao* 1: 209–210, 238.
3. Bozkurt, E. et al., 2012. Effects of *Thymus serpyllum* extract on cell proliferation, apoptosis and epigenetic events in human breast cancer cells. *Nutr. Cancer* 64: 1245–1250.
4. Sertel, S. et al., 2011. Cytotoxicity of *Thymus vulgaris* essential oil towards human oral cavity squamous cell carcinoma. *Anticancer Res.* 31: 81–87.
5. Miladi, H. et al., 2013. Essential oil of *Thymus vulgaris* L. and *Rosmarinus officinalis* L. Gas chromatography-mass spectrometry analysis, cytotoxicity and antioxidant properties and antibacterial activities against foodborne pathogens. *Nat. Sci.* (Irvine, CA, USA) 5: 729–739.

6. Fatimah, A.A., 2014. Chemical composition, antioxidant and antitumor activity of *Thymus vulgaris* L. essential oil. *Middle East J. Sci. Res.* 21: 1670–1676.

7. Nikolic, M. et al., 2014. Chemical composition, antimicrobial, antioxidant and antitumor activity of *Thymus serpyllum* L., *Thymus algeriensis* Boiss. and Reut and *Thymus vulgaris* L. essential oils. *Ind. Crops Prod.* 52: 183–190.

8. Amirghofram, Z. et al., 2001. Cytotoxic activity of thymus vulgaris, achillea millefolium and Thuja orientalis on different growth cell lines. *Med. J. Islam. Rep. Iran* (MJIRI), 15: 149–154.

9. Aazza, S. et al., 2014. Antioxidant, anti-inflammatory and anti-proliferative activities of Moroccan commercial essential oils. *Nat. Prod. Commun.* 9: 587–594.

10. Al-Menhali, A. et al., 2015. *Thymus vulgaris* (Thyme) inhibits proliferation, adhesion, migration, and invasion of human colorectal cancer cells. *J. Med. Food* 18: 54–59.

11. Ayesh, B.M. et al., 2014. In vitro inhibition of human leukemia THP-1 cells by *Origanum syriacum* L. and *Thymus vulgaris* L. extracts. *BMC Res.* 7: 612.

12. Ait M'Barek, L. et al., 2007. Cytotoxic effect of essential oil of thyme (*Thymus broussonettii*) on the IGR-OV1 tumor cells resistant to chemotherapy. *Braz. J. Med. Biol. Res.* 40: 1537–1544.

13. Wu, S. et al., 2013. Chemical composition of essential oil from *Thymus citriodorus* and its toxic effect on hepatoma cells. *Zhongyaocai* (5): 756–759.

14. Abdeslam, J. et al., 2007. Chemical composition and antitumor activity of different wild varieties of Moroccan thyme. *Rev. Bras. Farmacogn.* 17: 477–491.

15. Amirghofran, Z. et al., 2011. In vitro immunomodulatory effects of extracts from three plants of the Labiatae family and isolation of the active compound(s). *J. Immunotoxicol.* 8: 265–273.

16. *Thymus algeriensis* were collected from Zentan, Libya; *Thymus serpylum* is a commercial sample from a Greek local pharmacy; *Thymus vulgaris* were collected at the experimental field of the Institute for Medicinal Plant Research "Josif Pančić" in Pančevo, Serbia.'

17. Slamenova, D. et al., 2007. DNA-protective effects of two components of essential plant oils carvacrol and thymol on mammalian cells cultured in vitro. *Neoplasma* 54: 108–112.

18. Yin, Q.H. et al., 2010. Antitumor efficacy of thymol. *Prog. Mod. Biomed.* 10: 2073–2075.

19. Yin, Q.H. et al., 2012. Anti-proliferative and pro-apoptotic effect of carvacrol on human hepatocellular carcinoma cell line HepG2. *Cytotechnology* 64: 43–51.

20. Ozkan, A. et al., 2012. A comparative study of the antioxidant/prooxidant effects of carvacrol and thymol at various concentrations on membrane and DNA of parental and drug resistant H1299 cells. *Nat. Prod. Commun.* 7: 1557–1560.

21. Koparal, A. et al., 2003. Effects of carvacrol on a human non-small cell lung cancer (NSCLC) cell line, A549. *Cytotechnology* 43: 149–154.

22. Li, G. et al., 2014. Anti-prostate cancer effect of carvacrol via MAPK signaling pathway. *Dier Junyi Daxue Xuebao* 35: 285–290.

23. Mehdi, S.J. et al., 2011. Cytotoxic effect of carvacrol on human cervical cancer cells. *Biol. Med.* 3: 307–312.

24. Arunasree, K.M., 2010. Anti-proliferative effects of carvacrol on a human metastatic breast cancer cell line, MDA-MB 231. *Phytomedicine* 17: 581–588.

25. Al-Fatlawi, A.A. et al., 2014. Cytotoxicity and pro-apoptotic activity of carvacrol on human breast cancer cell line MCF-7. *World J. Pharm. Sci.* 2: 1218–1223.

26. Karkabounas, S. et al., 2006. Anticarcinogenic and antiplatelet effects of carvacrol. *Exp. Oncol.* 28: 121–125.

27. Liang, W.Z. et al., 2012. Carvacrol-induced [Ca2+]i rise and apoptosis in human glioblastoma cells. *Life Sci.* 90: 703–711.

28. Zeytinoglu, M. et al., 1998. Inhibitory effects of carvacrol on DMBA induced pulmonary tumorigenesis in rats. *Acta Pharm. Turcica* 40: 93–98.

29. Jayakumar, S. et al., 2012. Potential preventive effect of carvacrol against diethylnitrosamine-induced hepatocellular carcinoma in rats. *Mol. Cell. Biochem.* 360: 51–60.

30. Subramaniyan, J. et al., 2014. Carvacrol modulates instability of xenobiotic metabolizing enzymes and downregulates the expressions of PCNA, MMP-2, and MMP-9 during diethylnitrosamine-induced hepatocarcinogenesis in rats. *Mol. Cell. Biochem.* 395: 65–76.

31. Okumura, N. et al., 2012. Terpinolene, a component of herbal sage, downregulates AKT1 expression in K562 cells. *Oncol Lett.* 3: 321–324.

32. Aydin, E. et al., 2013. Anticancer and antioxidant properties of terpinolene in rat brain cells. *Arhiv. Za Higijenu Rada. i Toksikologiju* 64: 415–424.

33. Aydin, E. et al., 2014. The effect of carvacrol on healthy neurons and N2a cancer cells: Some biochemical, anticancerogenicity and genotoxicity studies. *Cytotechnology* 66: 149–157.

34. Wang, M.F. et al., 1999. Acetophenone glycosides from thyme (*Thymus vulgaris* L.) *J. Agric. Food Chem.* 47: 1911–1914.

35. Abaza, M.S.I. et al., 2015. Growth inhibitory and chemo-sensitization effects of naringenin, a natural flavanone purified from *Thymus vulgaris*, on human breast and colorectal cancer. *Cancer Cell Int.* 15: 1–35.

36. Pacifico, S. et al., 2016. A polyphenol complex from *Thymus vulgaris* L. plants cultivated in the Campania region (Italy): New perspectives against neuroblastoma. *J. Funct. Foods* 20: 253–266.

7 Cancer-Preventive Substances in Beverages

> 57. Coffee/*Coffea arabica, C. canephora, C. liberica*
>
> 58. Tea/*Camellia sinensis*

This chapter primarily addresses two basic beverages, coffee and tea, and their remarkable potential in cancer prevention, antioxidation, as well as several other health-improving functions. The approaches combined with phytochemistry and chemical biology have provided extensive and solid research evidences to support dietary intake of coffee and tea in human daily life. The biologically active substances in coffee and tea are helpful in eliminating pathogenic factors early and also serve in improving health conditions. For keeping an effective level of bioactive substances in the body, multiple cups of coffee and tea daily is indispensable. However, it is better to limit the consumption to 5 or 6 cups per day for most people, which also depends on personal conditions. Excess intake of the two beverages would induce negative health effects owing to caffeine content. Little or no sugar is also advised in coffee drinking because sugar is favorable for cancer development and excess weight gain. Fruit juices and the discussion of their health benefits are integrated in Chapter 5 together with fresh fruits.

Herbal teas are popular beverages in Eastern Asia, especially in China. Here, four kinds of oriental health upgrading herbal teas are introduced, which are individually made of dried wolfberry, dendrobe, honeysuckle flower, and white chrysanthemum. The first two can be used annually, whereas the latter two are commonly used in summer. The anticarcinogenic activities of the first three herbs have been extensively discussed in a book titled *Cancer Inhibitors from Chinese Medicines* (published by CRC Press in the end of 2016).

57. COFFEE

Café   Kaffee   Café

咖啡   コーヒー   커피

Coffea arabica, C. canephora, C. liberica

Rubiaceae

Coffee is one of the most popular beverages in the world and is derived from the seeds of berries from several *Coffea* plants. Roasted coffee beans are broadly consumed in nearly all zones and by all social classes of the population, especially in western countries. The coffee consumption with diverse modes of preparation reached approximately two billion cups per day despite the fact that coffee beans are not a nutrient-rich food and afford only small amounts of minerals and vitamins. Due to its higher caffeine content, coffee often gives humans a stimulating effect. Various clinical investigations suggest that moderate consumption of coffee is beneficial in healthy adults; however, caffeine can be harmful when consumed to excess.

SCIENTIFIC EVIDENCE OF CANCER PREVENTION

In recent decades, coffee has been subjected to research projects for evaluating the role of coffee intake on various types of carcinomas. The investigations revealed that coffee drinking is associated with a reduced risk of cancers in breast, colon/colorectal, liver, kidney, endometrial, head/neck, and so on.[1,2] The coffee-roasting process may enhance the chemopreventive activity of coffee beans against carcinogenesis.[3,4]

Coffer and colon/colorectal cancer: The protective effect of coffee drinking (4–5 cups/day) was demonstrated on colon carcinogenesis in a large U.S. cohort study and on colon adenomas (a precursor of colon cancer) in a middle-aged Japanese population.[5,6] Compared to intake of caffeinated coffee predominantly, the more significant prevention of colon and rectal cancers was observed for people drinking decaffeinated coffee predominantly.[6] Treatment with 2.5% (v/v) coffee for 24 h suppressed cytosolic estrogen sulfotransferase (SULT) activity and reduced SULT1E1 gene expression in human Caco-2 colon carcinoma cells but no significant changes in the expression of other SULT genes (SULT1A1 and SULT1A3) or UGT genes (UGT1A1 and UGT1A6). These findings indicated that daily intake of coffee can modify sulfo-conjugation reactions within intestinal epithelial cells and then enhance the estrogenic activity in the colon, thereby affecting the bioavailability of anticancer drugs and reducing the toxicity of environmental chemicals.[7,8] By blocking phosphorylation of ERKs and transactivation of AP-1 and NF-κB and notably inhibiting TPA-, EGF-, and H-Ras-induced neoplastic transformation of JB6 P+ epidermal cells, coffee drinking lessened ERKs phosphorylation in patients with colon cancer.[9] By strongly inhibiting mitogen-activated MEK1 and TOPK activities, the coffee deterred CT-26 colon cancer cell-induced lung metastasis.[9] However, diets with 1% coffee to rats failed to restrain the formation of azoxymethane (AOM)-induced aberrant crypt foci (ACF) in colon due to less fiber. By the same method, 10% coffer fiber obstructed AOM-induced colonic ACF in terms of total numbers of crypt multiplicity and numbers of ACF/cm^2 colon mucosa.[10] The findings revealed the coffee fiber to be an important agent for colon protection. According to a Spanish study, the soluble fiber in a single cup of coffee was 1.8 g for instant coffee, 1.5 g for espresso, and 1.1 g for filtered coffee. In addition, after diets containing 6% coffee given to mice for 5 days, glutamate cysteine ligase catalytic (GCLC) subunit and the mRNA levels of chemopreventive enzymes, that is, NAD(P)H:quinone oxidoreductase-1 (NQO1), glutathione S-transferase class-α1 (GSTA1), and UDP-glucuronosyl transferase 1A6 (UGT1A6) were enhanced by ~20-fold in the small intestine, leading to cancer prevention. These interactions were found to be mediated by Nrf2, a transcription factor.[11]

Coffee and endometrial/uterine cancer: A cup per day of coffee drinking can reduce the risk of endometrial cancer by 7%–10%, preventive effect of which appeared the greatest for women who are overweight. The potential mechanism in the decrease of endometrial cancer incidence by coffee drinking was mediated by the elevation of circulating sex hormone-binding globulin levels and/or improvement of insulin sensitivity.[12] According to Harvard University analyzed data in 67,470 women between the ages of 34 and 59, drinking 2–3 cups/day of coffee had 7% less chance of developing endometrial cancer, and 4 cups/day of coffee had a 25% lower risk of uterine cancer.[13]

Coffee and hepatoma: The studies revealed that 1–3 cups of coffee per day can decline the risk of developing hepatocellular carcinoma (HCC) by 29%. Compared to non-consumption of coffee per day, any coffee intake lessened the risk of HCC by 40%. Hence, coffee consumption reverses the incidence of liver carcinogenesis.[14,15] In a rat model, long-term coffee drinking restrained nitrosamine formation and repressed hepatocarcinogenesis caused by nitrosamine.[16] An *in vitro* assay exhibited that instant coffee powder (ICP) and ICP-loaded rat blood sera suppressed the proliferation and invasion of rat AH109A ascites hepatoma cells. The antiproliferative activity was correlated with the induction of cell-cycle arrest and apoptosis and the anti-invasive activity was mediated by decreasing oxidative stresses and scavenging ROS. In a male rat model with hepatoma, 0.1% ICP was fed in diet for 14 days hampered the proliferation of hepatoma cells and lessened the tumor metastases to lung and lymphatic nodes, associating with amelioration of abnormal lipoprotein profiles *in vivo*.[17] When diets containing 3% or 6% coffee are given to mice for 5 days, the mRNA levels of two chemopreventive enzymes, NQO1 and GSTA1 could be augmented for the cancer prevention in liver and small intestine by 4- and 20-fold.[11] Similarly, an increased coffee consumption also delayed the progression of fibrogenesis and mortality in patients with chronic and particularly alcohol liver diseases but without diabetes, HBV-, or HCV-negative cases, resulting in hindering the liver carcinogenesis and fibrogenesis.[15,18]

Coffee and breast cancer: A hospital-based, case-control study revealed that coffee intake can lead to decrease in the risk of breast cancer in premenopausal women, but showed no clear association between decaffeinated coffee consumption and breast cancer risk.[19] However, recent investigations signified that higher coffee drinking (≥5 cups/day), but not total caffeine, was able to decline the risk of estrogen receptor (ER) negative and postmenopausal breast cancers in independent CYP1A2 genotype.[20] Moderate (2–4 cups/day) to high (≥5 cups/day) coffee intake could diminish ER+ breast tumor proportion and repress primary breast tumor cell invasion. The moderate-to-high consumption also synergistically lowered the risk of breast cancer in tamoxifen-treated patients with the ER+ breast tumors (Tamoxifen is a drug for prevention and therapy of breast cancer).[21] The high intake of coffee not only impeded ER and cyclin D1 abundance in the ER+ cells prominently but also decreased insulin-like growth factor-I receptor (IGFIR) and pAkt levels in both ER+ MCF-7 cells and ER− MDA-MB-231 cells.[21] The observation implied that coffee drinking is helpful to lower the breast carcinogenesis and to enhance the bioavailability of tamoxifen to breast tumor cells.

Coffee and oral/head cancers: For testing the role of coffee on nasopharyngeal carcinoma (NPC), a case-control study was conducted in Taiwan with a total of 375 incident NPC cases and 327 controls. Daily coffee intake could significantly inverse the trend of NPC risk.[22] A prospective U.S. cohort study showed that >4 cups intake of caffeinated coffee each day lowered the risk of oral/pharyngeal cancer death by 49% compared to no/occasional coffee intake.[23] Similarly, another pooled analysis pointed out more than four cups of caffeinated coffee per day had a 39% lower risk of getting head/neck cancer.[24] In a hamster model, feeding whole roasted coffee exerted the inhibitory effect against the development of 7,12-dimethylbenz[a]anthracene (DMBA)-induced oral carcinomas by ≥50%.[25]

Coffee and brain cancer: A total of 335 incident cases of gliomas (men, 133; women, 202) were analyzed in three independent cohort studies, finding a statistically significant inverse association between caffeinated coffee and risk of glioma. The results suggest that at least five cups of coffee per day may prevent glioma by 40%. However, intake of decaffeinated coffee or total flavonoid from coffee did not affect the risk of glioma.[26]

Coffee and melanoma: A large U.S. cohort investigation resulted in higher coffee intake (≥4 cups/day) modestly lowering the risk of malignant melanoma, wherein caffeinated coffee was more statistically significant than decaffeinated coffee.[27] Orally giving coffee to SKH-1 mice for 2 weeks stimulated UVB-induced apoptosis and inhibited UVB-induced carcinogenesis in epidermis, but the treatment was safe for non-UVB treated normal epidermis.[28]

Coffee and prostate cancer: According to a report in 2009, a prospective investigation first found that drinking six cups of coffee each day had a 60% lower risk of aggressive prostate cancer compared to not drinking any coffee. The daily habit with six cups of coffee also led to a reduction in the risks of all forms of prostate cancer by 18% and of advanced prostate cancer by 53%.[29] In human-derived PC3 prostate cancer cells, coffee suppressed TNFα-induced NF-κB activity and DNA binding and then elicited apoptosis and modulated expression of a number of inflammation- and cancer-related genes in TNFα-treated PC3 cells. The anti-NF-κB and anti-inflammatory activities were deterred and the transcription of genes related to PC3 prostate cancer was hindered in mice receiving coffee. The findings further suggested the preventive mechanism links between coffee consumption and prostate cancer.[30]

Coffee and other cancers: A bone marrow micronucleus test revealed that pretreated gavage of decaffeinated or caffeinated instant coffee (140 mg/kg/day) to tested animals obviously inhibited genotoxicities caused by mitomycin C (MMC), cyclophosphamide (CP), benzo[a]pyrene (BAP), 7,12-dimethylbenz[a]anthracene (DMBA) or procarbazine (PCB), and moderately increase hepatic sulfhydryl (–SH) content and glutathione S-transferase (GST) activity.[31] In addition, the extract of spent coffee still exhibited more anticancer activity on P388 leukemia cells than the extract of low-grade green coffee beans (LCB), but the LCB extract had better radical-scavenging activity (92%) than spent coffee extract (82%–87%),[32] implying that the LCB and spent coffee also have chemopreventive effect.

1. Phenolic extract and compounds

Polyphenolic extract of coffee showed the inhibitory effects against human HeLa cervical cancer cells *in vitro*, activity of which was related to its prooxidant, proapoptotic, and antiproliferative activities but was less than the phenolic extract of green tea.[33] Two common phenolic acids, chlorogenic acid (**1**) and caffeic acid (**2**), were found in the isolates of coffee, both of which are also present in many foods and various herbs, showing anti-inflammatory, antioxidant, antidiabetic, and anticarcinogenic activities. Due to coffee beans containing high levels of chlorogenic acids (**1**), they are considered the richest dietary source of this phenolic acid. In the *in vivo* models, chlorogenic acid (**1**) in an oral dose of 150 mg/kg restrained nitrosamide formation and reduced a number of micronucleated cells in bone marrow and nuclear aberrations in colonic epithelial cells in mice, leading to reduction of mutagenic and carcinogenic risks.[34] 0.025% Chlorogenic acid (**1**) in a diet for 24 weeks obviously lowered numbers of hyperplastic liver cell foci and incidence of colon tumor caused by methylazoxymethanol acetate in hamsters.[35] Similarly, chlorogenic acid (**1**) exerted a regressive effect on the formation and development of ACF in AOM-prompted colorectal carcinogenesis in rats.[36] At a dose of 250 μM, chlorogenic acid (**1**) highly diminished miRNA 146A expression in HepG2 hepatoma cells (series 1886), presenting its potential in chemopreventive therapy on HCC.[37] In addition, from immature and green coffee beans, another six derivatives of chlorogenic acid (**1**, = 3-caffeoylquinic acid) were isolated, such as 4-caffeoylquinic acid, 5-caffeoylquinic acid, 5-feruloylquinic acid, 3,4-dicaffeoylquinic acid, 3,5-dicaffeoylquinic acid, and 4,5-dicaffeoylquinic acid. These derivatives exhibited weak antiproliferative effect against four carcinoma cell lines (U937, MCF-7, KB, and WI38-VA) in an *in vitro* assay, wherein KB cells were the most sensitive (IC_{50}s of 0.10–0.56 mM). However, these three dicaffeoylquinic acids exhibited 1.0–1.8-fold potent free–radical scavenging property than common antioxidants such as α-tocopherol and ascorbic acid.[38]

Compared to chlorogenic acid, caffeic acid (**2**) more effectively downregulated UVB-caused COX-2 expression at transcriptional level through inhibition of AP-1 and NF-κB transcription activities in mouse skin epidermal (JB6 P+) cells. In an *in vivo* test, caffeic acid (**2**) decrease of UVB-induced COX-2 expression by directly blocking Fyn kinase activity, leading to suppressed UVB-induced mouse skin carcinogenesis. Similarly, by directly targeting ERK1/2 activity, caffeic acid (**2**) exerted the chemopreventive activity against solar UV-induced skin carcinogenesis and the inhibitory effect against colony formation of human skin cancer cells in both *in vitro* and *in vivo* assays.[39–41] The antioxidant activity of caffeic acid was found to relate to its metal-chelating property so that it was able to prevent hydroxyl radical formation promoted by a classical Fenton reaction. In the test, caffeic acid (**2**) acted as an antioxidant through an iron-chelating mechanism, leading to prevention of free hydroxyl radical formation and suppression of Fenton-induced oxidative damage.[42] The findings could be explanation to its beneficial effects in the chemoprevention on skin cancer. Treatment with caffeic acid (**2**) resulted in the anti-growth effect against both human ER+ and ER− breast cancer cell lines but it was more sensitive to ER+ cells than to ER− cells.[23] Caffeic acid germanium could obstruct the growth of mouse U14 cervical cancer cells in association with induction of G2/M cell arrest and cell apoptotic death. The anti-growth rate (47.28%) in U14 cells was a little lower than that of cyclophosphamide (54.27%) in the same treatment condition.[41]

In addition, caffeic acid (**2**) was revealed to act as a dual mechanism on GSTP1/GSR1 and Nrf2/Keap1 pathways, that is, it can act both as inducers and inhibitors of GSTP1/GSR1 and Nrf2/Keap1, displaying that the effects of coffee on healthy humans and cancer patients are different, for example, healthy ovarian cells and cisplatin-resistant ovarian cancer cells. In healthy cells, caffeic acid (**2**) showed an ability to rescue healthy cells by preventing GST activity as a potential chemotherapeutic adjuvant, whereas in cisplatin-resistant A2780 cancer cells, it induced Nrf2 and phase-II enzymes and oxidation of Keap1 protein, events of which may enhance the cell resistance to the treatment.[43] The observation implied that the use of coffee in people under chemotherapeutic treatment should be monitored with care.

2. Alkaloids

Caffeine (**3**) is the major alkaloid component in caffeinated coffee. Overdose of caffeine is normally harmful to human health but it reduced the levels of insulin-like growth factor-I receptor (IGFIR) and pAkt and suppressed the growth of ER$^+$ ($P \leq 0.01$) and ER$^-$ ($P \leq 0.03$) human breast cancer cell lines in an *in vitro* assay, accompanied with stopped cell-cycle progression and enhanced cell death. It was also able to sensitize the ER$^+$ and ER$^-$ cells to tamoxifen (a FDA-approved preventive agent for breast tumor in women).[23] Oral administration of caffeine solution at a cancer-preventive level to mice for 2 weeks suppressed tumor formation and stimulated UVB-induced apoptosis in tumor cells but not in normal epidermis, subsequently obstructed UVB-induced skin carcinogenesis.[31] In a cotreatment, caffeine (**3**) augmented cisplatin-induced apoptotic death of both HTB182 and CRL5985 lung cancer cell lines and synergistically enhanced the lung cancer cell killings by cisplatin, together with inhibition of ATR and activation of ATM.[44]

Trigonelline (**4**), an inhibitor of nuclear factor E2-related factor 2 (Nrf2), is also found in coffee, especially in Arabica coffee, Nrf2 of which plays an essential role in cancer development and chemoresistance. By inhibition of Nrf2 transcription, trigonelline (**4**) restrained proteasome gene expression and its activity and then rendered the tested Panc1, Colo357, and MiaPaca2 pancreatic cancer cell lines that are more susceptible to apoptosis, showing beneficial in the improvement of cancer chemotherapy.[45] During the coffee-roasting process, the heat elicited a Maillard reaction between an amino acid and a reducing sugar to produce some carboxylic metabolites such as pyrazinoic acid (**5**) and methylpyrazinoic acids. At 0.05 and 1.0 mmol/L concentrations, pyrazinoic acid (**5**) and its mono-, di- and trimethylated derivatives could inhibit 10%–60% of invasion of human HepG2 hepatoma cells via Matrigel, wherein 3,5-dimethylpyrazinoic acid is the most potent inhibitor among these methylpyrazinoic acids, exhibiting significant anti-invasive effect at a concentration of 50 μmol/L.[46]

3. Diterpenoids

Cafestol (**6**) and kahweol (**7**) are the major and specific diterpenes in coffee beans. Both are present in coffee bean oil and unfiltered coffee drinks (such as French press coffee, Turkish coffee, and Greek coffee), but are negligible in filtered coffee drinks such as drip brewed coffee. Pharmacological approaches established the two diterpenes possessing antioxidant, hepatoprotective, anti-inflammatory, hypercholesterolemic, and anticarcinogenic properties. In several animal models, cafestol/kahweol mixture (C/K) and cafesol (**6**) exerted the chemopreventive effect against mutagenesis and carcinogenesis caused by carcinogens, including 2-amino-1-methyl-6-phenylimidazo [4,5-b]pyridine (PhIP), DMBA, and aflatoxin B1 (AFB1), effect of which was attributed to their abilities in regulation of several enzymes to detoxify carcinogens and modify xenobiotic metabolisms via enhancing conjugating enzymes (UDP-glucuronosyltransferase, GST, and/or glucuronosyl S-transferases), deactivating cytochrome P450 (CYP 2C11 and CYP 3A2), which are involved in carcinogen activation, activating hepatic O(6)-methylguanine-DNA methyltransferase for DNA repair, augmenting antioxidant enzymes (γ-glutamyl cysteine synthetase and heme oxygenase-1) for cellular defense, repressing sulfotransferase, and/or increasing quinone oxidoreductase-1 mRNA. By the induction of human GST, the C/K mixture was able to significantly obstruct covalent binding of AFB1 genotoxic metabolites to DNA.[13,47–52] These evidences have confirmed the cancer-preventive potential of cafestol (**6**) and kahweol (**7**), especially for protection of colon, liver, and kidney.

The anticancer and proapoptotic activities of cafestol (**6**) and kahweol (**7**) were further demonstrated by the *in vitro* experiments. In the treatment of human MSTO-211H malignant pleural mesothelioma cells, both the diterpenes increased sub-G1 population and nuclear condensation and induced the cell apoptosis via declining the expression levels of specificity protein 1 (Sp1), cyclin-D1, Mcl-1, and survivin proteins, leading to the antiproliferative and antiviability effects on the highly aggressive cancer cells. The $IC_{50}s$ (48 h) ranged between 56 and 82 µM in MSTO-211H and H28 mesothelioma cell lines.[53] By downregulation of antiapoptotic proteins and inhibition of phosphatidylinositol 3-kinase (PI3K)/Akt signal pathway, cafestol (6) stimulated the apoptosis of human Caki renal cancer cells. TRAIL is a marked apoptosis-inducing agent on a wide variety of neoplastic cells. Kahweol (7) was able to sensitize TRAIL-induced apoptosis in Caki renal carcinoma cells via downregulation of Bcl-2 and c-FLIP.[54,55] Moreover, kahweol (7) was capable of stimulating the apoptosis of human cancer cell lines such as HN22 and HSC4 (oral squamous cell), MDA-MB-231 (breast), HT-29 (colon), A549 (lung), U937 (promonocyte), and HL-60 (leukemic).[56–60] Its proapoptotic mechanisms were revealed to be mediated by (1) downregulation of antiapoptotic factors (Bcl-2, Bcl-xL, Mcl-1, and XIAP) and release of cytochrome c; (2) upregulation of caspases and poly(ADP-ribose) polymerase; (3) blockage of JNK and/or Akt signal pathways (such as in HT-29 and U937 cells); (4) increase in reactive oxygen species (such as in MDA-MB-231 cells); (5) downregulation of Sp1 (such as in HN22 and HSC4 cells), and (6) blockage of STAT3 signaling pathway (such as in A549 cells).[56–60] The anticancer activity of kahweol (7) in TH-29 cells was also contributed by its ability in suppression of heat shock protein 70 expression.[567] Its IC_{50} values were 60–82 µM in estrogen receptor-negative MDA-MB-231 breast carcinoma, HT-29 colon adenocarcinoma, HL-60 leukemia, and HT-1080 fibrosarcoma cell lines.[58] Together with lessening cyclin D1 protein level, kahweol (7) exerted a moderate antiproliferative effect against human HCT116 and SW480 colorectal cancer cell lines.[61] However, kahweol (7) was inactive to ZR75-1 and MCF-7 estrogen receptor-positive breast cancer and HepG2 hepatoma.[58]

Furthermore, the experimental researches further demonstrated that cafestol (6) and kahweol (7) are inhibitors of angiogenesis.[62,63] The antimigratory and anti-invasive properties of kahweol (7) were observed in various cancer cell lines *in vitro*. Kahweol (7) inhibited the migration and tube formation in endothelial cell model and obstructed the lung metastasis in B16–F10 melanoma metastasis model, the antimetastatic effect of which was mediated by repressing secretion and transcription of vascular endothelial growth factor (VEGF) and impairing MMPs-2 and -9 activities in the cancer cells concomitant with the suppression of STAT3 signaling pathways.[64] On the basis of these findings, it is clear that the unfiltered coffee intake may be more helpful in the prevention of certain cancers owing to having cancer inhibitors, cafestol (6) and kahweol (7), and both the diterpenes in coffee were proved to have potential in anticancer, anticarcinogenesis, apoptosis induction, and antimetastasis against a variety of human cancer cell lines.

CONCLUSION AND SUGGESTION

The emerging data from either chemical biology researches or cohort investigations consistently support a positive relationship between coffee drinking and cancer prevention. It is clearly determined that habitual coffee intake is especially helpful for persons to lower the cancer risk in liver, colon/colorectal, brain, oral/head, breast, prostate, endometrial, and skin. However, for being safe to human health, moderate coffee intake (corresponding to 3 to 4 cups/day with average strength) is recommended because coffee contains a higher level of caffeine. In general, less than 400 mg of caffeine from all sources per day would be a safe level for most healthy adults.[65] Caffeine in coffee was found to be a necessary substance for lessening the incidence of brain carcinogenesis for being inactive for the consumption of decaffeinated coffee, According to the observations from scientific tests, high coffee intake (>4–6 cups/day) would be required for the prevention of cancers in prostate, breast, oral/head, and shin, but it is not recommended for higher caffeine intake impacting the health balance. Moreover, coffee fiber plays an important role in the protection of colon and colorectal away from the cancer risk besides other bioactive substances in coffee. Therefore, intake of filtered coffee showed less activity than the coffee prepared by unfiltered processes.

Despite its simple appearance, a cup of coffee, in fact, is a complicated mixture of phytochemicals. The different contents of its chemical composition depend largely on the factors, including the coffee tree species and the growth environment. The diverse substances, such as phenolic acids (chlorogenic acid and caffeic acid), alkaloids (caffeine and trigonelline), and diterpenes (cafestol and kahweol) have been discovered from coffee. The studies of chemical biology and molecular biology demonstrated that these substances exert chemopreventive and bioactive potentials toward different cancers, hence helping to elucidate the health benefits of black coffee and unfiltered coffee in anticancer and cancer prevention.

REFERENCES

1. Nkondjock, A. et al., 2009. Coffee consumption and the risk of cancer: An overview. *Cancer Lett.* (Shannon, Ireland) 277: 121–125.
2. Nkondjock, A. et al., 2011. Coffee and cancers. In: Chu, Y.-F. (Ed.), *Coffee: Emerging Health Effects and Disease Prevention*, pp. 197–209. Ames, IA: IFT Press (Willy-Blackwell).
3. Turesky, R.J. et al., 1993. The pro- and antioxidative effects of coffee and its impact on health. *Colloque Scientifique International sur le Cafe 15th* (Vol. 2), pp. 426–432. Paris, France: ASIC.
4. Miller, E.G. et al., 1999. The anticancer activity of coffee beans. *ACS Symposium Series*, 754(Caffeinated Beverages), pp. 56–63. Washington, DC: American Chemical Society; Book of Abstracts, *217th ACS National Meeting*, Anaheim, CA, March 21–25, AGFD-083.
5. Budhathoki, S. et al., 2015. Coffee intake and the risk of colorectal adenoma: The colorectal adenoma study in Tokyo. *Int. J. Cancer* 137: 463–470.
6. Sinha, R. et al., 2012. Caffeinated and decaffeinated coffee and tea intakes and risk of colorectal cancer in a large prospective study. *Am. J. Clin. Nutr.* 96: 374–381.
7. Isshiki, M. et al., 2013. Coffee reduces SULT1E1 expression in human colon carcinoma Caco-2 cells. *Biol. Pharm. Bull.* 36: 299–304.
8. Okamura, S. et al., 2005. The effects of coffee on conjugation reactions in human colon carcinoma cells. *Biol. Pharm. Bull.* 28: 271–274.
9. Kang, N.J. et al., 2011. Coffee phenolic phytochemicals suppress colon cancer metastasis by targeting MEK and TOPK. *Carcinogenesis* 32: 921–928.
10. Rao, C.V. et al., 1998. Prevention of colonic aberrant crypt foci and modulation of large bowel microbial activity by dietary coffee fiber, inulin and pectin. *Carcinogenesis* 19: 1815–1819.
11. Higgins, L.G. et al., 2008. Induction of cancer chemopreventive enzymes by coffee is mediated by transcription factor Nrf2. Evidence that the coffee-specific diterpenes cafestol and kahweol confer protection against acrolein. *Toxicol. Appl. Pharmacol.* 226: 328–337.
12. Merritt, M.A. et al., 2015. Coffee drinking and endometrial cancer. *Curr. Nutr. Rep.* 4: 40–46.
13. Je, Y. et al., 2011. A prospective cohort study of coffee consumption and risk of endometrial cancer over a 26-year follow-up. *Cancer Epidemiol. Biomarkers Prev.* 20: 2487–2495.
14. Bravi, F. et al., 2013. Coffee reduces risk for hepatocellular carcinoma: An updated meta-analysis. *Clin. Gastroenterol. Hepatol.* 11: 1413–1421.e1.
15. Lai, G.Y. et al., 2013. The association of coffee intake with liver cancer incidence and chronic liver disease mortality in male smokers. *Br. J. Cancer* 109: 1344–1351.
16. Nishikawa, A. et al., 1986. An inhibitory effect of coffee on nitrosamine-hepatocarcinogenesis with aminopyrine and sodium nitrite in rats. *J. Nutr. Growth Cancer* 3: 161–166.
17. Miura, Y. et al., 2004. Inhibitory effect of coffee on hepatoma proliferation and invasion in culture and on tumor growth, metastasis and abnormal lipoprotein profiles in hepatoma-bearing rats. *J. Nutr. Sci. Vitaminol.* 50: 38–44.
18. Gressner, O.A. et al., 2009. Less Smad2 is good for you! A scientific update on çoffee's liver benefits. *Hepatology* (Hoboken, NJ, US) 50: 970–978.
19. Baker, J.A. et al., 2006. Consumption of coffee, but not black tea, is associated with decreased risk of premenopausal breast cancer. *J. Nutr.* 136: 166–171.
20. Lowcock, E.C. et al., 2013. High coffee intake, but not caffeine, is associated with reduced estrogen receptor negative and postmenopausal breast cancer risk with no effect modification by CYP1A2 genotype. *Nutr. Cancer* 65: 398–409.
21. Ann, H.R. et al., 2015. Caffeine and caffeic acid inhibit growth and modify estrogen receptor and insulin-like growth factor I receptor levels in human breast cancer. *Clin. Cancer Res.* 21: 1877–1887.
22. Hsu, W.L. et al., 2012. Lowered risk of nasopharyngeal carcinoma and intake of plant vitamin, fresh fish, green tea and coffee: A case-control study in Taiwan. *PLoS One* 7: e41779.

23. Hildebrand, J.S. et al., 2013. Coffee, tea, and fatal oral/pharyngeal cancer in a large prospective US cohort. *Am. J. Epidemiol.* 177: 50–58.

24. Galeon, G. et al., 2010. Coffee and tea Intake and risk of head and neck cancer: Pooled analysis in the international head and neck cancer epidemiology consortium. *Cancer Epidemiol. Biomarkers Prev.* 19: 1723–1736.

25. Miller, E.G. et al., 1993. Inhibition of oral carcinogenesis by roasted coffee beans and roasted coffee bean fractions. *15th Colloque Scientifique International sur le Cafe* (Vol. 2), pp. 420–425. Montpellier, France: ASIC.

26. Holick, C.N. et al., 2010. Coffee, tea, caffeine intake, and risk of adult glioma in three prospective cohort studies. *Cancer Epidemiol. Biomarkers Prev.* 19: 39–47.

27. Loftfield, E. et al., 2015. Coffee drinking and cutaneous melanoma risk in the NIH-AARP diet and health study. *J. Natl. Cancer Inst.* 107(2): dju421.

28. Conney, A.H. et al., 2007. Stimulatory effect of oral administration of tea, coffee or caffeine on UVB-induced apoptosis in the epidermis of SKH-1 mice. *Toxicol. Appl. Pharmacol.* 224: 209–213.

29. Coffee consumption associated with reduced risk of advanced prostate cancer. *Science News*, December 8, 2009.

30. Kolberg, M. et al., 2016. Coffee inhibits nuclear factor-kappa B in prostate cancer cells and xenografts. *J. Nutr. Biochem.* 27: 153–163.

31. Abraham, S.K. et al., 1999. Anti-genotoxicity and glutathione S-transferase activity in mice pretreated with caffeinated and decaffeinated coffee. *Food Chem. Toxicol.* 37: 733–739.

32. Ramalakshmi, K. et al., 2009. Bioactivities of low-grade green coffee and spent coffee in different in vitro model systems. *Food Chem.* 115: 79–85.

33. Krstic, M. et al., 2015. The anticancer activity of green tea, coffee and cocoa extracts on human cervical adenocarcinoma HeLa cells depends on both pro-oxidant and anti-proliferative activities of polyphenols. *RSC Adv.* 5: 3260–3268.

34. Wuerzner, H.P. et al., 1990. In vivo inhibition of nitrosamide formation by coffee and coffee constituents. *Proc. 13th ASIC Colloque* (Vol. date, 1989), pp. 73–81.

35. Tanaka, T. et al., 1990. Inhibitory effects of chlorogenic acid, reserpine, polyprenoic acid (E-5166), or coffee on hepatocarcinogenesis in rats and hamsters. In: Kuroda, Y. et al. (Eds.), *Basic Life Sciences*, Vol. 52 (Antimutagenesis and Anticarcinogenesis Mechanisms 2), pp. 429–440. Boston, MA: Springer.

36. Mori, H. et al., 2000. Chemopreventive effects of coffee bean and rice constituents on colorectal carcinogenesis. *BioFactors* 12: 101–105.

37. Sukohar, A. et al., 2013. Role of chlorogenic acid from lampung robusta coffee against gene expression of MIRNA (micro RNA) 146 A on hepatocellular carcinoma cells. *Int. J. Res. Pharm. Nano Sci.* 2: 776–784.

38. Iwai, K. et al., 2004. In vitro antioxidative effects and tyrosinase inhibitory activities of seven hydroxycinnamoyl derivatives in green coffee beans. *J. Agric. Food Chem.* 52: 4893–4898.

39. Kang, N.J. et al., 2009. Caffeic acid, a phenolic phytochemical in coffee, directly inhibits Fyn kinase activity and UVB-induced COX-2 expression. *Carcinogenesis* 30: 321–330.

40. Yang, G. et al., 2014. Caffeic acid directly targets ERK1/2 to attenuate solar UV-induced skin carcinogenesis. *Cancer Prev. Res.* 7: 1056–1066.

41. Zhang, Y. et al., 2010. Coffee acid germanium on growth of uterocervical carcinoma (U14) cell in mice. *Shiyong Yixue Zazhi* 26: 1912–1914.

42. Genaro-Mattos, T.C. et al., 2015. Antioxidant activity of caffeic acid against iron-induced free radical generation-a chemical approach. *PLoS One* 10(6): e0129963/1–e0129963/12.

43. Sirota, R. et al., 2015. The role of the catecholic and the electrophilic moieties of caffeic acid in Nrf2/Keap1 pathway activation in ovarian carcinoma cell lines. *Redox Biol.* 4: 48–59.

44. Wang, G. et al., 2015. The effect of caffeine on cisplatin-induced apoptosis of lung cancer cells. *Exp. Hematol. Oncol.* 4: 5.

45. Arlt, A. et al., 2013. Inhibition of the Nrf2 transcription factor by the alkaloid trigonelline renders pancreatic cancer cells more susceptible to apoptosis through decreased proteasomal gene expression and proteasome activity. *Oncogene* 32: 4825–4835.

46. Kagami, K. et al., 2008. Inhibitory effects of pyrazinoic acids on cell invasion of human hepatocellular carcinoma cells in matrigel cell-invasion assay. *Organ Biol.* 15: 57–64.

47. Huber, W.W. et al., 2003. Coffee and its chemopreventive components kahweol and cafestol increase the activity of O-6-methylguanine-DNA methyltransferase in rat liver—Comparison with phase II xenobiotic metabolism. *Mutat. Res.* 522: 57–68.

48. Cavin, C. et al., 2001. Protective effects of coffee diterpenes against aflatoxin B1-induced genotoxicity: mechanisms in rat and human cells. *Food Chem. Toxicol.* 39: 549–556.
49. Cavin, C. et al., 2002. Cafestol and kahweol, two coffee specific diterpenes with anticarcinogenic activity. *Food Chem. Toxicol.* 40: 1155–1163.
50. Cavin, C. et al., 1998. The coffee-specific diterpenes cafestol and kahweol protect against aflatoxin B1-induced genotoxicity through a dual mechanism. *Carcinogenesis* 19: 1369–1375.
51. Huber, W.W. et al., 2008. Effects of coffee and its chemopreventive components kahweol and cafestol on cytochrome P450 and sulfotransferase in rat liver. *Food Chem. Toxicol.* 46: 1230–1238.
52. Schilter, B. et al., 1996. Placental glutathione S-transferase (GST-P) induction as a potential mechanism for the anti-carcinogenic effect of the coffee-specific components cafestol and kahweol. *Carcinogenesis* 17: 2377–2384.
53. Lee, K.A. et al., 2012. Natural diterpenes from coffee, cafestol and kahweol induce apoptosis through regulation of specificity protein 1 expression in human malignant pleural mesothelioma. *J. Biomed. Sci.* (London, UK) 19: 60.
54. Choi, M.J. et al., 2011. Cafestol, a coffee-specific diterpene, induces apoptosis in renal carcinoma Caki cells through down-regulation of anti-apoptotic proteins and Akt phosphorylation. *Chem. Biol. Interact.* 190: 102–108.
55. Um, H.J. et al., 2010. The coffee diterpene kahweol sensitizes TRAIL-induced apoptosis in renal carcinoma Caki cells through down-regulation of Bcl-2 and c-FLIP. *Chem. Biol. Interact.* 186: 36–42.
56. Chae, J.I. et al., 2014. Anti-proliferative properties of kahweol in oral squamous cancer through the regulation specificity protein-1. *Phytother. Res.* 28: 1879–1886.
57. Choi, D.W. et al., 2015. The cytotoxicity of kahweol in HT-29 human colorectal cancer cells is mediated by apoptosis and suppression of heat shock protein 70 expression. *Biomol. Ther.* 23: 128–133.
58. Cardenas, C. et al., 2014. Insights on the antitumor effects of kahweol on human breast cancer: Decreased survival and increased production of reactive oxygen species and cytotoxicity. *Biochem. Biophys. Res. Commun.* 447: 452–458.
59. Oh, J.H. et al., 2009. The coffee diterpene kahweol induces apoptosis in human leukemia U937 cells through down-regulation of Akt phosphorylation and activation of JNK. *Apoptosis* 14: 1378–1386.
60. Kim, H.G. et al., 2009. Kahweol blocks STAT3 phosphorylation and induces apoptosis in human lung adenocarcinoma A549 cells. *Toxicol. Lett.* 187: 28–34.
61. Park, G.H. et al., 2016. The coffee diterpene kahweol suppresses the cell proliferation by inducing cyclin D1 proteasomal degradation via ERK1/2, JNK and GKS3β-dependent threonine-286 phosphorylation in human colorectal cancer cells. *Food Chem. Toxicol.* 95: 2–148.
62. Wang, S.Y. et al., 2012. Antiangiogenic properties of cafestol, a coffee diterpene, in human umbilical vein endothelial cells. *Biochem. Biophys. Res. Commun.* 421: 567–571.
63. Cardenas, C. et al., 2011. Anti-angiogenic and anti-inflammatory properties of kahweol, a coffee diterpene. *PLoS One* 6(8): e23407.
64. Kim, H.G. et al., 2012. The coffee diterpene kahweol inhibits metastasis by modulating expressions of MMPs and VEGF via STAT3 inactivation. *Food Chem.* 133: 1521–1529.
65. George, S.E. et al., 2008. A perception on health benefits of coffee. *Crit. Rev. Food Sci. Nutr.* 48: 464–486.

58. TEA

Thé   Tee   Té

茶葉   お茶   찻잎

Camellia sinensis

Theaceace

Tea, or *Camellia sinensis* (Theaceace), is the dried young leaves and leaf buds of a green plant, which is one of the most favorite and widely consumed plants for making beverages in the world. Tea was first used by the Chinese to prepare beverages and now the tea plants are cultured in many places, especially in East Asia such as China, Korea, Japan, India, and Sri Lanka. According to different processes, the tea leaves can be classified into five major varieties, that is, (1) green tea (dried while fresh), (2) red tea (fermented), (3) black tea (double fermented), (4) oolong tea (half fermented), and (5) jasmine tea (jasmine blossoms mixed with green tea, sometimes with red tea), that are most commonly found on the Chinese market. The famous Chinese red teas such as Qimen, Dianhong, Zhuancha as well as Pu-erh (*C. assamica*) are usually called black tea in the western countries. The green tea made of unopened buds and young leaves with fine silvery-white hairs is also termed white tea. Epidemiological observations and laboratory studies have proved that the tea possesses multiple bioactivities such as anti-inflammatory, anti-nitrite synthesis, diuretic, anticarcinogenic, antimutagen, hepatoprotective, antitrypanocidal, antipyretic, hypolipidemic, antiplatelet aggregation, antiallergic, anticataractogenic, antimicrobial, and other activities. Hence, the tea can diminish the risks of a variety of illnesses, such as cancers, cardiovascular, thrombus, coronary heart disease, hypertension, hyperlipidemia, atherosclerosis, and neurodegenerative.

SCIENTIFIC EVIDENCE OF CANCER-INHIBITORY AND CANCER-PREVENTIVE ACTIVITIES

The numerous *in vitro* and *in vivo* investigations substantiated that tea possesses the inhibitory activity against multiple neoplastic cell lines and carcinogenesis. The antiproliferative effect of green tea was observed in many *in vitro* human tumor cell lines, including BGC-823 (stomach), A498 and 769-P (renal), L7402 and QCY7703 (liver), as well as murine L1210 leukemia and Ehrlich ascites tumor.[1-11] The *in vitro* effects were consistent with the results obtained from in animal models. Intraperitoneal (I.p.) administration of green tea extract not only repressed the cell growth of sarcoma 180, Ehrlich ascites, and entity tumors and prolonged the survival duration of cancer-bearing mice, but also markedly promoted the immune function of the tested animals through increasing natural killer cell activity and interleukin-2 amount.[1-4] The growth inhibitory effects by green tea were revealed to correlate with (1) diminution of ornithine decarboxylase (ODC) activity and the cell viability (such as in Ehrlich ascites tumor cells); (2) arrest of cell cycle from G1 phase to S phase (such as in L1210 cells); and (3) blocking of protein synthesis (such as in BGC-823 cells). Besides the direct inhibition against cancer-cell proliferation, green tea also partially obstructed the tumor colony formation.[1-4] Decrease of ODC activity by green tea should be in association with cytochrome c release from mitochondria and caspase 3-like protease activation, events of which sequentially incited the neoplastic cells to apoptotic death.[5] In addition, the filtrates of green tea exhibited the antiproliferative effect against human A549 lung adenocarcinoma cell line *in vitro*.[12]

Moreover, three types of tea had been tested together with many carcinogens, providing various evidences in the significant ability of tea oral infusion on the chemoprevention of cancer. Both green tea and black tea could efficiently reduce the incidence rates of hepatoma induced by AFB1, fumonisin-B1 or diethylnitrosamine in rats,[6-8] and markedly deterred the genesis of papilloma in gastric mucosa and skin caused by benzyl methylamine, sodium nitrite, or DMBA with TPA in mice.[9-13] Green tea also demonstrated the antitumorigenic effect in rats against *N*-butyl-*N*-(4-hydroxybutyl) nitrosamine (BBN) caused urinary bladder tumor but black tea and oolong tea had no such effect. The antitumorigenic potency of green tea powder was great than that of green tea leaves.[6] Moreover, oral administration of black tea to tested animals could increase the apoptotic index by 100% in keratoacanthoma, by 95% in squamous cell carcinoma, and by 44% in squamous cell papilloma, and lessened the mitotic index by 42% in keratoacanthoma and 16% in squamous cell carcinoma.[10] The incidence of esophagus cancer was diminished obviously in rats by the oral infusion of either green tea or black tea.[14]

Black tea possesses a more marked antioxidative property compared to other types of tea. It exerted a dose-dependent protective effect against DMBA-induced oxidative stress via decrease in the antioxidant enzyme activities (such as GST, superoxide dismutase, glutathione reductase, and catalase) and exerted marked dose-dependent inhibition on DMBA-caused lipid peroxidation in three tissues (liver, kidney, and prostate) of mice.[15] In addition, green tea also demonstrated anti-genotoxic effect against genotoxic damage elicited by a steroid agent trenbolone or a chemotherapeutic agent docetaxel in human lymphocytes.[16] All the evidences clearly corroborated that green tea and black tea are able to afford the noticeable antioxidant and antigenotoxic protection against the carcinogenesis, the related oxidative damage, and the genotoxicity caused by many kinds of xenobiotics.[15]

Moreover, both green tea and black tea displayed the inhibitory effect on *N*-hydroxylated heterocyclic amines-induced *Salmonella* mutagenicity with more than 90% of antimutagenic rate. Due to the inhibitory effects on *N*,*O*-acetyl-transferase and microsomal NAD(P)H-cytochrome P450 reductase that closely related to the metabolic activation of heterocyclic amines, green tea and black tea can rapidly excrete heterocyclic amines to reduce the formation of colonic aberrant crypt *in vivo*.[17] Consequently, the preventive activity of tea consumption, especially green tea and black tea, has been demonstrated in many murine models with carcinogenesis in skin, lung, oral cavity, esophagus, liver, small intestine, forestomach, stomach, pancreas, duodenum, colorectal, bladder, prostate, and mammary gland.[18,19] The broad anticarcinogenic spectrum of tea encourages people not to miss the health benefit of tea in daily life.

SCIENTIFIC EVIDENCE OF CANCER-INHIBITORY AND CANCER-PREVENTIVE CONSTITUENTS

The bioactive constituents have been found in tea for cancer chemopreventive potential in polyphenols. The tea polyphenols (TP) normally have four types: (1) catechins such as gallate ((−)-Epigallocatechin-3-gallate [EGCG], **1**), (+)-gallocatechin, (−)-epicatechin, (−)-epigallocatechin, (−)-epicatechin, and gallate(−)-epgallocatechin; (2) theaflavins such as theaflavin (**2**), theaflavin-3-gallate, theaflavin-3′-gallate, and theaflavin-3,3′-digallate; (3) thearubigins; and (4) theasinensins. These constituents in the tea displayed marked diversity in biological chemistry owing to the structural differences caused by the dissimilar processes. Catechin polyphenols are the primary bioactive components in green tea, and the most abundant and the most active catechin in green tea is EGCG (**1**). Thearubigins and theaflavins are the two groups of polymeric polyphenols that are formed during the fermentation and enzymatic oxidation of the tea leaves. Thus, they are the principal active constituents in black tea and Chinese red tea. In oolong tea, dimers of EGCG such as theasinensin-A (**3**) became the major constituent by half fermentations. All these four types of TP exerted important health benefits for lowering the risk of carcinogenesis, and these characteristics behaving pharmacologically should be closely based on the structural diversity.

1. Total tea polyphenols

Anticarcinogenic activities: Green tea polyphenols (GTP) are able to impede the malignancy in various cancer cell lines *in vitro* and *in vivo*. In mice with bladder cancer established by BBN, GTP markedly inhibited the bladder tumor growth and angiogenesis.[20] Both GTP and black tea polyphenols (BTP) dose- and time-dependently obstructed the proliferation of human papilloma virus-16 positive SiHa cervical neoplastic cells concomitant with the increase of G2/M cell arrest and apoptosis.[21] Three clinical trials by using GTP had been performed in the treatment of prostate cancer patients, positive data of which corroborated that the GTP has affected as a chemopreventive agent to diminish the risk of prostate cancer.[22] Given 0.3% solution of GTP in drinking water exerted the preventive effect against lung preneoplasm lesions caused by 3,4-benzopyrene intrapulmonary injection in rats via enhancing p53 activity but reducing Bcl-2 expression, and exerted similar inhibitory effects against lung carcinogenesis elicited by benzo[a]pyrene in mice via alternating the expressions of p53-linked genes (Bax, Bcl-2, mdm2, p21, and p27) and H-ras, c-myc, and cyclin D1 at different time points.[23,24] The chemopreventive effects of GTP and BTP at tested doses (0.1% and 0.2% of both GTP and BTP) were observed against diethylnitrosoamine-induced lung tumors in mice and against 7,12-dimethylbenz[a]anthracene-triggered mammary tumorigenesis, associating with the inhibition of COX-2 expression and inactivation of phosphorylated forms of NF-κB and Akt.[25,26] Both the GTP and BTP effectively restrained their growth and the cumulative numbers of mammary tumors by ~92% and 77%, respectively.[26]

Moreover, TP are known to be strong antioxidant agents. The cancer-preventive mechanisms for the TP were suggested to be closely correlated with preclusion of oxidative stress, modulation of carcinoma cell metabolism, and deterrence of DNA damage.[16] Similarly, by obviously inhibiting ROS production and lactate dehydrogenase, the oxidative damage in human bronchial epithelial cells (BEAS-2B) induced by cigarette smoke condensate (CSC) was deterred remarkably, carcinogenesis of which can be protected by the TP.[27]

Anticancer activities: In the *in vitro* assay, TP demonstrated the inhibitory effects toward the proliferation of human cancer cell lines such as DU145 (prostate), SKVO3 (ovary), H460 (lung), LoVo and SW480 (colon), and PG (lung) cells, anticancer effects of which were selectively associated with induction of ROS-elevated apoptosis of SKVOS and H460 cells,[28] arrest of cell-cycle progression in H460 and PG cells,[29,30] upregulation of gap junction intercellular communication (GJIC) in highly metastatic PG cells,[30] repression of survivin expression in DU145 androgen-independent cells,[31] and downregulation of HES1, JAG1, MT2A, MAFA, and p38 in LoVo and SW480 cells.[32] In a nude mouse model, oral administration of GTP extract hampered the growth of androgen-dependent human LAPC4 prostate cancer cells and markedly lessened the tumor volume and size, anticancer effect of which on LAPC4 xenograft was due to GTP-mediated suppression of oxidative stress and angiogenesis.[33] The *in vivo* antitumor activity has also been demonstrated in hepatocellular carcinoma mice after treatment of TP (50, 100, and 150 mg/kg, body wt.) by gavage for 20 days, together with significant elevation of serum aspartate transaminase, alkaline phosphatase, alanine aminotransferase, and malondialdehyde levels and lessening of serum white blood cells, serum total protein, albumin, A/G, TNF-α, IFN-γ, and glutathione levels. The observations showed that the liver preventive activity of TP was largely attributed to its ability in augmenting the antioxidant enzyme levels.[34]

2. Catechin polyphenols

Anticancer activities of EGCG (**1**): EGCG is an abundant and valuable green tea catechin-type of polyphenol (GTP). The chemopreventive effects of EGCG (**1**) and GTP were demonstrated in the studies of epidemiology, cell culture, animal models, and clinics. *In vitro* assays with the carcinoma cell lines of KATO III (stomach), LoVo, and HT-29 (colon); HCT116 (colorectal), HeLa (cervix), HepG2, and Bel-7404 (liver); UACC-375 (skin), MCF-7 (breast), HEp-2 (larynx), CNE1-LMP1 (naso-pharynx), SPC-A1, and H1299 (lung); HL-60 (leukemic), Kaposi's highly vascular sarcoma, and spontaneously developed metastatic prostate cancer cells, GTP and EGCG (1) exerted marked pro-motion on the apoptosis and cell-cycle arrest and potent inhibition on the proliferation of the tumor cells but not in the normal cells.[35–48] The mechanism studied revealed that the anticancer activities of GTP and EGCG (1) were involved in multiple signaling pathways (such as mitogen-activated protein kinase-dependent pathway, growth factor-mediated pathway, and ubiquitin/proteasome degradation pathway) that were related with (1) eliciting oxidative stress and altering the different oxidative envi-ronments;[43,49] (2) blocking NF-κB constitutive expression;[25,50] and (3) reducing the enzyme activi-ties such as cyclin-dependent kinases, telomerase, MAP kinases, topoisomerase, tyrosine kinase, PKC, and MMPs.[41,51–56] In addition, the EGCG treatment caused the generation of intracellular ROS and mitochondrial ROS leading to the apoptosis-initiation of tumor cells. The prooxidant effects enhanced endogenous antioxidant systems in normal tissues that offer protection against carcino-genic insult.[48] By blocking E2- and Nic-induced α9-nAChR protein expression, EGCG also exerted a chemopreventive effect to hamper smoking-mediated breast tumorigenesis.[57]

The cancer-inhibitory activity of GTP and EGCG has been further verified by various animal models. Treatment with the polyphenols at a human achievable dose (equivalent to six cups of green tea per day) remarkably declined the tumor incidence in many organ sites such as skin, lung, liver, colon, stomach, and mammary gland, resulting in not only hampering the cell proliferation but also inhibiting the angiogenesis and metastasis.[19,48,58–64] For instance, *in vivo* treatments with GTP and EGCG (1) obviously cut the average number of metastatic foci on the lung surface in mice bearing Lewis lung carcinoma[55] and diminished the invasion of prostate cancer cells (spontaneously devel-ops metastasis CaP) in mice, thereby restraining the development, progression, and metastasis of cancer cells to other organ sites and prolonging survival of the tested animals.[37] The angiogenesis in mice bearing highly vascular Kaposi's sarcoma (KS) also could be obstructed during the inhibition of KS tumor growth by oral administration of GTP and EGCG (1).[40]

Synergic effect of EGCG (1): EGCG at >5 μmol/L concentrations was able to synergistically enhance the anti-tumor effect of 5-FU on Hep3B human hepatoma cells and to abrogate COX-2 overexpres-sion and PGE2 secretion induced by 5-FU, implying that the possibility of EGCG and 5-FU combi-nation inhibits chemoresistant cancer cells.[12] Cotreatment of doxorubicin (DOX) with EGCG (1) or epicatechin gallate (ECG) at lower doses notably suppressed chemoresistant BEL-7404/DOX hepa-toma cell proliferation *in vitro* and hepatoma growth in a xenograft mouse model. The cotreatment markedly augmented intracellular DOX accumulation and sensitized chemoresistant tumor cells to DOX via repression of *P*-glycoprotein efflux pump activity and suppression of MDR1 and HIF-1α mRNA expression, then directly or indirectly reversed the multidrug resistance.[65] The growth inhibi-tory effects of EGCG (1) could be augmented by 2- to 5-fold when cotreatment of human HT-29 colon cancer cells with genistein (a flavonoid from soy) in mice.[56] Similarly, a marked synergistic effect was achieved on the antiproliferation in mouse 4T1 breast cancer cells and HeLa cervical cancer cells *in vitro* when EGCG was combined with (–)-epicatechin, another GTP.[42,49] Prominently, the antioxidant capacities of GTP and EGCG (1) were demonstrated to involve significant reversal effects on doxorubicin-resistant cancer cell lines (S180-dox, SW620-dox, and KB-A-1), leading to the enhancement of DOX cytotoxic effect on the corresponding multidrug-resistant cancer cell lines. The MDR-reversal effect was figured out to be at least partly related to the potent amplification of intracellular ROS.[53,66,67]

Clinical treatment with EGCG (1): To breast cancer patients who were undergoing treatment with radiotherapy, oral administration of EGCG in 400 mg capsules three times per day for 2–8 weeks resulted in significantly lower serum levels of VEGF and hepatocyte growth factor (HGF) and inhi-bition of MMPs-9 and -2 compared to the patients who had no EGCG intake. The observed inter-actions indicated that EGCG potentiated the efficacy of radiotherapy in the breast cancer patients.

In addition, the sera were obtained from the breast cancer patients treated with a combination of radiotherapy and EGCG feeding for 2–8 weeks. Exposure of sera to cultures of highly-metastatic human MDA-MB-231 breast cancer cells *in vitro* interestingly exerted anti-proliferative and anti-invasive effects and elicited G0/G1 cell cycle arrest and stimulation of γ-radiation-induced apoptosis, anticancer activities of EGCG of which was found to be mediated by inactivation of MMPs-9, -2, lessening of NF-κB protein level and Akt phosphorylation, and decline of Bcl-2 and c-Met receptor expressions.[68] The results showed that the TP, especially ECGC, has potential in the chemotherapy of human metastatic breast cancer and hepatoma as a therapeutic adjuvant.

3. Theaflavins and thearubigins

Theaflavins and thearubigins, which are two groups of polymeric polyphenols, have been believed as the important contributors of the taste and bio-benefits for black tea and red tea. The major constituent in black tea is thearubigins while theaflavins are only 1%–2% in the water-extract of black tea.[69] These polymeric polyphenols are imperative for inhibiting tumor formation and proliferation in animal models. Some TP such as theaflavin (2) and a mixture of theaflavin-3-gallate and theaflavin-3′-gallate displayed moderate anti-proliferative activities on human U937 histolytic lymphoma cells with IC_{50}s around 12 μM, while theaflavin-3,3′-digallate and EGCG (1) showed lower suppressive effects on the U937 cells. These theaflavins were less effective on human Jurkat acute T-cell leukemia cells.[70–72] By restricting Akt signaling involved Hsp90 expression, Wnt/β-catenin signaling and FOXO1 (forkhead transcription factor-1) expression, theaflavins, thearubigins and black TP prompted G0/G1 cell cycle arrest in human leukemic U937 and K562 cell lines.[73] Theaflavins and EGCG (1) could sensitize human cervical cancer cells (HeLa and SiHa) to cisplatin to enhance cisplatin-induced anti-growth and proapoptotic effects by 3 ~ 4-folds, associated with inhibition of NF-κB and Akt signaling.[74] Similarly, by a ROS-involved and mitochondria related mechanism plus block of NF-κB and Akt pathway, theaflavins and EGCG (1) exerted a marked concentration- and time-dependent inhibition against the proliferation of HeLa human cervical cancer cells together with induction of the cell apoptosis and sub-G1 phase arrest,[75] and by modulation of self-renewal Wnt and hedgehog pathways, theaflavin (2) and EGCG (1) restricted mouse liver carcinogenesis-induced by CCl4/N-nitosodiethylamine together with marked suppression of the proliferation, induction of apoptosis, decrease of hepatocyte progenitor cell (AFP) prevalence and stem cell population (CD44).[76] Moreover, theaflavin (2) and EGCG (1) were also capable of markedly suppressing the invasion of highly metastatic HT1080 fibrosarcoma cells, accompanied with obvious inhibition on gelatin degradation mediated by MMPs-2 and -9.[77]

In comparison to EGCG (1), the antitumorigenic and anticancer potencies of thearubigins and theaflavins seem to be relatively lower in many cases, but the black tea polyphenols (BTP) exhibited greater antioxidative ability.[15] As superoxide scavengers, theaflavins, thearubigens as well as EGCG (1) could constrain the generation of reactive oxygen species (ROS) and xanthine oxidase (XO) to produce uric acid and to induce quinone reductase activity. The superoxide scavenging abilities were theaflavins < EGCG (1) but the H_2O_2 scavenging abilities were theaflavins > EGCG.[78,79] Similar to the actions of EGCG (1), theaflavins and thearubigins also could highly activate superoxide dismutase, glutathione peroxidase, glutathione-S-transferase and catalase. When *in vivo* treated with the polymeric polyphenols, a carcinogen (such as dimethylbenzanthracene) causing lipid peroxidation in the liver of mice could be obviously restricted,[80] indicating that the antioxidant effect of polymeric polyphenols/black TP is capable of live protection to block hepatomagenesis.

Interestingly, thearubigins and theaflavins as well as both black tea and GTP were also able to significantly *in vivo* retard the lung carcinogenesis induced by 4-(methylnitrosamino)-1-(3-pyridyl)-1-butanone (NNK), which is a potent nicotine-derived carcinogen found in tobacco, via block of 8-hydroxydeoxyguanosine (8-OHdG) formation in lung DNA of mice, in which 8-OHdG is a marker of oxidative DNA damage.[81–83] The findings recommended that the tea consumption may help to reduce the risk of lung carcinogenesis from smoking. However, the taste and bioactivity of black tea would be adversely affected when thearubigins are further oxidized if the tea is poorly stored.

4. Theasinensins

The polyphenols in oolong tea (half fermented) mainly present as a group of EGCG dimmers called theasinensins. As the effects of EGCG (**1**), theasinensins-A (**3**) and -D display strong growth inhibitory effects against human U937 histolytic lymphoma cells, and the two elicited the cell apoptosis as evidenced by DNA fragmentation, elevation of ROS production, chromatin condensation and activation of caspase-9.[71,72] In the treatment with theasinensins, human HL-60 promyelocytic leukemia cells not only promoted the dose- and time-dependent apoptosis but also induced the cell differentiation, accompanied with decrease of Bcl-2 and c-myc gene expressions, enhancement of c-fos gene expression and elevation of cAMP/cGMP ratio.[84,85] The theasinensins also significantly deterred the synthesis of DNA and protein in the HL-60 leukemia cells.[85] In addition, theasinensin-D and theaflavin-digallate only showed weak anti-invasive activity against highly metastatic HT1080 fibrosarcoma cells.[77]

CONCLUSION AND SUGGESTION

Tea has received much attention as a suitable health-promoting beverage because its antitumorigenic and antioxidant properties. The experimental discoveries have established the anticarcinogenic activities of GTP (e.g., epigallocatechin-3-gallate (EGCG), epigallocatechin (EGC), epicatechin-3-gallate, and epicatechin), and have evidenced remarkable antioxidant and antitumorigenic benefits of black/red tea and oolong TP oligomers (e.g., theaflavins, thearubigens, and theasinensins). The cancer preventive spectrum of the TP have been often proven in various cancer cells such as in gastrointestinal tract, lung, skin, liver, larynx, prostate, breast, nasopharynx, lymphocyte, and blood. Pleiotropic mechanistic studies disclosed that the TP are capable of lessening the total levels of early carcinogenesis biomarkers and amplifying the tumor inhibiting proteins. The chemopreventive effects of the TP should be also largely associated with the antioxidant and radical scavenging activities. In addition, the GTP, especially EGCG, has certain inhibitory potentials against the invasion, metastasis, and angiogenesis of carcinomas and has reversal effects against chemoresistance and radioresistance. Consequently, these scientific findings clearly demonstrated that tea drinking is helpful for the improvement of health and for cancer prevention and cancer therapy.

According to the necessity in medical efficacy for achieving the cancer-preventive effects, the TP are required to reach 10–20 µmol/L concentrations in blood plasma. However, the concentration of TP is usually much lower than the requirement. Therefore, to maintain a high level of TP in the human body for exerting the health benefits, it is necessary that intake of tea be frequent in large quantities. However, it is better to avoid heavy tea drinking in the evening and nighttime due to tea containing caffeine that impacts sleeping.

REFERENCES

1. Huo, Z.F. et al., 1991. The anticancer studies of green tea. *Jiangsu Yiyao* 17: 318.
2. Yan, Y.S. et al., 1989. Anticancer effect of green tea. *J. Nanjing Med. Coll.* 9: 301.
3. Yan, Y.S. et al., 1990. In vivo experiment on the anticarcinogenic activity and immune stimulation with the extract of Chinese green tea. *J. Tea Sci.* 10: 79–84.
4. Le, M.Z. et al., 1989. The anticancer effect of Longwu tea. *Jiangsu Yiyao* 15: 342–343.
5. Kennedy, D.O. et al., 2001. Growth inhibitory effect of green tea extract in Ehrlich ascites tumor cells involves cytochrome c release and caspase activation. *Cancer Lett.* 166: 9–15; Balasubramanian, K. et al., 2012. Study of antioxidant and anticancer activity of natural sources. *J. Nat. Prod. Plant Resour.* 2: 192–197.
6. Matsushima, M. et al., 1998. Antitumor effect of green tea on rat urinary bladder tumor induced by N-butyl-N-(4-hydroxybutyl) nitrosamine. *ACS Symposium Series* 701(Functional Foods for Disease Prevention I: Fruits, Vegetables, and Teas), pp. 191–197. Washington, DC: American Chemical Society; Chen, Z.Y. et al., 1987. Effect of six edible plants on the development of AFB1-induced gamma-glutamyltranspeptidase-positive hepatocyte foci in rats. *Zhonghua Zhongliu Zazhi* 9: 109–111.

7. Li, Y. et al., 1991. Comparative study on the inhibitory effect of green tea, coffee and levamisole on the hepatocarcinogenic action of diethyl nitrosamine. *Zhonghua Zhongliu Zazhi* 13: 193–195.

8. Marnewick, J.L. et al., 2009. Chemoprotective properties of rooibos (Aspalathus linearis), honeybush (Cyclopia intermedia) herbal and green and black (Camellia sinensis) teas against cancer promotion induced by fumonisin B1 in rat liver. *Food Chem. Toxicol.* 47: 220–229.

9. Han, C. et al., 1991. Chinese tea inhibits the occurrence of esophageal tumors induced by N-nitroso-methylbenzylamine and blocks its formation in rats. *IARC Sci. Publ.* 105: 541–545.

10. Lu, Y.P. et al., 1997. Inhibitory effect of black tea on the growth of established skin tumors in mice: Effects on tumor size, apoptosis, mitosis and bromodeoxyuridine incorporation into DNA. *Carcinogenesis* 18: 2163–2169.

11. Carvalho, M. et al., 2010. Green tea: A promising anticancer agent for renal cell carcinoma. *Food Chem.* 122: 49–54.

12. Yang, X.W. et al., 2012. Green tea polyphenol epigallocatechin-3-gallate enhances 5-fluorouracil-induced cell growth inhibition of hepatocellular carcinoma cells. *Hepatol. Res.* 42: 494–501.

13. Okai, Y. et al., 1998. Potent suppressive activity of nonpolyphenolic fraction of green tea (Camellia sinensis) against genotoxin-induced umu C gene expression in Salmonella typhimurium (TA 1535/pSK 1002), tumor promotor-dependent ornithine decarboxylase induction of BALB/c 3T3 fibroblast cells, and chemically induced mouse skin tumorigenesis. *Teratog. Carcinog. Mutagen.* 17: 305–312.

14. Gao, G.D. et al., 1990. Preventive effect of green tea. *Hebei Yiyao* 12: 84–86.

15. Kalra, N. et al., 2005. Antioxidant potential of black tea against 7,12-dimethylbenz(a)anthracene-induced oxidative stress in Swiss albino mice. *J. Environ. Pathol. Toxicol. Oncol.* 24: 105–114.

16. Gupta, J. et al., 2009. Protective role of green tea extract against genotoxic damage induced by anticancer drug and steroid compound, separately, in cultured human lymphocytes. *Pharmacologyonline* 3: 156–174.

17. Dashwood, R.H. et al., 1999. Cancer chemopreventive mechanisms of tea against heterocyclic amine mutagens from cooked meat. *Proc. Soc. Exp. Biol. Med.* 220: 239–243.

18. Mukhtar, H. et al., 2000. Tea polyphenols: prevention of cancer and optimizing health. *Am. J. Clin. Nutr.* 71(6 Suppl): 1698S–1702S.

19. Yang, C.S. et al., 2007. Tea and cancer prevention: Molecular mechanisms and human relevance. *Toxicol. Appl. Pharmacol.* 224: 265–273.

20. Sagara, Y.J. et al., 2010. Green tea polyphenol suppresses tumor invasion and angiogenesis in N-butyl-(-4-hydroxybutyl) nitrosamine-induced bladder cancer. *Cancer Epidemiol.* 34: 350–354.

21. Singh, M. et al., 2010. Regulation of cell growth through cell cycle arrest and apoptosis in HPV 16 positive human cervical cancer cells by tea polyphenols. *Invest. New Drugs* 28: 216–224.

22. Johnson, J.J. et al., 2010. Green tea polyphenols for prostate cancer chemoprevention: A translational perspective. *Phytomedicine* 17: 3–13.

23. Gu, Q.H. et al., 2013. Tea polyphenols prevent lung from preneoplastic lesions and effect p53 and bcl-2 gene expression in rat lung tissues. *Int. J. Clin. Exp. Pathol.* 6: 1523–1531.

24. Manna, S.J. et al., 2009. Tea polyphenols can restrict benzo[a]pyrene-induced lung carcinogenesis by altered expression of p53-associated genes and H-ras, c-myc and cyclin D1. *Nutr. Biochem.* 20: 337–349.

25. Roy, P. et al., 2010. Tea polyphenols inhibit cyclooxygenase-2 expression and block activation of nuclear factor-kappa B and Akt in diethylnitrosoamine induced lung tumors in Swiss mice. *Invest. New Drugs* 28: 466–471.

26. Roy, P. et al., 2011. Inhibitory effects of tea polyphenols by targeting cyclooxygenase-2 through regulation of nuclear factor kappa B, Akt and p53 in rat mammary tumors. *Invest. New Drugs* 29: 225–231.

27. Huang, B. et al., 2009. Tea polyphenols inhibiting oxidative damage of cigarette smoke condensate in BEAS-2B cells. *Nanhua Daxue Xuebao, Yixueban* 37: 150–152.

28. Fu, C.H. et al., 2012. Tea polyphenols induce apoptosis of ovarian cancer SKOV3 cells and its mechanism. *Yixue Yanjiusheng Xuebao* 25: 1146–1150.

29. Du, Y.M. et al., 2011. Tea polyphenols induces apoptosis of lung cancer cell line H460 and its effects on cell cycle. *Guangdong Yixue* 32: 1803–1805.

30. Li, X.Y. et al., 2012. Up-regulation of the gap junction intercellular communication by tea polyphenol in the human metastatic lung carcinoma cell line. *J. Cancer Ther.* 3: 64–70.

31. Liang, X. et al., 2013. Tea polyphenols inhibit the proliferation of prostate cancer DU145 cells. *Zhonghua Nankexue Zazhi* 19: 495–500.

32. Xu, Y.Y. et al., 2010. Tea polyphenol inhibits colorectal cancer with microsatellite instability by regulating the expressions of HES1, JAG1, MT2A and MAFA. *Zhongxiyi Jiehe Xuebao* 8: 870–876.

33. Henning, S.M. et al., 2012. Polyphenols in brewed green tea inhibit prostate tumor xenograft growth by localizing to the tumor and decreasing oxidative stress and angiogenesis. *J. Nutr. Biochem.* 23: 1537–1542.
34. Cui, B.K. et al., 2012. Effect of tea polyphenol on oxidative injury in S180 cells induced hepatocarcinoma mice. *Int. J. Mol. Sci.* 13: 5571–5583.
35. Hibasami, H. et al., 1998. Induction of apoptosis in human stomach cancer cells by green tea catechins. *Oncol. Rep.* 5: 527–529.
36. Borska, S. et al., 2003. Induction of apoptosis by EGCG in selected tumour cell lines in vitro. *Pol. Histochem. Cytochem. Soc.* 41: 229–232.
37. Gupta, S. et al., 2001. Inhibition of prostate carcinogenesis in TRAMP mice by oral infusion of green tea polyphenols. *Proc. Natl. Acad. Sci. USA* 98: 10350–10355.
38. Yamamoto, T. et al., 2003. Green tea polyphenol causes differential oxidative environments in tumor versus normal epithelial cells. *J. Pharmacol. Exp. Ther.* 307: 230–236.
39. Luo, F.J. et al., 2001. Effect of tea polyphenols and EGCG on nasopharyngeal carcinoma cell proliferation and the mechanisms involved. *Chin. J. Cancer Res.* 13: 235–242.
40. Fassina, G. et al., 2004. Mechanisms of inhibition of tumor angiogenesis and vascular tumor growth by epigallocatechin-3-gallate. *Clin. Cancer Res.* 10: 4865–4873.
41. Yokoyama, M. et al., 2004. The tea polyphenol, (–)-epigallocatechin gallate effects on growth, apoptosis, and telomerase activity in cervical cell lines. *Gynecol. Oncol.* 92: 197–204.
42. Uesato, S. et al., 2001. Inhibition of green tea catechins against the growth of cancerous human colon and hepatic epithelial cells. *Cancer Lett.* 170: 41–44.
43. Li, D.R. et al., 2003. Inhibitory effects of tea poly-phenols on telomerase and its ability to induce apoptosis of BEL-7404 human hepato-cellular carcinoma cells. *Zhongguo Yaolixue Tongbao* 19: 934–939.
44. Zhao, Y. et al., 1997. Apoptosis induced by tea polyphenols in HL-60 cells. *Cancer Lett.* 121: 163–167.
45. Sang, S.M. et al., 2006. Bioavailability and stability issues in understanding the cancer preventive effects of tea polyphenols. *J. Sci. Food Agric.* 86: 2256–2265.
46. Du, C.H. et al., 2004. Effects of tea polyphenols on proliferation and apoptosis of lung cancer cell line SPC-A1. *Qingdao Daxue Yixueyuan Xuebao* 40: 107–109, 111.
47. Valcic, S. et al., 1996. Inhibitory effect of six green tea catechins and caffeine on the growth of four selected human tumor cell lines. *Anti-Cancer Drugs* 7: 461–468.
48. Li, G.X. et al., 2010. Pro-oxidative activities and dose-response relationship of (–)-epigallocatechin-3-gallate in the inhibition of lung cancer cell growth: a comparative study in vivo and in vitro. *Carcinogenesis* 31: 902–910.
49. Morre, D.M. et al., 2002. Tea catechins in sustained release formulations as cancer specific proliferation inhibitors. U.S. 43 pp., US 2000-637840 20000810.
50. Ahmad, N. et al., 2000. Green tea polyphenol epigallocatechin-3-gallate differentially modulates NF-κB in cancer cells versus normal cells. *Archiv. Biochem. Biophys.* 376: 338–346.
51. Sachinidis, A. et al., 2000. Green tea compounds inhibit tyrosine phosphorylation of PDGF-receptor and transformation of A172 human glioblastoma. *FEBS Lett.* 471: 51–55.
52. Isemura, M. et al., 2000. Tea catechins and related polyphenols as anti-cancer agents. *BioFactors* 13: 81–85.
53. Stammler, G. et al., 1997. Green tea catechins (EGCG and EGC) have modulating effects on the activity of doxorubicin in drug-resistant cell lines. *Anti-Cancer Drugs* 8: 265–268.
54. Lambert, J.D. et al., 2003. Mechanisms of cancer prevention by tea constituents. *J. Nutr.* 133: 3262S–3267S.
55. Liu, S.H. et al., 2004. Effects of tea polyphenols on growth, metastasis and apoptosis of Lewis lung cancer in mice. *J. Qingdao Univ. Med. Coll.* 40: 104–106.
56. Lambert, J.D. et al., 2008. Effect of genistein on the bioavailability and intestinal cancer chemopreventive activity of (–)-epigallocatechin-3-gallate. *Carcinogenesis* 29: 2019–2024.
57. Ho, Y.S. et al., 2013. Tea extracts confer its antiproliferating effects through inhibition of nicotine- and estrogen-induced 9-nicotinic acetylcholine receptor upregulation in human breast cancer cells. *Special Publication - Royal Society of Chemistry*, 344(Nutrition, Functional and Sensory Properties of Foods), pp. 256–268. Cambridge, UK: RSC Publishing.
58. Lin, J.K. et al., 2009. Mechanisms of cancer chemoprevention by tea and tea polyphenols. *Nutraceutical Sci. Technol.* 8: 161–176.
59. Chen, D. et al., 2008. Tea polyphenols, their biological effects and potential molecular targets. *Histol. Histopathol.* 23: 487–496.
60. Xi, X.Y. et al., 2008. Advances in anti-tumor mechanisms of tea polyphenols and tea pigment. *Zhongguo Linchuang Yingyang Zazhi* 16: 62–65.

61. Yang, C.S. et al., 2009. Cancer prevention by tea: Animal studies, molecular mechanisms and human relevance. *Nat. Rev. Cancer* 9: 429–439.
62. Yang, C.S. et al., 2009. Antioxidative and anti-carcinogenic activities of tea polyphenols. *Archiv. Toxicol.* 83: 11–21.
63. Yang, G.Y. et al., 2000. Effect of black and green tea polyphenols on c-jun phosphorylation and H_2O_2 production in transformed and non-transformed human bronchial cell lines: Possible mechanisms of cell growth inhibition and apoptosis induction. *Carcinogenesis* 21: 2035–2039.
64. Kan, H. et al., 1996. Effect of green tea polyphenol fraction on 1,2-dimethylhydrazine (DMH)-induced colorectal carcinogenesis in the rat. *Nippon Ika Daigaku Zasshi* 63: 106–116.
65. Liang, G. et al., 2010. Green tea catechins augment the antitumor activity of doxorubicin in an in vivo mouse model for chemoresistant liver cancer. *Int. J. Oncol.* 37: 111–123.
66. Mei, Y.Y. et al., 2003. Reversal of cancer multidrug resistance by tea polyphenol in KB cells. *J. Chemother.* (Firenze, Italy) 15: 260–265.
67. Mei, Y.Y. et al., 2005. Reversal of multidrug resistance in KB cells with tea polyphenol antioxidant capacity. *Cancer Biol. Ther.* 4: 468–473.
68. Zhang, G. et al., 2012. Anticancer activities of tea epigallocatechin-3-gallate in breast cancer patients under radiotherapy. *Curr. Mol. Med.* 12: 163–176.
69. Yang, C.S. et al., 1998. Tea and cancer: What do we know and what do we need to know? *Carcinogenic and Anticarcinogenic Factors in Food, Symposium 3rd*, Kaiserslautern, Germany, October 4–7, pp. 334–347.
70. Leone, M. et al., 2003. Cancer prevention by tea polyphenols is linked to their direct inhibition of anti-apoptotic Bcl-2-family proteins. *Cancer Res.* 63: 8118–8121.
71. Pan, M.H. et al., 2000. Induction of apoptosis by the oolong tea polyphenol theasinensin A through cytochrome c release and activation of caspase-9 and caspase-3 in human U937 cells. *J. Agric. Food Chem.* 48: 6337–6346.
72. Saeki, K. et al., 1999. Apoptosis-inducing activity of polyphenol compounds derived from tea catechins in human histiolytic lymphoma U937 cells. *Biosci. Biotech. Biochem.* 3: 585–587.
73. Halder, B. et al., 2012. Black tea polyphenols induce human leukemic cell cycle arrest by inhibiting Akt signaling possible involvement of Hsp90, Wnt/β-catenin signaling and FOXO1. *FEBS J.* 279: 2876–2891.
74. Singh, M. et al., 2013. Tea polyphenols enhance cisplatin chemosensitivity in cervical cancer cells via induction of apoptosis. *Life Sci.* 93: 7–16.
75. Singh, M. et al., 2011. Tea polyphenols induce apoptosis through mitochondrial pathway and by inhibiting nuclear factor-κB and Akt activation in human cervical cancer cells. *Oncol. Res.* 19: 245–257.
76. Sur, S. et al., 2016. Tea polyphenols epigallocatechin gallete and theaflavin restrict mouse liver carcinogenesis through modulation of self-renewal Wnt and hedgehog pathways. *J. Nutr. Biochem.* 27, 32–42.
77. Yamamoto, M. et al., 1999. Effects of tea polyphenols on the invasion and matrix metalloproteinases activities of human fibrosarcoma HT1080 cells. *J. Agric. Food Chem.* 47: 2350–2354.
78. Lin, J.K. et al., 2000. Inhibition of xanthine oxidase and suppression of intracellular reactive oxygen species in HL-60 cells by theaflavin-3,3'-digallate, (–)-Epigallocatechin-3-gallate, and propyl gallate. *J. Agric. Food Chem.* 48: 2736–2743.
79. Qi, L. et al., 1997. Induction of NAD(P)H:quinone reductase by anticarcinogenic ingredients of tea. *Weisheng Yanjiu* 27: 323–326.
80. Saha, P. et al., 2003. Regulation of hazardous exposure by protective exposure: Modulation of phase II detoxification and lipid peroxidation by Camellia sinensis and Swertia chirata. *Teratog. Carcinog. Mutagen.* Suppl 1: 313–322.
81. Chung, F.L. et al., 1999. The prevention of lung cancer induced by a tobacco-specific carcinogen in rodents by green and black tea. *Proc. Soc. Exp. Biol. Med.* (NY, N.Y.) 220: 244–248.
82. Chung, F.L. et al., 1998. Inhibition of lung carcinogenesis by black tea in Fischer rats treated with a tobacco-specific carcinogen: Caffeine as an important constituent. *Cancer Res.* 58: 4096–4101.
83. Weisburger, J.H. et al., 2002. Mechanisms of chronic disease causation by nutritional factors and tobacco products and their prevention by tea polyphenols. *Food Chem. Toxicol.* 40: 1145–1154.
84. Xin, H.W. et al., 2001. Induction of apoptosis by theasinensin in HL-60 cells. *Zhongguo Yaolixue Tongbao* 17: 427–431.
85. Xin, H.W. et al., 2000. Induction of differentiation and its mechanism by theasinensin in HL-60 cells. *Zhongguo Yaolixue Tongbao* 16: 462–466.

8 Cancer-Preventive Substances in Mushrooms

59. Bamboo Fungus or Veiled Lady Mushroom/*Dictyophora (= Phallus) indusiatus, D. duplicata*

60. Golden Oyster Mushroom/*Pleurotus citrinopileatus*

61. Jew's Ear, Jelly Ear, or Judas's Ear/*Auricularia auricular, A. polytricha, A. delicata*

62. Lion's Mane Mushroom/*Heicium erinaceus, H. coralloides*

63. Maitake or Signorina Mushroom and Chestnut Mushroom/*Polyporus frondosus (= Grifola frondosa)*

64. Mongolia Tricholoma/*Tricholoma mongolicum*

65. Oyster Mushroom/*Pleurotus ostreatus*

66. Pine Mushroom/*Tricholoma matsutake*

67. Princess Matsutake or Brazilian Mushroom/*Agaricus blazei (= A. subrufescens, A. brasiliensis, A. rufotegulis)*

68. Ringless Honey Mushroom/*Armillaria tabescens (= Clitocybe tabescens)*

69. Shiitake or Sawtooth Oak Mushroom/*Lentinus edodes*

70. Snow Fungus/*Tremella fuciformis*

71. Split Gill Mushroom/*Schizophyllum commune*

72. Straw Mushroom/*Volvariella volvacea*

73. Winter Mushroom or Enokitake/*Flammulina velutipes*

The edible mushrooms have long been popular with people in many cuisines in East Asia and Europe. It is well known that the fleshy fruiting bodies of certain edible mushrooms have a lot to offer to both meal and human body. Currently, most mushrooms sold in food markets fresh, dried, and canned have been commercially grown on well-controlled mushroom farms. Thus, these mushrooms are safe to most people for consumption; however, wild-collected mushrooms must be very carefully identified because many are considered inedible due to the presence of poisons. This chapter introduces fifteen mushrooms for discussion of their health benefits in cancer prevention and body protection. Of them, the fourteen mushrooms are consumed as both nutritional and functional foods by Eastern Asians since ancient times. Due to their well-deserved reputation for delicious flavor, the selected mushrooms are traditionally used for cooking in both restaurant and home kitchens. While the desirable tastes and smells are enjoyable, consumption of these edible mushrooms also contributes to improving immune strength. Investigations integrating bioorganic chemistry and chemical biology in the last decades have established that these fifteen mushrooms possess a variety of biological properties including immunostimulation, anticancer, anticarcinogenesis, and antimutagenesis. Among these described mushrooms, six (Brazilian mushroom, maitake, shiitake, Lion's mane mushroom, winter mushroom, and oyster mushroom) have been extensively investigated and demonstrate prominent health-promoting and cancer-preventing potentials, while the other nine also display similar positive activities. All of these mushrooms are highly recommended by herbalists and nutritionists. Certainly, one kind of basidiomycete mushroom named *Agaricus bisporus* is the most common edible mushroom and is available in supermarkets worldwide. Its activities regarding human health have been observed in many scientific experiments, yet the mushrooms talked over in this chapter show medical function superior to *A. bisporus*.

59. BAMBOO FUNGUS OR VEILED LADY MUSHROOM

竹荪　衣笠茸

Dictyophora (= Phallus) indusiatus, D. duplicata

Phallaceae

Bamboo fungus is an edible mushroom that originated from two Phallaceae fungi *Dictyophora (= Phallus) indusiatus* and *D. duplicata*. The characteristic of bamboo fungus is a delicate lacy and net-like "white skirt" under its conical to bell-shaped cap fruiting body, thus, it is known as the "Queen of fungus" or "Snow Fairy." The fungus is distributed broadly in southern Asia, Africa, the Americas, and Australia, especially in tropical areas, and grows in woodlands and bamboo forests. The edible mushroom is featured as a precious ingredient in East Asian cuisine as it contains rich amounts of protein, polysaccharides, dietary fiber, zinc, manganese, and iron and has rather higher contents of vitamins C, E, B1, and B2, β-carotene, nicotinic acid, phosphate, and calcium. It has also been used to treat many gastric, inflammatory, and neural diseases as a folk medicine in China since ancient times. Pharmacological approaches established that bamboo fungus possesses some biological properties including antioxidant, antimutagenic, anticancer, antihyperglycemic, immunoregulating, anti-inflammatory, and antimicrobial effects. The cultivation of *D. indusiatus* has been a commercial success in China.

SCIENTIFIC EVIDENCE OF CANCER-INHIBITORY AND CANCER-PREVENTIVE CONSTITUENTS

The isolation and bioactivities of several micromolecules from bamboo fungus have been reported, such as dictyo-phorines-A and -B (nerve growth factor promotors), dictyoquinazols-A, -B, and -C (nerve protectors), hydroxylmethyl-furfural (inhibitor of tyrosinase and oxidant), albaflavenone (antibacterial agent), and five monoterpene alcohols. The antioxidant activity of the mushroom might be largely due to the presence of polyphenols, which could lessen the cellular damage from oxidative stress. However, the anticancer activity of these micromolecules has not been reported.[1] It is clear now that the major constituents in *D. indusiata* fungus were macromolecules such as protein-bound polysaccharides and polysaccharides, which were responsible for the certain levels of antitumor, antioxidant, antimutagenic, and immunoregulative activities.

1. Polysaccharides

Three crude polysaccharide extracts were isolated from the fungus *D. indusiata* by three water solutions with different pH degrees (acidic, neutral, and alkaline). The three extracts showed low antiproliferative effect against human HeLa cervical cancer and HepG2 hepatoma cell lines with the inhibitory rates of 34.15%–37.02% and 16.37%–22.62%, respectively, in an *in vitro* assay and displayed weak to moderate antioxidant activities in radical scavenging tests.[2] The macromolecule-rich hot water extract (HWE) from *D. indusiata* at 2 mg/mL concentration showed average scavenging effect on hydroxyl radical for 52.28%, superoxide anion scavenging effect for 48.64%, and DPPH radical for 97.35%.[3] The *D. indusiata* extracts also presented certain antimutagenicity against *Salmonella typhimurium* TA1535/pSK1002 (IC_{50} of 1.37 mg/mL).[4] The immunostimulating activities of *D. indusiata* polysaccharides were evidenced by the improvement of thymus and pancreatic indexes, elevation of $CD4^+$, CD16, CD57, and IL2 levels, and diminishing of $CD8^+$. Several polysaccharides have been isolated from the bamboo fungus, but most of them showed only lower levels of antitumor property except the two having marked cancer inhibition. Some chemical modification of the polysaccharide structures would amplify the suppressive rates on the carcinomas *in vitro* or *in vivo*.

PD1 and PD1-Zn: PDI (m.w. 1,132 kDa) was a polysaccharide separated from *D. indusiata* fruiting body, which is composed of mannose (29.7%), glucose (56.2%), and galactose (14.1%). In a mouse model with osteosarcoma s180, a dose-dependent viability inhibition and proapoptosis of osteosarcoma s180 were observed in response to treatment of PDI. The s180 cell apoptotic death elicited by PDI was associated with activation of caspase-3, a key executioner of apoptosis.[5] Except for the weak inhibition on MCF-7 cells, DP1 had no effect on other human cancer cells (HeLa, A549, HepG2, SCG-7901, and PC3) and human normal hepatocyte L02 cells.[6] When PDI was chelated with zinc chloride, the produced DP1-Zn complex at 250 μg/mL concentration could exert the antiviability effect against all the above tested cancer cell lines, especially against MCF-7 (breast) and A549 (lung) cell lines, together with the induction of the cell apoptosis.[6] DP1 also exhibited significant immunostimulating activities by enhancing the secretion of TNF-α, IL-6, and nitric oxide (NO) in murine RAW264.7 cells.[6]

DIP, S-DIP, and P-DIP: Although a water-insoluble polysaccharide (DIP) from *D. indusiata* exerted good antioxidant and weak anticancer effects on the tested two cell lines, *P*-DIP and S-DIP obtained from the phosphorylation and sulfation of DIP, respectively, exhibited a satisfactory water solubility and markedly promoted scavenging activity of hydroxyl radicals and DPPH and inhibitory activity against the proliferation of human MCF-7 breast carcinoma and mouse B16 melanoma cell lines.[7]

PD3 and RPD3: A triple helical (1-3)-β-D-glucan with (1-6)-β-D-glucosyl branch termed PD3 (m.w. 5.1×10^5) was isolated from *D. indusiata* fruiting body and another triple helical β-D-glucan assigned as RPD3 was obtained from treatment of PD3 with denaturation–renaturation process. Both PD3 and RPD3 had no direct suppressive effect on solid sarcoma 180 (S180) cells *in vitro* but showed *in vivo* antitumor activity. At i.p. doses of 100 and 250 mg/kg per day for ten days, the inhibitory rates of the S180 cells were 40.97% and 69.05% for RPD3 and 31.97% and 50.88% for PD3, respectively. RPD3 exhibited better antitumor activity than PD3 and even better than 5-FU (20 mg/kg, 51.11%) at the higher dose, suggesting that the process of denaturation–renaturation may be a good technique to improve the biological values of *D. indusiata* polysaccharides.[8]

Dd-S3P: A polysaccharide Dd-S3P (m.w. 380,000) was isolated from the dried fruiting bodies of *D. duplicata* by 2% Na_2CO_3 solution, which was composed of D-glucose, D-mannose, and D-xylose with a molar ratio of 1.83:1.00:1.21. In a mouse model, administration of Dd-S3P hindered the growth of s.c. implanted sarcoma 180 cells by 31.3%.[9]

U-3-A, T-5-N, and T-2-HN: Three water-soluble polysaccharides, that is, two (1-3)-β-D-glucan with β-(1-6)-D-glucosyl branch (T-4-N and T-5-N) and a partially O-acetylated (1-3)-α-D-mannan (T-2-HN, 620 kDa), were separated from aqueous ethanol and alkaline solution extracts of *D. indusiata*. T-5-N and T-2-NH in a mouse model obstructed the growth of sarcoma 180 cells by 77% in mice after, respectively, i.p. injection of 10 and 25 mg/kg per day for ten days, but T-4-N only showed 25% inhibition in the same model.[10] In addition, T-5-N also possesses anti-inflammatory property.

2. Protein-bound polysaccharides and glycoproteins

Six other types of soluble macromolecular fractions, D1–D6, were derived from fractionation of *D. indusiata* fruiting body by different solvents, whose m.w. ranged from 801 to 4656 kDa. D1 (4,656 kDa), D2 (2,118 kDa), D4 (2,919 kDa), and D6 (1,375 kDa) were natural protein-bound polysaccharides with protein–sugar ratios of 19.5:58.3; 1.1:98.8; 8.9:90.7; and 8.6:42.3, respectively, while D3 (801 kDa) and D5 were glycoproteins with protein–sugar ratios of 72.6:27.2 and 55.1:27.4, respectively. Myoinositol was the major residue in the saccharide parts of D1 (67.9%, in mole), D2 (76.5%), and D4 (92.5%), and it was the minor residue in D3 (9.4%) and D5 (5.3%) but undetectable in D6. Among the fractions, D3 displayed the most potent antioxidant capacities in the DPPH radical and hydroxyl radical scavenging tests, whereas D1 with the largest molecule had the weakest radical scavenging activity.[1] However, these soluble macromolecules have not reported their antitumor activity yet. The antioxidant activities should be conducive to exerting the anticarcinogenic, anti-inflammatory, and immunoenhancing effects. DIGP-2, a glycolprotein separated from the bamboo fungus, which consists of D-galactose, D-glucose, and D-mannose in a molar ratio of 0.78:2.12:1.00 in its saccharide part, showed 36.2% suppression against the viability of sarcoma 180 cells *in vitro*.[11]

Nanoformulation

DP1-SeNPs is a selenium nanoparticle of DP1 polysaccharide where DP1 is attached to the surface of selenium nanoparticles via Se–O bond. DP1-–SeNP could enhance selectively the antiproliferative activity on cancer cells via the cell apoptosis-induction and S cell cycle arrest. The proapoptotic mechanism was associated with overincrease of ROS, mitochondrial dysfunction, and activation of caspases-3, -8, and -9. This biofunctionalized nanoparticle technique may offer a better anticancer remedy with high efficiency and few side effects.[12]

Conclusion and Suggestion

On the basis of the experimental evidences, it can be concluded that the crude water extracts and macromolecules (such as polysaccharides, protein-bound polysaccharides, and glycoproteins) isolated from *Dictyophora indusiata* (bamboo fungus) possess antioxidant, anticancer, antimutagenic, and immunoregulative abilities. Although their potencies are not so prominent, consumption of bamboo fungus is still believed to bring various health benefits to humans. These bioactive ingredients including macromolecules and micromolecules in bamboo fungus may help synergistically to potentiate the immune responses and antioxidant functions, leading to the cancer-preventive potential.

REFERENCES

1. (a) Ker, Y.B. et al., 2011. Structural characteristics and antioxidative capability of the soluble polysaccharides present in Dictyophora indusiata (Vent. ex Pers.) Fish Phallaceae. *Evid.-Based Complement. Alternat. Med.* Article ID 396013: 9. (b) Zidan, A. 2014. A review on antitumor actions of polysaccharide isolated from medicinal mushrooms. *Int. J. Acad. Sci. Res.* 2(1): 14–20.
2. Li, X.Y. et al., a) 2012. In vitro antioxidant and antiproliferation activities of polysaccharides from various extracts of different mushrooms. *Int. J. Mol. Sci.* 13: 5801–5817; b) 2013. Antioxidant and antiproliferation activities of polysaccharides in edible fungi in vitro. *Shipin Keji* 38(3): 179–182.
3. Oyetayo, O.V. et al., 2009. Antioxidant and antimicrobial properties of aqueous extract from Dictyophora indusiata. *Open Mycol. J.* 3(1): 20–26.

4. Ishiharajima, E. et al., 2007. Investigation on bioactive substances contained in agricultural products produced in Tochigi prefecture-antimutagenicity of fungi. *Tochigi-ken Hoken Kankyo Senta Nenpo.* Volume Date 2006, 12: 43–47.

5. Zhong, B. et al., 2013. Induction of apoptosis in osteosarcoma S180 cells by polysaccharide from dictyophora indusiata. *Cell Biochem. Funct.* 31(8): 719–723.

6. Liao, W.Z. et al., a) 2015. Structure characterization of a novel polysaccharide from Dictyophora indusiata and its macrophage immunomodulatory activities. *J. Agric. Food Chem.* 63: 535–44; b) 2015. Preparation and characterization of Dictyophora indusiata polysaccharide-zinc complex and its augmented antiproliferative activity on human cancer cells. *J. Agricul. Food Chem.* 63(29): 6525–6534.

7. Deng, C. et al., 2015. Physiochemical and biological properties of phosphorylated polysaccharides from Dictyophora indusiata. *Int. J. Biol. Macromol.* 72: 894–899; 2015. Characterization, antioxidant and cytotoxic activity of sulfated derivatives of a water-insoluble polysaccharide from Dictyophora indusiata. *Mol. Med. Reports* 11: 2991–2998.

8. Deng, C. et al., 2013. Antitumor activity of the regenerated triple-helical polysaccharide from Dictyophora indusiata. *Int. J. Biol. Macromol.* 61, 453–458.

9. Lin, Y.M. et al., 1997. Isolation, purification and characterization of polysaccharide Dd-S3P from Dictyophora duplicata (Bose) Fischer. *Shengwu Huaxue Zazhi* 13(1): 99–102.

10. Ukai, S.G. et al., 1983. Polysaccharides in fungi. XIII. Antitumor activity of various polysaccharides isolated from Dictyophora indusiata, Ganoderma japonicum, Cordyceps cicadae, Auricularia auricula-judae, and Auricularia species. *Chem. Pharm. Bull.* 31(2): 741–744.

11. Ke, H.Z. et al., 2001. Studies on component analysis and antitumor of glycoprotein DIGP-2 from the submerged mycelium of Dityophora indusiata fish. *Strait Pharm. J.* 13(4): 1–3.

12. Liao, W.Z. et al., 2015. Biofunctionalization of selenium nanoparticle with Dictyophora indusiata polysaccharide and its antiproliferative activity through death-receptor and mitochondria-mediated apoptotic pathways. *Sci. Reports* 5: 18629.

60. GOLDEN OYSTER MUSHROOM

金顶蘑　榆木茸

Pleurotus citrinopileatus

Pleurotaceae

Golden oyster mushroom is the edible fruiting body of the Pleurotaceae fungus *Pleurotus citrino-pileatus*. The gilled mushroom is native to eastern Russia, northern China, and Japan. It is one of the most popular wild foods in its distributing region, and it is commercially cultivated in oriental countries now for cooking delicious cuisine. According to a report of the nutritional examination, the golden oyster mushroom collected in western Kenya is a great source of protein, fiber, vitamins B3 and B5, and potassium. The contents of vitamin B2, phosphorus, and magnesium in the mushroom are higher than those in other common mushrooms.[1] Biological approaches have evidenced the antioxidant, antihyperglycemic, blood-sugar-lessening, antidiabetic, and hypolipidemic properties.[2–5]

SCIENTIFIC EVIDENCE OF CANCER-INHIBITORY AND CANCER-PREVENTIVE CONSTITUENTS

1. Polysaccharides

A crude polysaccharide extract from liquid fermentation of *P. citrinopileatus* fed to mice at doses of 0.4 and 0.8 g/kg deterred the growth of sarcoma 180 (S180) cells by 35.84% and 40.93%, respectively. Meanwhile, the elevation of both indexes of thymus and spleen were observed in the tested mice, implying that the antitumor effect might be correlated to its immunoregulative activity.[6] Three polysaccharide extracts were obtained from the fractionation of *P. citrinopileatus* zymotic fluid, wherein the exopolysaccharide extract showed the strongest inhibitory effect against mouse S180 cells and human poorly differentiated colon adenocarcinoma cells *in vitro*, but the polysaccharide extracts from the whole zymotic fluid and the mycelia showed lower and lowest inhibition only on the colon cancer cells, respectively.[7] From *P. citrinopileatus* fruiting bodies, several polysaccharide extracts were isolated, FIII-1 and FIII-2 were two water-insoluble protein-bound β-(1-3)-D-glucans that were effective in restraining the proliferation of S180 cells with 79.5% and 93.5% inhibition, respectively. FIII-1a (m.w. 68×10^4) and FIII-1b (m.w. 40×10^4) were separated from the FIII-1, which consisted of glucan–protein 80:20 and 68:32 wt./wt. and showed 81.4% and 81.0% inhibitory rates on S180 cells, respectively. Likewise, FIII-2a (m.w. 19×10^5) and FIII-2b (m.w. 12×10^5) from the FIII-2 exerted 87.3% and 90.1% suppression on the S180 cells, both of which have the same ratios of glucan–protein as 87:13 wt./wt. However, the isolated water-soluble protein-bound polysaccharides FIs and water-insoluble protein-bound polysaccharides FIIs showed > 50% lower antiproliferative activities on the S180 cells than the FIII-1 and FIII-2.[8] PC-4 (189 kDa), a water-soluble homogeneous polysaccharide isolated from the fruiting bodies consists of β-(1-3)-linked glucopyranose as a main chain with (1–6) linked branches. Administration of PC-4 resulted in the antigrowth effect against sarcoma 180 in mice with 67% inhibitory rate. But, PC-4 showed no such inhibition *in vitro*.[9]

In addition, SPPC ($>10^5$ Da) was the water-soluble polysaccharide extract derived from the fermentation broth of *P. citrinopileatus* by alcohol precipitation, which mainly consists of glucose and mannose in higher percentages and presented obvious immunoregulating properties. Oral administration of SPPC in a daily dose of 50 mg/kg to tumor-bearing mice for 12 days could significantly amplify the numbers of T cells, CD4+ and CD8+ cells, and macrophages, subsequently delaying the proliferative rate of pulmonary sarcoma cells *in vivo*.[10] In addition, SPPC also exhibited antihyperglycemic effect in rats with streptozotocin (STZ)-induced diabetes.[4]

2. Glycoprotein

A glycoprotein termed PCP-3A was isolated from the fruit body of *P. citrinopileatus*, which is a nonlectin glycoprotein composed of 10 subunits (each approximately 45.0 kDa in size). At a concentration of $\approx$12.5 μg/mL, PCP-3A hampered the proliferation of human U937 myeloid leukemia cells *in vitro* in a time-dependent manner concomitant with induction of S cell cycle arrest and apoptotic death.[11] Further antibody neutralization test revealed that the growth inhibition on the U937 cells by PCP-3A was also related to the stimulation of human mononuclear cells to secrete cytokines TNF-α, IL-2, and IFN-γ. These cytokines subsequently participated in the growth suppression of U937 cells.[12] PCP-3A also showed an anti-inflammatory potential via down-regulation of certain pro-inflammatory mediators, including iNOS and NF-κB.[13] The findings suggested that PCP-3A has a potential for developing an antileukemia and anti-inflammatory ingredient in a health food combination.

3. Lectin

A homodimeric lectin (32.4 kDa) was prepared from fresh fruiting bodies of *P. citrinopileatus*, and its *N*-terminal amino acid sequence was assigned as QYSQMAQVME. In a mouse model implanted with sarcoma 180, intraperitoneal injection of the lectin at a daily dose of 5 mg/kg for 20 days exerted approximately 80% antigrowth effect *in vivo*. At a concentration of 2 μM, the lectin provoked a maximal mitogenic response from murine splenocytes, indicating that the immunostimulation was involved in the antitumor activity.[14] The lectin additionally displayed an inhibitory effect on HIV-1 reverse transcriptase without antifungal activity.[14]

CONCLUSION AND SUGGESTION

Golden oyster mushroom is rich in bioactive macromolecules such as protein-bound polysaccharides, glycoprotein, and lectin, all of which showed the antitumor effect against sarcoma 180 cells *in vivo*, and the cancer suppressive effect should mostly depend on their remarkable capacity of antitumor immunity. Of them, the isolated exopoly-saccharides showed the most potent *in vivo* and *in vitro* antitumor activity. Despite more evidences and more wide cancer suppressive potentials that need to be further investigated, golden oyster mushroom still is a safe and valuable health food being recommended for enhancement of human immune system and lowering the risk of cancer.

REFERENCES

1. Musieba, F. et al., 2013. Proximate composition, amino acids and vitamins profile of Pleurotus citrinopileatus Singer: An indigenous mushroom in Kenya. *Am. J. Food Technol.* 8: 200–206.
2. Rushita, S. et al., 2013. Effect of Pleurotus citrinopileatus on blood glucose insulin and catalase of streptozotocin-induced type 2 diabetes mellitus rats. *J. Animal & Plant Sci.* 23(6): 1566–1571.
3. Lee, Y.L. et al., 2007. Antioxidant properties of three extracts from Pleurotus citrinopileatus. *LWT–Food Sci. Technol.* 40(5): 823–823.
4. Hu, S.H. et al., 2006. a) Antihyperglycemic effect of polysaccharide from fermented broth of Pleurotus citrinopileatus. *Applied Microbiol. Biotechnol.* 70(1): 107–113; b) 2006. Antihyperlipidemic and antioxidant effects of extracts from Pleurotus citrinopileatus. *J. Agricul. Food Chem.* 54(6): 2103–2110.
5. Gunde-Cimerman, N. et al., 1995. Pleurotus fruiting bodies contain the inhibitor of 3-hydroxy-3-methylglutaryl-coenzyme A reductase-lovastatin. *Exp. Mycol.* 19(1): 1–6.
6. Xin, X.L. et al., 2009. Antitumor activity of polysaccharide from submerged fermentation liquid of Pleurotus citrinopileatus. *Shipin Kexue* 30(17): 324–325.
7. Wang, X.J. et al., 2005. A Study on the inhibition effect of polysaccharides extracted from Pleurotus citrinopileatus on tumor cells in vitro. *Acta Edulis Fungi* 12(1): 9–13.
8. Zhang, J. et al., 1994. Antitumor polysaccharides from a Chinese mushroom, Yuhuangmo, the fruiting body of Pleurotus citrinopileatus. *Biosci. Biotechnol. Biochem.* 58(7): 1195–2021.

9. Zhang, L.P. et al., 1995. Structural determination and study of antitumor activity of polysaccharide PC-4 from Pleurotus citrinopileatus. *Zhenjun Xuebao* 14(1): 69–74.

10. Wang, J.C. et al., 2005. Optimization for the production of water-soluble polysaccharide from Pleurotus citrinopileatus in submerged culture and its antitumor effect. *Appl. Microbial. Biotechnol.* 67(6): 759–766.

11. Chen, J.N. et al., 2009. A glycoprotein extracted from golden oyster mushroom Pleurotus citrinopileatus exhibiting growth inhibitory effect against U937 leukemia cells. *J. Agricul. Food Chem.* 57(15): 6706–6711.

12. Chen, J.N. et al., 2010. In vitro antitumor and immunomodulatory effects of the protein PCP-3A from mushroom Pleurotus citrinopileatus. *J. Agricul. Food Chem.* 58(23): 12117–12122.

13. Chen, J.N. et al., 2011. Inhibitory effect of a glycoprotein isolated from golden oyster mushroom (Pleurotus citrinopileatus) on the lipopolysaccharide-induced inflammatory reaction in RAW 264.7 macrophage. *J. Agricul. Food Chem.* 59(13): 7092–7097.

14. Li, Y.R. et al., 2008. A novel lectin with potent antitumor, mitogenic and HIV-1 reverse transcriptase inhibitory activities from the edible mushroom Pleurotus citrinopileatus. *Biochim. et Biophys. Acta.* 1780(1): 51–57.

61. JEW'S EAR, JELLY EAR, OR JUDAS'S EAR

黑木耳　黑キクラゲ　목이버섯

Auricularia auricular, A. polytricha, A. delicata

Auriculariales

Jew's ear originated from three edible fungi *Auricularia auricular*, *A. polytricha*, and *A. delicata*, as well as other fungi of the same genus (Auricularia). Jew's ear has been one of the favorite nutritional foods for the cuisines of Eastern Asia for many years. In the nutritional effects, it is shown that the Auricularia algae are a good source of vitamins B2 and D, niacin, and minerals (such as iron, magnesium, phosphorus, and calcium). Broad pharmacological studies demonstrated that Jew's ear possesses anti-inflammatory, antioxidant, hypoglycemic, hypolipemic, anticoagulant, antiatherosclerosis, antimutagenic, anticarcinogenic, antiulcerative, antiplatelet aggregation, immunoimproving, antifertile, antiaging, and nucleic acid/protein synthesis-enhancing properties.

SCIENTIFIC EVIDENCE OF CANCER-INHIBITORY AND CANCER-PREVENTIVE CONSTITUENTS

A dichloromethane fraction (DCMF) from 70% ethanol extract of *A. auricula-judae* was found to have potent inhibitory activity against the proliferation of broncheoalveolar cancer (IC_{50} of 57.2 μg/mL) and gastric cancer cells (IC_{50} of 73.2 μg/mL) concomitant with induction of the cell apoptosis via downregulation of Bcl-2 expression and upregulation of p53 expression.[1]

1. Protein-bound polysaccharides

Both HWE and 0.1 N NaOH extract of Jew's ear were rich in protein-bound polysaccharide, exhibiting 82.7%–90.8% inhibition against the growth of sarcoma 180 (S180) implanted in mice; the extracts consisted of four types of monosaccharides and 15 amino acids.[2] The extracts remarkably prolonged the life duration of mice bearing H22 hepatoma and suppressed the growth of entity S180 *in vivo*.[3] By i.p. injection to mice bearing sarcoma 180 for ten days, the water-soluble protein-bound polysaccharides at a dose of 200 mg/kg per day resulted in significant inhibitory effect against the growth of S180 cells with inhibitory ratio of 89%, whereas the alkali-soluble protein-bound polysaccharides showed lower tumor-inhibitory rate of 31% at the same dose.[4,5]

2. Polysaccharides

The polysaccharide component could be considered as the major constituent responsible for the *in vivo* antitumor property of Jew's ear. upon the basis of the different extraction techniques and a variety of the herb sources used in the investigations, many antitumor polysaccharides have been prepared from Jew's ear. APPs, a crude *A. polytricha* polysaccharide extract hindered the proliferation and DNA synthesis of A549 lung adenocarcinoma cells *in vitro* and *in vivo* in a dose-dependent manner. Simultaneously, APPs elicited the cell apoptosis and G0/G1 cell arrest via upexpression of cyclin-dependent kinase (CDK) inhibitors p53 and p21, downregulation of cyclins-A and -D and CDK2 expressions, release of cytochrome c from mitochondria to cytosol, activation of caspases-9 and -3, and cleavage of poly (ADP-ribose) polymerase.[6] From the isolation of APPs, several antitumor polysaccharides were obtained. Of them, APPIIA (110 kDa), which consists of xylose and mannose with both α- and β-glycosidic linkages, showed better suppressive effect against the growth of sarcoma 180 (S180) in a mouse model.[7] AAPS2 notably lowered sialic acid levels in S180 cell membrane and influenced the membrane glycoprotein and glycolipids chain terminal residues, leading to change in the membrane function and blockage of the S180 cell growth *in vivo*.[8]

Three β-(1-6)-branched (1-3)-β-D-glucans such as U-3-N (m.w. 6.1×10^5) and U-3-AP1 (m.w. 6.3×10^4) were isolated from the hot-water extract of Jew's ear and *N*-5P (m.w. 5.6×10^5) was derived from the alkali-soluble extract of the fruiting bodies. U-3-N and *N*-5P have similar backbone of β-(1-3)-linked D-glucosyl residues with single β-(1-6)-linked D-glucosyl groups attached as side chains; both displayed potent antitumor activity against the solid form of S180 in mice. U-3-AP1 was a β-(1-6)-branched (1-3)-β-D-glucan that only showed little effect against the S180 growth in the test.[9-11] Likewise, three acidic heteroglycans, U-3-A, MEA, and MHA, were also obtained from fractionation of Jew's ear extract. U-3-A, a glucuronoxyloglucomannan, displayed prominent antitumor activity against S180 in mice with 86% inhibitory rate by i.p. injection in a daily dose of 25 mg/kg for 10 days. Both MEA and MHA were glucuronoxylmannans with a core of partially O-acetylated-(1-3) linked D-mannosyl residues and only showed low suppression of S180 cells in vivo.[12] A water-soluble β-glucan coded as AAG was isolated by 70% ethanol extract of *A. auricular-judae*. AAG exhibited strong antiproliferative effect against acinar cell carcinoma. The in vivo tests showed that AAG markedly inhibited the growth of S180 cells in a dose-dependent fashion and augmented the ratios of tested animal body weight. In addition to the decrease of Bcl-2 expression and increase of Bax expression, AAG also obviously induced the apoptotic death of solid form of S180 cells.[13] AAFRC is a 0.05 M NaOH solution-soluble polysaccharide obtained from *A. polytricha*, which is a glucan consisting of a backbone of 1,3-β-glucan, 1,4-α-glucan, and 1,3-α-glucan with a single 1→)-α-D-glucopyranosyl side-branching unit on every six residues along the main chain. AAFRC (m.w. ≈ 1.2×10^6 Da) showed obvious antigrowth effect in mice implanted S180, with the inhibitory rate of 43.61%.[14] From *A. auricula-judae* grown in selenium medium, four selenium polysaccharides termed SeAP I-1, SeAP I-2, SeAP II, and SeAP III were prepared. All of them demonstrated antitumor activity against S180 cells. However, the activities of SeAP I-2 and SeAP II were significantly stronger than those of SeAP I-1 and SeAP III.[15]

Furthermore, in the experiments, the polysaccharide components prepared from Jew's ear also exerted anti-^{60}Co-γ radiation and immunoregulating activities including elevation of the spleen and thymus indexes, increase in phagocytosis and lymphocyte transformation, and activation of super oxide dismutase (SOD) and chloramhenicol acetyltransferase (CAT).[3,16-19] The Jew's ear polysaccharides are capable of diminishing chemotherapeutic drug (such as cyclophosphamide) induced toxic/side effects by reducing the raised micronucleus rate of bone marrow and promoting the declined leukocyte.[18]

The laboratory experiments further found that the structural modification by chemical methods was able to amplify the antitumor activities of polysaccharides. An aldehyde-type β-1,3-glucan was formed from modification of the Jew's ear polysaccharides, β-1,3-glucan (m.w. 9.5×10^5), which was effective on S180 cells in mice. After i.p. injection in a dose of 5 mg/kg per day for ten days, the inhibitory efficacy reached 99.8%,[20] and an alkali-insoluble and heavy-branched (1-3)-β-D-glucan was a major constituent of the fruiting body of Jew's ear, showing no inhibitory activity on the tumor. However, the numerous branched glucans of Jew's ear were degraded by a series of controlled chemical reactions including periodate oxidation, borohydride reduction, and mild acid hydrolysis. A degraded water-soluble glucan, having covalently linked polyhydroxy groups attached at O-6 of the (1-3)-linked-D-glucosyl residues, showed potent anti-neoplastic activity. The attachments of polyhydroxy groups to the (1-3)-β-D-glucan backbone altered the solubility in water, which enhanced the antitumor potency.[9]

Conclusion and Suggestion

On the basis of these encouraging research results, Jew's ear mushroom can be considered to be a nutritional and safe anticancer food; its polysaccharides are the most important functional components in the Auricularia algae. The scientific evidences revealed the biological capabilities of Jew's ear mushroom and its polysaccharides in both in vitro and in vivo anticancer, immunoenhancing, proapoptotic, antioxidant, and antiradiation effects without toxicity. Hence, these positive facts suggest that Jew's ear mushroom could be consumed as a functional additive and an antitumor supplement in human diet, being helpful in assisting cancer chemoprevention, chemo- and radiotherapies, besides the nutritional contribution.

REFERENCES

1. Reza, A. et al., 2014. Dichloromethane extract of the jelly ear mushroom auricularia Auricula-judae (higher Basidiomycetes) inhibits tumor cell growth in vitro. *Int. J. Med. Mushrooms* 16(1): 37–47.

2. Lee, S.A. et al., 1981. Studies on the antitumor components of Korean basidiomycetes. II. Antitumor components of Schizophyllum commune and Auricularia auricula-judae. *Han'guk Kyunhakhoechi* 9: 25–29.

3. Huang, B.N. et al., 2004. Study on antitumor effects of Auricularia auriculajudae polysaccharide. *Harbin Shangye Daxue Xuebao, Ziran Kexueban* 20: 648–651.

4. Qi, D.S. et al., 1994. Antitumor action of polysaccharides from Auricularia auricular. *Huazhong Nongye Daxue Xuebao* 13: 160–163.

5. Wu, C.M. et al., 1991. Cytoprotection action of the polysaccharide from Auricularia polytricha Sacc. *J. Zhongguo Pharm. Univ.* 22: 305–307.

6. Yu, J. et al., 2014. Auricularia polytricha polysaccharides induce cell cycle arrest and apoptosis in human lung cancer A549 cells. *Int. J. Biol. Macromol.* 68: 67–71.

7. Qing, Y. et al., 2009. Isolation, purification and structural characterization of bioactive polysaccharide APP II A from Auricularia polytricha. *Junwu Xuebao* 28(6): 813–818.

8. Song, G.L. et al., 2012. Research on change of S180 tumor cell membrane function by Auricularia polytricha polysaccharides. *Zhongguo Yaoxue Zazhi* 47(4): 255–261.

9. Misaki, A. et al., 1981. Studies on interrelation of structure and antitumor effects of polysaccharides: Antitumor action of periodate-modified, branched (1-3)-β-D-glucan of Auricularia auricula-judae, and other polysaccharides containing (1-3)-β-glycosidic linkages. *Carbohydr. Res.* 92: 121–135.

10. Kiho, T. et al., 1991. Polysaccharides in fungi. XXVI. Two branched (1-3)-β-D-glucans from hot water extract of Yuer. *Chem. Pharm. Bull.* 39: 798–800.

11. Kiho, T. et al., 1987. Polysaccharides in fungi. XX. Structure and antitumor activity of a branched (1-3)-β-D-glucan from alkaline extract of Yuer. *Chem. Pharm. Bull.* 35: 4286–4293.

12. Ukai, S. et al., 1983. Polysaccharides in fungi. XIII. Antitumor activity of various polysaccharides isolated from Dictyophora indusiata, Ganoderma japonicum, Cordyceps cicadae, Auricularia auricula-judae, and Auricularia species. *Chem. Pharm. Bull.* 31: 741–744.

13. Ma, Z.C. et al., 2010. Evaluation of water soluble β-glucan from Auricularia auricular-judae as potential antitumor agent. *Carbohydr. Polym.* 80: 977–983.

14. Song, G.L. et al., 2012. Structure characterization and antitumor activity of an α,β-glucan polysaccharide from Auricularia polytricha. *Food Res. Intl.* 45: 381–387.

15. Song, G.L. et al., 2010. Selenium polysaccharides from Auricularia auricula-judae and their effect on membrane mobility of ascite S180 tumor cells. *Junwu Xuebao* 29: 713–718.

16. Zhou, H.P. et al., 1989. Antihepatitis and antimutation of polysaccharides from the Mellella fuciormis and Auricularia auricular. *J. Zhongguo Pharm. Univ.* 20: 51–52.

17. Xia, E.N. et al., 1989. The bioactivity of Mu-Er polysaccharides. *J. Zhongguo Pharm. Univ.* 20: 227.

18. Misaki, A. et al., 1995. Kikurage (Tree-ear) and Shirokikurage (white Jelly-leaf): Auricularia auricula and Tremella fuciformis. *Food Review Int.* 11: 211–218.

19. Yu, M.Y. et al., 2009. Isolation of an antitumor polysaccharide from Auricularia polytricha (Jew's ear) and its effects on macrophage activation. *Eur. Food Res. Technol.* 228: 477–485.

20. Koiwa, S. et al., 1985. Modified polysaccharides as neoplasm inhibitors. Japanese Kokai Tokkyo Koho JP 83-245525 19831228.

62. LION'S MANE MUSHROOM

猴菇菌　山伏茸　노루궁뎅이버섯

Heicium erinaceus, H. coralloides

Hydnaceae

Lion's mane mushroom is the fruit body of edible fungi *Heicium erinaceus* and *H. coralloides* (Hydnaceae), which are native to North America, Europe and Asia. As a culinary–medicinal mushroom, it has been widely consumed for hundreds of years in some Asian countries (such as China, India, Japan, and Korea) to cook a wild gourmet food and treat digestive diseases. Nutritional analysis showed that each 100 g of the dried fungus provides 26.3 g protein, 4.2 g fat, 44.9 g carbohydrate, 6.4 g thin fiber, 0.89 mg vitamin B1, 1.89 mg vitamin B2, and 0.01 mg carotene as well as various amounts of nutritional minerals (calcium, chromium, cobalt, copper, iron, magnesium, manganese, molybdenum, phosphorus, selenium, sodium, sulfur, and zinc). Biological approaches demonstrated that *H. erinaceus* fruiting body and mycelia biomass possess many health-promoting properties such as antiulcer, hypolipemic, immunoenhancing, antioxidant, antihypertensive, antidiabetic, anti-inflammatory, neuroprotective, antiaging, and antimicrobial effects in addition to its antitumor and anticarcinogenic effects.[1]

SCIENTIFIC EVIDENCE OF CANCER-INHIBITORY AND CANCER-PREVENTIVE ACTIVITIES

Hot water (HWE) and microwaved 50% ethanol (MWE) extracts of *H. erinaceus* exerted strong promotion of the cell death of CT-26 murine colon cancer through proapoptosis. Daily i.p. injections of HWE or MWE (10 mg/kg/mice) for two weeks significantly reduced the tumor weights by 38% and 41%, together with simultaneous inhibition of COX-2, 5-LOX, and vascular endothelial growth factor (VEGF) and activation of natural killer (NK) cells and macrophages. Also, both HWE and MWE hampered lung metastasis by 66% and 69% in mice, respectively, along with blocking the expressions of MMPs-2, -9, and u-PA. Also, the downregulation of extracellular ERK, JNK, and p38 MAPK phosphorylations was found to involve in the antimigrative and anti-invasive effects on the CT-26 cells.[2,3] Another HEW obtained from *H. erinaceus* mycelia had markedly effective antioxidant activity. HEW prominently suppressed COX-2 expression in human HepG2 hepatoma cells.[4] Both its ethyl acetate extract and petroleum ether extract were effective in suppressing the proliferation of human SMMC-7221 and MHCC-97H hepatoma cell lines and their activities were comparable to those of 5-FU (a chemotherapeutic drug).[5]

Comparatively, the water extract (WEHE) of *H. erinaceus* exerted NK cell-based immunoregulatory anticancer activities. The immunopotentiative responses could be transferred to the effect of WEHE against the proliferation of tumor cells via activation of the cytolyticity of NK cells through the induction of IL-12 in total splenocytes and enhanced the cytolytic effect of total splenocytes toward Yac-1 cells (mouse T-lymphoma cells) in a dose-dependent manner.[6,7] *In vivo* studies confirmed its anticarcinogenetic property in the inhibition of aflatoxin-B-caused hepatoma.[1] Moreover, WEHE sensitized doxorubicin (Dox)-mediated apoptotic signaling by reducing c-FLIP expression via JNK activation and augmented intracellular Dox accumulation via blockage of NF-κB activity. The finding provided an effective tool that can be used for treating drug-resistant human hepatoma by combining the Lion's mane mushroom extract with Dox.[8]

Besides, two bioactive fractions labeled as HTJ5 and HTJ5A were isolated from the broth of *H. erinaceus* by multiple chromatographic fractionations. HTJ5 and HTJ5A showed concentration-dependent weak cytotoxic effect *in vitro* against human Huh-7 and HepG2 (liver), HT-29 (colon), and NCI-87 (stomach) cancer cell lines with IC_{50} values of 0.8–5.0 mg/mL. *In vivo* tumor xenograft studies further confirmed their antitumor efficacy in the four tumor models (HepG2, Huh-7, HT-29, and NCI-87). Their antitumor efficacy on the four tumors was greater than that of 5-FU and less toxic to the host. By using HPLC technique, twenty-two compounds were obtained from HTJ5 and HTJ5A including seven cyclodipeptides, five indoles, pyrimidines, amino acids and their derivative, one anthraquinone, three flavones, and six small aromatic compounds.[9]

SCIENTIFIC EVIDENCE OF CANCER-INHIBITORY AND CANCER-PREVENTIVE CONSTITUENTS

The chemical investigations on *H. erinaceus* led to isolation of various constituents such as volatile aromatics, mono- and diterpenes, alkaloids, polyphenols, steroids, fatty acids, vitamins, glycosphingolipids, and polysaccharides. Many different types of molecules have been found to be in charge of the cancer-inhibitory and -preventive activities as well as other diverse biological properties.

1. Polysaccharides

The total polysaccharides (HEPS) prepared from Lion's mane mushroom displayed prominent immunopotentiating activities. At a dose of 200 mg/kg in normal mice, HEPS stimulated NK cell activity and T-lymphocyte proliferation in mouse spleen and notably amplified phagocytosis rate and index.[10,11] Oral administration of HEPS to mice at doses of 50–400 mg/kg for 10–15 days notably enlarged the indexes of spleen and thymus and elevated the level of IFN-γ and IL-2 in serum as well as prompting the cell apoptosis through activation of caspase-3, thereby suppressing the growth of S180 *in vivo*. The best antigrowth rate (57.57%) was observed in the treatment with 50 mg/kg per day of HEPS for 10 days against xenograft sarcoma 180.[10–13] Similarly, intragastric administration of HEPS in doses of 100 and 200 mg/kg for 10 days resulted in the growth inhibitory effect against transplanted H22 hepatoma in mice by > 26% in mechanisms that closely correlated to the upregulation of immune function and antiangiogenic function in tumor tissue, that is, significantly amplified thymus index, elevated the serum levels of TNF-α and IL-2, reduced VEGF level, and augmented serum albumin.[14] The HEPS further demonstrated clinical benefits for the treatment of carcinomas of skin, esophageal, and stomach and for some other diseases in China; the established efficacy should be principally attributed to its positive capability on immune function.[15,16]

The water-soluble polysaccharides of Lion's mane mushroom are also rich in two complexes of mannogalactoglucoxylan–protein and galactomanno–glucoxylanxylan–protein.[17]

Fifteen individual polysaccharides have been separated from Lion's mane mushroom up to now. Among them, five of the polysaccharide fractions (FI0-a-β, FI0-a-β, FI-β, FII0-1, and FIII-2b) demonstrated prominent longevity effect in assays for anticancer activity.[15] Two water-soluble poly-saccharides (m.w. > 1 × 10[5] kDa), HEW and HLW, were separated from the cultivated broth of *H. erinaceus* and *H. laciniatum*, respectively. HEW was mainly composed of glucose, while HLW was composed of galactose. Both could markedly suppress pulmonary metastatic cancer via stimulation of T cells, CD4+ cells, and macrophages in mice. In addition, HEW was more effective than HLW *in vivo*, indicating that the β-glucan portion of the HEW is significant in the expression of immunoregulating and antitumor activities.[18,19]

2. A complex of polysaccharide protein

HEG-5, a polysaccharide protein purified from the fermentation of Hericium erinaceus mycelia CZ-2, could obviously elicit the tested human SGC-7901 gastric cancer cells to apoptotic death and cell cycle arrest at S phase along with downregulation of Bcl2, PI3K, and Akt1 expressions, upregulation of p53, CDK4, Bax, Bad, and capases-8 and -3 expressions, and lowering of a PI3k/Akt signaling pathway, subsequently impeding the proliferation and colony formation of the SGC-7901 cells *in vitro*.[20]

3. Fatty acids

Y-A-2 (**1**, = 9R*,10S*,12Z-9,10-dihydroxy-8-oxo-10-octadecenoic acid) is a fatty acid component obtained from the isolation of Lion's mane mushroom, which demonstrated moderate growth-inhibiting activity against human HeLa cervical carcinoma cells *in vitro*. When the concentration was increased to 100 μg/mL, Y-A-2 (**1**) was capable of fully killing the cervical cancer cells.[21–23]

4. γ -Pyrones and γ-pyridones

From the cultured mycelia of *H. erinaceum*, two γ-pyrones assigned as erinapyrones-A (**2**) and -B (**3**) were separated, showing antiproliferative effect against the HeLa cervical cancer cells *in vitro*. Their minimum concentrations giving complete death of HeLa cells were 0.88 μM for erinapyrone-A (**2**) and 1.76 μM for erinapyrones-B (**3**).[24,25] Four γ-pyridone alkaloids designated as erinacerins-M–P were isolated from the solid culture of *H. erinaceus*, displaying moderate cytotoxicity against human K562 leukemia cells with IC$_{50}$s in a range of 11.4–18.2 μM and weak cytotoxic effect against doxorubicin-resistant K562 cells. Among them, the most active alkaloid was assigned as erinacerin-P (**4**) in the *in vitro* assay with K562 cell line.[26]

5. γ -Lactams and γ-lactones

The bioassay-guided chemistry investigations led to the discovery of many isoindolinone alkaloids and the related lactones from the extracts of *H. erinaceum*. *In vitro* assays displayed that some lactams were contributors to the antitumor activity of *H. erinaceum*. Isohericenone (**5**), isohericerin (**6**), and erinacerin-A (**7**) were effective in the growth inhibition of a small panel of human neoplastic cell lines, A549 (lung), SKOV3 (ovary), SK-MEL-2 (skin), and HCT-15 (colon). The IC$_{50}$ values were 1.9–3.1 μM for isohericenone (**5**), 3.1–21 μM for isohericerin (**6**), and 7.7–14 μM for erinacerin-A (**7**). SK-MEL-2 melanoma cells were found to be most sensitive to the three tested compounds and isohericenone (**5**) was most active to the all tested cell lines.[25,27] Another antitumor active lactam designated as hericenone-B (**8**) was isolated from the acetone extract of *H. erinaceum* fruiting bodies and exhibited marked cytotoxic effect against HeLa cervical cancer cells. At a minimum concentration of 6.3 μg/mL, hericenone-B (**8**) completely obstructed the growth of HeLa cells *in vitro*.[25] A corresponding lactone was termed hericenone-A (**9**), whose minimum concentration that fully inhibited the growth of HeLa cells was 100 µg/mL, implying that the cytotoxic effect of hericenone-B (7) on HeLa cells was 15.8 times more potent than that of hericenone-A (9).[15,28–30]

Hericerin-A and hericerin (10) significantly reduced the proliferation of HL-60 leukemia cells (IC$_{50}$s 3.06 and 5.47 µM, respectively) and induced apoptosis of HL-60 cells, accompanied by time-dependent downregulation of p-Akt and c-myc levels. However, the effects of hericerin-A and hericerin (10) were weak on HEL-299 normal cells.[31] Eight similar γ-lactams extracts and two corresponding γ-lactones were separated from 70% ethanol extract of *H. erinaceus* fruiting bodies. All ten compounds exhibited prominent cell growth inhibition against human SMMC-7221 hepatoma cells and were more potent than 5-FU; among these, erinaceolactam-E, hericenone-A (9), and *N*-dephenyl-ethylisohericerin were also effective in deterring the proliferation of human MHCC-97H hepatoma cells in a dose-dependent manner. Of the ten tested compounds, hericenone-A (9) in 20 µg/mL concentration exerted the most potent obstruction against the proliferation of both SMMC-7221 and MHCC-97H cell line, which might be a novel efficient drug lead for further investigation.[5] Two other lactams, erinacerins-Q and -T, presented moderate to weak antiproliferative effects on human K562 leukemia cells and the weak effect on doxorubicin-resistant K562 cells *in vitro*, and these lactams were inhibitors of both protein tyrosine phosphatase-1B (PTP1B) and α-glucosidase.[26] Consequently, the evidences indicated that the introduction of a phenylethylamine to the lactone in the molecules for substitution of the oxygen would enhance the antineoplastic potency extensively, except for antihepatoma effect.[15,21–30]

6. Phenolic derivatives

Several phenolic derivatives were separated from the fruiting bodies of *H. erinaceum*. Among them, isohericenone-J, hericenone-J (11) and 4-[3',7'-dimethyl-2',6'-octadienyl]-2-formyl-3-hydroxy-5-methoxybenzylalcohol (12) exerted the similar levels of cytotoxicity to HL-60 leukemia cells (IC$_{50}$s 4.10–5.47 µM) and also to HEL-299 normal cells (IC$_{50}$s 5.07–8.46 µM).[31] Hericenone-I (13), hericenone-L (14), and hericene-D (15) showed the cytotoxicity against human EC-109 esophageal cancer cells, and the IC$_{50}$ value of hericenone-L (14) was 46 µg/mL.[32,33] 3,4-Dihydro-5-methoxy-2-methyl-2-(4'-methyl-2'-oxo-3'-pentenyl)-9(7H)-oxo-2H-furo-[3,4-h]benzopyran (16), which was isolated from the same edible mushroom, moderately hindered the proliferation of human A549 (lung), SKOV3 (ovary), SK-MEL-2 (skin), and HCT-15 (colon) cancer cell lines in the *in vitro* experiment. The IC$_{50}$s ranged from 11 to 17 µM.[27]

7. Ergosterols

Hericium fungi are rich in both ergosterol and ergosterol peroxide. Ergosterol and its derivatives, especially ergosterol peroxide (17), are key molecules that directly induce apoptosis in a variety of cell types, such as human lung adenocarcinoma cells, uterine cervical carcinoma cells, and tongue cancer cells.[34] Ergosterol at a concentration range of 50–200 µg/mL restrained the proliferation of human HepG2 hepatoma cells together with enhancing p21 activity.[35] At a concentration of 25 µM, ergosterol peroxide (17) completely inhibited the cell growth and induced apoptosis of human HL-60 leukemia cells *in vitro*.[36] The antiproliferative effect of ergosterol peroxide (17) was also demonstrated in human neoplastic cell lines such as K562 leukemia, prostate cancer cells (LNCaP androgen-sensitive line and DU-145 androgen-insensitive line), A549 lung cancer, XF498 glioma cells, and so on.[37–39]

Despite its weak inhibition of U266 multiple myeloma cells, ergosterol peroxide (17) at nontoxic concentrations effectively reduced the expression of STAT3 and CD34, significantly decreased VEGF, and blocked JAK2/STAT3 signaling pathway, thereby exerting the antiangiogenic and antigrowth effects in nude mice implanted with U266 cells.[40] Treatment with ergosterol peroxide (17) at concentrations lower than 20 µM also could inhibit the migration of human MDA-MB-231 breast cancer cells.[41] More research results revealed that ergosterol at nontoxic dose is capable of reversing multidrug resistance of SGCR7901/ADR human gastric cancer cells via accumulation of rhodamine 123 to amplify the concentration of chemotherapeutic agent in the tumor cells.[42]

8. Glycosphingolipid

A glycosphingolipid, labeled as cerebroside E, was isolated from the fruiting bodies of H. erinaceus and showed no antioxidant, anticancer, or acetylcholinesterase (AChE) inhibitory effects up to 200 μM, but it exhibited a significant inhibitory effect on angiogenesis of human umbilical vein endothelial cells (HUVECs) and considerably attenuated cisplatin-induced nephrotoxicity in LLC-PK1 pig kidney epithelial cells at high concentrations of 100 and 200 μM.[43]

OTHER BIOACTIVITIES

H. erinaceous fungus contains two characteristic micromolecules, hericenones and erinacines, which showed potent enhancing activity for nerve growth factor (NGF) synthesis, leading to the promotion of neuron repair and renewal, and also had inhibitory activity on prostaglandin-E2 production in the *in vitro* studies. These elicited pharmacological effects are able to provide a neuroprotection on focal cerebral ischemia and a healing effect in Alzheimer's dementia cases.[16,21,44]

CONCLUSION AND SUGGESTION

On the basis of these scientific evidences, the edible Lion's mane mushroom has been known to be rich in physiologically important components, especially polysaccharides, which are primarily responsible for anticancer, immunomodulating, and hypolipidemic properties of *H. erinaceous* fungus. The isolated secondary metabolites such as lactams, isoindolinone and pyridone alkaloids, polyphenols, fatty acids and ergosterols, and a complex of polysaccharide–protein were also demonstrated to have antiproliferative effects toward different tested cell lines derived from lung, cervix, ovarian, live, stomach, esophageal, colon, and skin carcinomas and leukemias in the *in vitro* systems. The polyphenols exerted remarkable antioxidant activities as well. These experimental evidences collectively reflect the beneficial effects of Lion's mane mushroom in cancer treatment and prevention. Of course, the anticarcinogenic and anticancer activities of the edible fungus should be also attributed to its immunoenhancing and antioxidant properties. Hence, it is no doubt that the culinary–medicinal Lion's mane mushroom is a health-promoting functional food that can be used to serve as an anticancer supplement and cancer-preventive dietary with high safety. In addition, a kind of pill prepared from *Hericium erinaceous* fungi has been clinically utilized in China to treat gastric ulcers and esophageal carcinoma.[45]

REFERENCES

1. Friedman, M. 2015. Chemistry, nutrition, and health-promoting properties of Hericium erinaceus (Lion's Mane) mushroom fruiting bodies and mycelia and their bioactive compounds. *J. Agricult. Food Chem.* 63: 7108–7123.
2. Kim, S.P. et al., 2013. Hericium erinaceus (Lion's Mane) mushroom extracts inhibit metastasis of cancer cells to the lung in CT-26 colon cancer-transplanted mice. *J. Agri. Food Chem.* 61: 4898–4904.
3. Kim, S.P. et al., 2011. Composition and mechanism of antitumor effects of Hericium erinaceus mushroom extracts in tumor-bearing mice. *J. Agric. Food Chem.* 59: 9861–9869.
4. Jin, K.S. et al., 2009. Modulation of Nrf2/ARE and inflammatory signaling pathways by Hericium erinaceus mycelia extract. *Food Sci. Biotechnol.* 18: 1204–1211.
5. Wang, X.L. et al., 2016. New isoindolinones from the fruiting bodies of Hericium erinaceum. *Fitoterapia* 111: 58–65.
6. Yim, M.H. et al., 2007. Soluble components of Hericium erinaceum induce NK cell activation via production of interleukin-12 in mice splenocytes. *Acta Pharmacol. Sinica* 28: 901–907.

7. Son, C.G. et al., 2006. Macrophage activation and nitric oxide production by water soluble components of Hericium erinaceum. *Intl. Immunopharmacol.* 6: 1363–1369.

8. Lee, J.S. et al., 2010. Hericium erinaceus enhances doxorubicin-induced apoptosis in human hepatocellular carcinoma cells. *Cancer Lett.* 297: 144–154.

9. Li, G. et al., 2014. Anticancer potential of Hericium erinaceus extracts against human gastrointestinal cancers. *J. Ethnopharmacol.* 153: 521–530.

10. Nie, J.S. et al., 2003. Hericium erinaceus polysaccharide and its antineoplastic activity and influence on immunity in mice. *Shanxi Yiyao Zazhi* 32: 107–109.

11. Xu, X. et al., 2001. Regulation of immunological functions by Hericium erinaceus polysaccharides. *Weisheng Dulixue Zazhi* 15: 165–166.

12. Jiang, Y. et al., 2015. Inhibitory effect of Hericium erinaceus polysaccharide on mice subcutaneous transplanted sarcoma and its mechanism. *Shandong Yiyao* 55: 8–10.

13. Xia, S.B. et al., 2014. Antineoplastic effect and influence on serum cytokine of Hericium erinaceus polysaccharides on S180 tumor-bearing mice. *Shiyong Yaowu Yu Linchuang* 17: 5–8.

14. Peng, Y. et al., 2012. Inhibitory effect of Hericium erinaceus polysaccharide on hepatoma-22 (H22) tumor bearing mice. *Shipin Kexue* (Beijing, China) 33: 244–246.

15. Mizuno, T. et al., 1998. Bioactive substances in Yamabushitake, the Hericium erinaceum fungus, and its medicinal utilization. *Foods Food Ingredients J. Jpn* 175: 105–114.

16. Fujiwara, M. et al., 2006. Neuroprotective effect of Hericium erinaceum. *Foods Food Ingredients J. Jpn* 211: 141–147

17. Mizuno, T. et al., 1993. Fungal antitumor polysaccharides and their isolation. Japanese Kokai Tokkyo Koho JP 91-306942 19911026.

18. Wang, J. et al., 2001. Antitumor and immunoenhancing activities of polysaccharide from culture broth of Hericium spp. *Kaohsiung J. Med. Sci.* 17: 461–467.

19. Mizuno, T. et al., 1992. Studies on the host-mediated antitumor polysaccharides. Part XVII. Antitumoractive polysaccharides isolated from the fruiting body of Hericium erinaceum, an edible and medicinal mushroom called yamabushitake or houtou. *Biosc. Biotech. Biochem.* 56: 347–348.

20. Zan, X.Y. et al., 2015. Hericium erinaceus polysaccharide-protein HEG-5 inhibits SGC-7901 cell growth via cell cycle arrest and apoptosis. *Int. J. Biol. Macromol.* 76: 242–253.

21. Kawagishi, H. et al., 1991. Biological active compounds from the mushroom *Hericium erinaceum*. *Tennen Yuki Kagobutsu Toronkai Koen Yoshishu* 33rd: 533–540.

22. Kawagishi, H. et al., 1990. Novel fatty acid from the mushroom *Hericium erinaceum*. *Agric. Biol. Chem.* 54: 1329–1331.

24. Kawagishi, H. et al., 1992. Erinapyrones A and B from cultured mycelia of *Hericium erinaceums*. *Chem. Lett.* 21: 2475–2476.

25. Kawagishi, H. et al., 1990. Hericenone A and B as cytotoxic principles from the mushroom *Hericium erinaceum*. *Tetrahedron Lett.* 37: 373–376.

26. Wang, K. et al., 2015. Eight new alkaloids with PTP1B and α-glucosidase inhibitory activities from the medicinal mushroom *Hericium erinaceus*. *Tetrahedron* 71(51): 9557–9563.

27. Kim, K.H. et al., 2012. Isohericenone, a new cytotoxic isoindolinone alkaloid from *Hericium erinaceum*. *J. Antibiotics* 65: 575–577.

28. Mizuno, T. et al., 1991. Isolation of octadecenoic acid derivatives for killing uterocervical cancer cells. Japanese Kokai Tokkyo Koho JP 89-295448 19891114.

29. Mizuno, T. et al., 1991. Isolation of phthalide derivative as uterocervical cancer inhibitor. Japanese Kokai Tokkyo Koho JP 89-295449 19891114.

30. Mizuno, T. et al., 1991. An isoindolinone derivative from *Hericium erinaceum* for treatment of uterine cancer. Japanese Kokai Tokkyo Koho JP 89-294415 19891113.

31. Li, W. et al., 2015. Isolation and identification of aromatic compounds in Lion's Mane mushroom and their anticancer activities. *Food Chem.* 170: 336–342.

32. Ma, B.J. et al., 2010. Cytotoxic aromatic compounds from *Hericium erinaceum*. *J. Antibiotics* 63: 713–705.

33. Ma, B.J. et al., 2012. Hericenone L, a new aromatic compound from the fruiting bodies of *Hericium erinaceums*. *Chin. J. Nat. Med.* 10: 363–365.

34. Kawai, J. et al., 2013. Apoptosis inducer containing ergosterol derivative for treatment of lung, tongue, or cervical cancer, and production thereof from Agaricus. *PCT Int. Appl.* WO 2013073085 A1 20130523.

35. Zhang, X. et al., 2010. Effect of ergosterol for inhibiting HepG2 proliferation by inducing p21 expression. *Zhongyao Yaoli Yu Linchuang* 27: 26–29.

36. Takei, T. et al., 2005. Ergosterol peroxide, an apoptosis-inducing component isolated from Sarcodon aspratus (Berk.) S. Ito. *Biosci. Biotechnol. Biochem.* 69: 212–215.

37. Ren, H. et al., 2010. Antitumor metabolites from marine-derived fungus Gliocladium catenulatum T31. *Zhongguo Yaoxue Zazhi* 45: 1720–1723.

38. Lee, I. et al., 2011. Cytotoxicity of ergosterol derivatives from the fruiting bodies of Hygrophorus russula. *Nat. Prod. Sci.* 17: 85–89.

39. Russo, A. et al., 2010. Proapoptotic activity of ergosterol peroxide and (22E)-ergosta-7,22-dien-5alpha-hydroxy-3,6-dione in human prostate cancer cells. *Chem. Biol. Interact.* 184: 352–358.

40. Rhee, Y.H. et al., 2012. Inhibition of STAT3 signaling and induction of SHP1 mediate antiangiogenic and antitumor activities of ergosterol peroxide in U266 multiple myeloma cells. *BMC Cancer* 12: 28.

41. Lee, D.Y. et al., 2009. Sterols isolated from Nuruk (Rhizopus oryzae KSD-815) inhibit the migration of cancer cells. *Microbiol. Biotechnol.* 19: 1328–1332.

42. Li, F.R. et al., 2002. Application of ergosterol in medicine for reversing multidrug resistance of tumor. Faming Zhuanli Shenqing CN 102552284 A20120711.

43. Lee, S.R. et al., 2015. A new cerebroside from the fruiting bodies of Hericium erinaceus and its applicability to cancer treatment. *Bioorg. Med. Chem. Lett.* 25(24): 5712–5715.

44. Sasa, T. et al., 2002. Cyathane derivatives from Hericium erinaceum as NGF inducers. Japanese Kokai Tokkyo Koho JP 2001-33369 20010209.

45. State Administration of Medicines in China, 1999. *Chinese Materia Medica*, vol. 1, pp 522, Published by Shanghai Press of Science and Technology, Shanghai, China.

63. MAITAKE OR SIGNORINA MUSHROOM AND CHESTNUT MUSHROOM

灰樹花　舞茸　회색 나무 꽃

Polyporus frondosus (= *Grifola frondosa*)

Meripilaceae

Maitake is the fruit body of a large grayish-brown fungus *Polyporus frondosus* (= *Grifola frondosa*) (Meripilaceae) whose mushroom was native to northeastern mountains of Japan and North America. Owing to its miraculous curative and sanitarian reputation, maitake has been valued as the "King of Fungi" since the ancient period. Because the fungus was rarely seen at that time, people would become extremely excited to dance when they discovered this mushroom. By this reason, its Japanese name is maitake, which means dancing mushroom. In traditional Chinese and Japanese herbology, the sclerotia of maitake are applied as a medicinal mushroom. The scientific investigations have proved that maitake is capable of augmenting both innate and adaptive immune systems and regulating the levels of glucose, insulin, and lipid in humans. Nutritionally, consumption of maitake provides a good source of proteins, polysaccharides, vitamins (such as B2, D2, E, B1, and C), dietary fibers, carotene, and minerals (such as calcium, potassium, iron, zinc, and magnesium); among these, the content of vitamins B1 and E is 10–20 times greater than that in other mushrooms. On the basis of these excellent nutritional and health-promoting properties, the popularity of maitake is growing in worldwide cuisines to improve body condition.

SCIENTIFIC EVIDENCE OF CANCER-INHIBITORY AND CANCER-PREVENTIVE ACTIVITIES

Pharmacological experiments demonstrated that maitake has marked anticarcinogenetic activity. When treatment with a carcinogen, *N*-butyl-*N'*-butanolnitrosoamine (BBN), together with a diet of maitake, the BBN-induced bladder carcinogenesis was noticeably diminished by 53.3%. The anticarcinogenic effect was associated with restoration of the chemotactic activity of macrophages and the cytotoxicity of lymphocytes and nature killer cells that were normally hampered by BBN in mice. Maitake treatment could keep the inhibition of lymphocytes against tumor cells such as Yac-1 lymphoma and P815 mastocytoma.[1] Maitake also markedly attenuated the side effects caused by cisplatin, which is used as a chemotherapy drug in clinics, and protected kidney and digestive organs to improve the treatment efficiency for cancer patients.[2] In addition, an ethyl acetate extract prepared from the supernatant of culture broth of *P. frondosus* established a modest cytotoxicity against human Hep3B and HepG2 (livers), CL1-1 (lung), and HeLa (cervix) neoplastic cell lines *in vitro*. The IC_{50} values were 78.4, 52.7, 71.0, and 77.6 µg/mL, respectively, whereas it was less active to normal human MRC-5 lung fibroblast cells (IC_{50} 233.3 µg/mL).[3]

SCIENTIFIC EVIDENCE OF CANCER-INHIBITORY AND CANCER-PREVENTIVE CONSTITUENTS

1. Phenols

A bioactive principal with a small molecule elucidated as O-orsellinaldehyde (**1**) was isolated from the ethyl acetate extract of *P. frondosus* culture broth. In the *in vitro* assay, O-orsellinaldehyde (**1**) displayed a selective cytotoxic effect against the Hep3B hepatoma and MRC-5 normal cell lines with IC_{50} values of 3.6 and 33.1 µg/mL, respectively.[3]

2. Polysaccharides

Crude polysaccharides of *P. frondosus* were prepared from different sources of the basidiomycete fungus such as its fruit bodies, cultured mycelium, and fermented broth. The polysaccharides are the major component in maitake fungi, demonstrating significant biological properties. Their anticancer potency was found to be dependent on the abilities to induce cell apoptosis and enhance immune system such as increase in delayed-type hypersensitivity and thymus index, rise in splenic lymphocyte proliferation and antibody formation in splenic cells, and speeding up of IgM hemolysin production. Oral administration of the polysaccharides to tumor-bearing mice noticeably suppressed the proliferation of sarcoma 180 cells and amplified the levels of TNF-α and IL-2.[4–7] In daily doses up to 3 g/kg, the inhibition ratio of the mycelium polysaccharides was ~80.5% and that of the fermented liquid polysaccharide was 58.4%–63% on the S180 cells.[6] Daily diet of 20% maitake led to significant lessening in the carcinogenesis and metastasis, but it was not as effective when administered as i.p. injection.[8] The polysaccharides also augmented the sensitivity of human HCT116 colon cancer cells to X-ray irradiation.[4] An acute toxic test further indicated that the maximal safe dose of maitake polysaccharides to mouse was >3 g/kg.[6] When *G. frondosa* polysaccharide combined with cisplatin, the co-treatment synergistically enhanced the tumor-inhibitory effect against H22 hepatoma cells together with additive stimulation of H22 cell apoptotic death via increase in caspase-8, release of cytochrome c and then activation of caspase-3.[9]

Moreover, phase I/II clinic trials with maitake polysaccharides were performed in the advanced malignant tumor patients. The clinic results revealed that the polysaccharides were able to rapidly and safely ameliorate the clinic symptoms and physical signs in patients with advanced malignant tumor by the immunoregulation, implying that the polysaccharides can be applied as an adjunctive agent in the cancer therapeutic treatment and prevention.[10,11]

Grifolan: Grifolan, a (1-3)-β-D-glucan with a β-glucosyl substitution at C-6 of every 3 units in its main chain, was derived from the fruit body and the mycelia of *G. frondosa*. Grifolan has two different solid-state conformations, that is, H (helix) and N (native).[12] In the pharmacological studies, grifolan was significantly effective in inducing cytokines (such as TNF-α, IL-1α, IL-6), activating peritoneal macrophage and Kupffer cells, amplifying nitric oxide in macrophage cells, and, subsequently, exerting notable immunoregulation-dependent inhibitory effect toward the cancer cells.[8,13]

MDF: D-fraction (MDF) isolated from the fruit body of *P. frondosus* has been extensively studied for 30 years. MDF (m.w. ~10^6 Da), a protein-bound β-(1-6)-glucan with β-(1-3)-glucosyl branches, presents obvious physiological benefits such as immunomodulatory, anticancer, and antiviral activities.[14] Daily i.p. injection of MDF at a dose of 1 mg/kg for ten days to mice implanted with hepatoma resulted in 90.3% and 91.3% inhibitions against the growth and metastasis of hepatoma cells, respectively.[15] The MDF at ≥480 μg/mL concentration near completely elicited human PC3 prostate cancer cells to death (> 95%) *in vitro*.[16] The inhibition was closely mediated by the induction of oxidative stress and oxidative membrane damage in the PC3 cells, forcing the cells to apoptosis. When combined with vitamin C (200 μM) in the treatment, MDF even at a low i.v. dose of 30–60 μg/mL could elicit >90% cytotoxic cell death as effectively as when MDF is used alone at a dose of 480 μg/mL, suggesting that the synergistic effect of MDF with vitamin C can beneficial for the cancer patients in clinics and the antioxidant activity involved in the promotion of PC3 cell apoptosis.[14,17] Treatment of human MCF-7 breast cancer cells with MDF in concentration of ≥18 μg/mL for 24 h notably diminished the cell viability and promoted the cell apoptosis via upregulation of BAK-1 and induction of cytochrome c transcripts and mitochondrial dysfunction.[18] When MDF (200 μg/mL) was combined with IFN-α2b (10,000 IU/mL), a synergistic suppression could be achieved against the proliferation of T24 bladder cancer cells by ≈75%, together with arrest of cell cycle at G1 phase.[19]

The anticancer effect of MDF was revealed also to importantly correlate with the host-mediated cellular immunoenhancing activity, which was associated with (1) increases in immunocompetent cell proliferation and differentiation, (2) activation of macrophages and dendritic cells; (3) enhancement of cytotoxicity of NK cells and T-cells; (4) extension of T-helper-1 dominant response; (5) promotion of IL-12, IL-18, and IFN-γ production; and (6) downregulation of tumor markers. On the basis of the potent cellular immunostimulation, MDF effectively exerted the inhibition of cell growth and metastatic progress in the *in vivo* cancer models.[20-27] Furthermore, MDF also notably enhanced the development of granulocyte-macrophage (CFU-GM) colonies in a dose range of 50–100 μg/mL and amplified non-adherent bone marrow cell (BMC) viability at doses of 12.5–100 μg/mL in mice. The protection of spleen weight and total number of nuclear cells occurred as well.[20,28,29] More studies revealed that MDF could directly cause bone marrow-derived dendritic cell (DCs) maturation via a C-type lectin receptor dectin-1 pathway. Oral intake of MDF markedly elicited the therapeutic response in association with (1) induction of systemic tumor-antigen-specific T-cell response via dectin-1-dependent activation of DCs; (2) increase in the activated T-cell infiltration into tumor; and (3) decrease in the tumor-caused immunosuppressive cells such as regulatory T cells and myomoeloid-derived suppressor cells.[30] If used in combinations cytosine-phosphate-guanine oligodeoxynucleotide (a Toll-like receptor agonist), MDF synergistically augmented the dendritic cell maturation and cytokine responses in a dectin-1-dependent pathway, resulting in a more effective tumor regression via an antitumor T-helper cell 1-type response.[31] Accordingly, MDF was capable of markedly restoring the cancer patient's systemic immune function, which was reduced by immunosuppressive effects caused from tumor and chemotherapeutic drugs, leading to improvement of the therapeutic quality and survival ratio prominently.[32]

Moreover, the suppressive effect of MDF on the cancer metastasis was impressive as well. The i.p. administration of MDF two days before tumor implantation significantly activated NK cells and triggered their cytotoxicity against YAC-1 T-lymphoma and colon-26 carcinoma. Simultaneously, MDF obstructed the lung metastasis of colon-26 cancer cells and B16/BL6 melanoma cells by augmenting NK cell activity and IL-12 production from antigen-presenting cells (APCs) and hindering intercellular adhesion molecule-1 (ICAM-1), leading to blockage of the cancer cell adhesion to vascular endothelial cells.[33] When used in combination with cisplatin, MDF not only efficiently improved the antigrowth and anti-metastatic activities but also attenuated the cisplatin-caused myelotoxicity and nephrotoxicity.[34]

In addition, by treatment with MDF in a dose >30 μg/mL, the inducible nitric oxide synthase (iNOS) mRNA expression in macrophage cells (RAW264.7) was activated and then the nitric oxide (NO) production was amplified, whereby the NO indirectly induced the cytotoxicity against human hepatoma-derived huH-1 cells.[35] MDF also displayed the highest scavenging rate on hypoxanthine-xanthine oxidase-generated superoxide anion radical (.bul. O^{2-}) and ferrous sulfate-hydrogen peroxide-generated hydroxyl radical (.bul. OH). These findings suggested that the iNOS induction and radical scavenging can partly contribute to the antitumor activity of MDF.[35,36]

MZF: MZ-Fraction (MZF, m.w. ≈ 23 kDa) is a β-glucan made up of β-(1-3)- and β-(1-6)-glucosyl bonds. Similar to MDF, MZF demonstrated both anticancer and immunostimulating activities. The experiments revealed that MZF obviously stimulated the productivity of TNF-α and IL-12 and augmented the antigen presentation of murine J774.1 macrophage cells *in vitro*.[13] In association with enhancing the cytotoxicity of NK cells and increasing the proliferation of splenocytes and peritoneal macrophages in spleen, MZF obviously repressed the growth of colon 26 cells in mice after MZF treatment.[37] Also, bone marrow-derived dendritic cells (DCs) pulsed with colon-26 lysate in the presence of MZF exerted both therapeutic and preventive effects against colon-26 tumor development in BALB/c mice. During the treatment, MZF enhanced the expression of CD80, CD86, CD83, and MHC II in the DCs and notably stimulated DCs to produce IL-12 and TNF-α. MZF-treated DCs noticeably augmented both allogeneic and antigen-specific and syngeneic T-cell responses and enhanced antigen-specific IFN-γ production by syngeneic $CD4^+$ T cells. The evidences suggest that MZF can be an effective adjuvant to potentiate DC-based immunotherapeutic antitumor activity against the colon cancer.[38]

S-GAP-P: A sulfated polysaccharide (S-GAP-P) was derived from the water-insoluble polysaccharides of *P. frondosus* mycelia by reaction with chlorosulfonic acid-pyridine, which has 2.8×10^4

of average molecular weight with 16.4% of sulfate content. *In vitro* studies showed that S-GAP-P retarded the growth of human SGC-7901 gastric cancer cells in a dose-dependent manner and induced the cell apoptosis. S-GAP-P also significantly inhibited the tumor growth and enhanced the peritoneal macrophages phagocytosis in S180-bearing mice. When S-GAP-P was combined with anticancer drugs such as 5-FU and CP, a synergic efficacy plus an improvement of immunocompetence could be significantly achieved for the cancer treatment.[39–41]

PET-F: PET-Fraction (PET-F) is a D-fraction-related polysaccharide component developed for veterinary use of maitake mushroom. In two types of canine carcinoma cell lines, PFT-F showed the obstructive effect associated with induction of cell apoptosis and G1 cell cycle arrest. PET-F at ≥500 μg/mL concentration provoked a maximum antigrowth effect for ~47% against CF33 mammary gland cancer cells and a maximum antigrowth effect for ~51% against CF21 soft tissue cancer cells *in vitro*. If PET-F is used in combination with vitamin C, a remarkable potentiative effect was achieved to prompt nearly complete cell death (> 95%) in both cancer cell lines.[42] Thus, PET-F may be one of the most promising products that have a developing potential for effectively and safely treating veterinary cancers.

3. Heteropolysaccharide

Several natural heteropolysaccharides with protein obtained from the isolation of *P. frondosus* are another kind of constituent displaying great antitumor activity similar to those of polysaccharides of maitake. The i.p. injection of this crude sugar–protein complex at a dose of 0.1 mg/kg per day to mice for ten times resulted in significant growth inhibition on MM-46 carcinoma cells for 83.4% *in vivo*, and it also showed the antitumor effect on sarcoma 180 cells *in vitro*.[43]

GFPS1b: An acid heteropolysaccharide assigned as GFPS1b (21 kDa) was purified from the cultured mycelia of *P. frondosus* (GF9801), which consisted of a polysaccharide unit (D-galactose, D-glucose, and L-arabinose), a protein (about 16.60%), and uronic acid (4.3%). The polysaccharide backbone is built up of α-(1-3)-linked D-glucosyl and α-(1-4)-linked D-galacosyl residues and branched at O-6 of glycosyl residues in the backbone with L-arabinosyl-(1-4)-α-D-glucose.[44,45] GFPS1b exhibited more potent antiproliferative activity on human MCF-7 (breast) and SGC-7901 (gastric) cancer cell lines than maitake polysaccharides, but it slightly influenced human L-02 normal liver cells.[44,46] After treatment with GFPS1b, typical apoptotic morphological features and G2/M cell cycle arrest were induced in the SGC-7901 cells.[46] By the similar antitumor mechanisms, GFPS1b was also effective in B16 mouse melanoma cells *in vivo*.[47]

GP11: A polysaccharide named GP11 was purified from *G. frondosa*, which was composed of D-mannose, D-glucose, and D-galactose. GP11 displayed indirect cytotoxic activity against HepG2 hepatoma cells, whose antitumor activity was found to be mediated by improvement of immune functions via TLR-4-mediated upregulation of TNF-α and nitric oxid.[48]

GFPW: GFPW (15.7 kDa), a water-soluble polysaccharide, was isolated from the fruit body of *G. frondosa*. Its backbone consists of α-(1-6)-linked galactopyranosyl residues, with branches attached to 2-OH of α-(1-3)-linked fucose residues and α-terminal mannose. By a chlorosulfonic acid-pyridine method, a sulfated derivative of GFPW was produced and the substitution was located at C-2 and C-3 positions in the Sul-GFPW with a substitution degree of 0.33. *In vitro* angiogenesis assay revealed that the Sul-GFPW notably inhibited the proliferation of endothelial cells in a dose- and time-dependent manner and diminished the migration and tube formation of endothelial cells.[49]

4. Exopolysaccharides

An exopolysaccharide (EPS) was separated from a liquid culture of *G. frondosa* and modified by selenising to give Se-EPS and by carboxymethylation to give CM-EPS. Both Se-EPS and CM-EPS showed enhanced antioxidant capacity and Se-EPS also exerted the more potent antiproliferative effect on HeLa cervical cancer cells compared with EPS, implying that the structure modification may have a great influence on augmenting the antioxidant and antitumor potencies of exopolysaccharides.[50] Likewise, a Se-enriched *G. frondosa* polysaccharide termed Se-GP11 (3.3×10^4 Da). Se-GP11 had no *in vitro* antitumor activity against HepG-2 hepatoma cells, but it obviously hindered HepG2 cell growth *in vivo*; antigrowth effect was also attributed to its abilities to promote immunity, such as increasing the thymus and spleen weights and elevating serum TNF-α and IL-2 levels.[51]

5. Glycoprotein

A glycoprotein component (30–90 kDa) was prepared from *G. frondosa* mycelium, whose polysaccharide moiety accounts for 2%–10% and consists of arabinose, fructose, mannose, and glucose, and its protein moiety accounts for 30%–90% and consists of 17 amino acids such as aspartic acid, methionine, and glutamic acid. In the *in vitro* assay, the glycoprotein exerted an inhibitory effect on the growth of human SGC-7901 (gastric) and MCF-7 (breast) cancer cell lines.[52] GFG-3a, a glycoprotein purified from the fermented mycelia of *G. frondosa*, could deter the proliferation of human SGC-7901 gastric cancer cells *in vitro* concomitant with induction of cell apoptosis and cell cycle arrest at S phase. During the apoptosis process, the events such as stress response, p53-dependent mitochondrial-mediated, caspases-8 and -3 activation, and PI3k/Akt pathways were observed in the GFG-3a-treated SGC-7901 cells, all of which should be involved in the tumor-inhibitory mechanisms.[53]

MPSP was a crude polysaccharide peptide extracted from *G. frondosa*. The MPSP and its three simply modified MPSP displayed the obvious growth inhibitory effect against C6 glioma cells but not on normal brain cells *in vitro*. In combination with cyclophosphamide (a chemotherapeutic drug), the MPSPs exerted a significant adjuvant effect to restrain the growth of C6 cells in a rat model. Interestingly, the phosphorylation of MPSP could notably potentiate the adjuvant effect and the growth inhibitory effect. The *in vivo* and *in vitro* assays substantiated the rank order of efficacy as phosphorylated MPSP > esterified MPSP ≥ acetylated MPSP ≥ crude MPSP.[54]

6. DNA extracts

A DNA extract isolated from *G. frondosa* exhibited nonspecific immunoenhancing activities, including significant augmentation of the activity of NK cells and the phagocytosis of macrophages and stimulation of the macrophages to produce TNF-α and IL-1 in mice. Due to the noticeable property, the DNA extract can be considered to be beneficial for humans indirectly by exerting the cancer-preventive effect and directly by enhancing the immune system.[55]

Conclusion and Suggestion

Maitake mushroom has attracted a great deal of attention by reason of many health benefits that have been demonstrated in both clinical practices and laboratory experiments, such as immunoregulation, cancer inhibition and prevention, treatment of cardiovascular diseases, antidiabetic, antiviral, and antimicrobial effects. A variety of bioactive macromolecules (such as glucans, heteropolysaccharides, glycoproteins, and DNA extract) have been discovered from maitake fruiting body, mycelium, and cultivated broth, and they all demonstrated the same corresponding health-promotive activities as obtained from maitake. Among those isolated from maitake, the most important macromolecules should be β-glucans, especially maitake D-fraction (MDF), which is the one being fully proven by various scientific approaches. Although some of them showed direct induction of antiproliferative and proapoptotic effects against cancer cells *in vitro*, their antitumor activities were found to be principally attributed to their prominent immunopotentiative capabilities. The remarkable immunoregulations were found mostly to present in these aspects, that is, (1) simulation of NK cells, T-lymphocyte, and macrophage functions and production; (2) augmentation of anticancer immunity effect concerned with secretion of cytokines (such as TNF-α, IFN-γ, ILs-1, -2, -12, and -18); (3) increase in thymus and spleen weights; (4) promotion of complement system; (5) induction of dendritic cell maturation; and so on.

Also, the potentials of maitake β-glucans in antimetastasis and antioxidation were observed in the experiments. Interestingly, the antioxidant and antitumor potencies of the β-glucans can be augmented by their combination with vitamin C, which is a very common agent obtained from many natural comestibles. The scientific data also evidenced that maitake macromolecules can afford more benefits to current conventional cancer therapies because they not only enhance the efficacy of anticancer drugs and radio-irritation but also mitigate/recover the damages/side effects (such as immune suppression, myelotoxicity, and nephrotoxicity) that are caused by these treatments. Undoubtedly, these findings provide the solid basis for frequent utilization of the health-improving advantages of maitake in diet. The consumption of maitake, therefore, is recommended as a nutritional and functional food supplement, which is useful for normal people to upgrade the immune system against the risk of cancer and is helpful for cancer patients to improve the therapy results and life quality and to lengthen overall survival based on the phenomenal antitumor immunity of maitake. In addition, the studies further found that the anticancer properties of maitake polysaccharides can be boosted chemically by structural modification, a finding that indicates a potential of maitake polysaccharides that may be developed as a new anticancer adjuvant agent.

REFERENCES

1. Kurashige, S. et al., 1997. Effects of Lentinus edodes, Grifola frondosa and Pleurotus ostreatus administration on cancer outbreak, and activities of macrophages and lymphocytes in mice treated with a carcinogen, N-butyl-N-butanolnitrosoamine. *Immunopharmacol, Immunotoxicol.* 19: 175–183.
2. Hong, S.B. et al., 2002. Grifola frondosa extracts for controlling side effect of cisplatin. Repub. Korean Kongkae Taeho Kongbo KR 2000-49043 20000823.
3. Lin, J. et al., 2006. O-Orsellinaldehyde from the submerged culture of the edible mushroom Grifola frondosa exhibits selective cytotoxic effect against Hep3B cells through apoptosis. *J. Agricul. Food Chem.* 54: 7564–7569.
4. Cao, W.T. et al., 2006. Promotion of X-ray induced apoptosis by polysaccharide from Grifola frondosa through upregulation of Bax in HCT116 cells. *Zhonghua Zhongxiyi Zazhi* 7: 580–583.
5. Li, X.D. et al., 2002. Effect of polysaccharide of Grifola frondosa (PGF-1) on immunological function in tumor-bearing mice. *J. Huazhong Agricul. Univ.* 21: 261–263.
6. Sun, Z. et al., 2001. Fractionation and antitumor activity of polysaccharide from Grifola frondosa. *Yaowu Shengwu Jishu* 8: 279–283.
7. Hou, X.Q. et al., 2007. Study on Grifola frondosa polysaccharide against S180 sarcoma in tumor-bearing mice. *Zhongguo Yaofang* 18: 180–181.
8. Ishibashi, K.I. et al., 2001. Relationship between solubility of grifolan, a fungal 1,3-β-D-glucan, and production of tumor necrosis factor by macrophages in vitro. *Biosci. Biotech. Biochem.* 65: 1993–2000.
9. Lu, D.X. et al., 2014. Tumor inhibitory action of Grifola frondosa polysaccharide combined with cisplatin on H22 liver cancer-transplanted mice. *Zhongguo Laonianxue Zazhi* 34(8): 2165–2166.
10. Deng, G. et al., 2009. A phase I/II trial of a polysaccharide extract from Grifola frondosa (Maitake mushroom) in breast cancer patients: immunological effects. *J. Cancer Res. Clin. Oncol.* 135(9): 1215–1221.
11. Liu, A. et al., 2008 Clinical observation of antitumor effect of Grifola frondosa polysaccharides. *Shandong Qinggongye Xueyuan Xuebao, Ziran Kexueban* 22: 43–45.
12. Ohno, N. et al., 1987. Conformational changes of the two different conformers of grifolan in sodium hydroxide, urea or dimethyl sulfoxide solution. *Chem. Pharm. Bull.* 35: 2108–2113.
13. Adachi, Y. et al., 1998. Activation of murine macrophages by grifolan. *Proc. Beltwide Cotton Conf.* in San Diego, CA, U.S.A. Jan. 5–9, 1998.
14. Masuda, Y. et al., 2006. Macrophage J774.1 cell is activated by MZ-fraction (Klasma-MZ) polysaccharide in Grifola frondosa. *Mycosci* 47: 360–366.
15. Nanba, H. et al., 1995. Activity of maitake D-fraction to inhibit carcinogenesis and metastasis. *Annals of the New York Academy of Sciences* 768(Cancer Prevention): 243–245.
16. Fullerton, S.A. et al., 2000. Induction of apoptosis in human prostatic cancer cells with β-glucan (Maitake mushroom polysaccharide). *Mol. Urol.* 4: 7–13.
17. Konno, S. 2009. Synergistic potentiation of D-fraction with vitamin C as possible alternative approach for cancer therapy. *Intl. J. General Med.* 2: 91–108.

18. Soares, R. et al., 2011. Maitake (D Fraction) mushroom extract induces apoptosis in breast cancer cells by BAK-1 gene activation. *J. Med. Food* 14: 563–572.
19. Louie, B. et al., 2010. Synergistic potentiation of interferon activity with maitake mushroom D-fraction on bladder cancer cells. *BJU Intl.* 105: 1011–1015.
20. Kodama, N. et al., 2005. Maitake D-Fraction enhances antitumor effects and reduces immuno-suppression by mitomycin-C in tumor-bearing mice. *Nutrition* (NY, NY, USA) 21: 624–629.
21. Kodama, N. et al., 2005. Enhancement of cytotoxicity of NK cells by D-fraction, a polysaccharide from Grifola frondosa. *Oncol. Reports* 13: 497–502.
22. Kodama, N. et al., 2003. Effect of maitake (Grifola frondosa) D-fraction on the activation of NK cells in cancer patients. *J. Med. Food* 6: 371–377.
23. Harada, N. et al., 2003. Relationship between dendritic cells and the D-fraction-induced Th-1 dominant response in BALB/c tumor-bearing mice. *Cancer Lett.* (Oxford, UK) 192: 181–187.
24. Kodama, N. et al., 2002. A polysaccharide, extract from Grifola frondosa, induces Th-1 dominant responses in carcinoma-bearing BALB/c mice. *Jpn. J. Pharmacol.* 90: 357–360.
25. Kodama, N. et al., 2002. Effects of D-Fraction, a polysaccharide from Grifola frondosa on tumor growth involved activation of NK cells. *Biol. Pharma. Bull.* 25: 1647–1650.
26. Konno, S. 2002. Anticancer and hypoglycemic effects of polysaccharides in edible and medicinal maitake mushroom (Grifola frondosa [Dicks.: Fr.] S. F. Gray). *Intl. J. Med. Mushrooms* 4: 185–195.
27. Inoue, A. et al., 2002. Effect of maitake (Grifola frondosa) D-fraction on the control of the T lymph node Th-1/Th-2 proportion. *Biol. Pharm. Bull.* 25: 536–540.
28. Lin, H. et al., 2004. Maitake β-glucan MD-fraction enhances bone marrow colony formation and reduces doxorubicin toxicity in vitro. *Int. Immunopharmacol.* 4: 91–99.
29. Ito, K. et al., 2009. Maitake beta-glucan enhances granulopoiesis and mobilization of granulocytes by increasing G-CSF production and modulating CXCR4/SDF-1 expression. *Intl. Immunopharmacol.* 9: 1189–1196.
30. Masuda, Y. et al., 2013. Oral administration of soluble β-glucans extracted from Grifola frondosa induces systemic antitumor immune response and decreases immunosuppression in tumor-bearing mice. *Intl. J. Cancer* 133: 108–119.
31. Masuda, Y. et al., 2015. Soluble β-glucan from Grifola frondosa induces tumor regression in synergy with TLR9 agonist via dendritic cell-mediated immunity. *J. Leukocyte Biol.* 98(6): 1015–1025.
32. Nanba, H. et al., 1997. Maitake D-fraction: Healing and preventive potential for cancer. *J. Orthomol. Med.* 12(1): 43–49.
33. Masuda, Y. et al., 2008. Inhibitory effect of MD-Fraction on tumor metastasis: involvement of NK cell activation and suppression of intercellular adhesion molecule (ICAM)-1 expression in lung vascular endothelial cells. *Biol. Pharm. Bull.* 31: 1104–1108.
34. Masuda, Y. et al., 2009. Maitake β-glucan enhances therapeutic effect and reduces myelo-supression and nephrotoxicity of cisplatin in mice. *Int. Immuno-pharmacol.* 9: 620–626.
35. Sanzen, I. et al., 2001. Nitric oxide-mediated antitumor activity induced by the extract from Grifola frondosa (Maitake mushroom) in a macrophage cell line, RAW264.7. *J. Experim. Clinical Cancer Res.* 20: 591–597.
36. Tazawa, K. et al., 2001. Evaluation of the radical scavenging activity of Grifola frondosa (Maitake). *Abstracts of Papers, 221st ACS National Meeting*, San Diego, CA, April 1–5, AGFD-046.
37. Masuda, Y. et al., 2009. Characterization and antitumor effect of a novel polysaccharide from Grifola frondosa. *J. Agricul. Food Chem.* 57: 10143–10149.
38. Masuda, Y. et al., 2010. A polysaccharide extracted from Grifola frondosa enhances the anti-tumor activity of bone marrow-derived dendritic cell-based immunotherapy against murine colon cancer. *Cancer Immunol. Immuno-Therapy* 59: 1531–1541.
39. Shi, B.J. et al., 2007. Anticancer activities of a chemically sulfated polysaccharide obtained from Grifola frondosa and its combination with 5-fluorouracil against human gastric carcinoma cells. *Carbohydr. Polym.* 68: 687–692.
40. Shi, B.J. et al., 2003. Preparation of Grifola frondosa polysaccharide sulfate and its antitumor activity. *Zhongguo Yiyao Gongye Zazhi* 34: 383–385.
41. Nie, X.H. et al., 2006. Preparation of a chemically sulfated polysaccharide derived from Grifola frondosa and its potential biological activities. *Intl. J. Biol. Macromol.* 39: 228–233.
42. Konno, S. et al., 2016. Potent anticancer effect of PET-fraction (PET-F) in comparison with other commercial products on canine cancer cells. *Open J. Veterinary Med.* 5(5): 101–110.
43. Nanba, H et al., 1997. Antitumor substance extracted from hen-of-the-woods. *PCT Intl. Appl.* WO 97-JP728 19970307.

44. Cui, F.J. et al., 2006. Structural analysis of antitumor acid heteropolysaccharide GFPS1b from the cultured mycelia of Grifola frondosa GF9801. *Shipin yu Shengwu Jishu Xuebao* 25: 66–71, 76.
45. Cui, F.J. et al., 2006. Structural analysis of antitumor heteropolysaccharide GFPS1b from the cultured mycelia of Grifola frondosa GF9801. *Bioresource Technol.* 98: 395–401.
46. Cui, F.J. et al., 2007. Induction of apoptosis in SGC-7901 cells by polysaccharide-peptide GFPS1b from the cultured mycelia of Grifola frondosa GF9801. *Toxicol. in Vitro* 21: 417–427.
47. Cui, F.J. et al., 2007. Antitumor activity of polysaccharide-peptide GFPS1b from the cultured mycelia of Grifola frondosa GF9801 in vivo. *Shipin yu Shengwu Jishu Xuebao* 26: 31–35.
48. Mao, G.H. et al., 2015. Antitumor and immunomodulatory activity of a water-soluble polysaccharide from Grifola frondosa. *Carbohydr. Polym.* 134: 406–412.
49. Wang, Y. et al., 2014. A heteropolysaccharide, L-fuco-D-manno-1,6-α-D-galactan extracted from Grifola frondosa and antiangiogenic activity of its sulfated derivative. *Carbohydr. Polym.* 101: 631–641.
50. Zhang, W.N. et al., 2016. Antioxidant and antitumor activities of exopolysaccharide from liquid-cultured Grifola frondosa by chemical modification. *Int. J. Food Sci. Technol.* 51(4): 1055–1061.
51. Mao, G.H. et al., 2016. Antitumor and immunomodulatory activity of selenium (Se)-polysaccharide from Se-enriched Grifola frondosa. *Int. J. Biol. Macromol.* 82: 607–613.
52. Cui, F.J. 2014. Grifola frondosa mycelium antitumor glycoprotein and preparation method thereof. Faming Zhuanli Shenqing CN 103509091 A 20140115.
53. Cui, F.J. et al., 2016. Grifola frondosa glycoprotein GFG-3a arrests S phase, alters proteome, and induces apoptosis in human gastric cancer cells. *Nutr. Cancer* 68(2): 267–279.
54. Chan, J.Y. et al., 2011. Enhancement of in vitro and in vivo anticancer activities of polysaccharide peptide from Grifola frondosa by chemical modifications. *Pharm. Biol.* (London, UK) 49: 1114–1120.
55. Yan, J.Z. et al., 2004. Effects of Grifola frondosa DNA on non-specific immunity of mice. *J. China Med. Univ.* 33: 203–204.

64. MONGOLIA TRICHOLOMA

蒙古口蘑　モンゴルキシメジ　몽골리아 버섯

Tricholoma mongolicum

Tricholomataceae

Mongolia tricholoma originates from the young fruiting body of the mushroom *Tricholoma mongolicum* (Tricholomataceae), an edible fungus that grows only in northern and northeastern areas of China during summer and autumn. Therefore, its production is limited and its consumption region is just around the mushroom distribution.

SCIENTIFIC EVIDENCE OF CANCER-INHIBITORY AND CANCER-PREVENTIVE CONSTITUENTS

1. Lectins

Two lectins, termed TML-1 and TML-2, were extracted from the mushroom *T. mongolicum*. The molecular weights of the two lectins are similarly close to 3.7×10^4 and structures of both are dimers that only differ in the contents of proline and tyrosine units. The two lectins showed the antiproliferative effect against mouse P815 mastocytoma and mouse PU5-1.8 monocyte-macrophage cell lines *in vitro*. *In vivo* studies demonstrated that the lectins were able to inhibit the proliferation of sarcoma 180 cells and prolong the life span of mice by 68.84% and 92.39%, respectively, concomitant with activation of macrophages and stimulation of nitrite ions production from macrophages in both normal and tumor-bearing mice, and then enhanced T-cell proliferation.[1-3] The results evidenced that the anticarcinoma activity of the two lectins are closely related to their marked immunoenhancing property.[3]

2. Polysaccharide–peptide complex

An immunoenhancing and anticarcinoma active polysaccharide–peptide complex (15.5 kDa) was isolated from the mycelial of the edible fungi. The ratio of carbohydrate and protein in the complex was about 8:1. By activating the effects of macrophages and stimulating macrophage antigen-presenting activity, the complex in turn augmented the proliferation of T cells and suppressed the growth of sarcoma 180 cells in tumor-bearing mice.[4]

3. Polysaccharide

The isolated Mongolia tricholoma polysaccharide (MOP) demonstrated antiproliferative effects against human cervical carcinoma and human hepatoma cell lines *in vitro*.[5]

4. Ergosterols

Ergosterol and ergosterol peroxide are the major constituents in the petroleum ether extract from the fruit bodies of *T. mongolicum*. Both sterols could promote the apoptosis of human HepG2 hepatoma cells and obstruct the cell division at the apoptotic early stage by 41.2% and 42.33%, respectively, *in vitro*. Administration with ergosterol peroxide at a dose of 5 mg/kg per day or the petroleum ether extract at a dose of 35 mg/kg per day resulted in suppressive effect against mouse H22 hepatoma cells by 67.15% and 69.61%, respectively, *in vivo*. Simultaneously, each treatment group showed higher thymus index, spleen index, and/or IL-2 level in serum compared with the control group, showing that the immunoenhancing effects were also importantly involved in the antihepatoma activity.[6]

CONCLUSION AND SUGGESTION

Although Mongolia tricholoma is not commonly an edible algae, the chemical biology studies disclosed the anticarcinoma potential and cancer-suppressive substances of the Mongolian mushroom. Its biological active components, including lectins, polysaccharides, polysaccharide–peptide complexes, and ergosterols, were demonstrated to be responsible for the anticancer-related activities such as antiproliferation, proapoptosis, immunoenhancement, antimutagenesis, antioxidation, and/or hematopoiesis.[7] Therefore, it is true that the consumption of Mongolia tricholoma can provide not only nutrients but also functional supplement for lowering the recidence of carcinogenesis. Actually, as a helpful functional food, the development of *Tricholoma mongolicum* cultivation is in progress in China to increase its production.

REFERENCES

1. Wang, H.X. et al., 1996. The immunomodulatory and antitumor activities of lectins from the mushroom Tricholoma mongolicum. *Immunopharmacol.* 31: 205–211.
2. Wang, H.X. et al., 1995. Isolation and characterization of two distinct lectins with antiproliferative activity from the cultured mycelium of the edible mushroom Tricholoma mongolicum. *Intl. J. Peptide Protein Res.* 46: 508–513.
3. Wang, H.X. et al., 1997. Actions of lectins from the mushroom Tricholoma mongolicum on macrophages, splenocytes and life-span in sarcoma-bearing mice. *Anticancer Res.* 17: 419–424.
4. Wang, H.X. et al., 1998. A polysaccharide-peptide complex from cultured mycelia of the mushroom Tricholoma mongolicum with immunoenhancing and antitumor activities. *Biochem. Cell Biol.* 74: 95–100.
5. Ge, S.M. et al. 2009. Study on the extraction and anti-tumor activity from Mongolia tricholoma polysaccharide. *Xiandai Yufang Yixue* 36: 3708–3711.
6. Bau, S. et al., 2012. Antitumor activity of Tricholoma mongolicum fruit bodies. *Shipin Kexue* (Beijing, China) 33: 280–284.
7. You, Q.H. et al., 2014. Extraction, purification, and antioxidant activities of polysaccharides from Tricholoma mongolicum Imai. *Carbohydr. Polym.* 99(2): 1–10.

65. OYSTER MUSHROOM

側耳　平茸　느타리 버섯

Pleurotus ostreatus

Tricholomataceae

Oyster mushroom is the fruiting body of the popular edible fungus *Pleurotus ostreatus* (Tricholomataceae), which is now grown commercially for nutritional purposes throughout the world. Compared to other mushroom species, it contains more vitamins B9, B1, and B3 but less vitamin B12 and has good contents of minerals such as copper, iron, potassium, phosphorous, magnesium, zinc, and sodium. Oyster mushroom has been frequently used in cooking all over the world due to its delicacy and rich nutritional and medicinal values, and it also has been reported to possess antihypercholesterolic, antiatherosclerotic, antidiabetic, antiarthritic, antioxidant, immunomodulatory, anticancer, antilipemic, antiviral, and antibacterial properties.[1]

SCIENTIFIC EVIDENCE OF CANCER-INHIBITORY AND CANCER-PREVENTIVE ACTIVITIES

Oyster mushroom has been demonstrated to have prominent anticarcinogenic activity *in vivo*. In a rat model with dimethylhydrazine-induced colon carcinogenesis, daily diet with 5% of dried oyster mushroom markedly lowered the incidence of lymphoid hyperplasia foci by <70%.[2] Feed of the edible fungi every day for 8 days significantly declined the incidence of urinary bladder carcinoma induced by *N*-butyl-*N'*-butanolnitrosoamine (BBN) from 100% to 65.0%. The BBN-elicited negative effects on chemotactic activity of macrophages and blastogenic response of lymphocytes could be reversed by intake of oyster mushroom.[3,4] Its water-soluble extract (POE) prepared from the fresh oyster mushroom induced a dose-dependent rapid apoptosis of PC3 cells in a concentration of 150 µg/mL and exhibited the cytotoxicity against human androgen-independent PC3 prostate cancer cells.[5] Its methanolic extract markedly repressed the survival rate of human HT-29 colon carcinoma cells *in vitro*. Interestingly, the extracts from its dark-gray and pink strains of the same fungi species showed higher suppressive effect against the HT-29 cells, but the extract from its yellow strain had higher radical scavenging activity.[6] The results clearly showed that the polar extracts of oyster mushrooms contain the main anticancer constituents with antineoplastic and anticarcinogenetic property and the different strains of *P. ostreatus* would influence the content of anticancer constituents. Either nonirradiated or UV-irradiated oyster mushroom extracts exerted the antigrowth effect on murine B16F10 melanoma cells with no cytotoxicity to keratinocytes.[7]

Furthermore, selenium- and zinc-enriched oyster mushrooms (SZMs) demonstrated both markedly improved antioxidant and antitumor capacities. After mice were fed with a diet supplemented with SZMs for six weeks, the activities of glutathione peroxidase (GPx) and superoxide dismutase were significantly enhanced and the levels of malondialdehyde and lipofuscin were declined; thereby showing that SZMs significantly attenuated the number of tumor nodes in a mouse model with lung neoplasms. The evidences implied that SZMs possess greater functions in the antioxidation and cancer prevention.[8] Also, the mushroom was capable of potentiating the cytotoxicity of lymphocytes against the tumor cell lines such as Yac-1 lymphoma and P815 lymphoblast-like mastocytoma,[3,4] inferring the antitumor immunity.

SCIENTIFIC EVIDENCE OF CANCER-INHIBITORY AND CANCER-PREVENTIVE CONSTITUENTS

1. Polysaccharides

Many polysaccharide components have been reported from the phytochemical studies of oyster mushroom and its cultivation by many research groups. Most polysaccharides isolated from

P. ostreatus demonstrated multiple biological activities including anticarcinogenesis, immunopotentiation, antioxidation, and so on.

Glucans and glycans: Two kinds of polysaccharides were extracted by hot water from fruiting bodies of *P. ostreatus* and its cultivated mycelium, respectively, which were both confirmed to be (1-3)- and (1-6)-β-D-glucans. Administration of a sublethal dose of the mycelial polysaccharides to mice-bearing solid Ehrlich cancer resulted in 87.67% growth-inhibitory ratio (T/C %) and significantly increased the percentage of survivors. The mycelial polysaccharides were more potent than the fruiting body polysaccharides in the *in vivo* test.[9] Both intracellular and extracellular polysaccharides isolated from *P. ostreatus* exhibited dose-dependent antiproliferative activity toward several tested human carcinoma cell lines in the *in vitro* assays, and the extracellular polysaccharides presented the highest suppressive effect toward RL95 endometrial cancer cells. The high superoxide dismutase-like activity exerted by the polysaccharides strongly supported the antigrowth effect against the tumor cells.[10]

Pleuran is a purified (1-3)-β-D-glucan that was isolated from oyster mushroom. A diet containing 10% pleuran to rats was found to obviously reduce the conjugated diene content in organs of erythrocytes (such as liver and colon). The dimethylhydrazine-triggered precancerous aberrant crypt foci (ACF) lesions and carcinogenic incidence in rats were lessened by >50% in a diet with 10% pleuran. Concurrently, pleuran increased superoxide dismutase (SOD) level and activated glutathione peroxidase (GPx) and glutathione reductase in liver, notably reduced glutathione levels in colon and GPx activity in erythrocytes, and enhanced catalase activity in erythrocytes. These findings revealed that the antioxidative effect of pleuran was obviously linked to its anticarcinogenetic activity.[9] Moreover, a highly branched (1-3)-β-glucan and a cold-alkali glucan were also isolated from oyster mushrooms; both glucans displayed the inhibitory activity against the growth of mouse-implanted sarcoma 180 cells *in vivo*, but the highly branched (1-3)-β-glucan showed more potent antitumor effect even at a dose of 0.1 mg/kg.[11,12] A low-molecular α-glucan was prepared from a hot-water soluble fraction of the cultured *P. ostreatus* mycelium. The α-glucan hindered the proliferation of HT-29 colon cancer cells *in vitro* in a dose-dependent manner concomitant with induction of cell apoptosis via upregulation of proapoptotic protein Bax and release of cytosolic cytochrome c, showing the promising anticarcinogenetic and anticancer properties.[13] Moreover, these glucans/glycans from either mycelia or fruit body of *P. ostreatus* were capable of enhancing immune functions such as lymphocyte proliferation, macrophage activation, and cytotoxicities of macrophage and NK cells. In a mice model with Dalton's lymphoma, the glucan/glycan treatments at 20 mg/kg doses exerted not only the tumor regression but also immunoenhancement, reaching the better antitumor activities for about 75% and 71.4%, respectively.[14] According to the results, it is clear that the antitumor property of glucans/glycans from oyster mushroom are primarily attributed to their multiple abilities in strengthening the immune system of the host, eliciting the apoptosis of cancer cells and inhibiting the proliferation of cancer cells.

Other polysaccharides: POPS-1, a water-soluble heteropolysaccharide (31 kDa) was prepared from the fruiting bodies by hot water extraction, which is composed of mannose, galactose, and glucose with a molar ratio of 1:2.1:7.9. Its structure comprised a β-(1-3)-linked glucose backbone that terminated with glucose and galactose residues and occasionally branched at O-6 of the hexose. POPS-1 presented marked dose-dependent suppressive effect against HeLa cervical cancer cells *in vitro*, but showed notably lower cytotoxic to human normal cells such as embryo kidney 293T cells.[15] Another water-soluble *P. ostreatus* polysaccharide did not trigger the apoptosis of human Caco-2 colon cancer cell line, but could inhibit the invasion of Caco-2 cells in association with downregulation of MMPs-2 and -9 expressions, upregulation of Hsp60 and Hsp90, and downregulation of Hsp70.[16] WPOP-N1 is an alkali-extracted water-soluble polysaccharide from *P. ostreatus*. In a mouse model implanted with sarcoma 180 cells, WPOP-N1 in doses of 100, 200, and 400 mg/kg displayed a prominent inhibitory effect on the growth of tumor cells through a mechanism that was found largely to relate to activating macrophages to secrete NO and TNF-α and augmenting the phagocytic activities of macrophages.[17] The anticancer activity of WPOP-N1 was further proved in the *in vivo* tests of mice engrafted with human BGC-823 gastric cancer cells.[18] Other data showed that the macrophage activation of WPOP-N1 was mediated by a NF-κB signaling pathway and the antitumor effect of WPOP-N1 was achieved by its immunostimulating property.[19] POMP2 (29 kDa) is a polysaccharide from *P. ostreatus* mycelium. Treatment with POMP2 at a concentration of 400 mg/L for 72 h showed 35.6% growth-inhibition and invasive-suppression against the BGC-823 cells *in vitro*.[18]

2. Proteoglycans

Four neutral proteoglycans were purified from water-soluble fractions of either the fruiting body or the mycelia. The ratios of polysaccharide moiety to protein moiety in the four proteoglycans were 3.46:1, 14.2:1, 18.3:1, and 26.4:1, respectively. The proteoglycans exerted marked immunoregulating effects including stimulation of cytotoxic NK cells, increase of thymocytes and splenocytes, promotion of IL-4 and IFN-γ production, and amplification of macrophages. By the proteoglycans treatment, the growth of sarcoma 180 cells was considerably hampered *in vivo* and *in vitro* together with cell cycle arrest in G0/G1 phase or pre-G0/G1 phase.[20,21]

A glycopeptide assigned as POGP was also separated from the oyster mushroom, which could enhance the cytotoxicities of LAK cells and NK cells to tumor cells. *In vivo* assay revealed that POGP not only inhibited the proliferation of sarcoma 180 cells but also led to the infiltration of lymphocytes and blockage of the tumor cell infiltration into the surrounding normal tissues. Also, the POGP was able to stimulate fiber formation in the tumor tissue, finally inducing the death of carcinoma tissue. The antineoplastic activity of the lower molecular POGP (POGP-L) was superior to its higher molecular POGP (POGP-H).[22,23]

3. Lectin

A dimeric lectin, which is composed of two subunits with m.w. 40 and 41 kDa, was isolated from fresh fruiting bodies of oyster mushrooms. This lectin component demonstrated potent *in vivo* antitumor activity against sarcoma 180 and hepatoma H22 in mice, and obviously lengthened the survival time of tumor-bearing mice after the lectin treatment.[24]

4. Protein

A functional nonlectin glycoprotein designated as PCP-3A was separated from the fresh fruiting body of *P. ostreatus*, which is composed of 10 subunits, each of whose size is approximately 45.0 kDa. PCP-3A at 12.5 μg/mL concentration impeded the proliferation of human U937 leukemic monocyte lymphoma cells in a time-dependent manner together with induction of S cell arrest and cell apoptosis.[25] Other studies revealed that the inhibition of PCP-3A on U937 cells was also associated with stimulation of human mononuclear cells to secrete cytokines such as TNF-α, IL-2, and IFN-γ.[26] Ostreolysin is a 16-kDa cytolytic protein isolated from *P. ostreatus* primordia and fruiting bodies, which was cytotoxic to mammalian tumor cells. Even at nanomolar concentrations, ostreolysin still could lyse erythrocytes by a colloid-osmotic mechanism.[27]

5. DNA component

A DNA component was isolated from the fruit body of oyster mushroom, whose DNA component could augment the cytotoxic activity of NK cells *in vitro* and significantly prolonged the life span of mice bearing solid Ehrlich carcinoma *in vivo*. The therapeutic effects of oyster mushroom DNA component probably were due to the presence of immunostimulatory unmethylated CpG motifs in DNA.[28]

6. Ribonuclease

A 15 kDa ribonuclease (RNase) was purified from a close species *Pleurotus djamor*, whose *N*-terminal amino acid sequence was different from other RNase sequences of mushrooms belonging to the genus of Pleurotus and other genera. At pH 4.6°C and 60°C, the RNase exhibited its maximal activity to inhibit proliferation of hepatoma cells and breast cancer cells. The active RNase generally carried metal ions and the ranking of inhibitory potencies for metal ions in the RNase were $Fe^{3+} > Al^{3+} > Ca^{2+} > Hg^{2+}$.[29] Similarly, RNase Po1, a guanylic acid-specific RNase (a RNase T1 family RNase) was derived from *P. ostreatus*. RNase Po1 at its optimum temperature of 20°C exerted higher anticancer activity than RNase T1. In an *in vitro* assay, RNase Po1 inhibited the proliferation of human neuroblastoma cell lines (IMR-32 and SK-N-SH) and human leukemia cell lines (Jurkat and HL-60).[30]

ADJUNCTIVE APPLICATION

When the oyster fungi were fermented by using corncob, the products demonstrated remarkable antitumorigenic activity. Diet of fermented corncob fiber significantly reduced the incidence of colon cancer induced by 1,2-dimethylhydrazine (DMH) in rats to 26%. Concurrently, the fungi-treated corncob significantly increased the content of p53 in the cell cytoplasm and elevated its serum levels to 33%–38% and lowered the cellular concentration of PCNA in tumor to 61% in the tumor-bearing rats. The anticarcinogenic mechanism was elucidated to be closely related to amplification of apoptosis, inhibition of proliferating cell nuclear antigen (PCNA) and activation of p53 protein.[31] By UV-B irradiation for 3 h, the ergosterol in oyster mushroom powder can be converted to vitamin D2 without obvious influences on the total polyphenolic content and antioxidative and tyrosinase inhibitory activities of the oyster mushroom.[7]

NANOFORMATION

By using a reduction of aqueous Ag^+ ions with culture supernatant from *P. ostreatus*, a kind of silver nanoparticles (AgNPs) were synthesized, whose size was in the range of 4–15 nm. The anticancer property of AgNPs was proved in the *in vitro* experiments. The AgNPs significantly diminished the viability and growth of human MCF-7 breast tumor cells. At ~640 μg/mL concentrations, the highest antigrowth rate reached 78%, showing a promising potential for application of the green synthesized nanomaterials in cancer therapy.[32]

CONCLUSION AND SUGGESTION

The earlier summary evidenced the high nutritional and biomedical importance of the edible oyster mushroom. The numbers of active substances discovered from the fruiting body and the cultured fungi/mycelium, especially macromolecules including polysaccharides, proteoglycans/glycopeptides, lectins, proteins, DNA components, and ribonuclease, demonstrated both direct and indirect suppressive effects against the proliferation and growth of cancer cells and against the development of carcinogenesis due to their safe and effective anticancer, immunoregulative, proapoptotic, antioxidant, and/or anti-inflammatory properties. On the basis of the remarkable therapeutic and nutritional values, the consumption of oyster mushroom can be expected to provide the potential for lowering the risk of cancer and the functional food supplement for augmenting the efficacy of cancer treatment. Therefore, frequent consumption of dietary oyster mushroom is highly encouraged to gain health benefits for cancer prevention, cancer therapy, and immune enhancement; the functional food is suitable for both healthy people and patients.

REFERENCES

1. Deepalakshmi, K. et al., 2014. Pleurotus ostreatus: an oyster mushroom with nutritional and medicinal properties. *J. Biochem. Tech.* 5(2): 718–26.
2. Bobek, P. et al., 1997. Effect of oyster mushroom (Pleurotus ostreatus) on dimethylhydrazine-induced colon carcinogenesis in the rat. *Ceska a Slovenska Gastroenterologie* 51: 128–32.
3. Kurashige, S. et al., 1997. Effects of Lentinus edodes, Grifola frondosa and Pleurotus ostreatus administration on cancer outbreak, and activities of macrophages and lymphocytes in mice treated with a carcinogen, N-butyl-N-butanolnitrosoamine. *Immunopharmacol. Immuno-toxicol.* 19: 175–83.

4. Petrova, R.D. et al., 2005. Potential role of medicinal mushrooms in breast cancer treatment: Current knowledge and future perspectives. *Intl. J. Med. Mushrooms* 7: 141–55.

5. Gu, Y.H. et al., 2006. Cytotoxic effect of oyster mushroom Pleurotus ostreatus on human androgen-independent prostate cancer PC-3 cells. *J. Med. Food* 9: 196–204.

6. Kim, J.H. et al., 2009. The different antioxidant and anticancer activities depending on the color of oyster mushrooms. *J. Med. Plants Res.* 3: 1016–20.

7. Banlangsawan, N. et al., 2016. Investigation of antioxidative, antityrosinase and cytotoxic effects of extract of irradiated oyster mushroom. *Songklanakarin J. Sci. and Technol.* 38(1): 31–9.

8. Yan, H.M. et al., 2013. Antioxidant and antitumor activities of selenium- and zinc-enriched Oyster mushroom in mice. *Biol. Trace Element Res.* 150: 236–41.

9. a) Jwanny, E.W. et al., 2002. Antitumor activity of polysaccharides extracted from Pleurotus ostreatus fruiting bodies and mycelia cultivated on date waste media. *Egypt. J. Biochem. Mol. Biol.* 20: 23–40; b) Yoshioka, Y. et al., 1985. Antitumor polysaccharides from P. ostreatus: isolation and structure of a β-glucan. *Carbohydrate Res.* 140: 93–100.

10. Silva, S. et al., 2012. Production, purification and characterisation of polysaccharides from Pleurotus ostreatus with antitumour activity. *J. Sci. Food Agric.* 92: 1826–32.

11. Misaki, A. et al., 1992. Chemical characterization and antitumor activities of the polysaccharide components of Simeji mushrooms (Pleurotus species). *Seikatsukagakubu Kiyo* 39: 1–8.

12. Bobek, P. et al., 2001. Effect of pleuran (β-glucan from Pleurotus ostreatus) on the antioxidant status of the organism and on dimethyl-hydrazine-induced precancerous lesions in rat colon. *British J. Biomed. Sci.* 58: 164–8.

13. Lavi, I. et al., 2006. An aqueous polysaccharide extract from the edible mushroom Pleurotus ostreatus induces antiproliferative and proapoptotic effects on HT-29 colon cancer cells. *Cancer Lett.* (Amsterdam, Netherlands) 244: 61–70.

14. Devi, K.S.P. et al., 2015. Immune augmentation and Dalton's lymphoma tumor inhibition by glucans/glycans isolated from the mycelia and fruit body of Pleurotus ostreatus. *Intl. Immunopharmacol.* 25: 207–17.

15. Tong, H.B. et al., 2008. Structural characterization and in vitro antitumor activity of a novel polysaccharide isolated from the fruiting bodies of Pleurotus ostreatus. *Bioresource Technol.* 100: 1682–6.

16. Cojocaru, S. et al., 2013. Water soluble Pleurotus ostreatus polysaccharide down-regulates the expression of MMP-2 and MMP-9 in Caco-2 cells. *Notulae Botanicae Horti Agrobotanici Cluj-Napoca* 41: 553–9.

17. Kong, F.L. et al., 2012. Inhibitory effect of water-soluble polysaccharide alkali-extracted from Pleurotus ostreatus and its mechanism. *Jilin Daxue Xuebao, Yixueban* 38: 1091–5.

18. Cao, X.Y. et al., 2015. Antitumor activity of polysaccharide extracted from Pleurotus ostreatus mycelia against gastric cancer in vitro and in vivo. *Mol. Med. Reports* 12: 2383–9.

19. Kong, F.L. et al., 2014. Antitumor and macrophage activation induced by alkali-extracted polysaccharide from Pleurotus ostreatus. *Intl. J. Biol. Macromol.* 69: 561–6.

20. Shah, S. et al., 2007. Immunomodulatory and antitumor activities of water-soluble proteoglycan isolated from the fruiting bodies of culinary-medicinal oyster mushroom Pleurotus ostreatus (Jacq.: Fr.) P. Kumm. (Agaricomycetideae). *Intl. J. Med. Mushrooms* 9: 123–38.

21. Sarangi, I. et al., 2006. Antitumor and immunomodulating effects of Pleurotus ostreatus mycelia-derived proteoglycans. *Intl. Immuno-pharmacol.* 6:1287–97.

22. Li, H. et al., 1994, Preparation and immunologic competence of glycopeptides components from Pleurotus ostreatus fungi. *Shandong Yike Daxue Xuebao* 32: 343–6.

23. Li, H. et al., 1994. Antitumor action of glycopeptide fraction from Pleurotus ostreatus fungi. *Yaowu Shengwu Jishu* 1: 35–8.

24. Wang, H.X. et al., 2000. A new lectin with highly potent antihepatoma and antisarcoma activities from the Oyster mushroom Pleurotus ostreatus. *Biochem. Biophys. Res. Communs.* 275: 810–16.

25. Chen, J.N. et al., 2009. A glycoprotein extracted from golden oyster mushroom Pleurotus citrinopileatus exhibiting growth inhibitory effect against U937 leukemia cells. *J. Agricul. Food Chem.* 57: 6706–11.

26. Chen, J.N. et al., 2010. In vitro antitumor and immunomodulatory effects of the protein PCP-3A from mushroom Pleurotus citrinopileatus. *J. Agric. Food Chem.* 58: 12117–22.

27. Sepcic, K. et al., 2003. Interaction of ostreolysin, a cytolytic protein from the edible mushroom Pleurotus ostreatus, with lipid membranes and modulation by lysophospholipids. *Eur. J. Biochem. FEBS* 270: 1199–210.

28. Shlyakhovenko, V. et al., 2006. Application of DNA from mushroom Pleurotus ostreatus for cancer biotherapy: a pilot study. *Experim. Oncol.* 28: 132–5.

29. Wu, X.L. et al., 2010. Isolation and characterization of a novel ribonuclease from the pink oyster mush-room Pleurotus djamor. *J. General Applied Microbiol.* 56: 231–9.
30. Kobayashi, H. et al., 2013. The inhibition of human tumor cell proliferation by RNase Po1, a member of the RNase T1 family, from Pleurotus ostreatus. *Biosci. Biotechnol. Biochem.* 77: 1486–91.
31. Zusman, I. et al., 1997. Role of apoptosis, proliferating cell nuclear antigen and p53 protein in chemically induced colon cancer in rats fed corncob fiber treated with the fungus Pleurotus ostreatus. *Anticancer Res.* 17: 2105–13.
32. Yehia, R.S. et al., 2014. Biosynthesis and characterization of silver nanoparticles produced by Pleurotus ostreatus and their anticandidal and anticancer activities. *World J. Microbiol. Biotechnol.* 30: 2797–803.

66. PINE MUSHROOM

松覃 松茸 송이

Tricholoma matsutake

Tricholomataceae

Pine mushroom is the fruiting body of the fungus *Tricholoma matsutake* (Tricholomataceae). The fungus usually forms a symbiotic relationship with the roots of pine and fir tree species. It normally grows in Asia, Northern Europe, and Northern America. Due to its characteristic flavor, odor, and functional properties, matsutake is a prized delicacy in Eastern Asian cuisines, especially in Japan. After being cooked, matsutake gives a pine-like fragrance. Two very close Tricholoma species, viz., Swedish matsutake (*T. nauseosum*) and American matsutake (*T. magnivelare*), are reported as substitutes of matsutake that are consumed in Asia. Nutritional analysis in Calorie Slism showed that matsutake is an excellent source of vitamins D, B3, and B complex, and some minerals (copper, potassium, iron, and zinc). Pharmacological studies showed that pine mushroom/matsutake possesses remarkable bioactivities such as antimutagenic, anticancer, antiradiation, immunopotentiating, antithrombotic, hypoglycemic, cholesterol-reducing, and skin-cosmetic effects.[1]

SCIENTIFIC EVIDENCE OF CANCER-INHIBITORY AND CANCER-PREVENTIVE ACTIVITIES

The anticancer activity of pine mushroom was demonstrated in *in vitro* and *in vivo* studies. The early studies showed that the inhibitory rates could reach 98.1% and 70% against the growth of sarcoma 180 and Ehrlich's ascites tumor *in vivo*, respectively, after administration of matsutake HWE.[1] Treatment with pine mushroom markedly inhibited the proliferation of human K562 leukemia cells *in vitro*, and it also induced differentiation of the K562 cells.[2] Pine mushroom juice (PMJ), which contains rich phenolic substances, demonstrated the growth inhibitory activity on human AGS (stomach), HeLa (cervix), HepG2 (liver), and HT-29 (colon) cancer cell lines. In addition, the PMJ could scavenge ABTS radicals, and the scavenging rates reached 81.7–91.8% at the concentration of 10–50 mg/mL.[3] Its water-soluble components were remarkably effective in the antitumor actions, while its oil-soluble components were weakly active. However, the different types of components exerted obvious antioxidant action in scavenging OH radicals.[4] Overall, these findings suggest that pine mushroom can be beneficial to body protection and promotion.

SCIENTIFIC EVIDENCE OF CANCER-INHIBITORY AND CANCER-PREVENTIVE CONSTITUENTS

Continuous chemical biology and molecular biology investigations have discovered three types of macromolecules such as proteins, glycoproteins, and polysaccharides in pine mushroom/matsutake as the major inhibitors responsible for the anticarcinogenic and cancer-preventive activities of matsutake.

1. Proteins

A tumoricidal protein termed TTM, which consisted of two subunits (m.w. 10,000–11,000 and 20,000–21,000), was purified from *T. matsutake*. TTM could induce the morphological changes and the cell apoptosis of various neoplastic cell lines *in vitro* at concentrations as low as 5–20 ng/mL, but it had no effect on normal cells. The IC_{50}s were 7 and 14 ng/mL in mouse transformed fibroblast and human HeLa cervical cancer cell lines, respectively.[5-7] Another two bioactive proteins, TMP and TMP-B, are derived from *T. matsutake* mycelium and demonstrated marked suppression against the proliferation of HeLa cells in the *in vitro* assay. Similar to TTM, the acceleration of the HeLa cell apoptosis by TMP and TMP-B was observed to be related to blocking of the cell cycle conversion from S to G2/M stage.[8,9]

2. Glycoproteins

Several bioactive glycoproteins, for example, M2 fraction, MTS03, and MTSGS1, were separated from the cultivated mycelia of *T. matsutake*. Their anticancer and anticarcinogenic potentials were demonstrated by both *in vitro* and *in vivo* experiments.

MTS03: Glycoprotein MTS03 (m.w. 2.37×10^4) comprises 86.53% of protein portion, which is composed of 17 amino acids and 12.46% of polysaccharide portion, which is composed of xylose, glucose, galactose, arabinose, and mannose in a molar ratio of 0.61:1.29:1.46:2.22:7.74. MTS03 showed very low cytotoxicity on human normal human liver L-02 cells, but it exhibited excellent inhibitory activity to carcinoma cells *in vitro*, especially to human BEL-7402 hepatoma, MCF-7 breast cancer, HL-60 leukemia, and C6 glioma cell lines. The IC_{50}s of MTS03 at 72 h were 8.18, 7.55, and 11.39 µg/mL in the MCF-7, BEL-7402, and sarcoma 180 cell lines, respectively. Moreover, in combination with chemotherapeutic drugs to treat the MCF-7 and Bel-7402 cancer cell lines *in vitro*, MTS03 at an appropriate concentration could remarkably improve the cytotoxicity of a therapeutic drug 5-FU and reduce its toxicity/side effects, resulting in significant synergistic anticancer effect. However, MTS03 would be decomposed at temperatures over 56°C, but it is stable at room temperature.[10]

MTSGS1: An isolated active glycoprotein, termed MTSGS1, demonstrated direct tumoricidal activity in the *in vitro* assays. Even in low doses (20–160 µg/mL), MTSGS1 still could deter the cell proliferation of human HeLa cervical cancer cells *in vitro* and induce cell apoptosis and cell cycle arrest. *In vivo* experiment further confirmed the inhibitory effect of MTSGS1 against sarcoma 180 cells in mice at a dosage of 50 mg/kg/day with 65% inhibitory rate. At the same time, the spleen weight and index in mice were augmented markedly, indicating an immunoenhancing action involved in the *in vivo* antitumor effect.[11]

M2 fraction: M2 fraction is a protein bound with α-glucan (38%), which is able to cure primary cancer and restrain the growth of metastatic carcinoma by intratumoral injection of M2 fraction. In addition, M2 fraction also remarkably stimulated the production of immunosuppressive acidic protein (IAP) from the activated macrophages transiently soon after intradermal administration of 5 mg M2 fraction.[12–14]

3. Polysaccharides

Polysaccharides isolated from pine mushroom could obviously suppress the proliferation of B16 human melanoma cells *in vitro* in a dose-dependent fashion; their inhibitory rate was 67% at the concentration of 10 mg/mL.[15] The *T. matsutake* polysaccharides were also effective in the growth inhibition against four human cancer cell lines (such as U87 glioma, HeLa cervical cancer, PANC-1 pancreatic duct cancer, and MCF-7 breast cancer) *in vitro* together with induction of S cell arrest and/or apoptosis.[16] Though the antiproliferative effects were moderate to weak in the HeLa, HepG2, and MCF-7 cells (IC_{50}s of 40.04, 53.77, and 100.65 µg/mL, respectively),[17] its maximum inhibition ratios to human HS766T (pancreas), MCF-7 (breast), HeLa (cervix), HepG2 (liver), and Tca8113 (tongue) cancer cells could reach 83.83%, 76.15%, 75.57%, 74.89%, and 67.71%, respectively, after 72 h exposure at a concentration of 100 µg/mL *in vitro*.[18] Three polysaccharide fractions labeled as TM-P1, TM-P2 and TM-P3 were separated from the *T. matsutake* polysaccharides. TM-P2 consisted of glucose, galactose, and mannose with a molar ratio of 5.9:1.1:1.0. The antigrowth activities of TM-P2 at 4.0 mg/mL concentration were 67.98% and 59.04% on the HepG2 and A549 cell lines, respectively.[19] TM-P1A, TM-P1B, TM-P2A, and TM-P2B were another four purified matsutake polysaccharide fractions. The molar ratios of glucose, galactose, and mannose were 8.7:1.8:1.0 for TM-P1A and 8.9:1.3:1.0 for TM-P2B, whereas the molar ratio of glucose, galactose, mannose, and fucose was 17.7:7.9:3.9:1.0 for TM-P2A. These three fractions were effective in hindering the proliferation of HepG2 hepatoma cells *in vitro*, and the antihepatoma rates at

1.0 mg/mL concentration were TM-P2B (90.23%) > TM-P2A (75.12%) > TM-P1A (29.11%). Also, TM-P2B showed the highest antioxidant activity among them. The structural character of TM-P2B was unbranched β-1,6-glucopyranosyl chain with small amounts of β-1,6-galactopyranosyl and β-1,6-mannopyranosyl units.[20]

Likewise, another polysaccharide-type component was prepared from the liquid fermentative production of pine mushroom. It demonstrated significant antigrowth effects against sarcoma 180, B16 melanoma, and hepatoma cell lines with the inhibitory rates of 47.7%, 75.0%, and 80.6%, respectively.[21] The matsutake polysaccharide extract also occurred in immune response in sarcoma 180-bearing mice. At two doses of 1 and 10 mg/kg/day for ten days, the polysaccharide extract significantly promoted TNF-α production and TNF-α mRNA expression but did not impact IL-2 level in serum, finally exerting both immunity potentiating and antitumor effects.[22]

Conclusion and Suggestion

Due to abundant bioactive substances presented, pine mushroom in the *in vitro* and/or *in vivo* assays was effective in fighting different types of cancer cells. The bioactive substances were revealed to be macromolecules such as proteins, glycoproteins, and polysaccharides, which were responsible for multiple biological activities of pine mushroom, including immunostimulatory, antitumor, antioxidation, antimutagenic, and/or hematopoietic properties. Other active substances in matsutake such as triterpenoids mainly displayed anti-inflammatory and antibacterial effects. All these substances are believed to act synergistically for playing an important role in cancer prevention and an adjuvant role in the cancer chemotherapy. Consequently, it is sure that the consumption of pine mushroom/matsutake is a great choice due to its natural protection from carcinogenesis and an adjuvant remedy combined with cancer treatment. Nevertheless, it is certainly not an economical choice if consumed frequently in diet.

REFERENCES

1. State Administration of Medicines in China, 1999. Chinese Materia Medica, vol. 1, 1–0258, pp. 584, Published by Shanghai Press of Science and Technology, Shanghai, China.
2. Wang, H. et al., 2007. Experimental studies on antitumor effect of Tricholoma matsutake polysaccharide on K562 cells. *Zhongguo Yaoshi* (Wuhan, China) 10: 1180–1181.
3. Kim, Y.E. et al., 2009. ABTS radical scavenging and antitumor effects of Tricholoma matsutake Sing. (Pine mushroom). *Han'guk Sikp'um Yongyang Kwahak Hoechi* 38: 555–560.
4. Liu, C.F. et al., 2015. Study on biological activities of active components obtained from Tricholoma matsutake. *Yaowu Fenxi Zazhi* 35(11): 1953–1957.
5. Kawamura, Y. et al., 2002. A novel antitumorigenic protein from a mushroom, Tricholoma matsutake, induces molecular alterations which lead to apoptosis to cancer cells. *J. Biol. Macromol.* 2: 52–58.
6. Kawamura, Y. et al., 1998. Action mechanism of antitumor protein of Tricholoma matsutake. *Kagaku to Seibutsu* 36: 77–79.
7. Kawamura, Y. et al., 1994. A noble antitumor protein from Tricholoma matsutake, its manufacture, and antitumor agent containing the protein as active ingredient. *Jpn. Kokai Tokkyo Koho* JP 92-260532 19920904.
8. Sun, Z. et al., 2002. Effect of protein from Tricholoma matsutake mycelium on apoptosis of HeLa cells. *Yingyang Xuebao* 24: 75–78.
9. Liu, P. et al., 2001. Apoptotic effect of active protein from Tricholoma matsutake mycelium. *Qinggong Daxue Xuebao* 20: 599–602, 607.
10. Wei, Y.Q. et al., 2005. Inhibition effect of glycoprotein MTS03 from the submerged mycelia of Tricholoma matsutake on proliferation in MCF-7 cells in vitro. *Zhongguo Yaoxue Zazhi* (Beijing, China) 40: 1545–1548.
11. Liu, P. et al., 2001. Antitumor effect and mechanism of active glycoprotein MTSGS1 from mycelium of Tricholoma matsutake. *Yaowu Shengwu Jishu* 8: 284–287.
12. Ebina, T. et al., 2005. Antitumor effects of intratumoral injection of Basidiomycetes preparations. *Gan to Kagaku Ryoho* 32: 1654–1656.

13. Ebina, T. et al., 2003. Activation of antitumor immunity by intratumor injection of biological prepara-
    tions. *Gan to Kagaku Ryoho* 30: 1555–1558.
14. Ebina, T. et al., 2002. Antitumor effect of a peptide-glucan preparation extracted from a mycelium of
    Tricholoma matsutake (S. Ito and Imai) Sing. *Biotherapy* (Tokyo, Japan) 16: 255–259.
15. Yang, S. et al., 2010. Preparation and the antitumor activity in vitro of polysaccharides from Tricholoma
    matsutake. *World J. Microbiol. Biotechnol.* 26: 497–503.
16. Zhang, Z.Y. et al., 2011. In vitro antitumor effects of Tricholoma matsutake polysaccharides on different
    tumor cell lines. *Shandong Yiyao* 51: 70–71.
17. Liu, G. et al., 2015. In vitro antitumor effect of extracts from different parts of Tricholoma matsutake
    Sing. *Zhongguo Yaoshi* 18(5): 701–704.
18. Liu, G. et al., 2013. Study of antitumor activities of polysaccharides from Tricholoma matsutake in vitro.
    Zhonghua Zhongyiyao *Xuekan* 31: 267–270.
19. You, L.J. et al., 2013. Structural characterisation of polysaccharides from Tricholoma matsutake and
    their antioxidant and antitumour activities. *Food Chem.* 138: 2242–2249.
20. You, L.J. et al., 2014. Identification and antiproliferative activity of polysaccharides from Tricholoma
    matsutake (mushroom). *Xiandai Shipin Keji* 30(8): 51–58.
21. Hu, S.Q. et al., 2006. Extraction and test of active metabolites from Tricholoma matsutake. *J. Anhui
    Agricul. Univ.* 33: 499–501.
22. Li, T. et al., 2014. Effect of polysaccharide from tricholoma matsutake on TNF-α and IL-2. *Appl. Mech.
    Mat.* 644-650: 5435–5438.

67. PRINCESS MATSUTAKE OR BRAZILIAN MUSHROOM

姫松茸　姫まつたけ　공주 송이

Agaricus blazei (= A. subrufescens, A. brasiliensis, A. rufotegulis)

Agaricaceae

Princess matsutake is an edible fruiting body of the Basidiomycete fungus *Agaricus blazei* that is native to southern Brazil and Peru and is now commonly cultivated in Japan, China, and Brazil as both nutritional and functional food. As noted in a wide range of research reports, it is capable of impacting the cells of the immune system, that is, not only bolstering the immunity but also attenuating the excessive immunoreactions to maintain a balance of immune function. Hence, it can be considered as a health food supplement and a complementary medicine for prevention of carcinogenesis, diabetes, hyperlipidemia, arteriosclerosis, chronic hepatitis, allergy, and inflammation and for the treatment of some types of cancers, AIDS, infection, and aging.[1,2] Today, the pharmacological properties and health benefits of *A. blazei* are gaining more and more focus.

Scientific Evidence of Cancer Prevention

Since the remarkable mushroom was discovered in 1960, numerous explorations on *A. blazei* fungus have been developed. The broad scientific evidences observed from *in vitro*, *in vivo*, and clinical experiments disclosed the health-promoting benefits of *A. blazei* mushroom in the nutraceutical and medicinal application. Especially, as a functional food, its antitumor immunity, immunoregulating, antimutagenic, and antioxidant potentials are attracting growing attention.

Immunoregulatory activities and antitumor immunities: The bioactive properties of *A. blazei* mushroom that first gained extensive attention were its remarkable immunoregulatory, phagocytic, and antigenotoxic effects. As we know, there are more than 130 subsets of white blood cells in the human immune system, and about 15% of these are NK cells. On the basis of the NK activity, the first line of defense is afforded for dealing with any form of invasion to the human body. In animal models, supplementation with the mushroom amplified monocyte proliferation and phagocytic capacity especially by pretreatment, simultaneous, and continuous pretreatments.[3] Administration of its aqueous extract to mice orally in doses of 4–100 mg/kg for 21 days promoted the NK cell activity and macrophage function, amplified the release of associated cytokines (IL-6, IFN-γ), but lessened the levels of IL-4.[4] All these immunoregulations would exert the cytotoxicity of NK cells and phagorytosis of macrophages against the cancer cell initiation and progression.

Synergetic antitumor immunities: The synergetic potential of *A. blazei* extracts was explored for improvement of their antitumor activity and antitumor immunity. Oral administration of a mixture of two HWEs from *A. blazei* and Chlorella (in a ratio of 1:0.3) to mice at doses of 200 and 300 mg/kg/day showed synergetic antiproliferative effects against sarcoma 180 and Meth-A sarcoma but not against B16 melanoma.[5] ABM-C, a similar mixture of *A. blazei* and Chlorella, could moderately impede the growth of *P-7423* pulmonary tumor in mice; its anticancer effect could be enhanced when ABM-C is used in combination with cyclophosphamide.[6] The treatment concurrently triggered multiple immunostimulating pathways, such as (i) augmenting degree of spleen cell-mediated sheep red blood cell hemolysis and indexes of spleen and liver, and amplifying amount of spleen cells; (ii) increasing peritoneal macrophages and the proportion of third component of complement (C3)-positive fluorescent cells; (iii) augmenting macrophage cells in spleen and Kupffer cells in liver and activating Kupffer cell phagocytosis; (iv) elevating levels of IFN-γ and IL-12 in blood and IFN-γ production; and (v) exerting cytotoxic T-lymphocyte (CTL) activity via activation or maturation of macrophages and dendritic cells; thereby, these prompted immunities lead to the antitumor effects.[5,6]

Moreover, the combination of *A. blazei* extract (246–984 mg/kg/day) with chitosan (5–20 mg/kg/day) for 6 weeks effectively hampered the formation of SK-Hep-1 hepatoma in mice. When treated with chitosan (5 mg/kg/day) and ABM-C (246 mg/kg/day) together, the levels of glutamic oxaloacetic transaminase (GOT) and VEGF were reduced.[7] The *A. blazei* extract plus lactoferrin (a globular glycoprotein) could reverse 5-FU-induced adverse reactions (such as myelotoxicity and body weight loss) and deter the tumor growth and metastasis to lung in osteosarcoma LM8-bearing mice. The protective activity of the combination was found to be mediated by positive induction of the numbers of red blood cells, leukocytes, and platelets, as well as the level of Hb and the hematocrit percentage without negatively affecting the antitumor and anti-metastatic effects of 5-FU.[8]

Antimutagenic and antitumor activities: Pretreatment but not posttreatment of Chinese hamster V79 cells with *A. blazei* extract was effective in deterring the mutagenesis and genotoxicity of a mutagen methyl methanesulfonate. The antimutagenic and antigenotoxic effects were also observed in male Swiss mice to obstruct cyclophosphamide-elicited clastogenicity in bone marrow and in peripheral blood besides the modulation of the immune system.[9,10] Both the direct and indirect protective effects are conducive to its anticarcinogenic effects. The broth of *A. blazei* was found to be cytotoxic to human prostate cancer cell lines (LNCaP, DU145, and PC3) with inhibitory rates of about 10%, 20%, and 15%, respectively, showing that the broth extract was relatively more cytotoxic to androgen-independent prostate cancer cell lines (DU145 and PC3). By targeting cell proliferation and angiogenesis, its *in vivo* antigrowth effect was demonstrated in hormone-refractory PC3 tumor xenografts in nude mice, in whom antiproliferative and antigrowth effects on prostate cancer were also mediated by a proapoptotic pathway without causing adverse effects in mice.[11] The *A. blazei* methanol extract at 0.5 mg/mL concentration hampered the proliferation of human AGS (stomach), HepG2 (liver), and HCT-116 (colon) cancer cell lines by 40%, 13%, and 12%, respectively, and also showed weak antioxidant effect in DHHP and hydroxyl radical scavenging assays.[12] The rats implanted W256 breast carcinoma were treated for 14 days by gavage (136 mg/kg) of the fungus extract, leading to lowering of tumor size and improvement of liver catalase and superoxide dismutase activity.[13] Oral administration of *A. blazei* water extract to mice led to a moderate tumor suppression against sp2 myeloma cells. When treated with a mixture of 0.5 mg/mL of water extract and 1.0 mg/mL squid phospholipid liposome (5 mL/day), the myeloma suppression was observed *in vivo*.[14] Also, *A. blazei* mushroom was evaluated in aberrant crypt foci assay, demonstrating a preventive effect against preneoplastic colorectal lesions.[3] A fraction (A-4) derived from a HWE of *A. blazei* mycelial cultures was able to block the abnormal collagen fiber formation in human hepatoma cells.[15]

Six polar extracts of *A. blazei* isolated by different mixtures of ethanol–water were effective in impeding the viability of human NB-4 myeloid leukemia cells with IC_{50}s < 250 μg/mL. Of these, the 50% and 70% ethanolic extract showed higher anticancer effects and JAB80E70 (a 70% ethanol extract at 80°C, which consists of 21.4% total carbohydrate, 1.27% total polysaccharide, and 1.8% total protein) displayed the most potent inhibition of NB-4 and K562 leukemia cells with the IC_{50}s of 109.6 and 138.3 μg/mL and the maximum inhibitory rates of 77.8 and 61.6%, respectively. The anti-leukemic activity of JAB80E70 was further proved in nude mice implanted with NB-4 cells.[45]

Influences on the production of proinflammatory cytokines: The water extract of *A. blazei* was able to activate NLRP3 inflammasome via multiple mechanisms, such as release of ATP, binding of extracellular ATP to purinergic receptor P2 × 7, generation of ROS, and efflux of potassium, then elicited IL-1β secretion (a proinflammatory cytokine) in human THP-1 macrophages.[16] Other studies also revealed that the *A. blazei* extract enhanced the production of proinflammatory cytokines (including IL-1β and IL-6) in human monocytes and umbilical vein endothelial cells in a dose-dependent manner, and enlarged cytokine production (IL-1β, IL-6, IL-8, TNFα, G-CSF, and MIP-1β) in monocyte-derived dendritic cells. In PMA-differentiated THP-1 cells, the *water* extract could have triggered the mRNA expressions of TNFα, IL-1β, and COX-2.[16] Taken together, these findings proposed that the abilities of *A. blazei* in the upregulation of IL-1β transcription and NLRP3 inflammasome-dependent caspase-1 activation may contribute to the suppressive effect against carcinogenesis and inflection.[16]

Clinical tests in the co-chemotherapies: The clinical trials by using the *A. blazei* mushroom in the chemotherapies of cancer patients have been conducted in China, Korea, Brazil, and other countries over the past 25 years. During the chemotherapies of ten cases of acute nonlymphocytic leukemia (ANLL), the HWE of *A. blazei* in a co-treatment promoted bone marrow hemopoiesis by increasing the concentration of Hb and the numbers of Wbc and Plt in peripheral blood, enhancing the concentrations of IgM and albumin and A/G ratio and lessening the concentration of globulin in plasma. It subsequently recovered the chemotherapy-caused bone marrow inhibition and promoted liquid immune function with no side effects.[17] Through the similar immune interactions, the co-treatment with the chemotherapeutic drugs plus the HWE improved the clinical symptoms in advanced digestive tract cancer patients, concomitant with augmentation of normal hematopoiesis and immune function.[18] Likewise, 100 patients with gynecological (cervical, ovarian, and endometrial) carcinoma and 30 patients with gastric carcinoma were treated with conventional chemotherapies. After oral consumption of the *A. blazei* extract together, obvious positive effects of relief in the anticancer drugs-associated side effects such as appetite, alopecia, emotional stability, and general weakness and improvement in quality of life experienced by the patients[19,20] were correlated with the stimulation of the immune system via marked augmentation in leukocyte amount, CD4/CD8 T-cell surface molecules, and NK cell cytoactivity by the treatment with *A. blazei* extract.

In addition, dietary supplementation with a closely related Brazilian mushroom *Agaricus sylvaticus* has been also employed in a clinical trial to treat twenty-eight postsurgical patients with colorectal cancer. The patients received *A. sylvaticus* (30 mg/kg/day) for six months, resulting in significant improvement in their immunological and hematological parameters such as hemoglobin, hematocrit, erythrocytes, mean cell volume, mean cell hemoglobin concentration, mean cell hemoglobin, and neutrophil levels. The platelet count was lowered obviously in the treatment, but still maintained the normal level range.[21] Collectively, these clinical investigations recommended that supplementation with the edible *Agaricus* fungi is beneficial for undergoing chemotherapy.

Scientific Evidence of Cancer-Preventive Constituents

Both the chemical biology and molecular biology studies have characterized the bioactive constituents of *A. blazei* crude extracts including macromolecules (polysaccharides [β-glucans, glucomannan, and mannogalactoglucan], proteoglucans and riboglucans) and micromolecules (ergosterol [provitamin-D2] derivatives and alkaloids). All these constituents demonstrated the antitumor-related activities in different degrees, but the polysaccharides consistently showed to be the major ingredients. Extensive investigations have elucidated the structures of polysaccharides and their relationship with antitumor immunity.

1. Polysaccharides

The major antitumor substances from *A. blazei* are polysaccharides and protein-bound polysaccharide complexes. Most of them showed remarkable abilities to exert the antitumor effects against various allogeneic and syngeneic tumors, and prevent oncogenesis and tumor metastasis indirectly via activation of specific and nonspecific immune responses and stimulation of immune cells, such as NK cells, macrophages, dendritic cells, and granulocytes (poly-morphonuclear leukocytes).[22] The *A. blazei* polysaccharides (ABP) included β-(1-6)-glucan, β-(1-3)-glucan, α-(1-6)- and α-(1-4)-glucan, glucomannan, and more. The chemical biology studies revealed that β-D-glucans are the major ABP, and the β-glucans exhibited varied immunomodulating abilities due to quite a diversity in size and structure. The significant antitumor immunity was largely served by the water-soluble β-(1-6)-(1-3)-glucans in the ABP.[2,23]

A purified (1-6)-β-D-glucan from the fruiting bodies of *A. blazei* was administered orally to female mice transplanted with highly metastatic pulmonary carcinoma (*P*-7423). The *P*-7423 tumor growth and the metastatic nodules in lung were restrained concomitant with the suppression of VEGF-induced neovascularization.[24] A similar (1-6)-β-D-glucan (10 kDa) from *A. blazei* in an *in vitro* assay prompted the antiproliferative and proapoptotic effects on human HRA ovarian cancer cells via promotion p38 MAPK activity and apoptosis cascade but it was inactive to murine Lewis lung cancer 3LL cells. In a mouse model, p.o. the glucan diminished pulmonary metastasis of 3LL cells and peritoneally disseminated metastasis of HRA cells by declining uPA expression but did not lessen the number of lung tumor colonies.[25] The β-glucan also showed a chemoprotective effect against DNA damage induced by benzo[a]pyrene (BAP).[26]

AbEXP1a, an extracellular polysaccharide, was derived from submerged cultural broth of *A. blazei*. It was composed of glucose and mannose in ratio 3:1. Its structure was revealed to be three β-(1-6)-glucoses linked as a main chain and a mannose linked with the chain by α-(1-6)- or β-(1-6)-glycosidic linkage. At doses of 10 and 20 mg/kg/day by i.p., AbEXP1a treatment affected spleen index significantly and thymus index obviously, and retarded the growth of sarcoma 180 cells in mice. The *in vivo* antitumor rate was 64.04% in 10 mg/kg/day dosage.[27] An exopolysaccharide extract, which was derived from the submerged fermentation of *A. blazei* LPS 03 strain, had no obvious cytotoxic effect on cell viability of Wistar mice macrophages but exerted 33% inhibition against the viability of Ehrlich tumor cells *in vitro* at a concentration of 20 mg/mL.[28] In recent years, several studies have reported the direct anticancer effect of *A. blazei* polysaccharides in *in vitro* assays. ABP-1a (4.2×10^5 Da), a heteropolysaccharide isolated from *A. blazei* fruiting bodies, consisted of galactose, glucose, and mannose in a molar ratio of 1:1:1, along with a trace of rhamnose. In a concentration range of 100–400 μg/mL, ABP-Ia promoted proapotosis and growth inhibition in HOS osteosarcoma cell line but no or minor inhibition of normal human osteoblast cells in dose-dependent manner.[29] Similarly, *A. blazei* polysaccharide extracts in the *in vitro* models showed the inhibitory effect against the proliferation of human SMMC-7721 hepatoma and HL-60 leukemic cells.

The antiproliferative effects were found to be associated with decline in total superoxide dismutase (T-SOD) and malondialdehyde (MDA) levels in SMMC-7721 cells and induction of mitochondrial caspase-3-dependent apoptotic death in HL-60 cells.[30,31] The antileukemia activity was further confirmed in tumor xenograft with HL-60 cells. The antihepatoma effect was obviously enhanced if *A. blazei* polysaccharides are combined with four other mushroom polysaccharide extracts (*Grifola frondosa, Coriolus versicolor*, and *Lentinus edodes*).[30,31]

Despite the detection of direct inhibitory effects against the cancer cells, the anticancer properties of *A. blazei* polysaccharides primarily emanated from their prominent capability of potentiating the host immune system. The mechanism of their immunomodulatory effects has been figured out to be mediated by (i) binding to receptors such as TLR2, dectin-1, and CR3 on innate immune cells and communication with T-helper cells to elicit an enhanced Th1 response and a reduction of Th2 response; (ii) activating NK cells and increasing infiltration of cells in tumor sites; (iii) prompting macrophages via surface receptors such as dectin-1 with or without TLR-2/6, and complement receptor-3, to elicit an immune response; (iv) impeding the function of Gr-1$^+$ CD11b$^+$ myeloid-derived suppressor cells (MDSCs) via upregulation of IL-6, IL-12, TNF, iNOS, CD86, MHC II, and pSTAT1 expressions, and selectively blocking TLR2 signal and enhancing M1-type macrophage characteristics; (v) amplifying iNOS production and deterring Arg1 production of Gr-1$^+$ CD11b$^+$ monocyte MDSCs; and (vi) inhibiting conversion from CD4$^+$ CD25$^+$ T cells to CD4$^+$ Foxp3$^+$ CD25$^+$ regulatory T cells.[22,32] In addition, probably by the immunomodulating processes, the *A. blazei* polysaccharides also demonstrated anti-inflammatory, antiallergic, antiasthmatic, and antidiabetic properties.

2. Low m.w. polysaccharides

LMPAB, a linear β-(1-3)-glucan with low m.w. (4.8×10^4 Da) was isolated from the *A. blazei* polysaccharides. In *in vitro* assays, LMPAB displayed the antiproliferative effect against human K562 (leukemic) and BGC823 (stomach) cancer cell lines and vascular endothelial cells and showed the anti-invasive effect against BGC823 (stomach) and Bel-7402 (liver) cancer cell lines.[33,34] At 1×10^{-4} g/mL concentration, the inhibitory rates on the viability and invasion of BGC-823 cells were 33.4% and 69.8%, respectively.[34] The anti-invasive effect and anti-metastatic potential were found to be associated with downregulation of MMP-9 and Telomerase-RNA mRNA expressions and upregulation of Nm23-H1.[33-35] In a concentration range of 5–20 mg/L, the LMPAB dose-dependently hindered the adhesion of HT-29 and LoVo colon cancer cells to HUVECs via downexpression of both sLex and α-1,3-fucosyl-transferase-VII (FucT-VII) in translation or transcription levels, inhibition of E-selectin protein and gene expression, and obstruction of NF-κB expression and nuclear translocation.[36-38] The *in vivo* model with sarcoma 180 (S180) showed the corresponding suppressive properties of LMPAB to the *in vitro* results on the carcinoma cell growth, invasion, and metastasis. After two weeks treatment of an animal model of S180 with LMPAB at doses of 100 and 200 mg/kg per day by i.p. injection, the antitumor rates were resulted in 23.9% and 33.0%, respectively, which anti-growth effect was accompanied with the induction of apoptosis.[39] LMPAB was also revealed to decrease lung metastatic foci in a mouse B16 melanoma model *in vivo*.[33] Two other *in vivo* assays further demonstrated antiangiogenic effect of LMPAB in models of chicken embryo chorioallantoic membrane (CAM) angiogenesis and Matrigel-induced mouse neovascularization; antiagiogenic effect in mice was in parallel with lowering of VEGF mRNA and protein levels.[39] In addition, i.p. injection of LMPAB (50–200 mg/kg/day) to S180 tumor-bearing mice simultaneously amplified splenic NK cell activity, splenocyte proliferation, index of spleen and thymus, expression of IFN-γ in spleen, and systemic levels of IL-12, IL-18, and TNF-α in a dose-dependent manner.[40] Accordingly, these findings confirmed the multiple antitumor-related properties of LMPAB, such as antiproliferation, anti-invasion, anti-metastasis, antiangiogenesis, and immunostimulation; however, the most important property of LMPAB is the immune-related positive antitumor activities. These evidences advocate a promising medicinal application of *A. blazei* LMPAB in the prevention and suppression of carcinoma cell viability and metastasis.

In addition, when the tested mice were immunized with ovalbumin (OVA, 100 μg) and LMPAB (50, 100 and 200 μg), the splenic lymphocyte proliferation and antigen-specific CD4+ T-cell activation could be markedly amplified and IgG2b antibody responses to OVA augmented, indicating that LMPAB significantly enhanced both humoral and cellular immune responses against OVA in the mice, thereby stimulating Th1-type immunity.[41] By a similar process, treatment with OVA mixed with *A. blazei* polysaccharide extract improved the immune functional status of mice, that is, the combination enhanced the indexes of spleen and thymus significantly and amplified the percentage of CD4+, CD8+ lymphocytes.[42] These findings established new adjuvant application for the polysaccharides to upgrade human body defense through immunostimulation.

3. Proteoglycans

Several chemical biology researches reported a group of antitumor proteoglycans discovered from *A. blazei* fungus. A soluble proteoglucans-rich and acid-treated fraction was prepared from the fruit body of *A. blazei*, and it showed natural tumoricidal effects in both *in vivo* and *in vitro* assays through infiltration of the distant tumor by NK cells with marked cytotoxicity and direct induction of growth suppression and apoptotic death. The proapoptosis in Meth-A sarcoma cells was found to be associated with upregulation of Apo2.7 antigen on mitochondrial membranes of tumor cells and arrest of cell cycle progression. By various chromatofocusing purification steps, two proteoglucans were detected. The one (170 kDa) contains (1-4)-α-D-glucan and (1-6)-β-D-glucan in a ratio of approximately 1:2 and another one (380 kDa, HM3-G) consisted of a backbone (1-4)-α-D-glucan with (1-6)-β-D-glucan in branch in a ratio of about 4:1, such that HM3-G contains more than 90% glucose.[43] ABE was a type of proteoglycan isolated from boiling water extract of *A. blazei*, followed by ethanol precipitation, dialysis, and protein depletion, which was comprised of polysaccharides and peptides in a ratio of 74:26. In *in vitro* models, ABE exerted antiproliferative effect on human AGS gastric epithelial cancer cells in a dose-dependent manner, together with proapoptosis and G2/M cell cycle arrest, and it also elicited the apoptosis of human U937 leukemia cells through decline in Bcl-2 expression and activation of caspase-3, associated with dephosphorylation of Akt signal pathway.[40,44]

An α-(1-4)-glucan-β-(1-6)-glucan–protein complex extracted from *A. blazei* had no direct cytotoxicity on tumor cells but showed *in vivo* antiviability effect against sarcoma 180 by host-mediated immunoenhancing mechanisms. When combined with 5-FU, the complex could prevent the 5-FU-caused leucopeny besides the antitumor effect.[46] In addition, an early investigation reported several types of glycan–protein complexes isolated from a hot-water-soluble extract of *A. blazei* fruiting body. Of them, heteroglycan–protein complexes (FII-a, -b, -c) had weak antitumor activities and a lycoprotein (FIII-2-b) exhibited obvious antigrowth activity against sarcoma 180 in mice by i.p. or p.o. administrations, which FIII-2-b contains 50.2% polysaccharide and 43.3% protein and consists of (1-6)-β-D-glucan in the sugar unit and rich Asx, Glx, Ala, Leu, and Pro amino acids in the protein unit. Meanwhile, a xyloglucan–protein complex (FIV-2-b) and a glucoxylan (FV-2-a) were also effective in deterring the sarcoma 180 in mice.[47]

4. RNA–protein complex

FA-2-b-β was an RNA–protein complex isolated from *A. blazei* mushroom. In an *in vitro* assay, FA-2-b-β induced HL-60 leukemia cell apoptosis concomitant with activation of caspase-3 mRNA and inhibition of telomerase activity, thereby exerting an *in vitro* suppressive effect against the viability and growth of HL-60 cells in a dose- and time-dependent manner. At 40 μg/mL and 80 μg/mL concentrations for 96 h, the inhibitory rates of FA-2-b-β were 54.5% and 86.3%, respectively, and its IC_{50} was 42.72 μg/mL (in 96 h).[48]

5. Ergosterol derivatives

Ergosterol (1) is contained in various mushrooms, including *A. blazei*. As an antitumor substance, ergosterol (1) was separated from a lipid fraction of *A. blazei*. Although ergosterol (1) had no cytotoxicity against sarcoma 180 and Lewis lung cancer cells *in vitro*, its antitumor property was shown in *in vivo* mouse models. Oral administration of ergosterol to mice at doses of 400 and 800 mg/kg per day for 20 days retarded the growth of sarcoma 180 cells by 70.9% and 85.5%, respectively, without side effects, whereas i.p. injection of ergosterol at doses of 100 and 200 mg/kg for 20 days resulted in 65.8% and 84.7% growth inhibition, respectively. In a mouse model, i.p. injection of ergosterol at doses of 5–20 mg/kg for 5 days hindered Lewis lung carcinoma-induced neovascularization. The suppressive effect against Matrigel-induced neovascularization was also shown in female mice.[49] Therefore, these experimental data designated that ergosterol (1) is an antitumor and antiangiogenic substance.

Blazein (2) and agarol (3) were two ergosterol derivatives isolated from *A. blazei*, showing proapoptotic activities in human cancer cell lines. Blazein (2) treatment triggered the apoptotic death in human lymphoid leukemia (Molt4B), lung cancer (LU99), gastric cancer (KATO-III), and colon cancer (Colo201) cell lines, leading to the cell growth inhibition.[50-52] Similarly, in parallel with proapoptosis, agarol (3) exerted the antiviability effect against two p53-wild MKN45 (stomach) and A549 (lung) cancer cells and p53-mutant HSC-3 and HSC-4 oral squamous cell carcinoma cells with IC_{50}s of 0.34, ~0.26, 1.72, and 1.79 µg/mL, respectively, but no such effect was observed on normal HNG-1 fibroblast cells. The proapoptotic mechanism in A549 cells was mediated by a mitochondrial pathway, including increase in ROS generation, loss of mitochondria membrane potential, release of AIF from mitochondria to cytosol, upregulation of Bax, and downregulation of Bcl-2 but independent of caspase. The *in vivo* anticancer activity of agarol (3) was further confirmed in a xenograft murine implanted with the A549 tumor.[53] An ethanolic extract of *A. blazei* fermentation product showed antiviability effect against two human hepatoma cell lines (Hep3B and HepG2). Further separation of the extract showed that blazeispirol-A (4), a unique biosynthesized molecule from ergosterol conversion, was the most active antihepatoma agent in the fermentation product. It deterred the proliferation of Hep3B cells together with induction of the cell apoptotic death via both caspase-independent and caspase-dependent cell death pathways, including downregulation of Bcl-2 and Bcl-xL expressions, upregulation of Bax expression, loss of the mitochondrial membrane potential, release of HtrA2/Omi and AIF from mitochondria into cytosol, and activation of caspases-9 and -3.[54] These findings revealed that the ergosterol derivatives from *A. blazei* and its fermentation have potential in chemoprevention and chemotherapy.

6. Alkaloids

From a diffusible fraction of *A. blazei* HWE, a hydrazine-containing alkaloid designated as agaritine (5) was discovered. It moderately impeded the proliferation of four different human leukemia cell lines (U937, Molt4, HL-60, and K562) with IC_{50}s of 2.7, 9.4, 13.0, and 16.0 µg/mL, respectively, *in vitro* and showed weak effect on normal lymphatic cells at 40 µg/mL.[55] After treatment of the U937 cells for 48 h, agaritine (5) at a concentration of 10 µg/mL moderately elicited nuclear damage, DNA fragmentation, and apoptosis by release of cytochrome c from mitochondria and activation of caspases-3, -8, and -9.[56] Also, agaritine (5) and its derivatives were proved to be inhibitors against HIV proteases.[57]

Moreover, two antiangiogenic substances (A-1 and A-2) were isolated from this fungal body, in which structure of A-1 was assigned as sodium pyroglutamate (6). At doses of 400 or 800 mg/mL, A-1 impeded the angiogenesis elicited by Matrigel supplemented with VEGF and heparin, while at doses of 30, 100, and 300 mg/kg/day for 30 days by oral, A-1 deterred the tumor growth and metastasis and induced the apoptosis in Lewis lung carcinoma-bearing mice. During the *in vivo* treatment, A-1 also reversed the reduced numbers of splenic lymphocytes, CD4+, and CD8+ T cells, and enhanced the numbers of CD8+ T and NK cells to attack the tumors.[58] Thus, the *in vivo* antitumor and antimetastatic actions of sodium pyroglutamate (6) should be contributed by its immunoregulative and antiangiogenic properties.

CONCLUSION AND SUGGESTION

All the broad scientific investigations clearly concluded that *Agaricus blazei* fungi (its fruiting body and fermentation broth) are capable of directly restraining the growth and/or metastasis of various cancer cells (such as liver, prostate, lung, gastric, colon, gynecological carcinomas, and leukemia) via induction of apoptotic and cell cycle arrest pathways and antiproliferative, anti-invasive, and antiangiogenic mechanisms and indirectly impeded the growth of these cancer cells via remarkable immunoregulative actions and stimulation of antitumor immunities. The macromolecules like polysaccharides and protein-bound polysaccharides (both of which mainly are β-glucans as the major components in the *A. blazei* fungus) served the prominent antitumor immunity on the carcinomas and carcinogenesis, not only to deter the cancer cell growth and viability but also to reverse the host immune suppression caused by tumor and chemotherapeutic drugs, leading to prolongation of the survival of cancer patients and improvement of the living quality. Although some macromolecules in *A. blazei* showed *in vitro* inhibition against the proliferation of cancer cells, the direct antigrowth and anti-invasive activities of *A. blazei* mushroom are primarily generated from its micromolecular constituents such as ergosterol derivatives, blazeispirol-A, agaritine, and sodium pyroglutamate. According to the research results and the scientific literatures, the frequent intake of Brazilian mushroom in diet is beneficial to health promotion both as medical and nutritional food. No doubt, the dietary intake of *A. blazei* fungus can provide efficient means for the prevention of cancer initiation and metastasis and for the important adjuvant treatment in the conventional chemotherapies. Hence, the princess matsutake is believed to be one of the ideal foods for people today.

REFERENCES

1. Hetland, G. et al., 2011. The mushroom *Agaricus blazei Murill elicits* medicinal effects on tumor, infection, allergy, and inflammation through its modulation of innate immunity and amelioration of Th1/Th2 imbalance and inflammation. *Adv. Pharmacol. Sci.* Vol. 2011, Article ID 157015.
2. Firenzuoli, F. et al., 2008. The medicinal mushroom *Agaricus blazei Murill*: Review of literature and pharmaco-toxicological problems. *Evid. Based Complem. Alternat. Med.* 5(1): 3–15.
3. Ishii, P.L. et al., 2011. Evaluation of Agaricus blazei in vivo for antigenotoxic, anticarcinogenic, phagocytic and immunomodulatory activities. *Regul. Toxicol. Pharmacol.* 59(3): 412–422.
4. Kang, I.S. et al., 2015. Effects of *Agaricus blazei Murill* water extract on immune response in BALB/c mice. *Han'guk Sikp'um Yongyang Kwahak Hoechi* 44(11): 1629–1636.
5. Arakawa, Y. et al., 2012. Antitumor activity mediated by immunopotentiation exerted by a mixture of Agaricus blazei and Chlorella hot water extracts. *Igaku to Seibutsugaku* 56(1): 26–34.
6. Itoh, H. et al., 2010. Antitumor effect of Agaricus blazei Murrill (Iwade strain 101) "Himematsutake" on mouse pulmonary tumor with special reference to activation of macrophage, Kupffer cell and complement system. *Biotherapy* (Tokyo, Japan) 24(6): 489–499.
7. Yeh, M.Y. et al., 2015. Chitosan oligosaccharides in combination with *Agaricus blazei Murill* extract reduces hepatoma formation in mice with severe combined immunodeficiency. *Mol. Med. Reports* 12(1, Pt. A): 133–140.
8. Kimura, Y. et al., 2015. Effects of Agaricus blazei extract plus lactoferrin or lactoferrin alone on tumor growth and UFT-induced adverse reactions in sarcoma 180- or highly metastatic osteosarcoma LM8-bearing mice. *Nat. Prod, J.* 5(1): 57–69.
9. Menoli, R.C. et al., 2001. Antimutagenic effects of mushroom Agaricus blazei Murrill extracts on V79 cells. *Mutat. Res.* 496(1–2): 5–13.
10. Delmanto, R.D., 2001. Antimutagenic effect of *Agaricus blazei Murrill* mushroom on the genotoxicity induced by cyclophosphamide. *Mutat Res* 496(1–2): 15–21.
11. Yu, C.H. et al., 2009. Inhibitory mechanisms of *Agaricus blazei Murill* on the growth of prostate cancer in vitro and in vivo. *J. Nutr. Biochem.* 20(10): 753–764.
12. Qi, Y.C. et al., 2013. Antioxidant and anticancer effects of edible and medicinal mushrooms. *Han'guk Sikp'um Yongyang Kwahak Hoechi* 42(5), 655–662.
13. Jumes, F.M.D. et al., 2010. Effects of *Agaricus brasiliensis* mushroom in Walker-256 tumor-bearing rats. *Canadian J. Physiol. Pharmacol.* 85(1): 21–27.

14. Murakawa K. et al., 2007. Therapy of myeloma in vivo using marine phospholipid in combination with *Agaricus blazei Murill* as an immune respond activator. *J. Oleo. Sci.* 56 (4): 179–188.

15. Sorimachi, K. et al., 2008. Inhibitory effect of *Agaricu blazei Murill* components on abnormal collagen fiber formation in human hepatocarcinoma cells. *Biosci Biotechnol Biochem.* 72 (2): 621–623.

16. Huang, T.T. et al., 2012. The anti-tumorigenic mushroom *Agaricus blazei Murill* enhances IL- 1β production and activates the NLRP3 inflammasome in human macrophages. *PLoS One* 7(7): e41383.

17. Tian, X. et al., 1994. Clinical observation on treatment of acute nonlymphocytic leukemia with Agaricus blazei Murill. *J. Lanzhou Univ. (Med. Sci.).* 20: 169–171.

18. Wang, J. et al., 1994. Clinical observation on treatment of digestive tract cancer with *Agaricus blazei Murill. Gansu Med. J.* (1): 5–6.

19. Ahn, W.S., 2004. Natural killer cell activity and quality of life were improved by consumption of a mushroom extract, *Agaricus blazei Murill Kyowa*, in gynecological cancer patients undergoing chemotherapy. *Int. J. Gynecol. Cancer.* 14(4): 589–594.

20. Fan, Y. et al., 2006. Agaricus blazei practical compound combined chemotherapy for gastric cancer patients. *Chinese Traditional Patent Med.* 28(9): 1314–1316.

21. Fortes, R.C. et al., 2009. Immunological, hematological, and glycemia effects of dietary supplementation with Agaricus sylvaticus on patients' colorectal cancer. *Experim. Biol. Med.* 234(1): 53–62.

22. Biedron, R. et al., 2012. *Agaricus blazei Murill*—Immunomodulatory properties and health benefits. *Funct. Foods Heal. Dis.* 2(11): 428–447.

23. a) Friedman, M. 2016. Mushroom polysaccharides: Chemistry and antiobesity, antidiabetes, anticancer, and antibiotic properties in cells, rodents, and humans. *Foods* 5(4), 80; b) Wisitrassameewong, K. et al., 2012. Agaricus subrufescens: A review. *Saudi J. Biol. Sci.* 19(2): 131–146.

24. Itoh, H. et al., 2012. Inhibitory actions of a (1-6)-β-D-glucan purified from the fruiting bodies of Agaricus blazei Murrill (Himematsutake) on lung metastasis and angiogenesis. *Igaku to Seibutsugaku* 156(2): 53–61.

25. Kobayashi H., 2005. Suppressing effects of daily oral supplementation of beta-glucan extracted from *Agaricus blazei Murill* on spontaneous and peritoneal disseminated metastasis in mouse model. *J. Cancer Res. Clin. Oncol.* 131 (8): 527–538.

26. Angeli, J.P. et al., 2009. Beta-glucan extracted from the medicinal mushroom Agaricus blazei prevents the genotoxic effects of benzo[a]pyrene in the human hepatoma cell line HepG2. *Arch. Toxicol.* 83 (1): 81–86.

27. Zhang, H. et al., 2013. Structure and antitumor activity of polysaccharide from Agaricus blazei Murr. *Dalian Gongye Daxue Xuebao* 32(4): 235–238.

28. Fernandes, M.B.A. et al., 2011. Influence of drying methods over in vitro antitumoral effects of exopolysaccharides produced by Agaricus blazei LPB 03 on submerged fermentation. *Bioproc. Biosyst. Eng.* 34(3): 253–261.

29. Wu, B. et al., 2012. A polysaccharide from Agaricus blazei inhibits proliferation and promotes apoptosis of osteosarcoma cells. *Int. J. Biol. Macromol.* 50(4): 1116–1120.

30. Li, X.H. et al., 2014. polysaccharide from the fruiting bodies of *Agaricus blazei Murill* induces caspase-dependent apoptosis in human leukemia HL-60 cells. *Tumor Biol.* 35(9): 8963–8968.

31. Zhu, Y.F. et al., 2011. Antioxidant and antitumor effects of four kinds of combined fungus polysaccharides. *Zhengzhou Daxue Xuebao, Yixueban* 46(2): 253–256.

32. Liu, Y. et al., 2015. Polysaccharide *Agaricus blazei Murill* stimulates myeloid derived suppressor cell differentiation from M2 to M1 type, which mediates inhibition of tumor immune-evasion via the Toll-like receptor 2 pathway. *Immunol.* 146(3): 379–391.

33. Niu, Y.C. et al., 2009. A low molecular weight polysaccharide isolated from Agaricus blazei Murill (LMPAB) exhibits its anti-metastatic effect by down-regulating metalloproteinase-9 and up-regulating Nm23-H1. *Am. J. Chinese Med.* 37(5): 909–921.

34. Chen, Q.X. et al., 2014. Influence of the low-molecule-weight polysaccharides of Agaricus blazei Murrill on proliferation and invasion in gastric cancer BGC823 cells. *Xiandai Shipin Keji* 30(7): 6–9, 73.

35. Niu, Y.C. et al., 2008. Effect of a low molecular weight antitumor polysaccharide isolated from Agaricus blazei Murill (LMPAB) on expression of Telomerase-RNA mRNA of Bel-7402 cells. *Shizhen Guoyi Guoyao* (2008), 19(11), 2630–2632.

36. Liu, J.C. et al., 2010. A polysaccharide isolated from *Agaricus blazei Murill* inhibits sialyl Lewis X/E-selectin-mediated metastatic potential in HT-29 cells through down-regulating α-1,3-fucosyltransferase-VII (FucT-VII). *Carbohydr. Polym.* 79(4): 921–926.

37. Yue, L.L. et al., 2012. A polysaccharide from *Agaricus blazei* attenuates tumor cell adhesion via inhibiting E-selectin expression. *Carbohydr. Polym.* 88(4), 1326–1333.

38. Zhang, C. et al., 2014. Inhibitive effect of low-molecular weight polysaccharide derived from Agaricus blazei on adhesion between Lovo cells and vascular endothelial cells and its mechanism. *Zhongguo Laonianxue Zazhi* 34(4): 968–970.

39. Niu, Y.C. et al., 2009. A low molecular weight polysaccharide isolated from Agaricus blazei suppresses tumor growth and angiogenesis in vivo. *Oncol. Rep.* 21(1): 145–52; 2009. Antitumoral effect of low-molecular-weight polysaccharide isolated from *Agaricus blazei Murill* on sarcoma 180 in mice and its mechanism. *Zhongliu Fangzhi Yanjiu* 36(3): 180–182.

40. Niu, Y.C. et al., 2009. Immunostimulatory activities of a low molecular weight antitumoral polysaccharide isolated from *Agaricus blazei Murill* (LMPAB) in Sarcoma 180 ascitic tumor-bearing mice. *Pharmazie* 64(7): 472–476.

41. Cui, L.R. et al., 2013. A polysaccharide isolated from *Agaricus blazei Murill* (ABP-AW1) as a potential Th1 immunity-stimulating adjuvant. *Oncol Lett.* 6(4): 103910–44.

42. Jiang, L.Y. et al., 2014. Co-administration of *Agaricus blazei Murill* polysaccharide with OVA improve the immunity of E. G7-OVA tumor-bearing mice. *Shizhen Guoyi Guoyao* 25(5): 1056–1057.

43. Fujimiya, Y. et al., 1998, Selective tumoricidal effect of soluble proteoglucan extracted from the basidiomicete, Agaricus blazei Murill, mediated via natural killer cell activation and apoptosis. *Cancer Immunol. Immunother.* 46: 147–159.

44. Jin CY. et al., 2006. Induction of G2/M arrest and apoptosis in human gastric epithelial AGS cells by aqueous extract of Agaricus blazei. *Oncol. Rep.* 16(6): 1349–1355; 2007. Bcl-2 and caspase-3 are major regulators in *Agaricus blazei*-induced human leukemic U937 cell apoptosis through dephoshorylation of Akt. *Biol Pharm Bull.* 30(8): 1432–1437.

45. Kim, C.F. et al., 2009. Inhibitory effects of Agaricus blazei extracts on human myeloid leukemia cells. *J. Ethnopharmacol.* 122(2): 320–326.

46. Gonzaga, ML. et al., 2009. In vivo growth-inhibition of Sarcoma 180 by an α-(1-4)-glucan-β-(1-6)-glucan-protein complex polysaccharide obtained from Agaricus blazei *Murill. Nat. Med.* (Tokyo). 63(1): 32–40.

47. Mizuno, T. et al., 1990. Antitumor activity and some properties of water-insoluble hetero-glycans from "Himematsutake," the fruiting body of *Agaricus blazei Murill. Agricul. Biol. Chem.* 54(11): 2889–2896.

48. Gao, L. et al., 2007. Primary mechanism of apoptosis induction in a leukemia cell line by fraction FA-2-b-ss prepared from the mushroom *Agaricus blazei Murill. Braz J Med Biol Res.* 40(11): 1545–1555.

49. Takaku, T. et al., 2001. Isolation of an antitumor compound from *Agaricus blazei Murill* and its mechanism of action. *J. Nutr.* 131: 1409–1413.

50. Itoh, H. et al., 2013. Blazein induces apoptosis by a generation of active oxygen in human lymphoid leukemia molt 4B cells. *Igaku to Seibutsugaku* 157(5): 597–602.

51. Itoh, H. et al., 2008. Blazein of a new steroid isolated from *Agaricus blazei Murrill* (himematsutake) induces cell death and morphological change indicative of apoptotic chromatin condensation in human lung cancer LU99 and stomach cancer KATO III cells. *Oncol. Rep.* 20(6): 1359–1361.

52. Itoh, H. et al., 2010. Induction of apoptosis by blazein of a new steroid isolated from *Agaricus blazei Murrill* (himematsutake) in human colon cancer Colo201 cells. *Igaku to Seibutsugaku* 154(7): 310–316.

53. Shimizu, T. et al., 2016. Agarol, an ergosterol derivative from *Agaricus blazei*, induces caspase-independent apoptosis in human cancer cells. *Int. J. Oncol.* 48(4): 1670–1678.

54. Su, Z.Y. et al., 2011. Blazeispirol A from Agaricus blazei fermentation product induces cell death in human hepatoma Hep3B cells through caspase-dependent and caspase-independent pathways. *J. Agricul. Food Chem.* 59(9): 5109–5116.

55. Endo, M. et al., 2010. Agaritine purified from *Agaricus blazei Murrill* exerts antitumor activity against leukemic cells. *Biochimica et Biophysica Acta* 1800(7): 669–673.

56. Akiyama, H. et al., 2011. Agaritine from *Agaricus blazei Murrill* induces apoptosis in the leukemic cell line U937. *Biochimica et Biophysica Acta*, 1810(5): 519–525.

57. Gao, W.N. et al., 2007. Agaritine and its derivatives are potential inhibitors against HIV proteases. *Med. Chem.* 3(3): 21–26.

58. Kimura, Y. et al., 2004. Isolation of an anti-angiogenic substance from *Agaricus blazei Murrill*: Its antitumor and antimetastatic actions. *Cancer Sci.* 95: 758–764.

68. RINGLESS HONEY MUSHROOM

亮菌　楢茸モドキ

Armillaria tabescens (= Clitocybe tabescens)

Tricholomataceae

Ringless honey mushroom is the mycelia or fruit body of a Tricholomataceae mushroom *Armillaria tabescens (= Clitocybe tabescens)*. It commonly grows in North America and Europe, and its white mycelium presents light blue fluorescence in the dark. The mushroom is a functional food in eastern Asia, as the mushroom extract has been reported to have hepatoprotective, anti-inflammatory, antiradiation, leucocyte-evaluating, immunoenhancing, and anticancer activities. Also, it is able to accelerate DNA synthesis in hematopoietic tissue. *A. tabescens* has been found to be poisonous; however, its fruiting body would be edible and delicious after cooking.

Scientific Evidence of Cancer-Inhibitory and Cancer-Preventive Constituents

The extract of *A. tabescens* in a mouse model restrained the growth of sarcoma 180 cells by 53% when consumed in a daily dose of 30 mg/kg for ten consecutive days.[1] According to the chemical biology studies, the anticancer-related properties of ringless honey mushroom were mostly attributed to its polysaccharide components.

ATM3, a polysaccharide component prepared from a HWE of *A. tabescens*, exhibited antigrowth activity against sarcoma 180 and Ehrlich ascites tumor in mice with inhibitory ratio of 26.6 and 37.7%, respectively.[2,3] Two polysaccharides termed AT-HW and AT-AL were isolated from the hot water and alkaline extracts, respectively. AT-HW (m.w. 105,000) is a water-soluble heteroglycan consisting of D-fucose, D-glucose, D-galactose, D-mannose, and small amounts of peptide moieties, whereas AT-AL (m.w. 93,000) is a water-insoluble (1-3)-α-D-glucan with small amounts of other sugar residues. Both AT-HW and AT-AL were effective in inhibiting the growth of sarcoma 180 cells *in vivo*. The anticancer rates were 77% and 71% at an early i.p. administration schedule (300 µg/mouse/day) for 5 days and 85% and 45% at late i.p. administration schedule with the same dose and days, respectively. Furthermore, AT-HW and AT-AL also notably augmented immune and reticuloendothelial systems, including amplification of peritoneal exudates cell proliferation, activation of macrophage and acidic phosphatase, increase of glucose consumption and superoxide anion production, and promotion of mitogenic reaction.[4,5] ATPSII and ATPSII-2 were two other kinds of polysaccharides isolated from *A. tabescens*, both of which obstructed the growth of sarcoma 180 in mice by 46.7% and 51.7%, respectively, at a high dose (80 mg/kg/day for 10 days) and whose antitumor potencies were comparable to those of cyclophosphamide in the test.[6] Likewise, an intracellular polysaccharide IPS-B2 with antitumor effect was derived from HWE of cultured *A. tabescens* mycelia, which was an α-(1-6)-D-glucan (49.5 kDa). In the experiments, IPS-B2 was able to activate macrophage via induction of nitric oxide (NO) and cytokines (TNF-α, IL-1β, and IL-6) production and expression, thereby exerting the antitumor effect.[7,8]

Further investigations demonstrated that the extract and its polysaccharide component isolated from ringless honey mushroom could obviously lessen the damages caused by ^{60}Co-γ radiation and chemotherapy via restoration of hematopoiesis function, enhancement of DNA synthesis in hematopoiesis system, and elevation of leukocytes.[9,10] In addition, oral administration of ringless honey mushroom liquid was able to obviously improve the quality of life in cancer patients who were on cisplatin chemotherapy.[10] After treatment for 2–3 days, the middle doses (9.67–11.45 g/day) of *A. tabescens* extract could efficiently deter a chemotherapeutic drug cisplatin-induced pica response and ameliorate cisplatin-induced gastrointestinal tract reaction in animal models.[11]

OTHER BIOACTIVITIES

Armillarisin-A, a major component with coumarine skelecone in ringless honey mushroom, has been employed in China clinically to treat cholecystitis, chronic gastritis, and hepatitis.

CONCLUSION AND SUGGESTION

According to the bioactivities-related chemical investigations, ringless honey mushroom has been recognized as a potential functional food and natural medicine having multiple anticarcinogenesis-related properties such as obvious immunoenhancing, antiradiation, leucocyte-evaluating, anti-inflammatory, and hepatoprotective activities. Several polysaccharides isolated from ringless honey mushroom have primarily shown potential successes in cancer prevention and treatment as health-beneficial agents that stimulate the immune system to arrest cancer initiation and development, protect the body from radiation damages, and reverse the toxicity/side effects caused by chemo- and radiotherapies. Thus, dietary cooked fruiting body of *Armillaria tabescens* can consistently show remarkable functional effects in cancer prevention.

REFERENCES

1. Kim, B.K. et al., 1983. Studies on constituents of Korean basidiomycetes (L). Antitumor components extracted from cultured mycelia of several basidiomycetes. *Archiv. Pharm. Res.* 6(2): 141–142.
2. Fang, J.N. et al., 1984. Studies on polysaccharides of Liangjun I. Isolation and identification of ATM3. *Acta Biochimica et Biophysica Sinica* 16: 222–229.
3. Zhang, L.H. et al., 1992. Research progress of bioactive polysaccharides in medicinal fungi. *Zhongcaoyao* 23: 95–99.
4. Kiho, T. et al., 1992. Antitumor and immunomodulating activities of two polysaccharides from the fruiting bodies of Armillariella tabescensi. *Chem. Pharm. Bull.* 40: 2110.
5. Kiho, T. et al., 1992. Polysaccharides in fungi. XXIX. Structural features of two antitumor polysaccharides from the fruiting bodies of Armillariella tabescens. *Chem. Pharm. Bull.* 40: 2212–2214.
6. Cai, F. et al., 2013. Study on the isolation, purification and antitumor activity in vivo of polysaccharide extracted from Armillariella tabescens. *Jiyinzuxue Yu Yingyong Shengwuxue* 32: 767–770.
7. Luo, X. et al., 2008. Effects of Armillariella tabescens polysaccharide IPS-B2 on activity of mouse peritoneal macrophages and transcription of related gene. *China J. Chin. Materia Med.* 33(11): 1305–1308.
8. Luo, X. et al., 2008. Characterisation and immunostimulatory activity of an α-(1-6)-D-glucan from the cultured *Armillariella tabescens mycelia*. *Food Chem.* 111: 357–363.
9. Yu, R.R. et al., 1999. *Chinese Materia Medica* Vol. 1, Published by Shanghai Science Technology Express, 1-0241, pp. 569.
10. Sun, T. et al., 2012. A comparative study of oral liquid of *Armillaria tabescens* on improving the quality of life in patients with cancer. *J. Chin. Oncol.* 18: 290–293.
11. Du, J. et al., 2011. Ameliorative effect of *Armillariella tabescens* on cisplatin-induced gastrointestinal tract reaction in the rat. *Chinese J. Oncol.* 33(8): 579–582.

69. SHIITAKE OR SAWTOOTH OAK MUSHROOM

香菇   椎茸   표고 버섯

Lentinus edodes

Marasmiaceae

Shiitake is the fruiting body of the edible fungus *Lentinus edodes* (Marasmiaceae). This East Asia-native fungus has been broadly applied in Eastern Asia as a gourmet food and medicinal herb for thousands of years. Nowadays, the fungus is commonly cultivated as a popular cuisine material in many countries around the world and is often found in Asian supermarkets and grocery stores. Nutritional facts show that shiitake has good content of vitamin B complex and moderate levels of some dietary minerals (manganese and phosphorus). Each 100 g of shiitake affords 5.7 mg of selenium, which is an extremely vital mineral for human health. Pharmacological approaches have proven shiitake to have a variety of health benefits such as immunopotentiating, anticarcinogenic, antioxidative, anti-allergic, antiobesity, antilipemic, antidiabetic, antiplatelet aggregation, cardiovascular-improving, antihepatitic, and skin-caring properties.[1]

SCIENTIFIC EVIDENCE OF CANCER-INHIBITORY ACTIVITIES

An ethyl acetate fraction derived from shiitake concentration-dependently hindered the proliferation of human breast carcinoma (MDA-MB-453 and MCF-7) and myeloma (RPMI-8226 and IM-9) cell lines, concomitant with the induction of apoptosis and cell cycle arrest.[1] According to recent reports, the ethyl acetate fraction of shiitake powder in 1 g/L concentration exhibited marked cytotoxicity in human A549 (lung), Hep3B (liver), AGS (stomach), MCF-7 (breast), and HeLa (cervix) cancer cell lines *in vitro* with the respective inhibitory rates of 56.7%, 64.6%, 71.5%, 84.9%, and 85.1%, but it also had some cytotoxicity on human transformed primary embryonal kidney cells (293).[2,3] In the *in vitro* tests, the extract of shiitake obviously diminished the incidence of bladder cancer induced by *N*-butyl-*N'*-butanol-nitrosoamine (BBN) from 100% to 52.9% and recovered the BBN-depressed macrophage and NK cell cytotoxicity and enhanced blastogenic response to normal levels.[4] Shiitake mycelium extract in a co-treatment noticeably augmented the 5-fluorouracil-mediated upregulation of p53, p21/Cip1, and p27/Kip1 proteins in human Colo 205 colon cancer cells, subsequently sensitizing the Colo 205 cells going to G0/G1 cell arrest and apoptosis *in vitro* and *in vivo*.[5] Moreover, its ethyl acetate fraction also showed the antimutagenic and DPPH radical scavenging properties.[6] These findings experimentally evidenced that the shiitake can play roles in cytotoxicity, antimutagenesis, anticarcinogenesis, and anticancer.

SCIENTIFIC EVIDENCE OF CANCER-INHIBITORY AND CANCER-PREVENTIVE CONSTITUENTS

1. Polysaccharides

In the recent decade, many polysaccharides derived from nature and cultures of *Lentinus edodes* have been reported to possess valuable tumor-inhibitory activity and immunoregulating functions. The shiitake polysaccharides have been mostly evaluated for the antitumor and immunomodulation effects. A polysaccharide component extracted from the edible fungi could repress the proliferation of human SMMC-7721 hepatoma cells *in vitro* and inhibit the growth of mouse sarcoma 180 (S180) *in vivo*. In concentration of 50 μg/mL, the mitosis index and the mitochondria activity of SMMC-7721 cells were obviously obstructed by the polysaccharide. The inhibition rates on S180 cells in mice were 56.6% in a dose of 24 mg/kg.[7] Daily delivery of the polysaccharide component in doses of 6–24 mg/kg to tested mice markedly restrained the growth of lymphoma cells and U14 cervical cancer cells and also showed synergistic effect *in vivo* when combined with γ-ray treatment.[8]

An acidic polysaccharide prepared from the mycelia of oak mushroom consisted of xylose, arabinose, mannose, galactose, glucose, and uronic acid in a molar ratio of 1.4:0.7:2.0:0.9:1.0:1.5. The i.p. administration of the acidic polysaccharide markedly suppressed the growth of solid sarcoma 180 cells by 87.9% in mice given doses of 100 mg/kg per day for ten days.[9] A polysaccharide L-2 (2.03×10^5 Da) purified from shiitake was composed of only D-glucose. In the S180-bearing mice, L-2 significantly promoted the production of TNF-α and IFN-γ and enhanced the immunity in dose of 10 mg/kg per day. It also notably increased the weights of spleen and thymus and promoted the responses of delayed-type hypersensitivity (DTH), macrophage phagocytosis, and NO production, leading to hampering of the tumor formation markedly.[10,11] Likewise, the *L. edodes* polysaccharides at doses of 100 and 200 mg/kg dose-dependently suppressed the growth of hepatoma cells and augmented the indexes of spleen and thymus.[12] The observations clearly revealed that the antitumor effect of shiitake polysaccharides was principally mediated by immunoregulating effects such as enhancement of macrophage-dependent immune system responses and TNF-α mRNA expression at the transcriptional level.

Many polysaccharides have been separated from shiitake and its mycelia. Among them, the most important anticancer polysaccharide purified from shiitake was assigned as lentinan (LNT). Its biological properties have been extensively investigated. In addition, the sulfated modification and triple helix conformation usually are the important factors in the enhancement of antitumor potentials of shiitake polysaccharides.[13]

Lentinan: Lentinan (LNT), a finely purified β-(1-3)-glucan with β-(1-6) branches every five glucose residues, was demonstrated to have anticancer and immune adjuvant activities *in vivo* with no mutagenicity. Since 1985, LNT has been especially applied in the treatment of inoperable and recurrent gastric cancer patients.[14,15] In the mouse models, LNT by various administration routes exerted the inhibitory effect against the growth of MH-134 ascites hepatoma, S908D2 sarcoma, and K36 leukemia in a dose- and time-dependent fashion and the suppressive rates could reach 94.44%, 88.59%, and 83.14%, respectively.[16-18] LNT also displayed the life-prolongation effect and quality of life (QOL) improvement effect in animal models and cancer patients via augmenting host immune systems.[15,17] LNT in both *in vitro* and *in vivo* assays prompted the apoptosis of H22 hepatoma cells and G2/M cell arrest through a mitochondria pathway and increases of intracellular ROS and free calcium concentrations and hampered the growth of H22 cells via obstruction of NF-κB, Stat3, and survivin signalings.[19,20] At concentrations of 10–20 μg/mL, LNT markedly impeded the growth of human oral squamous cell cancer cell lines (KB and HSC3) *in vitro*. Compared to HSC3 cells, the preferential antigrowth effect of LNT occurred in KB cells. Co-treatment with LNT (10 μg/mL) and 5-FU (1 μg/mL) resulting in significant suppressive effect against the growth of KB cells *in vitro* and *in vivo* due to LNT may lead to enhancement of chemosensitivity to 5-FU.[21] In addition to the synergistic suppressive effect with oxaliplatin against HepG2 hepatoma cells, LNT also attenuated the side effects caused by oxaliplatin (a chemotherapeutic drug).[20] In an *in vivo* test, LNT showed a profound inhibition ratio of ~75% against S180 tumor growth, wherein the effect was obviously greater than that of a chemotherapeutic drug cytoxan (~54%). During the treatment, LNT not only elicited the cell apoptosis and growth-inhibition via initiating p53-dependent signaling pathway and caspase-dependent pathway but also sharply promoted the accumulation of immune cells into tumors, indicating that LNT played both important roles, that is, direct antitumor effect and indirect immune cell cytotoxic effect, in fighting the sarcoma 180.[22] Interestingly, a triple-helix LNT with m.w. of 1.49×10^6 presented the highest *in vivo* antitumor activity against sarcoma 180.[23] Besides, LNT also was able to deter angiogenesis in the S180 tissue by blocking VEGF expression, thereby retarding the sarcoma progression.[22]

The remarkable antitumor immunity and immunopotentiation of LNT were principally associated with stimulation of cytokines production from immunocytes, that is, highly raising the levels of lymphocytokines (such as IL-1, IL-2, IFN-γ, and TNF-α) and the levels of macrophages and activating B-lymphocytes and T-lymphocytes.[24-26] Therefore, the immunotherapy with LNT was able to promote the chemotherapeutic actions induced by MMC, 5-FU, or cytosine arabinoside.[18] By activating NRF2-ARE signaling pathway and limiting ROS accumulation, LNT alleviated cisplatin-triggered nephrotoxicity in human kidney 2 (HK-2) cells.[27] From these observations, it is recognized that LNT is able to act as a unique class of host defense potentiators to protect the hosts from the side effects of conventional therapies and to improve various kinds of immunological parameters with no toxicity and side effects.[23] This chemoimmunotherapy should be highly recommended in clinics for the co-treatment of neoplastic patients instead of chemotherapy or radiotherapy alone.[28]

In addition, the structural modification with sulfation and carboxymethylation could augment the antitumor effect of LNT,[29] where sulfated LNT showed significant antiproliferative effect against human hepatoma HepG2 cell line *in vitro*, wherein lower sulfated LNT exerted more marked anti-HepG2 activity than the higher sulfated ones.[30]

(1-3)-α-D-Glucans: Water-insoluble α-(1-3)-D-glucans from shiitake normally exhibited no direct inhibitory effect on tumor cells. After reacting with sulfur trioxide–pyridine complex, the sulfated α-(1-3)-D-glucan derivatives (such as SL-FV-II and SL-II) were derived with substitution degrees from 0.9 to 2.1. The O-sulfonated derivatives, which present having an expanded flexible chain in aqueous solution and holding intramolecular hydrogen bonding or interaction formed between charge groups, exerted significantly enhancement on the antitumor activity against solid sarcoma 180 cells *in vitro* and *in vivo*. For instance, SL-FV-II at 20 μg/mL concentration obstructed the proliferation of four human and murine cancer cell lines *in vitro* and the inhibitory rate reached 52% in human MCF-7 breast cancer cells. *In vivo* experiment by gavage of SL-FV-II to mice in a dose of 50 mg/kg/day effectively restrained the growth of solid sarcoma 180 cells by 42%.[31,32]

WPLE-Ns and S-WPLEs: One (1-6)-β-D-glucan (WPLE-N-1) and two mannogalactoglucans (WPLE-N-2 and WPLE-N-3) were isolated from *Lentinus edodes* by hot water extraction. WPLE-N-1 (757.5 kDa) was composed of glucose (92%) with small contents of galactose (3.9%) and mannose (4.1%), while WPLE-N-2 (20.9 kDa) and WPLE-N-3 (4.7 kDa) contained mannose, galactose, and glucose in the molar ratios of 10:27:63 and 5:12:83, respectively. *In vitro* assay displayed the three polysaccharides exerting antitumor effect against sarcoma 180 and colon carcinoma (HCT-116 and HT-29) cell lines.[33]

SLNT1 and JLNT1: SLNT1, SLNT2, JLNT1, JLNT2, and JLNT3 were isolated from *L. edodes* fruit body. These five polysaccharides consist of β-D-glucose, with a main chain of (1-3)-glucose and branch chains of (1-6)-glucose with different molecular weights, and their structures appear triple-helical conformation. In a mouse model, SLNT1 and JLNT1 treatments remarkably deterred the growth of mouse H22 hepatoma by 65.41% and 61.07%, respectively, and significantly increased serum IL-2 levels, TNF-α production, and the cell apoptotic death in the H22-bearing mice, implying that the antihepatoma activity was mediated by two different mechanisms, that is, stimulation of the host's immunity and promotion of tumor cell apoptosis.[34]

LMP2: LMP2 (m.w. 2.27×10^4 Da) was isolated from the mycelia of *L. edodes*, consisting of mannose, arabinose, xylose, galactose, and rhamnose in a relative molar ratio of 1:0.74:1.18:3.23:10.98. At 200 mg/mL concentration, LMP2 could hinder the proliferation of HEp-2 laryngeal squamous cancer cells by 37.2 % after 72 h in *in vitro* treatment. Simultaneously, the colony formation and invasion of HEp-2 cells were significantly diminished by LMP2.[35]

LT1: A water-soluble polysaccharide LT1 (642 kDa) was isolated from the basidiocarps of *L. edodes* by hot water extraction. Its backbone is composed of (1-4)-linked and (1-3)-linked glucopyranosyl residues and its branches of single glucosyl are attached at C-6 of β-(1-4)-linked glucopyranosyl. In 0.10 M NaOH solution or distilled water, LT1 existed as a triple helix chain. *In vivo* studies showed that LT1 presented obvious antitumor activities on solid type of sarcoma 180 cells implanted in mice.[36]

JLNT: JLNT was a purified polysaccharide (m.w. 605.4 kDa) from the fruiting bodies of *L. edodes*, whose structure contains β-(1-3)-D-glucose as a main chain and β-(1-6)-D-glucose as side chains. In both *in vitro* and *in vivo* assays, JLNT showed direct antitumor effects on human MCF-7 breast cancer cells and mouse sarcoma 180 cells. JLNT also elicited the cell apoptosis of S180 tumor in mice through a mitochondria pathway, that is, increase in p53 expression and Bax/Bcl-2 ratios by upregulating Bax and downregulating Bcl-2, activating caspase-3, and amplifying Smac expression.[37]

LTN: An alkali-soluble polysaccharide termed LTN was isolated from the *L. edodes*. It was able to provoke the apoptosis and G2/M cell cycle arrest of H22 hepatoma cells through induction of microtubule depolymerization, stimulation of ROS, loss of mitochondrial membrane potential, and increase in Ca^{2+} intracellular concentration.[38]

MPSSS: MPSSS (577.2 kDa) derived from the *L. edodes* is composed of glucose (75.0%), galactose (11.7%), mannose (7.8%), and xylose (0.4%). In the experiments, MPSSS was capable of stimulating the differentiation of myeloid-derived suppressor cells (MDSCs) and reversing the immunosuppressive functions of MDSCs on CD4+ T-cells via a MyD88-dependent NF-κB signaling pathway, including upregulation of MHC II and F4/80 expressions on MDSCs. The *in vivo* antigrowth effect of MPSSS occurred against McgR32 tumor, an action that was found to be mediated by targeting MDSCs to reduce percentage of MDSCs in peripheral blood.[39]

Chitosans: Chitin was obtained from shiitake stripes with no antitumor activity. However, from the chitin, several chitosans were yielded by alkaline N-deacetylation. In an *in vitro* assay, the shiitake chitosans moderately impeded the proliferation of human IMR 32 neuroblastoma and HepG2 hepatoma cell lines. At 5 mg/mL, the viability of IMR 32 cells was lessened to 68.8–85.0%, while that of HepG2 cells was lessened to 60.4–82.9%, wherein chitosans B120 and C120, which presented high degrees of N-deacetylation, exerted relatively higher inhibitory effect on the growth of IMR32 and HepG2 cells. The discoveries pointed out the medicinal potentials of shiitake chitin and chitosan in cancer prevention, health food processing, and cosmetics.[40]

2. Protein-bound polysaccharides

Several bioactive protein-bound polysaccharides were separated from the shiitake. Their cancer-inhibitory activities were elucidated to be mainly based on an immunoregulation type of antitumor mechanism. LAP1, a xylose-rich proteoglycan prepared from a water-soluble extract of shiitake mycelium, showed no direct effect on the proliferation of hepatoma cells *in vitro*, but i.p. administration in a dose of 3 mg/kg per day obviously prolonged the survival rates of hepatoma-bearing rats by 50%, together with marked enlargement of the productions of IFN-γ and nitrite and augmentation of the macrophage-migration inhibitory activity of splenic cells *in vivo*.[41,42] A fraction-E (1.05×10^5 Da) prepared from the cultured mycelia exerted 88–90% inhibition against solid sarcoma 180 in mice at a dose of 20 mg/kg per day.[43,44] This fraction-E contains 87% polysaccharide and 1.3% protein, and its saccharide portion is composed of mannose (48.35%), galactose (30.79%), xylose (19.05%), and fucose (1.79%) and its protein portion comprised of 14 amino acids including L-threonine and L-serine as well as 0.37% hexosamine.[43] Six water-soluble protein-bound heteroglucans labeled as S-WPLE-I-a, S-WPLE-I-b, S-WPLE-II-a, S-WPLE-II-b, S-WPLE-III-,a and S-WPLE-III-b were separated from *L. edodes*, all of which were composed of glucose, galactose, mannose, and a small portion of protein in various ratios. These S-WPLEs in an *in vitro* assay hampered the proliferation of solid sarcoma 180 cells and human colorectal cancer cell lines (HT-29 and HCT-116) at the same dose of 5 mg/mL. The potent inhibition was observed in sarcoma 180 cells treated by S-WPLE-I-b and S-WPLE-I-a.[45]

Four other (1-3)-β-D-glucans with 4.6–15.2% proteins (m.w. 1.47×10^6 to 1.67×10^6) were isolated from four kinds of fruiting bodies of *L. edodes* and coded as L-I1, L-I2, L-I3, and L-I4. Both *in vivo* and *in vitro* antitumor assays revealed that these proteoglucanes with native triple helical conformation exerted notable antigrowth effect against solid sarcoma 180 cells. The highest *in vivo* inhibitory ratio reached 70.0% for L-I3, and the antitumor potency should be correlated with the bound protein and the molecular size closely.[44] LEPs is a crude polysaccharide bound with a small amount of protein, which is obtained from *L. edodes* by enzyme-assisted extraction at 54°C and pH 5.0. LEPs in an *in vitro* test exhibited antiproliferative effect on HCT-116 and HeLa cancer cell lines. Further separation led to two distinct fractions, LEP-1 (152.33 kDa) and LEP-2 (644.7 kDa). At a concentration of 1.79 mg/mL, the proliferation ratios were reduced to 32.5% and 26.7% in HeLa cervical cancer cells and 36.4% and 28.9% in HCT-116 colon cancer cells, respectively, for LEP-1 and LEP-2.[46]

3. Proteins

Lentin: A protein component designated lentin (27.5 kDa) was isolated from the fruiting bodies of shiitake, which possesses a similarity to endoglucanase in its *N*-terminal sequence. The shiitake lentin manifested the inhibitory activity not only against HIV-1 reverse transcriptase and mycelial growth in a variety of fungal species but also against the proliferation of leukemia cells.[47]

LFP91-3: LEP91-3 are proteins isolated from *L. edodes* C91-3 fermentative liquid. The proteins are water-soluble light-brown powder (m.w. 1–90 kD) that comprised of 18 kinds of amino acids and showed pH of 5.0–8.0 in its aqueous solution. *In vitro* assay showed that LEP91-3 was able to promote the apoptosis of mouse tumor cell lines such as H22 hepatoma and sarcoma 180, subsequently restraining the cell proliferation. *In vivo* treatment of mice bearing S180 with oral administration of LFP91-3 liquid retarded the tumor growth and prolonged the survival time of mice in addition to notable stimulation of the host immune functions, including amplification of spleen lymphocyte proliferation and NK cell cytotoxicity and increase in serum IL-2 and TNF-α levels. The remarkable immunopotentiating ability definitely contributed to its anticancer efficacy *in vivo*.[48-52]

Lentinus edodes C91-3 apoptosis protein 24414 and latcripin-1: An apoptosis protein 24414 was extracted from *L. edodes* C91-3, which was expressed successfully in *Pichia pastoris* GS115. The apoptosis protein 24414 could induce the cell apoptosis of human A549 lung carcinoma and mouse Hca hepatoma *in vitro* in concentrations of 7.5, 15, and 30 μg/mL. At its three concentrations, the treatment gave the maximum inhibitory rates of 70.03%, 82.02%, and 74.66% against the Hca hepatoma cells, respectively, without toxic effect on normal cells, where the strongest proapoptosis was found in 30 μg/mL concentration of the protein.[53,54] Similarly, latcripin-1 was also a protein prepared from the same *L. edodes* C91-3 that was expressed and characterized in *Pichia pastoris* GS115. *In vitro* exposure of latcripin-1 could markedly trigger the apoptotic death of human A549 lung cancer cell line.[55]

Adjunctive Application

The fungus of *Lentinus edodes* has been used to enzymically ferment rice bran. From the treated rice bran, two polysaccharides with effective biological response modification were separated and assigned as RBEP (a rice bran exobiopolymer) and MGN-3 (an arabinoxylan). Both could dose-dependently induce the activation of NK cells *in vivo*. RBEP prolonged the life span of mice bearing sarcoma 180 cells and inhibited the growing tumor cells by i.p. injection and suppressed the cell growth of B16 melanoma by oral administration, where the anticancer activity by i.p. injection was more effective than oral administration, which indirectly induced an immune response. MGN-3 augmented the apoptosis of human HUT 78 leukemic cells induced by death ligands (anti-CD95 antibody), an action that might be relevant for the antitumor activity. The induction of apoptosis in the HUT 78 cells was accompanied by downregulation of Bcl-2 expression, increase in mitochondrial membrane potential depolarization, and activation of caspases-3, -8, and -9.[47,56,57]

Conclusion and Suggestion

Although several bioactive micromolecules such as eritadenines and ergosterols were separated from shiitake and the micromolecule-rich ethyl acetate fraction of shiitake were detected to have the inhibitory effect in the *in vitro* assays with various cancer cell lines, the macromolecules such as polysaccharides and proteins prepared from shiitake have attracted a great deal of attention in the scientific studies for cancer prevention and therapy due to their many health benefits and predominant contents in shiitake. Most of the biological macromolecules from the shiitake, especially lentinan, demonstrated remarkable immunostimulating and cancer-suppressive properties in both *in vitro* and *in vivo* experiments. These facts designated that frequent consumption of shiitake can receive both direct and indirect anticancer and anticarcinogenic advantages. The immunoregulatory properties of shiitake polysaccharides also provide more health benefits to humans such as upgrading and/or recovering immune systemic function and protecting and abrogating or attenuating the toxicities and side effects triggered by chemotherapy, radiotherapy, and some harmful chemicals from environmental pollution. Owing to the prominent biological features, it is sure that shiitake should be commended as a natural functional food and healthy food additive in human diet for potentiation of the body's protection capacity and prevention of carcinogenesis and mutation in the early stage.

REFERENCES

1. Fang, N. et al., 2006. Inhibition of growth and induction of apoptosis in human cancer cell lines by an ethyl acetate fraction from shiitake mushrooms. *J. Altern. Complement Med.* 12(2):125–132.
2. Kim, B.K. et al., 1996. Development of new basidiomycetes by protoplast fusion and nuclear transfer II. The effects of the components of the protoplast fusants on mouse immune cells. *Saengyak Hakhoechi* 27: 231–237.
3. Petrova, R.D. et al., 2005. Potential role of medicinal mushrooms in breast cancer treatment: Current knowledge and future perspectives. *Int. J. Med. Mushrooms* 7: 141–155.
4. Kurashige, S. et al., 1997. Effects of Lentinus edodes, Grifola frondosa and Pleurotus ostreatus administration on cancer outbreak, and activities of macrophages and lymphocytes in mice treated with a carcinogen, N-butyl-N-butanolnitrosoamine. *Immunopharmacol. Immunotoxicol.* 19: 175–183.
5. Wu, C.H. et al., 2007. Antitumor activity of combination treatment of Lentinus edodes mycelium extracts with 5-fluorouracil against human colon cancer cells xenografted in nude mice. *J. Cancer Mol.* 3: 15–22.
6. Yoo, S.J. et al., 2007. Antioxidative, antimutagenic and cytotoxic effects of natural seasoning using Lentinus edodes powder. *Han'guk Sikp'um Yongyang Kwahak Hoechi* 36: 515–20.
7. Jiang, S.M. et al., 1999. Inhibitory activity of polysaccharide extracts from three kinds of edible fungi on proliferation of human hepatoma SMMC-7721 cell and mouse implanted S180 tumor. *World J. Gastroenterol.* 5: 404–407.
8. Xu, W.Q. et al., 2006. Studies on antitumor and synergism combined with γ-rays of polysaccharide from Tremella fuciformis ferment in mice. *Zhongguo Shenghua Yaowu Zazhi* 27: 254.
9. Togami, M. et al., 1982. Studies on Basidiomycetes. I. Antitumor polysaccharide from bagasse medium on which mycelia of Lentinus edodes (Berk.) Sing. had been grown. *Chem. Pharma. Bull.* 30: 1134–1140.
10. Ruan, Z. et al., 2006. Effect of polysaccharide L-2 from Lentinus edodes on TNF-α and IL-2. *Shipin Kexue* 27: 223–226.
11. Ruan, Z. et al., 2005. Characterization and immunomodulating activities of polysaccharide from Lentinus edodes. *Intl. Immunopharmacol.* 5: 811–820.
12. Fu, H. et al., 2011. Inhibition of Lentinus edodes polysaccharides against liver tumor growth. *Intl. J. Phys. Sci.* 6: 116–120.
13. Surenjav, U. et al., 2005. Structure, molecular weight and bioactivities of (1-3)-β-D-glucans and its sulfated derivatives from four kinds of Lentinus edodes. *Chinese J. Polymer Sci.* 23: 327–336.
14. Odagiri, Y. et al., 2006. Mutagenicity test for functional food containing superline dispersed lentinan (β-1,3-glucan): reverse mutation test, chromosomal aberration test and mouse micronucleus test. *Biotherapy* 20: 557–567.

15. Oka, M. et al., 2006. Safety and availability of functional food containing superfine dispersed lentinan (β-1,3-glucan) in cancer patients: multi-central unified protocol clinical trial. *Biotherapy* (Tokyo, Japan) 20: 590–606.

16. Yap, A. et al., 2005. An improved method for the isolation of lentinan from the edible and medicinal shiitake mushroom, Lentinus edodes (Berk.) Sing. (agaricomycetideae). *Intl. J. Med. Mushrooms* 3: 9–19.

17. Maruyama, S. et al., 2006. Antitumor activities of lentinan and micellapist in tumor-bearing mice. *Gan to Kagaku Ryoho* 33: 1726–1729.

18. Moriyama, M. et al., 1981. Antitumor effect of polysaccharide lentinan on transplanted ascites hepatoma-134 in C3H/He mice. *Intl. Congress Series* 576(Manipulation Host Def. Mech.), 207–218.

19. You, R.X. et al., 2015. Preliminary study on apoptosis mechanisms of mouse hepatocarcinoma H22 cells induced by polysaccharides derived from Lentinus edodes. *Zhongguo Yiyuan Yaoxue Zazhi* 35(9): 776–781.

20. Zhang, Y. et al., 2016. Polysaccharide from Lentinus edodes combined with oxaliplatin possesses the synergy and attenuation effect in hepatocellular carcinoma. *Cancer Lett.* (NY, NY, US) 377(2): 117–125.

21. Harada, K. et al., 2010. Effects of Lentinan alone and in combination with fluoro-pyrimidine anticancer agent on growth of human oral squamous cell carcinoma in vitro and in vivo. *Intl. J. Oncol.* 37: 623–631.

22. Xu, H. et al., 2016. Antitumor effect of β-glucan from Lentinus edodes and the underlying mechanism. *Scientific Reports* 6: 28802.

23. Zhang, L. et al., 2005. Correlation between antitumor activity, molecular weight, and conformation of lentinan. *Carbohydrate Res.* 340: 1515–1521.

24. Yap, A.T. et al., 2003. Immunopotentiating properties of lentinan (1-3)-β-D-glucan extracted from culinary-medicinal shiitake mushroom Lentinus edodes (berk.) singer (agaricomycetideae). *Intl. Med. Mushrooms* 5: 339–358.

25. Mizuno, M. et al., 2001. Antitumor polysaccharides from edible and medicinal mushrooms and immunomodulating action against murine macrophages. *Int. J. Medicinal Mushrooms* 3: 355–360.

26. Suga, Y. et al., 2005. Analysis of binding of β-glucan to mouse peripheral blood leukocytes. *Biotherapy* (Tokyo, Japan) 19: 197–203.

27. Chen, Q. et al., 2016. Activation of the NRF2-ARE signalling pathway by the Lentinula edodes polysaccharose LNT alleviates ROS-mediated cisplatin nephrotoxicity. *Int. Immunopharmacol.* 36: 1–8.

28. Mitamura T et al., 2000. Effects of lentinan on colorectal carcinogenesis in mice with ulcerative colitis. *Oncol. Reports* 7: 599–601.

29. Zhu, X.R. et al., 2008. Inhibitory effect of chemical modified Le-2 from Lentinula edodes on SP-2 ascitic tumor of mice. *Shihezi Daxue Xuebao, Ziran Kexueban* 26: 603–607.

30. Ma, B.J. et al., 2010. Study on antitumor activity of sulfated fractional lentinan in vitro. *Zhongguo Yaoshi* (Wuhan, China) 13: 451–453.

31. Zhang, P.Y. et al., 2002. Evaluation of sulfated Lentinus edodes α-(1-3)-D-glucan as a potential antitumor agent. *Biosci. Biotech. Biochem.* 66: 1052–1056.

32. Unursaikhan, S. et al., 2006. Antitumor activities of O-sulfonated derivatives of (1-3)-α-D-glucan from different Lentinus edodes. *Biosci. Biotech. Biochem.* 70: 38–46.

33. Jeff, I.B. et al., 2013. Purification and in vitro anti-proliferative effect of novel neutral polysaccharides from Lentinus edodes. *Intl. J. Biol. Macromol.* 52: 99–106.

34. Wang, K.P. et al., 2013. Structure and inducing tumor cell apoptosis activity of polysaccharides isolated from Lentinus edodes. *J. Agric. Food Chem.* 61: 9849–9858.

35. Cao, X.Y. et al., 2013. A novel polysaccharide from Lentinus edodes Mycelia exhibits potential antitumor activity on laryngeal squamous cancer cell line HEp-2. *Applied Biochem. Biotech.* 171: 1444–1453.

36. Zhang, Y. et al., 2010. Structure, chain conformation and antitumor activity of a novel polysaccharide from Lentinus edodes. *Fitoterapia* 81: 1163–1170.

37. Zhang, Y. et al., 2015. Induction of apoptosis in S180 tumour bearing mice by polysaccharide from Lentinus edodes via mitochondria apoptotic pathway. *J. Functional Foods* 15: 151–159.

38. You, R.X. et al., 2014. Alkali-soluble polysaccharide, isolated from Lentinus edodes, induces apoptosis and G2/M cell cycle arrest in H22 cells through microtubule depolymerization. *Phytother. Res.* 28: 1837–1845.

39. Wu, H. et al., 2012. Polysaccharide from Lentinus edodes inhibits the immunosuppressive function of myeloid-derived suppressor cells. *PLoS One* (2012), 7: e51751.

40. Chen, R.C. et al., 2016. Antimicrobial and antitumor activities of chitosan from shiitake stipes, compared to commercial chitosan from crab shells. *Carbohydr. Polym.* 138: 259–264.

41. Hibino, Y. et al., 1994. Productions of interferon-γ and nitrite are induced in mouse splenic cells by a heteroglycan-protein fraction from culture medium of Lentinus edodes mycelia. *Immunopharmacology* 28: 77–85.

42. Sugano, N. et al., 1985. Anticarcinogenic action of an alcohol-insoluble fraction (LAP1) from culture medium of Lentinus edodes mycelia. *Cancer Lett.* (Shannon, Ireland) 27: 1–6.

43. Jin, M. et al., 1991. Studies on constituents of the higher fungi of Korea. (LXIX). Antitumor components of the cultured mycelia of Lentinus edodes. *Soul Taehakkyo Yakhak Nonmunjip* 16: 766–796.

44. Surenjav, U. et al., 2006. Effects of molecular structure on antitumor activities of (1-3)-β-D-glucans from different Lentinus Edodes. *Carbohydr. Polym.* 63: 97–104.

45. Zheng, Y. et al., 2015. Relationship of chemical composition and cytotoxicity of water-soluble polysaccharides from Lentinus edodes fruiting bodies. *Pakistan J. Pharm. Sci.* 28(3, Suppl.): 1069–1074.

46. Zhao, Y.M. et al., 2016. Extraction, purification and antiproliferative activities of polysaccharides from Lentinus edodes. *Int. J. Biol. Macromol.* 93(Part-A), 136–144.

47. Ghoneum, M. et al., 2003. Modified arabinoxylan rice bran (MGN-3/Biobran) sensitizes human T cell leukemia cells to death receptor (CD95)-induced apoptosis. *Cancer Lett.* (Oxford, UK) 201: 41–49.

48. Wang, X.L. et al., 2009. Primarily isolation of Lentinus edodes C91-3 broth proteins and its antitumor effect in vitro. *Shandong Yiyao* 49: 73–74.

49. Wu, Y.H. et al., 2012. Isolation and purification of effective proteins from fermentative liquor of Lentinus edodes C91-3 and its antitumor effect. *Shizhen Guoyi Guoyao* 23: 538–542.

50. Zhong, M. et al., 2011. Antitumor effect of proteins from Lentinus edodes C91-3 mycelium's fermentative liquid in vivo. *Dalian Yike Daxue Xuebao* 33: 551–553, 557.

51. Zhao, Y. et al., 2009. Immuno-mechanism of antitumor effect of proteins (LFP91-3C) from lentinus edodes C91-3 mycelium's fermentation liquid. *Zhongguo Weishengtaixue Zazhi* 21: 226–228.

52. Huang, M. et al., 2009. Antitumor pure protein LFP91-3-A prepared by Lentinus edodes fermentation, method for extracting said protein, and preparation containing said protein. *Faming Zhuanli Shenqing* CN 101343651 A 20090114.

53. Liu, B. et al., 2012. Apoptosis mechanism of Lentinus edodes C91-3 apoptosis protein 24414 on human lung cancer cell line A549. *Zhonghua Zhongliu Fangzhi Zazhi* 19: 428–431.

54. Liu, B. et al., 2012. Study of biological function of Lentinus edodes C91-3 apoptosis protein 24414 on mouse hepatoma Hca cell line. *Dalian Yike Daxue Xuebao* 34: 30–35.

55. Liu, B. et al., 2012. A novel apoptosis correlated molecule: expression and characterization of protein Latcripin-1 from Lentinula edodes C91-3. *J. Mol. Sci.* 13: 6246–6265.

56. Kim, H.Y. et al., 2007. A polysaccharide extracted from rice bran fermented with Lentinus edodes enhances natural killer cell activity and exhibits anticancer effects. *J. Med. Food* 10: 25–31.

57. Ngai, P.H.K. et al., 2003. Lentin, a novel and potent antifungal protein from shiitake mushroom with inhibitory effects on activity of human immunodeficiency virus-1 reverse transcriptase and proliferation of leukemia cells. *Life Sci.* 73: 3363–3374.

70. SNOW FUNGUS

銀耳　白キクラゲ　은이버섯

Tremella fuciformis

Tremellaceae

Snow fungus is the fruit body of *Tremella fuciformis* (Tremellaceae), which is found worldwide in subtropical regions. As a health-improving and high nutrition food, snow fungus has been consumed in east Asia for over 2,000 years. According to the nutrition facts in Calorie Slism, snow fungus is a rich source of vitamins D and B2, potassium, calcium, iron, and zinc, and a good source of dietary fiber, vitamin B complex, vitamin A, magnesium, diverse nutrients, and so on, and it also affords selenium, an important healthy mineral. In the pharmacological tests, snow fungus showed various health beneficial features such as immunostimulating, hepatoprotective, cholesterol and low-density lipoprotein decreasing, atherosclerosis preventing, anti-inflammatory, antiallergic, antidiabetic, skin-beautifying, and antiaging properties. However, current commercialized snow fungus is mostly produced by using cultivation techniques. The cultivational quality would largely influence the nutritive and medicinal values of snow fungus.

SCIENTIFIC EVIDENCE OF CANCER-INHIBITORY AND CANCER-PREVENTIVE CONSTITUENTS

The organic solvent fractions (i.e., n-hexane, chloroform, and ethyl acetate) derived from the cultivated snow fungus exhibited cytotoxicity in human DLD-1 colon adenocarcinoma cells *in vitro* (IC_{50}s of 150–450 ppm). The most potent cytotoxicity was showed in its ether extract (IC_{50} of 150 ppm), followed by the ethyl acetate and chloroform fractions.[1] Nonetheless, the polysaccharides isolated from snow fungus water extract have received more attention in the scientific investigations.

1. Polysaccharides

Polysaccharides are the major component in snow fungus, which normally has no direct effect on tumor cells such as mouse ascites type sarcoma 180 and human K562 chronic myelogenous leukemia,[2] but only a polysaccharide (BII) showed *in vitro* cytotoxicity to human HeLa cervical cancer cells.[3] The polysaccharides from an alkali-soluble fraction and from a water-soluble fraction of the fruit bodies displayed *in vivo* anticancer activity in mice against transplanted sarcoma 180 ascites cells.[4,5] A polysaccharide (TSP) from spores of the fungi demonstrated *in vivo* growth inhibitory effect against sarcoma C57BL/6 in a dose of 200 mg/kg/day by i.p., [6] and against hepatoma 22 and sarcoma 180 in a dose of 25–100 mg/kg/day by i.p.[7] The best inhibition rate in H22 hepatoma cells reached 72.3% when polysaccharide was given to mice in a daily dose of 6 mg/kg.[8] During the treatment, the NK cell activity and lymphocyte transformation were notably augmented in the tumor-bearing mice. TSP also is able to amplify the number of nucleated splenocytes and the weight of spleen and markedly augment the spontaneous incorporation rate of thymocytes *in vivo*.[6,7] Similarly, another polysaccharide termed TP derived from snow fungus showed notable *in vivo* immunostimulating effects, that is, enhancing phagocytotic clearance of C particles in doses of 12.5–25 mg/kg and increasing hemolysin formation in a dose of 50 mg/kg in mice.[9] A (1-3)-β-glucan was separated from the snow fungus polysaccharides, exerting both activities of cancer cell growth inhibition and immunoenhancement *in vivo*.[10] The results evidently signified that the cancer-inhibitory effect of snow fungus polysaccharides is principally mediated by their immunopotentiating property.

Furthermore, the immune system and its functions are usually damaged by chemotherapy and radio irradiation. The snow fungus polysaccharides have distinct benefits in promoting the immunity of tumor-suffering animals such as enhancing NK cell activity and phagocytotic function of reticuloendothelial system and restoring the cytotoxic immunity of humoral and cellular.[6-13] Hence, co-treatment with snow fungus polysaccharides would obviously improve the anticancer efficacy of chemotherapies and radiotherapies. For instances, TSP was combined with 5-fluorouracil or cyclophosphamide for treatment of rats or mice transplanted with hepatoma 22 or sarcoma 180. The tumor suppressive rates, immune organ index, and carbon granule clearance index were remarkably promoted, displaying additive inhibitory effect.[11,12] A polysaccharide derived from *T. fuciformis* ferment was also reported to have the suppressive effect against the growth of lymphoma cells and U14 cervical cancer cells in mice at the doses of 6–24 mg/kg. When treatment of this polysaccharide at a dose of 6 mg/kg was combined with γ-ray irritation, the *in vivo* inhibitory rates were notably elevated to 72.6% on the lymphoma and to 71.2% on the U14 cervical carcinoma.[13]

2. Sulfated polysaccharides

When the polysaccharides from snow fungus were reacted with chlorosulfonic acid and pyridine, three sulfated polysaccharides designated as S-I, S-II, and S-III (m.w. 84,000, 90,000, and 96,000, respectively) were produced. The structural sulfation markedly potentiated the antiproliferative activity of the polysaccharides. S-I and S-III at a dose of 12 mg/kg significantly repressed the growth of lymphoma cells *in vivo* with inhibitory rates of 59.8% and 69.9%, respectively.[14]

OTHER BIOACTIVITIES

The multiple medical advantages of snow fungus polysaccharides have been demonstrated by pharmacological approaches, including antimutagenic, leukocytotic, antioxidant, immunopotentiating, antiulcerative, anticoagulative, antithrombotic, hypoglycemic, hypolipemic, hepatoprotective, antiaging, membrane-protecting, and protein/nucleic acid synthesis-promoting properties. The facts designated that the rich polysaccharide components mostly represent the snow fungus in the biological benefits.

CONCLUSION AND SUGGESTION

The extensive research results scientifically confirmed the anticancer property of snow fungus. Although the organic solvent extracts from the fungus showed certain *in vitro* cancer inhibition, the major and abundant ingredient was assigned as polysaccharides in snow fungus, which was prominently responsible for variety of biological properties of snow fungus, especially the *in vivo* anticancer and immunopotentiating effects. The cancer-suppressive activity of *T. fucirormis* polysaccharides was revealed to be primarily attributed to their capacity of boosting host immune system and cytotoxic immune function. The immunostimulation was also helpful for diminishing the toxicity and side effects caused by chemotherapies and radiotherapies, leading to augmentation of the efficacy of current cancer treatments and improvement of the quality of life of cancer patients. Consequently, the positive data further suggested that snow fungus as a safe and nontoxic functional food should be encouraged to be used frequently in human dietary for upgrading human immunity and reducing incidence of diseases including carcinogenesis, especially for adjuvant to clinical cancer therapies.

REFERENCES

1. Kim, K.A. et al., 2006. Cytotoxic effects of extracts from Tremella fuciformis strain FB001 on the human colon adenocarcinoma cell line DLD-1. *Food Sci. Biotechnol.* 15: 889–895.
2. Tong, L. et al., 1994. Effects of plant polysaccharides on cell proliferation and cell membrane contents of sialic acid, phospholipid and cholesterol in S180 and K562 cells. *Zhongguo Zhongxiyi Jiehe Zazhi* 14: 482–484.

3. Gao, Q.Q. et al., 1991. Polysaccharides and their antitumor activity of Tremella fucirormis berk (I). *Tianran Chanwu Yanjiu yu Kaifa* 3: 43–48.

4. Irikura, T. et al., 1972. Antitumor polysaccharides A and B from Tremella. *Jpn. Kokai Tokkyo Koho* JP 72-712498 19720127.

5. Ukai, S. et al., 1972. Antitumor activity on sarcoma 180 of the polysaccharides from Tremella fuciformis. *Chem. Pharm. Bull.* 20: 2293–2294.

6. Zheng, S.Z. et al., 1992. A preliminary survey on the enhancing effect of Tremella fuciformis spore polysaccharides (TSP) on radiotherapy. *J. Nanjing Med. College* 12: 384–387.

7. Xu, H.L. et al., 2008. Effect of tremella fuciformis spores polysaccharides on transplanted tumor and immunological function in mice. *Zhongguo Xiandai Yingyong Yaoxue* 25: 93–95.

8. Han, Y. et al., 2011. Tumor-inhibitory effect and mechanism of polysaccharide from Tremella fuciformis in mice. *Yiyao Daobao* 30: 849–952.

9. Deng, W.L. et al., 1984. Immunopharmacological study on the polysaccharide of tremella (Tremella fuciformis). *Zhongcaoyao* 15: 23–26, 22.

10. Yang, X.T. et al., 2003. Quantification of (1-3)-β-glucan in edible and medicinal mushroom polysaccharides by using limulus G test. *Junwu Xitong* 22: 296–302.

11. Li, Y.C. et al., 2008. Antitumor effect of Tremella polysaccharide and 5-fluorouracil combination in mice implanted with sarcoma 180 and hepatocarcinoma 22. *Zhongguo Yiyuan Yaoxue Zazhi* 28: 209–11.

12. Xu, H.L. et al., 2008. Synergistic effect of Tremella fuciformis spores polysaccharides on tumor bearing mice treated by cyclophosphamide. *Zhongguo Yaoshi* (Wuhan, China) 11: 493–495.

13. Xu, W.Q. et al., 2006. Studies on antitumor and synergism combined with γ-rays of polysaccharide from Tremella fuciformis ferment in mice. *Zhongguo Shenghua Yaowu Zazhi* 27: 351–354.

14. Xu, W.Q. et al., 2007. Studies on synthesis of sulfated Tremella fuciformis polysaccharides and its inhibition effect on tumor. *Zhongguo Yaoxue Zazhi* 42: 630–632.

71. SPLIT GILL MUSHROOM

樹花　末広茸　나무 꽃

Schizophyllum commune

Schizophyllaceae

Split gill mushroom is the fruiting body of the edible fungus *Schizophyllum commune* (Schizophyllaceae), which is one of the most widely distributed and common mushrooms on the Earth. Although small and leathery, the tiny fruiting bodies are frequently consumed as a culinary food in Mexico, India, and Southeast Asia. The fungus has good nutritional contents of vitamin B3, potassium, calcium, and magnesium, and comprises bioactive components such as alkaloids, flavonoids, phenols, saponins tannins, and proteins in varying quantities, but the flavonoids and proteins occur in relatively higher contents.[1]

Scientific Evidence of Cancer-Inhibitory and Cancer-Preventive Constituents

1. Alkaloids

Two iminolactone-type alkaloids assigned as schizine-A (**1**) and schizine-B (**2**) were separated from the fruiting bodies of *S. commune*; the two showed obvious antiproliferative effect against human EL4 (leukemic), MCF-7 (breast), and PC3 (prostate) cancer cell lines but no inhibitory effect on three benign cell lines (McCoy, 3T3, and MCF 10A). The IC_{50} values were 3.7 and 4.0 μM in EL4 cells, 4.9 and 6.7 μM in MCF-7 cells, and 14.7 and 13.4 μM in PC3 cells, respectively.[2] Also, a group of indole derivatives such as schizocommunin (**3**), indigotin (**4**), indirubin (**5**), isatin (**6**), and tryptanthrin (**7**) were isolated from the culture broth of *S. commune*. These indole derivatives were found to possess growth-inhibitory properties on tumors. Treatment with schizocommunin (**3**) resulted in strong cytotoxicity against murine lymphoma cells.[3]

2. Polysaccharides

Schizophyllan: The most important anticarcinoma and immunomodulatory agent in split gill mushroom is a β-(1-6)-branched β-(1-3)-D-glucohexaose with m.w. around 10^6, which is designated as schizophyllan (SPG) or sizofiran.[4] Since the 1970s, SPG has been used as a biological response modifier in combination with radiotherapies and chemotherapies, especially for patients with gastric or cervical carcinomas, to decrease cancer recurrence rate and improve survival duration.[5] In animal models, SPG at a dose of 1 mg/kg per day for ten days diminished the tumor weight by 99% in mice bearing sarcoma 180 and inhibited the growth of BC-47 bladder cancer cells in rats,[6,7] but SPG did not exert direct effect on the cancer cells. The i.p. administration of SPG to rats could activate the antitumor antigen formation in T cells and elicit macrophages in the tumors directly or indirectly. The results designated that the antitumor property of SPG should be strictly mediated by host immunomodulating effects to enhance the resistance of the host against tumors. Further investigation revealed that the immunoactivity-dependent anticancer mechanism of SPG was triggered by (i) binding of the (1-3)-β-D-glucan to dectin-1 receptors in the macrophages and other cells, (ii) stimulating macrophages to secrete large amounts of lysosomal enzymes, (iii) significantly motivating to produce bone marrow stimulating factors in serum, (iv) stimulating a lymphoid T-cell cascade with subsequent increased production of cytokines such as (ILa-1, -2, and -3) and TNF-α, and (v) augmenting the levels of IFN-γ and IL-2 from the mitogen-stimulated peripheral blood mononuclear cells, leading to final restraint on the tumor cell growth and amplification of the survival rate of tested animals.[8-11] Interestingly, an ultrasonic treatment could significantly improve the immunoenhancing and antitumor activities of SPG in tests with splenic lymphocytes, macrophages RAW264.7, and human breast carcinoma T-47D cells.[12]

Combination therapy with SPG: The combination of SPG with current therapeutic drugs resulted in remarkable improvement in the anticancer immune responses at tumor site. A co-treatment with SPG and tamoxifen effectively inhibited the development of breast and hepatic cancers caused by 7,12-dimethylbenz[a]anthracene (DMBA) in mice together with the cell proapoptosis.[13] Administration of SPG combined with recombinant human rIL-2 was effective in suppressing lymphoma cells and prolonging the survival time of mice implanted with EL-4 lymphoma. At the same time, the immune-response cells in the peritoneal cavity such as T lymphocytes, macrophages, and NK cells were clearly activated.[14] When the SPG were integrated with radiotherapy and immunotherapy, the antigrowth effect could be accomplished from an early stage. Daily i.m. injection in doses of 5 or 10 mg/kg of SPG and local irradiation with pion or electron given to mice for consecutive days not only exerted the inhibitory and life-prolonging effects against NR-S1 and SCCVII squamous cell cancer cell lines but also showed pulmonary metastasis-suppressing effect.[15,16]

Structural modification of SPG: SPG was modified to produce formylmethylated and amino-ethylated derivatives. The degree of the formylmethyl substitution was about 0.19 and the formyl-methyl group locations in the derivative were predominantly located at C-6 and C-4 positions in glucose residues. The derivatives still showed the similar helical stereostructure to SPG and only slightly increased molecular weight. The i.p. administration of the formylmethylated or amino-ethylated derivatives at a same dosage of 10 mg/kg per day for 7 days to mice bearing sarcoma 180 exhibited 1.5–2 times more potent antitumor activity than SPG alone in a dose of 100 mg/kg, and the two derivatives also were cytotoxic to mouse L929 fibrosarcoma cells. The derivatives could potentiate the reticuloendothelial system, as SPG did but simulated more secretion of cyto-toxic factors (such as superoxide anion and TNF-α) from macrophages, appearing to be more efficient than schizophyllan (SPG).[17]

Another active derivative, carboxymethylated schizophyllan (CMSPG), linked SPG to mitomycin-C (MMC) as a conjugate. The conjugate exerted two times higher activity at 50% growth-inhibitory concentration against L1210 leukemia cells *in vitro* compared to MMC alone. The *in vivo* antineoplastic activity of the conjugate was similar to that of MMC in mice implanted with solid sarcoma 180; however, CMSPG showed the remarkable ability to induce the tumor-regressing factor and the neutrophil chemotactic factors in the serum, which then significantly attenuated the MMC caused side effects.[18]

3. Lectin

A homodimeric lactose-binding lectin (64 kDa) was isolated from the fresh fruiting bodies of split gill mushroom. The lectin demonstrated antiproliferative activity toward L1210 leukemia,

MBL2 leukemia, and HepG2 hepatoma cell lines *in vitro* in association with marked blockage of methylthymidine uptake by these cancer cells. It also exerted potent mitogenic activity toward mouse splenocytes and suppressive activity toward HIV-1 reverse transcriptase (IC_{50} of 1.2 μM).[19]

4. Protein

Hydrophobin-SC3 is a fungal protein prepared from *S. commune*, which had no direct cytotoxicity on sarcoma cells and certain cytotoxicity toward melanoma cells at a high concentration. Incubation of spleen cells with hydrophobin-SC3 could augment the levels of interleukin-10 and TNF-α mRNA by 1.5–2.5-fold. Daily i.p. injection of hydrophobin-SC3 to mice for 12 days resulted in tumor-suppressive activity on sarcoma and melanoma via immunomodulation without causing any signs of toxicity, where the tumor size and weight were reduced more significantly in the skin cancer than in the sarcoma.[20] Therefore, hydrophobin-SC3 may have a beneficial value as an adjuvant in the co-treatments with chemotherapy and radiation.

NANOFORMULATION

The extracellular and intracellular synthesis of silver nanoparticles was succeeded by shaking broth cultures of split gill mushroom (*S. commune*) with 1 mM silver nitrate at 25 ± 2°C and pH 7. The created silver nanoparticles at the concentrations of 10 and 100 μg/mL induced 27.2% and 64% mortality of human HEp-2 epidermoid larynx cancer cells, respectively.[21]

CONCLUSION AND SUGGESTION

Although the fruiting body of *Schizophyllum commune* is not a popular mushroom as a food source, the biology-linked phytochemical researches found its medicinal potential in lowering the risk of cancer through regular consumption. A group of iminolactones and indole derivative alkaloids and a homodimeric lactose-binding lectin isolated from the split gill mushroom demonstrated moderate antiproliferative effects against leukemic, breast, and prostate cancer, leukemia, and hepatoma cell lines *in vitro*, respectively. The isolated schyzophyllan glucan (schizophyllan) and protein (hydrophobin-SC3) exerted *in vivo* suppressive effects against the cancer cell growth in murine animal models; these anticancer properties were principally dependent on their remarkable immunoregulative capacities. Owing to the immunoenhancing activities, the two macromolecules amplified the cancer-inhibitory potencies and diminished the toxicity/side effects elicited by chemotherapy and radiotherapy when in combined treatments. Accordingly, split gill mushroom can be considered as a functional food not only for the cuisine application but also for the development of nutraceuticals and pharmaceuticals to exert its potential in cancer prevention and adjuvant remedy.

REFERENCES

1. Okwulehie, I.C. et al., 2007. Pharmaceutical and nutritional prospects of two wild macro-fungi found in Nigeria. *Biotechnol.* 6: 567–572.
2. Liu, X.M. et al., 2015. Iminolactones from Schizophyllum commune. *J. Nat. Prod.* 78: 1165–1168.
3. Hosoe, T. et al., 2000. Isolation of a new potent cytotoxic pigment along with indigotin from the pathogenic basidiomycetous fungus Schizophyllum commune. *Mycopathologia* Volume Date 1999, 146: 9–12.
4. Chen, J.Z. et al., 2007. Medicinal importance of fungal β-(1-3),(1-6)-glucans. *Mycological Res.* 111: 635–652.

5. Hobbs, C.R. et al., 2005. The chemistry, nutritional value, immunopharmacology, and safety of the traditional food of medicinal split-gill fungus Schizophyllum commune Fr. *Intl. J. Med. Mushrooms* 7: 127–139.
6. Kinoshita, M. 1986. Histological and cytochemical studies on the distribution of schyzophyllan glucan (SPG) in cancer-bearing animals. II. Difference in distribution of SPG and biochemical and cytochemical difference in lysosomal enzyme activity between responders and nonresponders. *Ochanomizu Igaku Zasshi* 34: 221–237.
7. Franz, G. 1987. Structure-activity relation of polysaccharides with antitumor activity. *Farmaceutisch Tijdschrift voor Belgie* 64: 301–311.
8. Miyazaki, K. et al., 2002. Sizofiran. *Biotherapy* (Tokyo, Japan) 16: 35–43.
9. Tsuchiya, Y. et al., 1989. Cytokine-related immunomodulating activities of an antitumor glucan, sizofiran (SPG). *J. Pharmacobio-Dynamics* 12: 616–625.
10. Sakagami, Y. et al., 1988. Effects of an antitumor polysaccharide, schizophyllan, on interferon-γ and interleukin 2 production by peripheral blood mononuclear cells. *Biochem. Biophys. Res. Commun.* 155: 650–655.
11. Suzuki, M. et al., 1982. Cooperative role of T lymphocytes and macrophages in antitumor activity of mice pretreated with schizophyllan (SPG). *Jpn J. Experimental Med.* 52: 59–65.
12. Zhong, K. et al., 2015. Immunoregulatory and antitumor activity of schizophyllan under ultrasonic treatment. *Int. J. Biolog. Macromol.* 80, 302–308
13. Mansour, A. et al., 2012. Schizophyllan inhibits the development of mammary and hepatic carcinomas induced by 7,12 dimethylbenz(α) anthracene and decreases cell proliferation: comparison with tamoxifen. *J. Cancer Res. Clin. Oncol.* 138: 1579–1596.
14. Kano, Y. et al., 1996. Augmentation of antitumor effect by combined administration with interleukin-2 and sizofiran, a single glucan, on murine EL-4 lymphoma. *Biotherapy* (Dordrecht, Netherlands) 9: 241–247.
15. Ogawa, Y. et al., 1990. Combination therapy of pions and SPG (sonifilan, schizophyllan), a biological response modifier for mouse tumor systems. *Intl. J. Radiation Oncol. Biol. Physics* 18: 1415–1420.
16. Arika, T. et al., 1992. Combination therapy of radiation and Sizofiran (SPG) on the tumor growth and metastasis on squamous-cell carcinoma NR-S1 in syngeneic C3H/He mice. *Biotherapy* (Dordrecht, Netherlands) 4: 165–170.
17. Usui, S. et al., 1995. Preparation and antitumor activities of β-(1-6) branched (1-3)-β-D-glucan derivatives. *Biol. Pharm. Bull.* 18: 1630–1636.
18. Usui, S. et al., 1994. Preparation and antitumor activities of mitomycin C β-(1-6)-branched (1-3)-β-D-glucan conjugate. *Biol. Pharma. Bull.* 17: 1165–1170.
19. Han, C.H. et al., 2005. A novel homodimeric lactose-binding lectin from the edible split gill medicinal mushroom Schizophyllum commune. *Biochem. Biophys. Res. Communic.* 336: 252–257.
20. Akanbi, M. et al., 2013. The antitumor activity of hydrophobin SC3, a fungal protein. *Applied Microbiol. Biotechnol.* 97: 4385–4392.
21. Arun, G. et al., 2014. Green synthesis of silver nanoparticles using the mushroom fungus Schizophyllum commune and its biomedical applications. *Biotechnol. Bioprocess Eng.* 19(6): 1083–1090.

72. STRAW MUSHROOM

草菇   袋茸   버섯의-일종

Volvariella volvacea

Pluteacea

Straw mushroom is the fruiting body of the edible fungus *Volvariella volvacea* (Pluteacea). The wild straw mushroom grows mainly on rice strew beds in tropical and subtropical climates. Today, it is cultivated throughout East and Southeast Asia region and used extensively in Asian cuisines and in Indian medicine system. The straw mushroom is a good nutritional source of protein, fibers (chitin), vitamins C, B2, B7, and B1, essential amino acids, and dietary minerals (potassium, sodium, and phosphorus).[1] The phytochemicals in *V. volvacea* were, identified as polypeptides, terpenes, steroids, flavonoids, phenolic acids, and tannins. The phenolic components in straw mushroom are the major contributors to the antioxidant activities, and the macromolecules such as polysaccharides and proteins are in charge of the immunomodulatory effects of *V. volvacea*.[1]

SCIENTIFIC EVIDENCE OF CANCER-INHIBITORY AND CANCER-PREVENTIVE CONSTITUENTS

An aqueous ethanolic extract of cultured *V. volvacea* mycelium displayed prominent hydroxyl and DPPH radical scavenging and lipid peroxidation-inhibiting activities. In two mouse models, this extract had profound antitumor activity against both Ehrlich cell-induced ascites and Dalton's lymphoma cell-induced solid tumors.[2] Meanwhile, the crudest triterpenoid content (17%) was in the petroleum ether extract of *V. volvacea* mycelium, while the most flavonoid content (9.31%) and triterpenoid content (15.4%) was in the ethyl acetate extract. The mycelia extracts of ethyl acetate and ethanol showed the highest antioxidative activities. At concentrations of 200–800 µg/mL, the three organic extracts impeded the proliferation of human BGC gastric cancer cells *in vitro*.[3] Remarkably, two types of macromolecules, that is, glucans and lectins, have been claimed to primarily respond to the antitumor properties of straw mushroom.

1. Glucans

Bioactive (1-6)-branched (1-3)-β-D-glucans were purified from alkali-soluble extract of the fruiting body and cultured mycelium of *V. volvacea*. The glucan from the cultured mycelium exhibited strong suppressive effect against the growth of cancer cells in mice implanted with sarcoma 180 with an inhibitory ratio of 87.8%; the tumoricidal activity was found to closely depend on its triple helical backbone conformation, molecular shape, and distribution of side chains in the glycon.[4-7] If the glucosyl groups were modified into the corresponding polyhydroxyl groups at its branches of (1-3)-β-D-glucose, the anticancer activities could be significantly potentiated on both allogeneic and syngeneic tumors *in vivo*.[6,7]

2. Lectins

An antiproliferative fungal lectin (VVL) was also prepared from straw mushroom. VVL at a concentration of 0.32 μM markedly reduced thymidine incorporation into tumor cells and activated the expressions of p21, p27, p53, and Rb whose proteins act as cyclin-dependent kinase inhibitors. At a concentration range from 0.32 to 0.8 μM, VVL could induce prominent blebs on the surface of sarcoma cells and large vacuoles in the cytoplasm but not apoptotic bodies. By these interactions, VVL finally arrested cell cycle progression at G2/M phase and hampered the proliferation of sarcoma 180 cells.[8]

CONCLUSION AND SUGGESTION

From the scientific information as presented in this section, straw mushrooms are known to show several biological properties including noticeable antioxidant and radical scavenging activities and anticancer and immunomodulatory potentials. The isolated macromolecules, glucans and lectins, were shown to exert the cancer-inhibitory activities *in vivo* and/or *in vitro*. In addition to showing prominent antioxidant effects, the organic solvent extracts of *Volvariella volvacea*, which are rich in polyphenolics and triterpenoids, were also effective in hindering the proliferation of a gastric cancer cell line, but no antitumor micromolecule has been reported yet in phytochemical investigation. Altogether, the investigations provided scientific evidences for straw mushroom being a healthy dietary food, which is propitious to cancer prevention. The rich antioxidative activities of straw mushroom are believed also to help in the prevention of multiple diseases caused by malignant, cardiovascular, neurodegeneration, and aging-induced degeneration.[1]

REFERENCES

1. Amit, Roy et al., 2014. Volvariella volvacea: A macrofungus having nutritional and health potential. *Asian J. Pharm. Tech.* 4(2): 110–113
2. Mathew, J. et al., 2008. Antioxidant and antitumor activities of cultured mycelium of culinary-medicinal paddy straw mushroom volvariella volvacea (Bull.: Fr.) Singer (Agaricomycetideae). *Int. J. Med. Mushrooms* 10(2): 139–148.
3. Zhao, J.X. et al., 2007. Analysis of crude triterpenoids and flavonoids contents, antioxidative and antitumor activities of crude extracts from culture broth of Volvariella volvacea. *Junwu Xuebao* 26(3), 426–432.
4. Kishida, E. et al., 1989. Purification of an antitumor-active, branched (1-3)-β-D-glucan from Volvariella volvacea, and elucidation of its fine structure. *Carbohydrate Res.* 193: 227–239.
5. Kishida, E. et al., 1992. Structures and antitumor activities of polysaccharides isolated from mycelium of Volvariella volvacea. *Biosci. Biotech. Biochem.* 56: 1308–1309.
6. Misaki, A. et al., 1993. Antitumor fungal (1-3)-β-D-glucans: Structural diversity and effects of chemical modification. *Frontiers in Biomed. Biotech.* 1: 116–129.
7. Kishida, E. et al., 1991. Effects of branch distribution and chemical modifications of antitumor (1-3)-β-D-glucans. *Carbohydrate Polymers* 17: 89–95.
8. Liu, W.K. et al., 2000. Suppression of cell cycle progression by a fungal lectin: activation of cyclin-dependent kinase inhibitors. *Biochem. Pharmacol.* Volume Date 2001, 61: 33–37.

73. WINTER MUSHROOM OR ENOKITAKE

冬菇　榎茸　팽이버섯

Flammulina velutipes

Marasmiaceae

Winter mushroom is the edible fruit bodies of the Marasmiaceae fungus *Flammulina velutipes*. The delicious fungi are one of the common mushrooms often used in Asian cuisines, especially in China, Japan, Korea, and Vietnam. Every 100 g of dried enokitake contains various B-vitamins (61 mg B3, 10.9 mg B5, 1.69 mg B2, and 0.35 mg B1) and dietary minerals (14 mg calcium, 8.3 mg iron, 0.61 mg copper, 54 µg selenium, and large amounts of potassium) without cholesterol, vitamins A, and C.[1] In pharmacological studies, winter mushroom showed multiple biological properties such as antioxidant, hepatoprotective, hypolipidemic, hypoglycemic, immunopotentiating, anti-inflammatory, antidiabetic, antihypercholesterolemic, and antiweary effects. The biologically responsible active components in winter mushroom were assigned to be dietary fiber, polysaccharides, protein-bound polysaccharide, glycoprotein, proteins, norsesquiterpenes, and sterols. Winter mushroom is also a rich source of antioxidants, particularly ergothioneines. The hydrophilic antioxidants in the mycelium substrate are richer than in the harvested fruiting body mushrooms.[2]

SCIENTIFIC EVIDENCE OF CANCER-INHIBITORY AND CANCER-PREVENTIVE CONSTITUENTS

Aqueous extract of winter mushroom demonstrated significant anticarcinogenic and antitumor properties.[3] Its cold-water extracts (~800 µg/mL) markedly stimulated the inhibitory activity of human peripheral blood mononuclear cells against the proliferation of human U937 leukemic cells.[4] The water-based extract also exerted its dose-dependent antiproliferative and cytotoxic activities on two human estrogen-receptor negative breast cancer cell lines (MDA-MB-231 and BT-20) *in vitro*, with a IC_{50} of 30 µg/mL in BT-20 cells. The aqueous extract treatment also reduced colony formation of human MCF-7 breast cancer by 99%. The extract could induce an exceptionally rapid apoptosis in both estrogen-receptor positive (MCF-7) and negative (MDA-MB-231) breast cancer cell lines.[5] An unsaponifiable extract of *F. velutipes* fruiting body showed the suppressive effects against the proliferation of other human cancer cell lines (HepG2, SGC, U251, and A549) *in vitro*.[6] These results designated that the aqueous extract of winter mushroom contains potential chemotherapeutic and chemopreventive components such as polysaccharides, protein-bound polysaccharide, glycoproteins, proteins, and so on.

1. Polysaccharides

FVP, a polysaccharide extract from the edible fungi could inhibit the proliferation of human hepatoma SMMC-7721 cells *in vitro* at a concentration of 50 µg/mL and repress the growth of sarcoma 180 cells by 52.8% in mice at a dose of 24 mg/kg as well as Lewis lung tumor and H22 hepatoma *in vivo*.[7-9] CFVP (crude polysaccharides), DCFVP (deproteinized polysaccharides), and FVP2 (a polysaccharide fraction) were obtained from the fractionation of the edible winter mushroom. *In vitro* co-incubated with neoplastic cell lines for 72 h resulted in the antiproliferation effect of CFVP, DCFVP, and FVP2. Among them, the higher inhibitory ratio was achieved by CFVP at a concentration of 500 µg/mL, such as 64.6% in A375 melanoma cells and 55.3% in HEp-2 throat cancer cells. But it displayed only 29.3% inhibition of B16 melanoma cells, whereas FVP2 retarded 69.2% of B16 cells at the same concentration (500 µg/mL).[10] Similarly, FvP-2 (crude polysaccharides) and FvP-3 (deproteinized polysaccharides) were prepared from the mycelia of *F. velutipes*. FvP-2 at 640 µg/mL concentration displayed 45% suppression against human BEL-7402 hepatoma cells, while FvP-3 at a concentration of 200 µg/mL showed noticeable radical scavenging activity.[11]

Two polysaccharides termed PA5DE (m.w. 4.71×10^5) and PA3DE (m.w. 5.4×10^6) with β-glycoside linkage were isolated from the mushroom. Both PA5DE and PA3DE were composed of D-glucose, D-mannose, and L-fucose in the molar ratios of 15.83:1.70:1.00 and 22.31:1.46:1.00, respectively, and their inhibitory rates were 50.2% and 46.7% on solid sarcoma 180 implanted in mice, respectively.[12,13] Two other polysaccharides, that is, EA3 and EA5 also prepared from winter mushroom exhibited remarked *in vivo* antitumor rates at 82% and 84%, respectively, on sarcoma 180 model in mice. The EA3 was elucidated as a β-(1-3)-glucan.[14] In addition, from the mushroom cell wall, an alkali-soluble polysaccharide (ASP, m.w. $\approx$ 200 kD) was isolated. The backbone of ASP is primarily composed of β-(1-3)-D-linked glucose. When i.p. injection to mice, ASP triggered the proliferation of splenic lymphocytes and enhanced vascular dilation and hemorrhage (VDH) response in addition of potent antitumor activity against SC-180 sarcoma *in vivo*.[15] Likewise, during the treatment of sarcoma 180 *in vivo*, FVP (100, 50, 25 mg/kg) was able to regulate murine immune function by promoting the serum levels of TNF-α, INF-γ, and IL-2.[16]

On the basis of the research results, it is revealed that the *in vivo* antitumor effect of these polysaccharides should be principally contributed by their high levels of immunomodulating functions, such as increase in lymphocyte T-cell subsets. All the data suggested that the polysaccharides of winter mushroom may be useful for cancer prevention as a functional food additive.

2. Protein-bound polysaccharides

A bioactive protein-bound polysaccharide assigned as EA6 was isolated from a HWE of winter mushroom. EA6 was effective in increasing the life duration in mice bearing Lewis lung carcinoma or B16 melanoma and proadministration of EA6 orally in a dose of 10 mg/kg/day after surgery markedly displayed antitumor effect against the Meth-A tumor secondary inoculated in mice, but it showed no inhibitory effect on the intradermally inoculated Meth-A fibrosarcoma. The antigrowth effect was found to attribute to the enhancement of both humoral and cell-mediated immunity and IL-2 production by EA6 via mediation of CD4-positive T cells.[17] Similarly, administration of EA6 to mice bearing sarcoma 180 (cryosurgery) could augment the host's humoral immunity, cellular immunity, and IL-2 production in situ freeze-destruction.[18-20] When co-treatment with a vaccine, EA6 in a dose of 40 mg/kg markedly prolonged the life span (ILS of 223%) of mice bearing L1210 leukemia.[21] These observations evidenced that the EA6 protein-bound polysaccharide and the other polysaccharides are the important bioconstituents in winter mushroom, having immuno-potentiation-dependent antitumor functions.

3. Proteins

A *F. velutipes* protein component was extracted and patented in China, which demonstrated marked growth-inhibitory and apoptosis-promoting effects against the tested human HepG2 (liver), MCF-7 (breast), and A549 (lung) cancer cell lines *in vitro*. The IC_{50}s were the same as 8 μg/mL in the three cancer cell lines and the cancer-inhibitory rates could be amplified with time-extension and concentration increase.[22] Two proteins, flammulin (2.37×10^4) and Zb (3.0×10^4), were purified from the aqueous extract of the mushroom fruiting body, and flammulin is composed of 235 amino acidic residues. Both proteins showed direct growth inhibition against tumor cells *in vitro* and the IC_{50} of Zb was 0.75 μg/mL against MGC80-3 gastric carcinoma cell line. In mouse models, flammulin markedly obstructed the growth of sarcoma 180 and Ehrlich ascites tumor *in vivo*.[23-25]

An immunomodulatory protein designated as FVE was purified from winter mushroom, which is documented as an activator for human T lymphocytes. Oral administration of FVE to mice in dose of 10 mg/kg markedly augmented the tumoricidal capacity of peritoneal macrophages and elevated tumor-specific splenocytes to highest levels against the growth of murine BNL hepatoma cells, resulting in the significant increase in the life span and decrease in the size of BNL hepatoma and angiogenesis in mice.[26] FIP-fve, an immunomodulatory and anti-inflammatory protein also from *F. velutipes* that in an *in vitro* assay suppressed the proliferation of human A549 lung cancer cells after 48 h treatment, together with induction cell cycle arrest and cell migration arrest but no apoptosis. The antiproliferation in A549 cells was mediated by a p53 activation pathway and the antimigration in A549 cells was correlated to reduction of RacGAP1 mRNA and protein levels.[27] A hemagglutinin isolated from the fruiting bodies of *F. velutipes* showed similar molecular mass to FIP-fve (12 kDa), but its *N*-terminal sequence was different from that of FIP-fve. The hemagglutinin of *F. velutipes* in the tests stimulated methylthymidine uptake by mouse splenocytes and hindered the proliferation of leukemia L1210 cells (IC_{50} of 13 μM), which was stable between pH 4 and pH 11 and <60°C.[28]

4. Glycoprotein

Proflamin (PRF), an antitumor glycoprotein with the molecular weight about 1.3×10^4, was isolated from the cultured mycelium of the mushroom, which contains more than 90% protein and less than 10% carbohydrate but has weak acidic nature. Oral administration of PRF significantly augmented various immunoresponses in mice bearing tumors with no lethal or any other apparent adverse effect. By the host-mediated antitumor activities, PRF at a dose of 10 mg/kg per day greatly prolonged the life span of mice implanted with syngeneic B16 melanoma and adenocarcinoma 755 by 86% and 84%, respectively, and inhibited the growth of the solid type of sarcoma 180 *in vivo*. When combined with surgery and PRF, the co-treatment could result in strong antiproliferative effect in mice bearing Meth-A fibrosarcoma. Likewise, in combination with cryosurgery, PRF worked as an immunopotentiator to augment the immunity and to maintain the immunocompetence at a high level in the cancer cells for a long duration; the immunocompetence was usually decreased in patients after cryosurgery.[29,30]

FMG1, another glycoprotein prepared from winter mushroom mycelia, presented immunostimulation-related antitumor activity in the assays. FMG1 could significantly enhance phagocytosis by reticuloendothelial system and amplify the thymus index and body weight of mice bearing tumor, and it could remarkably potentiate the proliferation of T lymphocyte in mouse spleen; immunoenhancing actions subsequently elicited the prominent suppressive effect on sarcoma 180 *in vivo* after oral administration of FMG1.[31]

5. Norsesquiterpenes

Six isolactarane-related norsesquiterpenes assigned as flammulinolides-A–G were isolated from the solid culture of *F. velutipes* together with other sesquiterpenes. *In vitro* experiments showed that flammulinolide-A (**1**), flammulinolide-B (**2**), flammulinolide-F (**3**) obviously restrained the proliferation of human KB nasopharyngeal carcinoma cell line (IC_{50}s ranged from 3.6 μM to 4.7 μM) and inhibited human HepG2 hepatoma cell line (IC_{50}s ranged from 34.7 μM to 123.0 μM) in lower degree. Flammulinolide-C (**4**) exerted the cytotoxicity against human HeLa (cervix) and KB (nasopharynx) cancer cell lines, with IC_{50}s of 3.0 and 12.4 μM, respectively, while flammulinolide-E (**5**) and flammulinolide-G (**6**) only displayed moderate to weak inhibitory effect against the proliferation of HeLa cells with IC_{50}s of 25.8 and 59.5 μM, respectively.[32]

6. Ergosterols

A sterol fraction (FVS) from *F. velutipes* consisted of mainly ergosterol (54.78%), 22,23-dihydroergosterol (27.94%), ergost-8(14)-ene-3β-ol, and ergosta-5,8,22-triene-3-ol, ergost-8(14)-ene-3-ol. *In vitro* treatment with FVS by 72 h could obviously restrain the growth of human HepG2 hepatoma, SGC gastric cancer, A549 lung cancer U251 glioma cell lines with respective IC_{50}s of 9.3, 11.99, 20.4, and 23.42 μg/mL, but performed poorly against human LoVo colon (IC_{50} of > 40.0 μg/mL) and HeLa cervix cancer cell lines. To improve the solubility and bioavailability of FVS, the mixed microemulsion formulation and micellar nanoformulation of FVS have been developed. Both prepared liposomes and nanomicelles of FVS showed a significant promising delivery system for enhancing oral bioavailability and selective biodistribution of FVS as compared to the free FVS suspension.[33-35]

CONCLUSION AND SUGGESTION

As described earlier, the anticancer and anticarcinogenic potentials of winter mushroom *F. velutipes* have been demonstrated. The antitumor-related active substances in the mushroom *F. velutipes* are revealed to be two types of chemicals, that is, macromolecules such as polysaccharides, protein-bound polysaccharides, glycoproteins and proteins, and micromolecules such as ergosterols and norsesquiterpenes. These macromolecules as the major bioactive ingredients of *F. velutipes* were reported to have significant functions such as antitumor, antioxidation, enhancing immunity, hepatoprotection, lowering cholesterol, relieving fatigue, improving the memory and antiviral, and so on. However, it is now confirmed that the four types of macromolecules showed antiproliferative and antigrowth effects against a group of cancer cells *in vivo* and/or *in vitro* and their antitumor activities principally involve host-mediated immunopotentiation, though the *F. velutipes* proteins also exerted obvious *in vitro* suppressive effects against the tested liver, breast, lung, and gastric and leukemic neoplastic cell lines concomitant with cell apoptosis promotion. The anticancer activities of *F. velutipes* micromolecules, norsesquiterpenes and sterols, were observed in the *in vitro* assays against some human solid tumor cell lines with moderate to weak degrees. Overall, the winter mushroom (enokitake) has great development potential to be used in the fields of food and medicine. The consumption of the mushroom *F. velutipes* is recommended as a safe and helpful dietary supplement for cancer prevention and cancer therapies.

REFERENCES

1. Stamets, P.E., 2005. Notes on nutritional properties of culinary-medicinal mushrooms. *Int. J. Med. Mushrooms* 7(1/2): 103–110.
2. Bao, H.N. et al., 2010. Antioxidative activities of hydrophilic extracts prepared from the fruiting body and spent culture medium of Flammulina velutipes. *Bioresour Technol.* 101(15): 6248–6255.
3. Kohama, H. et al., 2003. Antitumor activity of extract of edible mushrooms (EEM), Flammulina velutipes and Hypsizigus marmoreus in mice. *Oyo Yakuri* 65: 73–77.
4. Ou, H.T. et al., 2005. The antiproliferative and differentiating effects of human leukemic U937 cells are mediated by cytokines from activated mononuclear cells by dietary mushrooms. *J. Agricul. Food Chem.* 53: 300–305.
5. Gu, Y.H. et al., 2006. In vitro effects on proliferation, apoptosis and colony inhibition in ER-dependent and ER-independent human breast cancer cells by selected mushroom species. *Oncol. Reports* 15: 417–423.
6. Yu, J.N. et al., 2013. Unsaponifiable extract from Flammulina velutipes with antitumor effect and its application. *Faming Zhuanli Shenqing* CN 103054908 A 20130424.
7. Jiang, S.M. et al., 1999. Inhibitory activity of polysaccharide extracts from three kinds of edible fungi on prolife-ration of human hepatoma SMMC-7721 cell and mouse implanted S180 tumor. *World J. Gastroenterol.* 5: 404–407.
8. Zeng, Q.T. et al., 1991. *Zhongguo shiyong Zhenjun* 10: 11; 1999. Chinese Materia Medica Vol. 1, Published by Shanghai Science Technology Express, 1-0242, pp. 570.
9. Mizuno, M. et al., 2001. Contents of antitumor polysaccharides in certain mushrooms and their immunomodulating activities. *Food Sci. Technol. Res.* 7: 31–34.
10. Zou, Y.X. et al., 2013. Effect of purification processing on antitumor activity of polysaccharides from Flammulina velutipes in vitro. *Zhongguo Shipin Xuebao* 13: 9–14.
11. Zhao, C. et al., 2013. In vitro antioxidant and antitumor activities of polysaccharides extracted from the mycelia of liquid-cultured Flammulina velutipes. *Food Sci. Technol. Res.* 19: 661–667.
12. Cao, P.R. et al., 1989. Isolation and characterization of polysaccharide PA5DE from the fruiting bodies of Flammulina velutipes (Curt. ex Fr.) Sing. *Shengwu Huaxue Zazhi* 6: 176–180.
13. Cao, P.R. et al, 1989. Isolation, purification and analysis of a polysaccharide PA3DE from the fruit bodies of Flammulina velutipes (Curt. ex Fr.) Sing. *Shengwu Huaxue yu Shengwu Wuli Xuebao* 21: 152–156.
14. Ikekawa, T et al., 1982. Studies on antitumor polysaccharides of Flammulina velutipes (Curt. ex Fr.) Sing. II. The structure of EA3 and further purification of EA5. *J. Pharmaco-biodynamics* 5: 576–581.

15. Leung, M.Y.K. et al., 1997. The isolation and characterization of an immunomodulatory and antitumor polysaccharide preparation from Flammulina elutipes. *Immunopharmacology* 35: 255–563.
16. Chang, H.L. et al., 2009. Effect of Flammulina velutipes polysaccharides on production of cytokines by murine immunocytes and serum levels of cytokines in tumor-bearing mice. *Zhongyaocai* 32(4): 561–563.
17. Maruyama, H. et al., 2005. Combination therapy of transplanted meth-A fibrosarcoma in BALB/c mice with protein-bound polysaccharide EA6 isolated from enokitake mushroom Flammulina velutipes (W.Curt.:Fr.) singer and surgical excision. *Intl. J. Med. Mushrooms* 7: 213–220.
18. Ohkuma, T. et al., 1983. Augmentation of host's immunity by combined cryodestruction of sarcoma 180 and administration of protein-bound polysaccharide, EA6, isolated from Flammulina velutipes (Curt. ex Fr.) Sing. in ICR mice. *J. Pharmacobiodynamics* 6: 88–95.
19. Ohkuma, T. et al., 1982. Augmentation of antitumor activity by combined cryodestruction of sarcoma 180 and protein-bound polysaccharide, EA6, isolated from Flammulina velutipes (Curt. ex Fr.) Sing in ICR mice. *J. Pharmacobiodynamics* 5: 439–444.
20. Maruyama, H. et al., 2007. Immunomodulation and antitumor activity of a mushroom product, pro-flamin, isolated from Flammulina velutipes (W. Curt.: Fr.) Singer. *Int. J. Medicinal Mushrooms* 9: 109–122.
21. Otagiri, K. et al., 1983. Intensification of antitumor-immunity by protein-bound polysaccharide, EA6, derived from Flammulina velutipes (Curt. ex Fr.) Sing. combined with murine leukemia L1210 vaccine in animal experiments. *J. Pharmacobiodynamics* 6: 96–104.
22. Zhao, S. et al., 2013. Flammulina velutipes protein extracts and antitumor applications thereof. *Faming Zhuanli Shenqing* CN 103272214 A 20130904.
23. Fu, M.J. et al., 2005. Change in protein content of Flammulina velutipes and biological activities of one protein. *Yingyong Yu Huanjing Shengwu Xuebao* 11: 40–44.
24. Zhou, K.S. et al., 2003. A new method of separation and bioactivity assay of flammulin. *Zhongguo Shengwu Huaxue yu Fenzi Shengwu Xuebao* 19: 234–239.
25. Zhou, K.S. et al., 2003. Purification and crystallization of flammulin, a basic protein with antitumor activities from Flammulina velutipes. *Chin. Chem. Lett.* 14: 713–716.
26. Chang, H.H. et al., 2010. Oral administration of an Enoki mushroom protein FVE activates innate and adaptive immunity and induces antitumor activity against murine hepatocellular carcinoma. *Intl. Immunopharmacol.* 10: 239–246.
27. Chang, Y.C. et al., 2013. Interruption of lung cancer cell migration and proliferation by fungal immuno-modulatory protein FIP-fve from Flammulina velutipes. *J. Agric. Food Chem.* 61(49): 12044–12052.
28. Ng., T.B. et al., 2006. An agglutinin with mitogenic and antiproliferative activities from the mushroom *Flammulina velutipes. Mycologia* 98(2): 167–171.
29. Ikekawa, T. et al., 1985. Proflamin, a new antitumor agent: preparation, physicochemical properties and antitumor activity. *Jpn J. Cancer Res.* 76: 142–148.
30. Maruyama, H. et al., 2005. Antitumor effect of combination therapy of proflamin with cryosurgery with cryosurgery of Meth-A fibrosarcoma in BALB/c mice. *Intl. J. Med. Mushrooms* 7: 539–545.
31. Liu, Y. et al., 1998. Antitumor activity and effect on immunocompetence of Flammulina velutipes mycelia glycoprotein. *Zhongguo Shenghua Yaowu Zazhi* 19: 369–371.
32. Wang, Y.Q., et al., 2012. Two new sesquiterpenes and six norsesquiterpenes from the solid culture of the edible mushroom Flammulina velutipes. *Tetrahedron* 68: 3012–3018.
33. Yi, C.X. et al., 2013. Cytotoxic effect of novel Flammulina velutipes sterols and its oral bioavailability via mixed micellar nanoformulation. *Intl. J. Pharm* (Amsterdam, Netherlands). 448: 44–50.
34. Yi, C.X. et al., 2013. Enhanced oral bioavailability and tissue distribution of a new potential anticancer agent, Flammulina velutipes sterols, through liposomal encapsulation. *J. Agric. Food Chem.* 61(25): 5961–5971.
35. Yi, C.X. et al., 2012. Enhanced oral bioavailability of a sterol-loaded microemulsion formulation of Flammulina velutipes, a potential antitumor drug. *Int. J. Nanomed.* 7: 5067–5078.

9 Cancer-Preventive Substances in Seaweeds

74. Alga Gloiopeltidis/*Gloiopeltis furcata, G. tenax*

75. Chipolata Weed/*Scytosiphon lomentarius*

76. Dried Moss of Enteromorphites or Hutai/*Enteromorpha prolifera, E. clathrata*

77. Hijiki/*Sargassum fusiforme*

78. Kelp/*Laminaria japonica, L. angustata, L. angustata* var. *longissima*

79. Kurome/*Ecklonia kurome*

80. Laver or Nori/*Porphyra haitanensis, P. yezoensis, P. tenera, P. umbilicalis*

81. Sea Mustard/*Undaria pinnatifida*

82. Umitoranoo/*Sargassum thunbergii*

Seaweeds have a variety of purposes. Some are consumed as a kind of food by coastal population (especially in East and Southeast Asia) and some are used as materials for food additives and food/emollient-related products. Seaweeds are chock-full of vitamins, minerals (iodine, calcium, zinc, magnesium, iron, and selenium), fibers, omega-3 fatty acids (DHA and EPA), and odd types of carbohydrates. Some possess anti-inflammatory, antioxidant, and antimicrobial properties. Some cancer-fighting agents isolated from seaweeds elicit a desire for their application in the treatment of malignant tumors. This chapter primarily discusses the potential of edible seaweeds/marine algae in both cancer prevention and health improvement, and covers the bioactive components involved in anticancer, anticarcinogenic, antimutagenic, anti-angiogenic, and immunostimulating activities of seaweeds. Although, some isolated constituents with small molecules exert certain inhibitory effect against the proliferation of cancer cells, and the macromolecules such as polysaccharides, sulfated polysaccharides, sulfated protein polysaccharides, and glycoproteins largely contribute to the cancer-inhibitory effects of the seaweeds.

This chapter introduces nine kinds of seaweeds for their positive health benefits in anticarcinogenesis and body protection. Six of them are largely popular in East and Southeast Asia. Impressively, nori is consumed every day and at every meal by all Japanese families and is used to make cookies and sushi to improve overall health. In addition, consumption of other seaweeds such as dulse and arame may also contribute to lowering cancer risk and improving health. Owing to the high level of iodine in the seaweeds, intake of seaweed is best limited and served with foods such as cruciferous vegetables and/or soybean products to avoid thyroid problems from excess iodine.

74. ALGA GLOIOPELTIDIS

海蘿

Gloiopeltis furcata, G. tenax

Endocladiaceae

Alga Gloiopeltidis, or *Gloiopeltis furcata* and *G. tenax* (Endocladiaceae), is the dried edible red–brown seaweed. The two species of Gloiopeltis are distributed only in the North Pacific Ocean, that is, broadly being grown along the shorelines of China, Taiwan, Korea, Japan, and far east of Russia, as well as from the Aleutian Islands south to Baja California. The seaweeds have long been utilized as a healthy food source in Eastern Asia. Modern pharmacological studies revealed that the seaweed extracts are able to significantly lower the glucose level in the blood and inhibit the growth of several human cancer cell lines.

SCIENTIFIC EVIDENCE OF CANCER-INHIBITORY AND CANCER-PREVENTIVE CONSTITUENTS

Pharmacological evidences have proven that *G. furcata* possesses potential antineoplastic activity. Its methanolic extract inhibits the growth of several human carcinoma cell lines *in vitro*. For instance, the extract markedly reduced the viability of human HepG2 hepatoma cells and arrested cell cycle at the G2/M phase in a concentration-dependent manner together with an increase in cyclin-dependent kinase (Cdk) inhibitor p21 activity, downregulation of cyclin-A and COX-2 expressions, and dephosphorylation of Cdc25C. The IC_{50}s were 35.7 and 38.2 µg/mL in KB (oral epidermoid) and HT-29 (colon) cancer cells for its methanol extract, 39.3 and 12.2 µg/mL in KB and HT-29 cells for its ethyl acetate extract, respectively, and 11.8 µg/mL in KB cells for its ethanol extract.[1–3] Two compounds isolated from the seaweed were identified as zeaxanthin (**1**) and fucosterol. In an *in vitro* assay, zeaxanthin (**1**) showed moderate cytotoxicity in human KB (oral) and Bel-7402 (liver) cancer cell lines with IC_{50}s of 8.31 and 7.06 µg/mL, respectively, but had no such effect in A549 lung cancer cells and HELF normal cells, whereas fucosterol had no activity in all the tested cell lines.[2] Moreover, a sulfated polysaccharide prepared from *G. furcata* displayed antitumor activity *in vitro* against the proliferation of MKN45 (gastric) and DLD (intestinal) cancer cell lines and antioxidant activity in superoxide radical assay, ABTS assay, and DPPH assay.[4]

Funoran, a polysaccharide purified from *G. tenax*, exerted significant suppressive effect against the growth of Ehrlich ascites and solid tumors, Meth-A fibrosarcoma and sarcoma 180. When intraperitoneal (i.p.) injection is given to tumor-bearing mice, funoran augmented the spleen weight of mice and improved the transformation from lymphocytes to plasma cells in the spleen. Concurrently, percentages of L3T4+ and Lyt2+ T-cells were markedly increased in the peripheral blood, and the percentages of asialo CM1+ cells in thymus and peripheral blood were significantly amplified. The results clearly revealed that the antineoplastic effect of funoran is closely attributed to its immuno-potentiating properties such as an increase in T-helper, T-cytotoxic, and NK cells.[5]

CONCLUSION AND SUGGESTION

These evidences conferred scientific support for the consumption of Alga Gloiopeltidis as a healthy food. The edible red–brown seaweed was demonstrated to possess antitumor, antioxidant, and immunoenhancing properties. Some extracts with small molecules mainly exerted antiproliferative activity against several types of cancer cells, whereas the polysaccharide extract showed immuno-regulative and *in vivo* antitumor properties. The isolated sulfated polysaccharide was found to be responsible for both antitumor and antioxidant activities. Although the cancer-inhibitory potencies ranged from moderate to weak, dietary Alga Gloiopeltidis should be a good choice for lessening the risk of cancer safely.

REFERENCES

1. Bae, B.J. et al., 2007. Methanol extract of the seaweed Gloiopeltis furcata induces G2/M arrest and inhibits cyclooxygenase-2 activity in human hepato-carcinoma HepG2 cells. *Phytother. Res.* 21: 52–57.
2. Xu, N.J. et al., 2004. Screening marine algae from China for their antitumor activities. *J. Applied Phycol.* 16: 451–456.
3. Xu, N.J. et al., 2001. Screening marine algae from Shandong coast for antitumor activity. *Haiyang Yu Huzhao* 32: 408–413.
4. Shao, P. et al., 2013. In vitro antioxidant and antitumor activities of different sulfated polysaccharides isolated from three algae. *Intl. J. Biol. Macromol.* 62: 155–161.
5. Ren, D.L. et al., 1995. The effects of an algal polysaccharide from Gloiopeltis tenax on transplantable tumors and immune activities in mice. *Planta Med.* 61: 120–125.

75. CHIPOLATA WEED

萱藻

Scytosiphon lomentarius

Scytosiphonaceae

1

Chipolata weed, or *Scytosiphon lomentarius*, is the dried Scytosiphonaceae algae. This species is widely found in temperate waters around the world, the seaweed of which has an olive brown color and generally grows on shells and stones in rock pools and in near-shore waters. The edible seaweed is a source of health food, forage, and folk medicine. Chipolata weed is rich in amino acids, wherein the content of aspartic acid and glutamic acid is more than 20% of the total amino acids, and the content of arginine and histidine is higher. Pharmacological approaches proved that the algae extract can markedly augment cardiac coronary flow and the contained fucosterol exerted estrogen-like action and cholesterol-lowering activity.

SCIENTIFIC EVIDENCE OF CANCER-INHIBITORY AND CANCER-PREVENTIVE ACTIVITIES

The brown algae Scytosiphon showed significant antigrowth activity against Ehrlich cancer with an inhibitory rate of 69.8%. Its extract displayed appreciable suppressive activity on Meth-A fibrosarcoma in mice and cytotoxic effect on human KB (oral epidermoid), HT-29 (colon), Bel-7402 (liver), and A549 (lung) neoplastic cell lines *in vitro*.[1,2] Its ethanol extract exhibited the most potent inhibitory effects on the KB and HT-29 cells with IC_{50}s of 12.6 and 1.49 µg/mL, respectively, compared to its methanol extract (IC_{50}s of 32.3–45.3 µg/mL). However, the two extracts were also effective in hindering human normal NIH-3T3 cells (IC_{50}s of 35.3–48.7 µg/mL).[2] Treatment with the methanolic extract in human A549 (lung) and (HL-60 leukemic) cancer cell lines received cell growth inhibitory rates of over 80%.[3] The ethanolic extract of chipolata weed exhibited marked selective cytotoxicity on KB nasopharynx cancer cells (LD_{50} < 4.40 µg/mL) and HT-29 colon cancer cells (LD_{50} 1.49 µg/mL) *in vitro*.[4] Zeaxanthin (1) and fucosterol were the two compounds reported from the isolation of *S. lomentarius* and *Gloiopeltis furcata*. Zeaxanthin (1) was shown as a cancer inhibitor against Bel-7402 (liver) and KB (oral) human cancer cell lines (IC_{50}s of 7.06–8.31 µg/mL).[2]

Treatment of human HL-60 leukemia cells with an ethyl acetate (EtOAc) fraction derived from chipolata weed appeared to have remarkable apoptotic characteristics such as DNA fragmentation, chromatin condensation, and an increase in the population of sub-G1 hypodiploid cells. During the apoptosis provoked by the EtOAc fraction, c-myc and Bcl-2 expressions were reduced, and Bax and caspase-3 activation were augmented followed by the cleavage of poly(ADP-ribose) polymerase to 85 kDa. These interactions might importantly reflect the antitumor mechanism on the HL-60 cells treated by the EtOAc fraction.[5,6]

OTHER BIOACTIVITIES

In biological studies, the extract of algae Scytosiphon demonstrated the activities in inducing the differentiation and promoting the proliferation of osteoblasts, leading to the development of bone formation. Fucoxanthin is one of the bioactive constituents in chipolata weed, possessing anti-inflammation and antioxidant activity.[7]

Conclusion and Suggestion

Chipolata weed is one of the popular seaweeds in the littoral areas of Eastern Asia. Despite that it has not yet been commercialized, the chemical biology studies suggested that chipolata weed has a developing potential as a healthy and economic food for nutrition supplement and cancer prevention. The seaweed extract was recommended by a Korean patent to be prepared for preventing and treating carcinomas such as leukemia, gastric cancer, breast cancer, colon cancer, lung cancer, ovarian cancer, and so on.[8] Up to now, only one cancer inhibitor assigned as zeaxanthin was isolated from both seaweeds *Scytosiphon lomentarius* and *Gloiopeltis furcata*. However, their extracts showed more potential in cancer prevention.

REFERENCES

1. Noda, H. et al., 1990. Antitumor activity of marine algae. *Hydrobiologia* 204–205: 577–584.
2. Xu, N.J. et al., 2004. Screening marine algae from China for their antitumor activities. *J. Applied Phycol.* 16: 451–456.
3. Niu, R.L. et al., 2003. Anticancer and antibacterial activities of methanol extracts from Chinese algae. *Zhongguo Haiyang Yaowu* 22: 1–4.
4. Xu, N.J. et al., 2001. Screening marine algae from Shandong coast for antitumor activity. *Oceanologia et Limnologia Sinica* 32: 408–413.
5. Kim, S.C. et al., 2004. The Cytotoxicity of Scytosiphon lomentaria against HL-60 promyelocytic leukemia cells. *Cancer Biother. Radio-pharm.* 19: 641–648.
6. Hyun, J.H. et al., 2005. Pharmaceutical composition preventing and treating cancer and HL-60 leukemia cell containing scytosiphon lomentaria extract. Repub. Korean Kongkae Taeho Kongbo KR 2003-79494 20031111.
7. Park, M.H. et al., 2016. Effects of Scytosiphon lomentaria on osteoblastic proliferation and differentiation of MC3T3-E1 cells. *Nutr. Res Pract.* 10: 148–153.
8. Hyun, J.H. et al., 2005. A Scytosiphon lomentaria extract having cancer preventing and treating effects. Repub. Korean Kongkae Taeho Kongbo KR 2005045429 A 20050517.

76. DRIED MOSS OF ENTEROMORPHITES OR HUTAI

浒苔　スジ青のり

Enteromorpha prolifera, E. clathrata

Ulvaceae

Hutai, or *Enteromorpha prolifera*, *E. clathrata*, and others, is the simplest name to call the dried moss of Enteromorphites, which generally originated from the green seaweeds of the same genus (Ulvaceae). These green algae were extensively distributed along seashores around the world. Hutai is rich in proteins, iron, and calcium and other nutrients and trace minerals. Dietary hutai can decrease the total amount of cholesterol in serum. In addition, the green algae are a common source of free fertilizer in the coastal areas, in addition to a healthy food supplement.

SCIENTIFIC EVIDENCE OF CANCER-INHIBITORY AND CANCER-PREVENTIVE CONSTITUENTS

In vivo experiments with mouse models exhibited that the green seaweeds (*E. prolifera*) markedly restrained the growth of Ehrlich carcinoma cells by 51.7% and potently suppressed 7,12-dimethylbenz[a]anthracene-initiated and TPA-promoted mouse skin tumorigenesis.[1–4] The methanolic extract of *E. prolifera* exerted obvious antimutagenic effect against the induction of TPA-dependent ornithine decarboxylase in BALB/c 3T3 fibroblast cells and mutagen-induced umu C gene expression in *Salmonella typhimurium*, indicating the antimutagenic and anticarcinogenic activities.[5] The ethanolic extract prepared from *E. clathrata* showed selective cytotoxicity against transformed mouse embryonic fibroblast 3T3 cells (SV-T2). Two fractions showing anticancer properties, one holding a higher molecular weight and another one having a low molecular weight (around 500 Da), were reported in the isolation of the ethanolic extract.[6]

1. Pheophytin-a

Hutai is rich in a chlorophyll-related compound assigned as pheophytin-a (**1**), which was partially responsible in the *in vivo* antigenotoxic and anticarcinogenic effects of hutai. Pheophytin-a (**1**) could potently hamper the initiation and promotion phases of chemical-induced mouse skin tumorigenesis.[2] Pheophytin-a was also shown to have a certain level of antioxidant activity in a test with the 2,2-diphenyl-1-picrylhydrazyl (DPPH) method.[7]

2. Peptides

Three peptides with low molecular weight were prepared from pepsin hydrolysates of the seaweed (*E. prolifera*). Peak-1 peptide and peak-3 peptide demonstrated the inhibitory activity on the proliferation of cancer cells, whereas peak-2 and peak-3 peptides exerted anti-tyrosinase effect.[8]

3. Polysaccharides

Several polysaccharide components were extracted with cold, hot, and acidic water from hutai (*E. clathrata*). Photoimmobilized phycocyanin obtained from *E. clathrata* effectively repressed the growth of SW1990 pancreatic cancer cells *in vitro*.[9] The polysaccharides from *E. prolifera* inhibited the growth of hepatoma in mice by 49.1% and 53.1% at doses of 400 and 800 mg/kg, respectively, together with an increase of IL-2 and decreases in TGF-β and VEGF. The *in vivo* antihepatoma activity was superior to an antitumor agent 5-FU, the inhibitory rate of which was 21.2%.[10] ESR1-2 and ESR2-2 are the two antitumor polysaccharides that were separated from water-extracted crude polysaccharides and NaOH-extracted polysaccharides of hutai, respectively. Both could retard the proliferation of human HL-60 leukemia cells, where EPS1-2 has better activity than EPS2-2.[11] In addition, the polysaccharides from *E. prolifera* displayed the hydroxyl radical-scavenging capacity and protective effects against injury of rat adrenal pheochromocytoma PC12 cells induced by H_2O_2 at concentrations of 100, 200, and 300 μg/mL.[11,12]

Moreover, from a hot water extract of a closely related green algae *E. intestinalis*, two polysaccharides, WEA and WEB, were isolated. WEA (72.03 kDa) consisted of rhamnose, xylose, mannose, and glucose in a molar ratio of 1.39:1.00:0.13:3.23, and WEB (60.12 kDa) comprised rhamnose, xylose, galactose, and glucuronic acid in a molar ratio of 7.32:1.00:0.51:1.28. Both the polysaccharides had no direct *in vivo* cytotoxicity on sarcoma 180 but enhanced the immune system remarkably via stimulated lymphocyte proliferation and macrophages, promoted TNF-α expression in serum, and enlarged spleen and thymus weights, thereby exerting immunoenhancement to obstruct the growth of sarcoma 180 in tumor-burdened mice.[13]

CONCLUSION AND SUGGESTION

Based on the scientific findings, it is clear that its two types of bioactive components, pheophytin-a (1) and polysaccharides, primarily contributed the antitumor and anticarcinogenic properties of hutai. Impressively, *E. prolifera* polysaccharides demonstrated much better *in vivo* antihepatoma effect than a chemotherapeutic drug 5-fluorouracil (5-FU), cancer suppressive effect of the polysaccharides was revealed to be also correlating with the immunoenhancing and angiogenesis-hindering activities. In addition, the hydroxyl radical-scavenging capacity of the polysaccharides might be helpful in brain protection. Therefore, these experimental results provided a suggestion for the application and development of a safe and feasible diet of hutai in cancer prevention and immunity stimulation.

REFERENCES

1. Noda, H. et al., 1990. Antitumor activity of marine algae. *Hydrobiologia* 204–205: 577–84.
2. Kiyota, H.O. et al., 1999. Potent suppressive effect of a Japanese edible seaweed, Enteromorpha prolifera (Sujiao-nori) on initiation and promotion phases of chemically induced mouse skin tumorigenesis. *Cancer Lett.* 140: 21–25.
3. Okai, Y. et al., 1994. Suppressive effects of the extracts of Japanese edible seaweeds on mutagen-induced umu C gene expression in Salmonella typhimurium (TA 1535/pSK 1002) and tumor promotor-dependent ornithine decarboxylase induction in BALB/c 3T3 fibroblast cells. *Cancer Lett.* 87: 25–32.
4. Okai, Y. et al., 1997. Pheophytin a is a potent suppressor against genotoxin-induced umu C gene expression in Salmonella typhimurium (TA 1535/pSK 1002). *J. Sci. Food Agric.* 74: 531–535.
5. Okai, Y. e al., 1994. Suppressive effects of the extracts of Japanese edible seaweeds on mutagen-induced umu C gene expression in Salmonella typhimurium (TA 1535/pSK 1002) and tumor promotor-dependent ornithine decarboxylase induction in BALB/c 3T3 fibroblast cells. *Cancer Lett.* 87: 25–32.
6. Tang, H.J. et al., 2004. Anti-tumorigenic components of seaweed, Enteromorpha clathrata. *BioFactors* 22: 107–110.
7. Lai, K. et al., 2015. Identification, isolation and antioxidant activity of pheophytin from green tea (Camellia Sinensis Kuntze). *Procedia Chem.* 14: 232–238.

8. Lee, J.M. et al., 2005. Functional activities of low molecular weight peptides purified from enzymatic hydrolysates of seaweeds. *Han'guk Sikp'um Yongyang Kwahak Hoechi* 34: 1124–1129.
9. Guan, Y.Q. et al., 2002. Isolation, purification and antitumor activities of polysaccharides from Enteromorpha clathrata Grev. *J. Funct. Polym.* 15: 19–23.
10. Lin, W.T. et al., 2011. Inhibitory effect of Enteromorpha prolifera polysaccharide on tumor-bearing mice. *Zhongguo Gonggong Weisheng* 27: 457–458.
11. Tian, H. et al., 2013. Extraction and bioactivity of polysaccharides from Enteromorpha prolifera. *Shipin Keji* 38: 205–209.
12. Shi, D.H. et al., 2012. Protective effects of polysaccharides from Enteromorpha prolifera on the PC12 cells injury induced by H_2O_2. *Zhongguo Shenghua Yaowu Zazhi* 33: 40–42.
13. Jiao, L.L. et al., 2010. Antitumor and immunomodulating activity of polysaccharides from Enteromorpha intestinalis. *Biotechnol. Bioprocess Eng.* 15: 421–428.

77. HIJIKI

羊栖菜 ヒジキ 녹미채

Sargassum fusiforme

Sargassaceae

Hijiki is a Japanese name for the dried brown seaweed *Sargassum fusiforme* (Sargassaceae), which is one of the most commonly consumed healthy seafood vegetables in Japan due to its richness in dietary fiber and essential minerals (such as calcium, iron, and magnesium). Hijiki was also reported to have multiple biological functions such as immuno regulating, hypotensive, anticoagulant, hypolipemic, antifatigue, organism-protecting, anti-infection, and antiviral effects. Since the 1960s, hijiki has spread broadly to western countries being available at natural food stores and oriental culinarians.

SCIENTIFIC EVIDENCE OF CANCER-INHIBITORY AND CANCER-PREVENTIVE CONSTITUENTS

Although the methanolic extract of hijiki has no *in vitro* inhibitory effect on human KB (oral) and HT-29 (colon) cancer cell lines,[1] its polysaccharide components have been reported to be responsible for both *in vitro* and *in vivo* anticancer activities of hijiki.

1. Sulfate protein-polysaccharides

Sulfate protein-polysaccharides (SFPS) prepared from hijiki demonstrated significant antitumor effect and marked survival prolongation of mice-borne cancer *in vivo* against sarcoma 180 (S180), Ehrlich ascites carcinoma (EAC), and reticulocytic leukemia (L615). The SFPS treatment also resisted thymus and adrenal gland atrophy in mice caused by vaccination of cancer cells and obviously enhanced erythrocyte immune function in mice-inoculated S180, EAC, or L615 leukemia. The results evidenced that SFPS plays an important role in immunopotentiation for the antitumor effect. Similarly, in L615 leukemia-implanted mice, SFPS remarkably attenuated the content of lipoid peroxide and amplified the activities of catalase and superoxide dismutase in whole blood, liver, and spleen, suggesting that free-radical scavenging and lipid peroxidation-eliminating effects are the important action in the antileukemia mechanisms of SFPS against L615 tumor.[2–4]

Moreover, SFPS also displayed *in vitro* inhibitory effect on nine kinds of human cancer cell lines, such as HepG2 and Bel-7405 (liver), cc801 (cervix), MCF-7 (breast), Colo205 (rectum), LoVo (colorectal), SGC-7901 (stomach), HL-60 (leukemic), Eca109 (esophagus), DU-145 (prostate), and SPC-A1 (liver) cells, of which, the most obvious results were observed in SGC-7901 and Colo205 cell lines.[4–15] The anticancer activities in the SCG-7901 and Colo205 cells were found to be accompanied with an increase in intracellular calcium level and induction of cell apoptosis and G0/G1 cell arrest.[5–9] By the activation of caspases-3 and -9, SFPS provoked the apoptosis of LoVo cells and then retarded the proliferation of LoVo cells moderately (IC_{50} of 60 μg/mL, in 72 h).[11–13]

An acidic sulfate protein-polysaccharide (SFPP) with molecular weight of 13,000 and a composition of mannuronic acid and glucuronic acid was isolated from the hot water extract of hijiki. In the *in vivo* models, SFPP prominently lengthened the life span of mice-implanted murine ascetes sarcoma 180 by 63.44%.[16] SFP2 is a similar type of polysaccharide, which could markedly increase the weight index of thymus and spleen and obviously enhance the activity of NK cells and the function of macrophages *in vivo*, showing remarkable immunoenhancing function.[17]

2. Polysaccharides

From *S. fusiforme*, a polysaccharide component was isolated by hot water extraction and ethanol preparation. These polysaccharides not only noticeably inhibited the growth of human A549 lung adenocarcinoma cells *in vivo* and *in vitro*, but also markedly promoted immune responses, such as enhancement of splenocyte proliferation, IL-1 and TNF-α production from peritoneal macrophage, and serum TNF-α level in mice bearing A549 carcinoma.[18] The polysaccharides also acted as a PI3K inhibitor to protect pancreatic beta cells against H_2O_2 injury and to enhance SOD activity.[19] SFPS-B2, a polysaccharide fraction isolated from the seaweed, exhibited antiproliferative and proapoptotic effects against human SGC-7901 gastric cancer cells *in vitro*, proapoptosis of which was mediated by a mitochondrial-mediated pathway.[20] An isolated fraction 04S2P was structurally composed of β-D-mannuronic acid residues and α-L-glucuronic acid residues with a ratio of 9:1. Two sulfated polysaccharides 04S2P-S and Alg–S were separated from 04S2P. In the *in vitro* assay, Alg–S showed marked antiproliferative effects on human SMMC7721 and Bel-7402 (liver) and HT-29 (colon) cancer cell lines, whereas 04S2P-S showed antitumor effect only in the Bel-7402 cells.[21] Besides, Alg–S obviously restrained the angiogenesis of human microvascular endothelial cells (HMEC-1).

Similarly, a fucoidan termed FP08S2 was isolated from the boiling water extract of *S. fusiforme*, which consisted of fucose, xylose, galactose, mannose (Man), glucuronic acid (GlcA), and 20.8% sulfate, and the sulfate groups attached to diverse positions of the first four sugar residues, the backbone of which was composed of alternate 1,2-linked α-D-Man and 1,4-linked β-D-GlcA. FP08S2 could significantly inhibit tube formation and migration of HMEC-1 cells in a dose-dependent manner, indicating its antiangiogenic property.[22] Two polysaccharides DEI and DEII were purified from a hijiki-like seaweed *S. pallidum*, contents of total sugar (including xylose, fucoidan, galactose, fructose, mannose, and the glucose) of which in DEI and DEII were 52.40% and 38.8%, respectively, and the fucoidan was the major component in the polysaccharides. In an *in vitro* assay, DEI and DEII exerted the inhibitory activities against a murine P388 leukemia cell line.[23]

CONCLUSION AND SUGGESTION

Hijiki as the most popular seaweed in the Japanese diet was discovered richly to comprise proteins and polysaccharides. Prominently, the sulfate protein-polysaccharides (SFPP) and polysaccharides derived from the fractionation of hijiki demonstrated to be in charge of the anticancer properties of hijiki. Although showing moderate-to-weak degrees of inhibitory activity on human cancer cell lines *in vitro*, more *in vivo* findings suggested that the anticancer activity is contributed by the remarkable abilities in enhancing the immune responses and repressing oxidation. These findings revealed that intake of hijiki would potentiate human immune defense and subsequently exert cancer prevention.

However, recent investigations found hijiki also containing potentially toxic quantities of inorganic arsenic. Thus, due to food safety, the frequency and quantity of hijiki consumption should be limited. The food safety agencies of major western countries have informed against its consumption but such results do not influence the dietary habits in Japan.

REFERENCES

1. Xu, N.J. et al., 2004. Screening marine algae from China for their antitumor activities. *J. Applied Phycol.* 16: 451–456.
2. Ji, Y.B. et al., 1995. Effects of SFPS on erythrocytic immune function in mice inoculated with tumor. *Zhongguo Haiyang Yaowu* 14: 10–14.
3. Ji, Y.B. et al., 1994. An experimental study of the anticancer effect of compound herbal polysaccharide preparation. *Zhongguo Haiyang Yaowu* 13: 20–24.
4. Ji, Y.B. et al., 1994. Effects of SFPS on contents of LPO and enzyme activities of GR, GSH-PX, CAT and SOD in mice with leukemia L615. *Zhongguo Haiyang Yaowu* 13: 20–23.
5. Ji, Y.B. et al., 2005. Antitumor effects and mechanism of Sargassum fusiforme polysaccharide in vitro. *Zhongguo Linchuang Kangfu* 9:190–192.
6. Ji, Y.B. et al., 2003. Studies on antitumor activities and apoptosis induction of Sargassum fusiforme polysaccharide *in vitro*. *Zhongcaoyao* 34: 638–640.

7. Ji, Y.B. et al., 2003. Studies on antitumor activities of Sargassum fusiforme polysaccharide in vitro and its mechanism. *Zhongcaoyao* 34:1111–1114.

8. Ji, Y.B. et al., 2004. Influence of Sargassum fusiforme polysaccharide on apoptosis of tumor cells. *Zhongguo Zhongyao Zazhi* 29: 245–247.

9. Ji, Y.B. et al., 2004. Studies on antitumor activities of Sargassum fusiforme polysaccharide (SFPS) and its mechanism. *Zhongguo Haiyang Yaowu* 23: 7–10.

10. Yan, L.L. et al., 2006. Apoptosis in Lovo cells induced by SFPS was associated with an activation of caspase-3 mediated by caspase-9. *Xibao Shengwuxue Zazhi* 28: 193–200.

11. Zhang, R. et al., 2006. Study on the isolation, purification and component property of fucoidan from Sargassum fusiforme. *Zhongguo Shipin Xuebao* 6: 22–27.

12. Yan, L.L. et al., 2005. Study on the apoptosis and its mechanism in Lovo human colorectal cancer cells induced by SFPS. *Shiyan Shengwu Xuebao* 38: 447–455.

13. Zhang, H.F. et al., 2006. Apoptosis in tumour cells induced by polysaccharides from Sargassum fusiforme. *Shizhen Guoyi Guoyao* 17: 1124–1125.

14. Liang, Q. et al., 2004. Study on the apoptosis of HL-60 human promyeloid leukemia cells induced by SFPS. *Shiyan Shengwu Xuebao* 37: 125–132.

15. Cen, Y.Z. et al., 2005. Preparation of polysaccharides from Sargassum fusiforme and its inhibitory effect on the HepG2 cells. *Zhongguo Haiyang Yaowu* 24: 21–24.

16. Gu, Q.Q. et al., 1998. Studies on the chemical composition and antitumor activity of the acid polysaccharide from alga Sargassum fusiforme. *Nat. Prod. Sci.* 4: 88–90.

17. Yan, Q.N. et al., 2008. Isolation of polysaccharides from Sargassum fusiforme and their immune regulation effects in mice. *Shiyong Yixue Zazhi* 24: 2046–2048.

18. Chen, X.M. et al., 2012. Antitumor and immunomodulatory activity of polysaccharides from Sargassum fusiforme. *Food Chem. Toxicol.* 50: 695–700.

19. Ni, X.F. et al., 2009. Effect of PI3K inhibitor and protection and mechanism of Sargassum fusiforme polysaccharides for pancreatic beta cells. *Zhonghua Zhongyiyao Xuekan* 27: 1506–1058.

20. Ji, Y.B. et al., 2014. Human gastric cancer cell line SGC-7901 apoptosis induced by SFPS-B2 via a mitochondrial-mediated pathway. *Bio-Med. Mater. Eng.* 24: 1141–1147.

21. Cong, Q.F. et al., 2014. Structure and biological activities of an alginate from Sargassum fusiforme, and its sulfated derivative. *Intl. J. Biol. Macromol.* 69: 252–259.

22. Cong, Q.F. et al., 2016. Structural characterization and effect on anti-angiogenic activity of a fucoidan from Sargassum fusiforme. *Carbohydr. Polym.* 136, 899–907.

23. Li, J.Q. et al., 2005. Study on isolation, purification, structure and anti-cancer activity of polysaccharides from Sargassum pallidum. *Tianran Chanwu Yanjiu Yu Kaifa* 17: 564–567.

78. KELP

Varech   Seetang   Quelpo

海带   昆布   다시마

Laminaria japonica, L. angustata, L. angustata var. longissima

Laminiariaeae

Kelp, or *Laminaria japonica, L. angustata,* and *L. angustata* var. *longissima*, is a dried large dark brown algae. These seaweeds are beneficial as a healthy food widely in East Asia and have been a folk medicine in China for more than 1700 years. Kelp has been used to treat goiter over long history due to its high concentration of iodine. Now, kelp is an important ingredient used in Eastern Asian cuisines. Nutrition analysis showed that kelp is a rich source of vitamin K and folate and a good source of vitamin B2 and edible minerals (such as magnesium, manganese, calcium, iron, and zinc). A fibrous material called alginate in kelp was found to be good for reducing fat absorption. Pharmacological studies have already proven that kelp possesses extensive biological activities such as antithrombotic, anticoagulant, anti-inflammatory, antioxidant, radioprotective, hypoglycemic, immunopotentiating, hypotensive, hypolipemic, and antibacterial properties.

SCIENTIFIC EVIDENCE OF CANCER-INHIBITORY AND CANCER-PREVENTIVE ACTIVITIES

In mouse models, the brown seaweed *L. japonica* was found to possess appreciable suppressive activity against the growth of Ehrlich carcinoma and Meth-A fibrosarcoma with a 57.6% inhibitory rate on Ehrlich.[1] The hot water extracts prepared from the three sources of kelp exhibited great *in vivo* anti-growth effect against sarcoma 180 cells in a dose of 100 mg/kg per 2 days (i.p.) for 5 times, inhibitions of which were 13.6% for *L. japonica* and 92.3%–94.8% for *L. angustata* and its variety.[2] The kelp derived from *L. angustata* and its variety also showed *in vivo* antileukemia effect on mouse L1210 cells.[3] Dietary kelp could obviously restrain 7,12-dimethylbenz[a]anthracene-induced mammary tumorigenesis and 1,2-dimethylhydrazine-induced intestinal carcinogenesis.[4–6] Its antitumor-promoting activity was testified by an assay of teleocidin B-4-promoted Epstein–Barr virus early antigen induction.[7]

   Moreover, the organic solvent extracts of *L. angustata* in 10–100 mg concentration range greatly suppressed a carcinogen 2′-dimethyl-4-aminobiphenyl-induced mutagenicity in both *Salmonella typhimurium* strains TA98 and TA100 (80%–96% inhibition) and restrained DMBA-caused mutagenic effect in TA100 (about 82%), whereas both hot-water and cold-water extracts exhibited a moderate inhibition on both the strains in a dose-related manner.[8] These experimental studies in murine animal models confirmed the anticarcinogenic and antimutagenic properties of kelp.

Scientific Evidence of Antitumor Constituents and Activities

Diverse chemical components, including proteins, fats, carbohydrates, cellulose, alginic acid and its salts, chlorophylls, phenols, steroids, nucleic acids, and minerals have been determined in the health-beneficial marine algae. Its steroids, polysaccharides, and carotenoids have been reported to exert the suppressive effect toward cancer growth and carcinogenic initiation *in vitro* and/or *in vivo*.

1. Steroids

Two steroidal ketones, ergosta-4,24(28)-diene-3,6-dione (**1**) and stigmasta-4,24(28)-diene-3,6-dione (**2**) isolated from the holdfast of cultivated *L. japonica* demonstrated significant cytotoxic activity on human MCF-7 breast cancer cells *in vitro*. The anti-growth rates in MCF-7 cells were 96% and 79%, respectively, at a concentration of 10 μg/mL.[9]

2. Alkaloids

Bioassay guided separation of the EtOAc extract from *L. japonica* led to the discovery of two antitumor active alkaloids assigned as 6-bromo-1H-indole-3-carbaldehyde (**3**) and 1H-indole-3-carbaldehyde (**4**). Both exhibited moderate cytotoxicity against two human prostate cancer PC-3M and LNCaP cell lines with IC_{50} value ranging between 18 and 35 μM, but there was no cytotoxicity to normal human HEK293 embryonic kidney cells up to 100 μM concentrations.[10] Another isolated alkaloid designated as 2,6-dibromo-4-(2-(methylamino)ethyl)phenol showed only weak cytotoxicity in the assay against PC-3M and LNCaP cell lines (IC_{50}s of 72.5 and 66.1 μM, respectively).[10]

3. Polysaccharides

Polysaccharides as a major anticancer component in kelp could obviously prolong the survival duration of tumor-bearing mice and suppress the growth of EAC, L615 reticulocytic leukemia, and sarcoma 180 in mice.[11] A polysaccharide fraction labeled as FGS, which was derived from the kelp, markedly deterred the proliferation of human SMMC hepatoma and NKM myeloid leukemia cell lines and blocked the incorporation of TdR, UR, and Leu into the two cell lines *in vitro*.[12] *Laminaria japonica* polysaccharides (LJP) displayed obvious antiproliferative effect against human HONE1 and CNE2 nasopharyngeal cancer cell lines (NPC) and stimulated the HONE1 cell apoptosis *in vitro*. In a nude mice model, the significant suppression of the growth of HONE1 xenografts was observed following the administration of LJP in a dose-dependent manner, and the inhibition ratios were 33.7% and 47.0%, respectively, after treatment with 25 mg/kg and 50 mg/kg LJP.[13] The anti-NPC potency of LJP could be potentiated notably when combined with tea polyphenols.[14] I.p. injection of LJP (50, 100, and 150 mg/kg) to mice-implanted H22 hepatoma led to not only tumor growth inhibition but also decrease in the serum vascular endothelial growth factor level together with the elevation of serum IL-2 and TNF-α levels.[15]

A water-soluble crude polysaccharide (WPS) was obtained from *L. japonica* by hot-water extraction. From the WPS, four polysaccharide fractions labeled as WPS-1, WPS-2, WPS-2-1, and WPS-3 were separated. The analyzed data indicated that galactose was the predominant monosaccharide in WPS-3 (54.11%), whereas fucose was predominant in WPS-1 and WPS-2, accounting for 46.91% and 45.1%, respectively.[16] WPS-2-1 (80 kDa) was composed of mannose, rhamnose, and fucose with a molar ratio of 1.0:2.3:1.2 and with a backbone array by (1-4)-glycosidic linkages.[17] *In vitro* assay showed that WPS-1, WPS-2, and WPS-2-1 significantly inhibited the growth of human A375 melanoma cells, and WPS-2-1 also presented marked anti-growth effect against BGC823 gastric cancer cells and augmented the apoptosis of A375 cells via a mitochondrial apoptotic pathway, including downregulation of Bcl-2 expression, loss of mitochondrial membrane, and activation of caspases-3 and -9. Besides, WPS-2 and WPS-2-1 exerted low antiproliferative effect on vascular smooth muscle cells (VSMCs) and significant function of scavenging hydroxyl free radicals, whereas WPS-1 exhibited marked inhibitory effects on superoxide radicals.[17,18]

Sodium alginate (m.w. 112,200) derived from *L. japonica* contains 80.2% sugars without nucleic acid and protein. Na alginate could clearly stimulate lymphocyte transformation, induce red cell agglutination through potentiation of phagocytosis by macrophage, and increase hemolysin content in the serum of mice. These actions resulted in a definite antitumor immunoenhancing effect toward sarcoma 180 in mice.[19]

4. Sulfated polysaccharides

A sulfated polysaccharide (LJSP) prepared from *L. japonica* exhibited marked growth inhibitory and proapoptotic effects on mouse U14 cervical cancer cells *in vitro* and *in vivo* with little toxicological effects on hepatic function and renal function. The treatment concurrently enhanced the indexes of spleen and thymus and enlarged the body weight of U14 tumor-bearing mice.[20] In association with increasing SOD and GPx activities and decrease in MDA level in the tumor cells, LJSP obviously restrained the proliferation of sarcoma 180 cells in mice, implying that the capabilities of LJSP in antioxidant and immunoregulation would help in its anticancer activity.[21,22]

Fucoidan is a sulfated polysaccharide purified from *L. japonica*, which is a highly branched and partially acetylated galactofucan, built up of (1-3)-α-L-fucose residue. *In vitro* experiments showed that the fucoidan distinctly inhibited proliferation and colony formation in human T-47D (breast), AGS (stomach), and SK-MEL-28 (skin) cancer cell lines in a dose-dependent manner.[23,24] The fucoidan treatment could elicit both apoptotic and autophagic cell death of the AGS cells. The apoptosis induced by the fucoidan was mediated by downregulation of Bcl-2 and Bcl-xL expressions, loss of mitochondrial membrane potential, activation of caspases, and degradation of poly(ADP-ribose) polymerase protein, whereas the autophagy was mediated by the conversion of microtubule-associated protein light chain-3 (LC3)-I to LC3-II and accumulation of beclin-1.[24] Moreover, the radioprotective effect of fucoidan was proved in normal human HS68 newborn foreskin fibroblast cells. In a viability assay, fucoidan could recover 8Gy radiation-induced damage in all the tested doses (10, 50, and 100 μg/mL). Pretreatment with fucoidan increased the survival rate of the HS68 cells by two times more than the untreated HS68 cells. Fucoidan also protected the blood cells such as recovery of the irradiated thrombocyte counts and hematocrit level and elevation of erythrocyte level.[25]

Similarly, two fucoidans assigned as L-fucoidan and GA-fucoidan were purified from the holdfast of *L. japonica*. The L-fucoidan is rich in fucose and sulfate, whereas GA-fucoidan is rich in fucose and uronate. Their anticancer properties were demonstrated in mice-transplanted 755 adenocarcinoma after injection of the two fucoidans by i.p. or p.o.[26] In addition, when the fucoidans were sulfated, their suppressive effect against the growth of MCF-7 breast carcinoma cells was significantly amplified due to the effect of sulfate groups on DNA replication, causing decrease of replication protein A (RPA)'s DNA-binding activity.[27] Overall, these results suggested that the application of sulfated polysaccharides from kelp may be a potential choice for cancer treatment and prevention.

5. Glycoprotein

LJGP was a glycoprotein separated from the brown algae *L. japonica*, which could dose-dependently hamper the proliferation of human AGS (stomach), HepG2 (liver), and HT-29 (colon) cancer cell lines *in vitro*. The antiproliferative effect of LJGP on the HT-29 cells was found to be correlated with apoptosis induction, which may be mediated via multiple pathways, including Fas signaling and mitochondrial pathways and sub-G1 cell-cycle arrest.[28]

6. Carotenoids and chlorophylls

Several pigments such as fucoxanthin, chlorophyll-a, chlorophyll-c, and β-carotene were detected from fertilized *L. japonica*. Fucoxanthin, a natural carotenoid, has been reported to have antitumorigenic activity in mouse colon, skin, and duodenum models.[29] Treatment of human EJ-1 bladder cancer cells with fucoxanthin markedly reduced cell viability in a dose- and time-dependent manner and induced apoptosis over 93% (in 72 h with a dose of 20 μM).[30] At 25 and 50 μM concentrations, it could arrest the cell cycle in the G0/G1 phase and induce the apoptotic death of human colon adenocarcinoma cells by the upregulation of p21WAF1/Cip1.[31] The antitumor effect of fucoxanthin was also observed in other two human carcinoma cells, HepG2 (liver) and DU-145 (prostate), concomitant with marked upexpression of GADD45A (a cell cycle-related gene) and induction of G1 cell-cycle arrest. Nonetheless, fucoxanthin induced no apoptosis of HepG2 and DU-145 cells during the treatment. These findings evidenced that fucoxanthin can act as a chemopreventive carotenoid in certain cancer cells by inhibiting tumor-cell viability.[32]

CONCLUSION AND SUGGESTION

Kelp is the most common edible seaweed in the diet of Eastern Asians. The chemical biology investigations *in vitro* and *in vivo* have evidenced the anticancer, anticarcinogenic, and antimutagenic activities of kelp and have disclosed that micromolecules (such as sterols, alkaloids, and carotenoids) and macromolecules (such as polysaccharides, sulfated polysaccharides, and glycoproteins) in kelp are synergistically responsible for the cancer-suppressive and preventive effects. The moderate-to-weak degrees of anticancer activities afforded from the intake of kelp are suitable for safe protection of stomach, colon, liver, breast, prostate, skin, and so on from the risk of cancer. Hence, frequent consumption of kelp as both nutritional and functional diet should be highly recommended.

REFERENCES

1. Noda, H. et al., 1990. Antitumor activity of marine algae. *Hydrobiologia* 204–205: 577–584.
2. Yamamoto, I. et al., 1986. The effect of dietary or intraperitoneally injected seaweed preparations on the growth of sarcoma-180 cells subcutaneously implanted into mice. *Cancer Lett.* 30: 125–131.
3. Yamamoto, I. et al., 1982. Antitumor activity of crude extracts from edible marine algae against L-1210 leukemia. *Bot. Mar.* 25: 455–457.
4. Yamamoto, I. et al., 1985. Effect of dietary seaweed preparations on 1,2-dimethyl lhydrazine-induced intestinal carcinogenesis in rats. *Cancer Lett.* 26: 241–251.
5. Yamamoto, I. et al., 1990. Inhibition by dietary seaweed of carcinogen DMBA absorption through intestinal tract. *J. Cancer Res. Clin. Oncol.* 16: 352.
6. Yamamoto, I. et al., 1987. The effect of dietary seaweeds on 7,12-dimethyl-benz[a]anthracene-induced mammary tumorigenesis in rats. *Cancer Lett.* 35: 109–118.
7. Park, Y.B. et al., 1998. Elucidation of an antitumor initiator and promoter derived from seaweed. *Han'guk Susan Hakhoechi* 31: 587–593.
8. Reddy, B.S. et al., 1984. Effect of Japanese seaweed (Laminaria angustata) extracts on the mutagenicity of 7,12-dimethylbenz[a]anthracene, a breast carcinogen, and of 3,2′-dimethyl-4-aminobiphenyl, a colon and breast carcinogen. *Mutation Res.* 127: 113–118.
9. Nishizawa, M. et al., 2003. Cytotoxic constituents in the holdfast of cultivated Laminaria japonica. *Fisheries Sci.* 69: 639–643.
10. Wang, C. et al., Cytotoxic compounds from Laminaria japonica. *Chem. Nat. Compds.* 49: 699–701.
11. Ji, Y.B. et al., 1994. An experimental study of the anticancer effect of compound herbal polysaccharide preparation. *Zhongguo Haiyong Yaowu* 13: 20–24.
12. Xu, Z.P. et al., 2006. Anticancer effect of FGS, polysaccharide fraction from Laminaria japonica Aresch in vitro and in vivo. *J. Qufu Normal Univ. (Nature Sci.)* 32: 103–106.
13. Zeng, M.L. et al., 2012. Inhibition of human nasopharyngeal carcinoma cell proliferation and xenograft growth in nude mice by Laminaria japonica poly-saccharides. *Zhongguo Zhongliu Linchuang* 39: 634–638.
14. Sun, W.Z. et al., 2013. Effects of tea polyphenols and Laminaria japonica polysaccharides on nasopharyngeal carcinoma cell HONE1 and CNE2. *Linchuang Er-Bi-Yanhou Tou-Jing Waike Zazhi* 27: 425–428.
15. Zhu, Q.W. et al., 2016. Antitumor activity of polysaccharide from Laminaria japonica on mice bearing H22 liver cancer. *Int. J. Biol. Macromol.* 92: 156–158.
16. Peng, Z.F. et al., 2012. In vitro antioxidant effects and cytotoxicity of polysaccharides extracted from Laminaria japonica. *Int. J. Biol. Macromol.* 50: 1254–1259.
17. Peng, Z.F. et al., 2012. Composition and cytotoxicity of a novel polysaccharide from brown alga (Laminaria japonica). *Carbohydr. Polym.* 89: 1022–1026.

18. Peng, Z.F. et al., 2013. In vitro antiproliferative effect of a water-soluble Laminaria japonica polysaccharide on human melanoma cell line A375. *Food Chem. Toxicol.* 58: 56–60.
19. Fanal, M.F. et al., 1988. Isolation, analysis, and biological activities of sodium alginate. *J. China Pharm. Univ.* 19: 279–281.
20. Zhai, Q.Z. et al., 2014. Antitumor activity of a polysaccharide fraction from Laminaria japonica on U14 cervical carcinoma-bearing mice. *Tumor Biol.* 35: 117–122.
21. Teng, X. et al., 1998. Study on the antioxidative and antitumor effects of sulfated polysaccharides from seaweeds. *Acta Nutr. Sinica* 20: 48–52.
22. Wang, C.Z. et al., 2010. Purification of sulfated polysaccharide from Laminaria Japonica and studies of its anti-tumor mechanism. *Jiefangjun Yaoxue Xuebao* 26: 283–286.
23. Vishchuk, O.S. et al., 2011. Sulfated polysaccharides from brown seaweeds Saccharina japonica and Undaria pinnatifida: isolation, structural characteristics, and antitumor activity. *Carbohydr. Res.* 346: 2769–2776.
24. Park, H.S. et al., 2011. Antiproliferative activity of fucoidan was associated with the induction of apoptosis and autophagy in AGS human gastric cancer cells. *J. Food Sci.* 76: T77–T83.
25. Lee, K. et al., 2009. Fucoidan protects human skin fibroblast cell line HS68 against γ-radiation-induced damage. *Open Nat. Prod. J.* 2: 38–41.
26. Ozawa, T. et al., 2006. Two fucoidans in the holdfast of cultivated Laminaria japonica. *J. Nat. Med.* 60: 236–239.
27. Park, J.S. et al., 2002. Increased anticancer activity by the sulfated fucoidan from Korean brown seaweeds. *J. Korean Chem. Soc.* 46: 151–156.
28. Go, H. et al., 2010. A glycoprotein from Laminaria japonica induces apoptosis in HT-29 colon cancer cells. *Toxicol. in Vitro* 24: 1546–1553.
29. Hosokawa, M. 2004. Fucoxanthin induces apoptosis in cancer cells. *Bio-Industry* 21: 52–57.
30. Zhang, Z.Y. et al., 2008. Potential chemoprevention effect of dietary fucoxanthin on urinary bladder cancer EJ-1 cell line. *Oncol. Reports* 20: 1099–1103.
31. Das, S.K. et al., 2005. Fucoxanthin induces cell cycle arrest at G0/G1 phase in human colon carcinoma cells through up-regulation of p21WAF1/Cip1. *Biochimica et Biophysica Acta, General Subjects* 1726: 328–335.
32. Yoshiko, S. et al., 2007. Fucoxanthin, a natural carotenoid, induces G1 arrest and GADD45 gene expression in human cancer cells. *In Vivo* 21: 305–310.

79. KUROME

黑昆布

Ecklonia kurome

Lessoniaceae

Kurome, *Ecklonia kurome*, is a Japanese/Okinawan name for an edible black–brown algae. In Eastern Asian countries, kurome is a long-time common substitute for kelp as a nutritional food and a remedial herb. Normally, kurome is used in Okinawan and Chinese cuisines. According to pharmacological studies, kurome possesses various biological and nutritional benefits similar to kelp. In addition, other Ecklonia algae are also edible seaweeds, for instance, three closely related algae *E. stolonifera*, *E. cava*, and *E. bicyclis* are widely consumed in Korea and Japan. Seanol, a polyphenolic extract from the seaweeds *E. cava* is also utilized as an herbal remedy.

SCIENTIFIC EVIDENCE OF CANCER-INHIBITORY AND CANCER-PREVENTIVE CONSTITUENTS

The bioactive components such as chlorophyllin, phenols, lutein, and α-cryptoxanthin in black algae were found to be responsible for the inhibition of mutagenesis caused by mutagens, 2-amino-1-methyl-6-phenylimidazo[4,5-b]-pyridine (PhIP), or 2-amino-3,8-dimethylimidazo[4,5-f]-quinoxaline (MeIQx).[1]

1. Polysaccharides

A polysaccharide isolated from *E. kurome* obviously suppressed the proliferation of neoplastic cells and prolonged the survival duration of mice-implanted EAC, L615 reticulocytic leukemia, or sarcoma 180.[2] Alginates are the acidic polysaccharides separated from kurome, which are composed of L-guluronic acid and D-mannuronic acid. The antitumor activity of alginates was demonstrated in mice-transplanted ascites sarcoma 180.[3] Alginate hydrolysates derived from a close alga (*E. stolonifera*) in Korea displayed the antimutagenic effect against the PhIP and MeIQx but at high doses.[1] Fucoidan, a kind of polysaccharide prepared from *E. stolonifera* exerted the anti-growth effect against human MCF-7 breast cancer cells. If the fucoidan were sulfated, the growth-inhibitory effect would be obviously augmented.[4]

2. Polyphenols

Compared to other types of seaweeds, Ecklonia algae contain higher amounts of polyphenol component, which confer stronger antioxidant and radical-scavenging properties. Phlorotannins separated from *Ecklonia kurome* are potent inhibitors toward hyaluronidase, the enzyme of which appears to have biological activities related to tumor proliferation, progression, invasion, and metastasis in some carcinomas such as ovarian, endometrial, breast, and bladder. However, acetylation of the phlorotannins would markedly decrease the anticancer potency.[5–7] Phlorofucofuroeckol-A (**1**, PFF-A) is a phlorotannin isolated from the brown algae species such as *E. bicyclis*, *E. kurome*, *E. stolonifera*, and *E. cava*, which showed potent inhibition on AKR1B10 (a biomarker of several cancers). The inhibitory rate was 61.41% against AKR1B10 cells at a concentration of 10 μM (IC$_{50}$ of 6.22 μM). The findings suggested that PFF-A (**1**) may be a potential agent to deserve further investigation in cancer prevention.[8] Five phlorotannins isolated from the methanol extract of *E. cava* showed weak cytotoxicity against four cultured human carcinoma cell lines (HeLa, HT1080, A549, and HT-29) and one cultured human normal cell line (MRC-5). Only at higher concentrations (100–400 μM), these phlorotannins exerted the anticancer effect on these cell lines.[9] The five phlorotannins also showed angiotensin-converting enzyme (ACE)-inhibitory activity.[10]

Both chloroform and ethyl acetate fractions of *E. stolonifera* extract in 20 μg/mL concentration exhibited a high antitumor-promoting effect of 88.0% and 85.9%, respectively, against Epstein–Barr virus early antigen (EBV-EA) activation caused by a tumor promoter teleocidin-B-4, suggesting that the algae possesses notable inhibitory property against carcinogenesis. Bromophenol and phloroglucinol, two major phenols isolated from the brown seaweed, exhibited 57%–66% inhibitory effects on tumor promotion at a concentration of 20 μg/mL.[11] Oral administration of phloroglucinol effectively disrupts VEGF-induced neovessel formation and EPCs-induced capillary-like tube formation and hindered CD45$^-$/CD34$^+$ progenitor mobilization into peripheral blood, thereby significantly inhibiting tumor growth and angiogenesis *in vivo* in the Lewis lung carcinoma-bearing mouse model.[12]

3. Photodithiazines and carotenoids

Pheophorbide-a (**2**) and chlorophyll-a (**3**) from *E. kurome* at a concentration of 5 μM/mL could impede the EBV-EA activation by 66.6% and 77.4%, respectively. Two bioactive carotenoids from *E. stolonifera* such as lutein and α-cryptoxanthin (**4**) also exerted remarkable EBV-EA inhibition of 76.9% and 84.4% at a concentration of 20 μg/mL, respectively, indicating anticarcinogenic and anticancer preventive activities.[11]

CONCLUSION AND SUGGESTION

Kurome and its closely related Ecklonia algae are common edible seaweeds in East Asian countries and widely consumed throughout China, Korea, and Japan because of their nutritional importance and medicinal values. The biology integrated phytochemical studies provide valuable insights concerning the anticancer potential of these Ecklonia algae and their effective ingredients. The results disclosed that the isolated phlorotannins, photodithiazines, carotenoids, or polysaccharides have not only anticarcinogenic, antitumor-promoting, and/or antimutagenic activities but also prominent antioxidant, immunoregulating, and/or antiangiogenic potentials. The phloroglucinol may be used to develop new antiangiogenic drugs as a starting material. Following these findings, it is necessary to extensively utilize Ecklonia algae as functional foods into human healthy diet menu for lessening cancer threat. In the recent decade, adding the dried kurome created a new natural herb prescription for the treatment of patients with some types of chronic diseases and cancers.[13]

REFERENCES

1. Park, Y.B. et al., 1998. Elucidation of antitumor initiator and promoter derived from seaweed-4: desmutagenic principles of Ecklonia stolonifera extracts against carcinogenic hetero-cyclic amines. *Han'guk Sikp'um Yongyang Kwahak Hoechi* 27: 537–542.
2. Ji, Y.B. et al., 1994. An experimental study of the anticancer effect of compound herbal polysaccharide preparation. *Zhongguo Haiyang Yaowu* 13: 20–24.
3. Fujihara, M. et al., 1992. The effect of the content of D-mannuronic acid and L-guluronic acid blocks in alginates on antitumor activity. *Carbohydrate Res.* 224: 343–347.
4. Park, J.S. et al., 2002. Increased anticancer activity by the sulfated fucoidan from Korean brown seaweeds. *J. Korean Chem. Soc.* 46: 151–156.
5. Shibata, T. et al., 2002. Inhibitory activity of brown algal phlorotannins against hyaluronidase. *Int. J. Food Sci. Technol.* 37: 703–709.
6. Tamakoshi, K. et al., 1997. Hyaluronidase activity in gynaecological cancer tissues with different metastatic forms. *Breast J. Cancer* 75: 1807–1811.
7. Lokeshwar, V.B. et al., 2005. HYAL1 Hyaluronidase: A molecular determinant of bladder tumor growth and invasion. *Cancer Res.* 65: 2243–2250.
8. Lee, J.Y. et al., 2012. Phlorofucofuroeckol-A, a potent inhibitor of aldo-keto reductase family 1 member B10, from the edible brown alga Eisenia bicyclis. *J. Korean Soc. Appl. Biol. Chem.* 55: 721–727.
9. Li, Y. et al., 2011. Cytotoxic activities of phlorethol and fucophlorethol derivatives isolated from Laminariaceae Ecklonia cava. *J. Food Chem.* 35: 357–369.
10. Wijesinghe, W.A.J.P. et al., 2011. Effect of phlorotannins isolated from Ecklonia cava on angiotensin I-converting enzyme (ACE) inhibitory activity. *Nutr. Res. Pract.* 5(2): 93–100.
11. Park, Y.B. et al., 1998. Elucidation of an antitumor initiator and promoter derived from seaweed. *Han'guk Susan Hakhoechi* 31: 587–593.
12. Kwon, Y.H. et al., 2012. Phloroglucinol inhibits the bioactivities of endothelial progenitor cells and suppresses tumor angiogenesis in LLC-tumor-bearing mice. *PlosOne* 7(4): e33618.
13. Xu, J.P. 2017. *Cancer Inhibitors from Chinese Natural Medicines*, Boca Raton, FL: CRC Press/Taylor & Francis Group, p. 488.

80. LAVER OR NORI

Laituc   rouge   Porphyrtang

紫菜 ノリ 김

Porphyra haitanensis, P. yezoensis, P. tenera, P. umbilicalis

Bangiaceae

Laver or nori is the purple or green–purple algae of several *Porphyra* species (Bangiaceae). Currently, the commercial laver/nori originated from four *Porphyra* algae such as *P. haitanensis*, *P. yezoensis*, *P. tenera*, and *P. umbilicalis*. The popular edible seaweeds have been used particularly in East Asian region and north European coast as a dietary food for long time. Laver/nori has a good content of vitamins such as B-complex, A, and C and dietary minerals (such as iodine, manganese, phosphorus, iron, and zinc). The dried laver/nori is also a good source of vitamin B12, carotene, ektachrome, and *n*-3 polyunsaturated fatty acids. It affords rich common amino acids.[1] In recent decades, laver/nori has attracted great attentions for its remarkable health benefits, including immunopotentiating, hepatoprotective, hypoglycemic, hypolipemic, radioprotecting, antileucopenic, antifatigue, and antiaging properties.

SCIENTIFIC EVIDENCE OF ANTICARCINOGENIC ACTIVITY

Significant suppressive effect of nori (*P. yezoensis*) was found against the growth of Ehrlich carcinoma and Meth-A fibrosarcoma.[2] The methanolic extract of nori (*P. tenera*) displayed relatively better inhibitory activities against a tumor promoting agent (TPA)-dependent ornithine decarboxylase in BALB/c 3T3 fibroblast cells and against a mutagen (Trp-P-1)-induced umu-C gene expression in SOS response of *Salmonella typhimurium*, indicating that the edible seaweeds have antimutagenic and antitumor-promotion properties, which are closely related to anticarcinoma property.[3] Nori (*P. tenera*) exerted preventive effects against diethylnitrosamine-elicited hepatocarcinogenesis via marked decrease in glutathione *S*-transferase placental form (GST-P)-positive foci in the liver of male F344 rats.[4] Daily fed with the nori (*P. tenera*) for 12 weeks obviously lessened the incidence of intestinal tumors induced by a carcinogen 1,2-dimethylhydrazine in rats.[5] Moreover, the extract of *P. tenera* at 200 and 400 µg/mL dose-dependently restrained the adhesion, invasion, and migration of human SK-Hep1 hepatoma cells in association with downexpression of MMPs-2 and -9 in addition to the cell-growth inhibition.[6] The immunostimulatory effects of dried *P. yezoensis* were demonstrated *in vitro* and *in vivo* and the augmented IFN-γ production and NK cell cytotoxic activity could prolong the survival of mice bearing melanoma after multiple oral administrations.[7] These preliminary data afforded strong scientific evidences to support the healthy laver becoming a potential adjuvant/supplement in the diet for carcinoma therapy and prevention for long-term use.

SCIENTIFIC EVIDENCE OF CANCER-INHIBITORY AND CANCER-PREVENTIVE CONSTITUENTS

1. Pigments

Several photosynthetic pigments such as chlorophylls and carotenoids (lutein and β-carotene) were purified from laver/nori (*P. tenera*). Those pigments demonstrated obvious anticarcinogenic activities and a suppressive effect on the mutagenesis of *Salmonella typhimurium* in in vitro assays.[8]

2. Sulfolipid

Telomerase presents one of the promising tumor therapeutic targets because the higher telomerase activity is always detected in most cancer cells. A sulfolipid component assigned as sulfoquinovosyl diacylglycerols (SQDG, **1**) isolated from laver (*P. yezoensis*) noticeably and dose-dependently diminished the activity of telomerase in the test. A fatty acid component of SQDG identified as eicosapentaenoic acid could act as a potent telomerase inhibitor, implying that the sulfate groups and fatty-acid component in the SQDG play an important role in the inhibition of telomerase. Therefore, SQDG (**1**) has potential value for targeting telomerase to prevent carcinogenesis.[9]

3. Polysaccharides

At 1000 μg/mL concentration, the polysaccharides from *P. haitanensis* could retard HeLa cervical carcinoma cells by 35.64% and induce cell apoptosis through activation of caspases-10 and -3.[10] A polysaccharide fraction obtained from *P. yezoensis* significantly restrained the growth of sarcoma 180 by 47.55% and increased the average survival time of the tested mice by 1.8-fold when i.p. injected with the polysaccharides in a dose of 150 mg/kg to tumor-bearing mice. The polysaccharide fraction also could noticeably protect mice from ^{60}Co γ-radiation and obviously antagonize 79.60% leucopenia induced by tumor or radiation. By reducing the frequency of micronuclei caused by an anticancer agent cyclophosphamide, the polysaccharide fraction was able to markedly diminish the toxicity caused by chemotherapies.[11]

Two polysaccharide components designated as PY-D1 and PY-D2 were isolated from laver/nori (*P. yezoensis*). The PY-D2 in 0.5 mg/mL concentration restrained the growth of human HO-8910 (ovary), MCF-7 (breast), SMMC-7721 (liver), and K562 (leukemic) cancer cell lines with 19.8%–23.6% inhibitory rates *in vitro*, associated with blockage of G0/G1 or G2/M period cells in the cell cycle. From the PY-D2, two polysaccharides (PY-G1 and PY-G2) were separated, two of which demonstrated antiproliferative effect on human MCF-7 breast tumor cell line *in vitro*.[12–14] PY3, a polysaccharide purified from *P. yezoensis*, was assayed in both human K562 leukemia cells and murine immunocytes *in vitro*. The experiments demonstrated that PY3 was capable of suppressing the growth of K562 cells and enhancing the mixed lymphocyte reaction and proliferation of murine bone marrow cells and spleen cells. These evidences substantiated that PY3 possesses remarkable anticancer and immunopotentiating properties that are useful for cancer prevention.[15]

Another purified polysaccharide assigned as porphyran derived from *P. yezoensis* is a sulfate galactan, which showed appreciable suppressive effects on Ehrlich carcinoma *in vivo* and on HT-29 (colon) and AGS (gastric) cancer cell lines *in vitro* without influencing the viability of normal human BJ cells. Even at low concentration (5 or 10 μg/mL), the porphyran was able to hamper the growth of HT-29 cells and AGS cells by 50% in correlation with the promotion of caspase-3–activated apoptotic death.[16–18] When fixation of 5-FU to porphyran at 6-position of galactose units, the created water-soluble conjugate achieved the enhancement of antitumor activity of 5-FU and improvement of immunocompetence damaged by 5-FU in a mice model with sarcoma 180.[19] Moreover, by a digestive reaction of the porphyran with an enzyme of *Arthrobacter sp.*, several neutral and anionic oligosaccharide fractions were derived. Among them, a sulfated disaccharide fraction OSP1 exhibited considerable antitumor activity against EAC and Meth-A fibrosarcoma *in vivo* when administered to mice by i.p. Simultaneously, the OSP1 treatment augmented the phagocytosis of macrophages.[16] In addition, ultrasound degradation could amplify the antiproliferative effect of the *P. yezoensis* polysaccharides against human SGC7901 gastric cancer cells.[20]

4. Phycobiliproteins

Two phycobiliproteins termed R-phycoerythrin (R-PE) and R-phycocyanin (R-PC) have been isolated from laver (*P. haitanensis*), both of which demonstrated remarkable photodynamic inhibition against human Bcap-37 breast cancer cells *in vitro* in a dose-dependent manner. At a concentration of > 25 µg/mL, the intensity of photodynamic effect of R-PE in the Bcap-37 cells was more potent than that of R-PC,[21] and the combination treatment with R-PE and photodynamic therapy (PDT) significantly obstructed the growth of human HeLa cervical cancer cells up to 81.5% and promoted the HeLa cell apoptosis.[22] R-PC markedly repressed the growth of human HL-60 leukemia cells together with the induction of G0/G1 cell arrest in dose- and time-dependent fashions.[23] A C-phycocyanin was prepared from laver/nori (*P. yezoensis*) and it exerted dose-dependent growth inhibition on human HEp-2 (larynges) and A375 (skin) carcinoma cells *in vitro* when its concentrations are higher than 5 µg/mL.[15]

In a mouse model, R-PE injection at a dose of 300 mg/kg not only markedly inhibited the growth of sarcoma 180 (S180) up to 41.3%, but also notably improved the immunity and antioxidant abilities of mice bearing S180. At the same time, the indexes of spleen and thymus, proliferation of lymphocyte, activities of NK cells and SOD, and secretion of TNF-α were increased, whereas the level of malondialdehyde (MDA) in mouse liver declined. These interactions must contribute to the antitumor effect of R-PE *in vivo*.[22] The enzymic hydrolysis of R-PE by papain remarkably enhanced the hydroxyl radical-scavenging ability and augmented the antiproliferative effect of R-PE by 2–3 times against human HepG2 hepatoma and U2O sarcoma cell lines.[24]

5. Peptides

From pepsin hydrolysates of laver (*P. tenera*), two peptides, A and B with low molecular weight were purified. Peptides-A and -B were demonstrated to possess significant antioxidative, anti-tyrosinase, and ACE-inhibitory activities, suppressive activities of which might be beneficial to the anticarcinogenic effect.[25] Treatment of human MCF-7 breast cancer cells with 500 ng PPY (a peptide derived from *P. yezoensis*) for 24 h could induce cell autophagy via activation of a mTOR signaling pathway and prompt the cell apoptosis via regulation of Bcl-2 family members and modulation of p53/NF-κB and PI3K/Akt/mTOR pathways and insulin-like growth factor-I receptor signaling pathway, eventually impeding the growth of breast cancer cells.[26,27]

Conclusion and Suggestion

Laver or nori is a major component of Japanese foods and also a favorite food in China and Korea that contains many attractive functional constituents, including micromolecules (sulfolipid, chlorophylls, and carotenoids) and macromolecules (polysaccharides, sulfated polysaccharides, and phycobiliproteins). All the isolated bioactive constituents from laver/nori have been substantiated to possess anticarcinogenic, antitumor-promoting, and antimutagenic activities in different degrees. Particularly, polysaccharides such as porphyran (a sulfated galactan) and phycobiliproteins such as phycoerythrin and phycocyanins are the major constituents in Porphyra algae, which are capable of stimulating immunity, additively augmenting the anticancer activities of chemotheraphy and radiotheraphy, and attenuating the toxicity/side effects caused by chemotherapy and radiation, in addition to their cancer-inhibitory activities. Moreover, the hydrolysates of phycobiliproteins by pepsin or papain displayed better antioxidant and antiproliferative potentials. Based on the scientific evidences, it is shown that frequent consumption of laver/nori as functional foods can switch on the safe and effective option for the improvement of the human defense system and the inhibition of cancer initiation and proliferation. In addition, due to pollution and mildew, some toxicity of laver/nori would be formed. A simple examination can be used to identify the quality of laver/nori, that is, if a water infusion presents blue–purple color, the laver/nori must be prohibited as a food.

REFERENCES

1. Watanabe, F. et al., 2014. Vitamin B12-containing plant food sources for vegetarians. *Nutrients* 6: 1861–1873.
2. Noda, H. et al., 1990. Antitumor activity of marine algae. *Hydrobiologia* 204–205: 577–584.
3. Okai, Y. et al., 1994. Suppressive effects of the extracts of Japanese edible seaweeds on mutagen-induced umu C gene expression in Salmonella typhimurium (TA 1535/pSK 1002) and tumor promotor-dependent ornithine decarboxylase induction in BALB/c 3T3 fibroblast cells. *Cancer Lett.* (Shannon, Ireland) 87: 25–32.
4. Ichihara, T. et al., 1999. Inhibition of liver glutathione S-transferase placental form-positive foci development in the rat hepatocarcino-genesis by Porphyra tenera (Asakusanori). *Cancer Lett.* (Shannon, Ireland) 141: 211–218.
5. Yamamoto, I. et al., 1985. Effect of dietary seaweed preparations on 1,2-dimethylhydrazine-induced intestinal carcinogenesis in rats. *Cancer Lett.* 26: 241–251.
6. DoThi, N. et al., 2014. Effects of laver extracts on adhesion, invasion, and migration in SK-Hep1 human hepatoma cancer cells. *Biosci. Biotechnol. Biochem.* 78: 1044–1051.
7. Kitajima, H. et al., 2013. Immunostimulatory effects of extract from Nori (Porphyra yezoensis) in vitro and in vivo. *Kagaku Kogaku Ronbunshu* 39: 359–362.
8. Kiyoka, H.O. et al., 1995. Protective role of Japanese edible seaweeds against carcinogenesis. Association with antimutagenic photosynthetic pigments. *Osaka Kun'ei Joshi Tanki Daigaku Kenkyu Kiyo* 30: 93–101.
9. Eitsuka, T. et al., 2004. Telomerase inhibition by sulfoquinovosyl diacylglycerol from edible purple laver (Porphyra yezoensis). *Cancer Lett.* 212: 15–20.
10. Xie, H.G. et al., 2013. Synergistic antitumor activity in vitro of polysaccharides from three different matrices. *Shipin Kexue* (Beijing, China) 34(5): 289–294.
11. Zhou, H.P. et al., 1989. The cytoprotection by polysaccharide from Porphyra yezoensis Ueda. *Zhongguo Yaoke Daxue Xuebao* 20: 340–343.
12. Gu, J.W. et al., 2007. Isolation, purification and antitumor activity of polysaccharides from Porphyra yezoensis. *Zhongguo Shengwu Gongcheng Zazhi* 27: 50–54.
13. Zhang, L.X. et al., 2007. Effect of Porphyra yezoensis polysaccharide PY-D2 on the growth of four human tumor cell lines. *Shengwu Jishu Tongxun* 18: 608–611.
14. Zhang, L.X. et al., 2011. Anticancer effects of polysaccharides and phytocyanin from Porphyra yezoensis. *J. Marine Sci. Technol.* 19: 377–382.
15. Zhang, W.Y. et al., 2002. Effects of polysaccharide from Porphyra yezoensis on murine immunocytes and human leukemia K562 cells. *Shengming Kexue Yanjiu* 6: 167–170.
16. Osumi, Y. et al., 1998. Antitumor activity of oligosaccharides derived from Porphyra yezoensis porphyran. *Nippon Suisan Gakkaishi* 64: 847–853.
17. Min, H.K. et al., 2008. Growth-inhibitory effect of the extract of porphyran-Chung kook jang on cancer cells. *Han'guk Sikp'um Yongyang Kwahak Hoechi* 37: 826–833.
18. Kwon, M.J. et al., 2007. Chromatographically purified porphyran from Porphyra yezoensis effectively inhibits proliferation of human cancer cells. *Food Sci. Biotechnol.* 16: 873–878.
19. Wang, X.M. et al., 2014. The antitumor activity of a red alga polysaccharide complexes carrying 5-fluorouracil. *Intl. J. Biol. Macromol.* 69: 542–545.
20. Yu, X.J. et al., 2015. Effect of ultrasonic treatment on the degradation and inhibition cancer cell lines of polysaccharides from Porphyra yezoensis. *Carbohydr. Polym.* 117: 650–656.
21. Chen, X.Q. et al., 2005. Photodynamic effect of three kinds of phycobiliproteins on human mammary cancer line Bcap-37. *J. Zhejiang Univ, Science Edit.* 32: 438–441, 447.
22. Pan, Q.W. et al., 2013. Antitumor function and mechanism of phycoerythrin from Porphyra haitanensis. *Biol. Res.* 46: 87–95.
23. Liu, Y.F. et al., 2000. Inhibitory effects of red-phycocyanin from Porphyra haitanensis on growth of human leukemia HL-60 cells. *Zhongguo Haiyang Yaowu* 19: 20–24.
24. Fang, Y. et al., 2012. Preparation of enzymatic hydrolysate of R-phycoerythrin from Porphyra yezoensis and its antioxidant and tumor cell proliferation inhibiting activities. *Zhongguo Nongye Kexue* (Beijing, China) 45: 3222–3230.
25. Lee, J.M. et al., 2005. Functional activities of low molecular weight peptides purified from enzymatic hydrolysates of seaweeds. *Han'guk Sikp'um Yongyang Kwahak Hoechi* 34: 1124–1129.
26. Park, S.J. et al., 2015. Activation of the mTOR signaling pathway in breast cancer MCF-7 cells by a peptide derived from Porphyra yezoensis. *Oncol. Reports* 33: 19–24.
27. Park, S.J. et al., 2014. Induction of apoptosis by a peptide from Porphyra yezoensis: regulation of the insulin-like growth factor I receptor signaling pathway in MCF-7 cells. *Int. J. Oncol.* 45: 1011–1016.

81. SEA MUSTARD

Wakame   Wakame   Wakame

裙帶菜   ワカメ   미역

Undaria pinnatifida

Alariaceae

Sea mustard is the dried green–brown seaweed *Undaria pinnatifida* (Alariaceae). The edible algae are commercially produced in China, Japan, and Korea as both health food supplement and folk medicine. Nowadays, sea mustard (wakame) is often used in soups and salad in Eastern Asia and Europe. In nutrition, sea mustard is a rich source of eicosapentaenoic acid (an omega-3 fatty acid). It contains high levels of folate, manganese, and magnesium, and it is a good source of iodine, calcium, iron, vitamin B-complex, and fiber. The protein and iron are richer in sea mustard than in kelp. Similar to kelp, the sea mustard possesses extensive bioactivities, including antioxidative, hypotensive, immunomodulating, antithrombotic, radiation-protecting, hypolipemic, hypoglycemic, and anticoagulant effects.

SCIENTIFIC EVIDENCE OF CANCER-INHIBITORY AND CANCER-PREVENTIVE ACTIVITIES

In vitro and *in vivo* tests demonstrated sea mustard extract possessing marked anticancer- and antitumor-promoting activities, especially against the proliferation of breast cancer cells.[1] The sea mustard extract accelerated intracellular signaling and activated caspases-3, -6, and -8 for inducing apoptosis of human MDA-MB-231 breast cancer cells.[2] Fed with a diet containing sea mustard prominently augmented the activity of NK cells for > 2-fold and suppressed the proliferation of sarcoma 180 cells *in vivo*.[3] Through the transportation of the organic iodine from serum into mammary tissues and induction of apoptosis by TGF-β expression, sea mustard enriched with organic iodine efficiently obstructed the rat breast carcinogenesis induced by 7,12-dimethylbenz[a]anthracene (DMBA).[4] A crude extract of sea mustard (collected in New Zealand and containing 0.2% fucoxanthin) in an *in vitro* assay showed moderate antiproliferative effects against nine human cancer cell lines, including LoVo and WiDr (colon), NCI-H522 and A549 (lung), SiHa (cervix), SK-N-SH (brain), HepG2 (liver), MCF-7 (breast), and Malma-3M (skin) carcinoma cells with IC_{50}s in a range of 8.84–25.13 μM (in 72 h). It also hindered the proliferation of HUVEC (IC_{50} of 7.64 μM in 72 h), implying the antiangiogenic potential. However, its crude extract moderately retarded human dermal fibroblast (HDFb) cells and weakly deterred human embryonic kidney (HEK293) cells *in vitro*.[5]

SCIENTIFIC EVIDENCE OF CANCER-INHIBITORY AND CANCER-PREVENTIVE CONSTITUENTS

Sea mustard (Wakame) contains a wide range of biologically active phytochemicals such as carotenoids, phycobilins, fatty acids, polysaccharides, vitamins, sterols, tocopherol, and phycocyanins, wherein fucoxanthin and fucoidan are the major components in *U. pinnatifida* in charge of anticancer-related activities.

1. Carotenoids

A chemopreventive and chemotherapeutic carotenoid assigned as fucoxanthin (**1**) is one of the most abundant carotenoids found in wakame. It was shown to inhibit the proliferation of human HL-60 leukemia cells *in vitro* with proapoptotic effect.[6] In human colon carcinoma cell lines (Caco-2, HT-29, and DLD-1) and human hepatoma cell lines (SK-Hep-1 and HepG2), fucoxanthin (**1**) remarkably restrained the viability of tumor cells together with the induction of cell-cycle arrest, apoptotic death, and DNA fragmentation.[6–8] The investigations further revealed that the antiproliferative effect against SK-Hep-1 hepatoma cells by fucoxanthin was associated with the enhancement of gap junction intercellular communication (GJIC) via upregulation of Cx32 and Cx43. The enhanced GJIC was responsible for an increase in intracellular calcium level and accumulation Ca^{2+}, leading to promotion of cell-cycle arrest and apoptosis in the cancer cells.[7] Fucoxanthin (**1**) was also reported to be effective in the inhibition of prostate cancer cells. When three types of prostate cancer cell lines were cultured in a carotenoid-supplemented medium for 72 h, fucoxanthin (**1**) at 20 μmol/L concentration significantly diminished the viability of prostate cancer cells to 14.9% for PC3 cells, 5.0% for DU-145 cells, and 9.8% for LNCaP cells.[9] The antiproliferative effects of fucoxanthin (**1**) were also found in the *in vitro* assays with other types of cell lines such as MGC-803 gastric cancer, GOTO, and SK-N-SH neuroblastoma, WiDr and LoVo colon adenocarcinoma, A549 and NCI-H522 lung carcinoma, MCF-7 breast adeno-carcinoma, SiHa cervix squamous cancer and Malme-3M malignant melanoma, and noncancer cell lines (HUVEC, HDFb, and HEK293).[5] In addition, a combinational treatment with fucoxanthin (**1**) (3.8 μM) and troglitazone (10 μM) could efficiently obstruct the proliferation of human Caco-2 colon cancer cells *in vitro*.[10] The results hinted that ingestion of the edible seaweeds rich in fucoxanthin may have a potential to decrease the risk of cancers in prostate, colon, and liver. Impressively, the crude extract with low level of fucoxanthin was more effective in inhibiting the growth of lung cancer, colon cancer, and neuroblastoma, compared to pure fucoxanthin,[5] indicating that sea mustard comprises other more interesting bioactive components.

2. Polysaccharides

Crude polysaccharides (UPPS) prepared from sea mustard displayed obvious inhibitory effect on HepG2 hepatoma cells *in vitro* in concentrations of 10–15 mg/mL and against Hca-f hepatoma in mice in doses of 200–400 mg/kg. The inhibitory ratios were 51.79%–57.20% on HepG2 cells *in vitro* and 42.11%–69.13% on Hca-f cells *in vivo*; anticancer potencies of UPPS were comparable to those of 5-FU, an anticancer drug.[11] A separated polysaccharide termed UPPS-B1 exerted inhibitory effect against the proliferation of human SGC-7901 gastric adenocarcinoma and HepG2 hepatoma cell lines. When the treated concentration was up to 1000 μg/mL, UPPS-B1 could reach the inhibitory rates of 69.45% on SGC-7901 cells and 71.36% on HepG2 cells.[12] After treatment with PUP (a wakabe polysaccharide extract) in a dose of 100 μg/mL for 48 h, the apoptosis of human TE-13 esophageal carcinoma cells and BGC-823 gastric cancer cells were enhanced by 52.19% and 69.91%, respectively, thereby deterring the proliferation of cancer cells. The proapoptotic mechanism was found to be associated with the blockage of cell-cycle progression and downregulation of survivin mRNA expression.[13,14]

3. Sulfated polysaccharides

Fucoidans were fucose-enriched sulfated polysaccharides derived from sea mustard, consisting of (1-3)- or (1-3) (1-4)-α-L-fucose residues and exerting a variety of biological potentials, such as anticancer, antiangiogenic, and anti-inflammatory effects. The anticancer activity was observed in several types of neoplastic cell lines, including human leukemia, breast carcinoma, and lung adenocarcinoma and murine Ehrlich carcinoma. Dietary 1% of the fucoidan (34 mg/mouse/day) for 50 days could repress murine A20 leukemia cell growth by 65.4% in mice.[16] If the fucoidans were administered for 4 days before the tumor-cell inoculation, the survival duration could be prolonged in mice bearing P388 leukemia.[17] Oral administration of the fucoidans to sarcoma 180-implanted mice in daily doses of 100 and 50 mg/kg for 7 days resulted in the tumor-inhibitory rates of 56.17% and 65.71%, respectively.[18] Besides, when the fed with the fucoidans, the cytotoxicities mediated by T-cells and NK cells were augmented notably in mice, indicating that the anticancer activity exerted by fucoidan was partially related to its abilities in enhancing the immune responses such as activations of Th1 cells, NK cells, and IFN-γ and decrease in human neutrophil apoptosis.[16–20]

The continuing investigations provided positive evidences in the fucoidans isolated from *U. pinnatifida*. In *in vitro* models, the fucoidans distinctly hindered the proliferation and colony formation in both T-47D breast cancer cells and SK-MEL-28 melanoma cells in a dose-dependent manner.[21,22] The fucoidans promoted both intrinsic and extrinsic apoptosis of human PC3 (prostate) and A549 (lung) carcinoma cells through inactivation of p38 MAPK and PI3K/Akt signaling pathway, activation of ERK1/2 MAPK, and downregulation of Wnt/β-catenin signaling pathway.[23,24] The fucoidan-induced apoptosis of human SMMC-7721 hepatoma cells was associated with an increase in intracellular ROS levels, depletion of reduced glutathione, downregulation of Livin and XIAP mRNA expressions, damage of mitochondrial ultrastructure, loss of mitochondrial membrane potential, and activation of caspase, where the increase in ROS played a critical role for trigging the proapoptotic process.[25]

Moreover, the fucoidan isolated from sporophyll of cultured Korean *U. pinnatifida* contained β-galactose (44.6 mol %) and α-fucose (50.9 mol %) as the main neutral sugar units with sulfate (0.97 mol/mol) and acetate (0.24 mol/mol) esters, defining this fucoidan to be *O*-acetylated and sulfated galactofucan. The fucoidan exerted the antitumor effect against PC3 (prostate), HeLa (cervix), A549 (lung), and HepG2 (liver) cancer cell lines in a similar cancer-inhibitory pattern to the common sea mustard fucoidan.[26] When hydrolyzed in boiling water with HCl for 5 min, the obtained shortened fucoidans (m.w. 490 kDa) showed significant double-augmented anticancer activity compared to the native fucoidans.[27] Similarly, a crude sulfated xylogalactofucan with minor contents of mannose, glucose, uronic acid, and protein was isolated from New Zealand-cultured sporophyll of *U. pinnatifida*. Treatment with 1 mg/mL of the sulfated xylogalactofucan for 72 h exerted reducing capacity effects against WiDr, MCF-7, and A549 cancer cells for 96.22%, 98.32%, and 99.96% and also against HEK-293 and HDFb normal cells for 63.7% and 79.8%, respectively.[28] SPUP, a sulfated polysaccharide extract was isolated from *U. pinnatifida* (produced in Yantai, China) with 19.42% yield. SPUP (m.w. 97.9 kDa) was composed of fucose, glucose, and galactose in a molar ratio of 27.15:19.34:53.51. The contents of total saccharide, uronic acid, protein, and sulfate radical in the SPUP were 80.48%, 3.21%, 7.12%, and 29.14%, respectively. In DMBA-triggered breast cancer rat model, the SPUP notably hampered abnormal breast enlargement and reduced tumor incidence.[29] Consequently, the approaches have provided evidences for supporting the uses of sulfated *polysaecharides* and polysaccharides (such as fucoidans) from sea mustard in cancer chemotherapy and chemoprevention.

NANOFORMULATION

The sea mustard polysaccharides have been fabricated as selenium nanoparticles, which were more effective in the suppression of human A375 melanoma, CNE2 nasopharyngeal cancer, HepG2 hepatoma, and MCF-7 breast cancer cell lines with IC_{50}s ranging from 3.0 to 14.1 μM. In the A375 cells, the selenium nanoparticles could dose-dependently trigger more apoptosis concomitant with the involvement of oxidative stress and mitochondrial dysfunction *in vitro*.[15]

CONCLUSION AND SUGGESTION

According to the chemical biology and phytochemical investigations, sea mustard (wakame) has been demonstrated to have positive potentials in anticarcinogenesis, antiproliferation, proapoptosis, and antiangiogenesis. The anticancer activities of sea mustard are broadly presented in various types of carcinomas such as in colon, lung, liver, breast, stomach, prostate, brain, cervix, skin, and blood. The major components in sea mustard were proved to be fucoidans (polysaccharides), sulfated polysaccharides, and fucoxanthin (**1**), all of which, especially the sulfated polysaccharides are primarily responsible for the anticancer-related activities of sea mustard. Even though it also showed certain inhibition on hDFb dermal fibroblasts and HEK293 embryonic kidney cells, the great potential of sea mustard still can be recommended as a functional food for lessening the cancer incidence or cancer treatment supplements.

REFERENCES

1. Ohigashi, H. et al., 1994. Antitumor promoters from edible plants. *ACS Sympos. Series* 547 (Food Phytochemicals for Cancer Prevention II): 251–261.
2. Sekiya, M. et al., 2005. Intracellular signaling in the induction of apoptosis in a human breast cancer cell line by water extract of Mekabu. *Intl. J. Clin. Oncol.* 10: 122–126.
3. Fujii, M. et al., 2000. Effects of sporophyll of Undaria pinnatifida on spleen natural killer activity, and on the growth of implanted cancer cells in mice. *Food Style 21* 4: 67–69.
4. Funahashi, H. et al., 1999. Wakame seaweed suppresses the proliferation of 7,12-dimethyl-benz(a)-anthracene-induced mammary tumors in rats. *Jpn. J. Cancer Res.* 90: 922–927.
5. Wang, S.K. et al., 2014. Extracts from New Zealand Undaria pinnatifida containing fucoxanthin as potential functional biomaterials against cancer in vitro. *J. Funct. Biomater.* 5: 29–42.
6. Hosokawa, M. et al., 1999. Apoptosis-inducing effect of fucoxanthin on human leukemia cell line HL-60. *Food Sci. Technol. Res.* 5: 243–246.
7. Liu, C.L. et al., 2009. Inhibition of proliferation of a hepatoma cell line by fucoxanthin in relation to cell cycle arrest and enhanced gap junctional intercellular communication. *Chemico-Biol. Interactions* 182: 165–172.
8. Li, D.T. et al., 2012. Study on extraction, isolation of fucoxanthin of Undaria pinnatifida and the inhibitory effect on proliferation of HepG2. *Liaoning Shifan Daxue Xuebao, Ziran Kexueban* 35: 383–389.
9. Kotake-Nara, E. et al., 2001. Carotenoids affect proliferation of human prostate cancer cells. *J. Nutr.* 131: 3303–3306.
10. Hosokawa, M. et al., 2004. Fucoxanthin induces apoptosis and enhances the antiproliferative effect of the PPAR ligand, troglitazone, on colon cancer cells. *Biochim. Biophys. Acta, Gene. Subjects* 1675: 113–119.
11. Wang, X. et al., 2006. Studies on antitumor activities of Undaria pinnatifida polysaccharides (UPPS). *J. Dalian Med. Univ.* 28: 98–100.
12. Wang, E.M. et al., 2011. Separation, purification and antitumor activity of Undaria pinnatifida polysaccharides. *Shipin Keji* 36: 199–202.
13. Shang, X.L. et al., 2011. The effects of polysaccharides from the Undaria pinnatifida on human esophageal carcinoma cell TE-13 and relating mechanisms. *Xiandai Yufang Yixue* 38: 1017–1019.
14. Shang, X.H. et al., 2011. Effect of polysaccharides from Undaria pinnatifida on gastric carcinoma BGC-823 cells. *Zhongliu Fangzhi Yanjiu* 38: 134–136, 140.
15. Chen, T.F. et al., 2008. Selenium nanoparticles fabricated in Undaria pinnatifida polysaccharide solutions induce mitochondria-mediated apoptosis in A375 human melanoma cells. *Colloids Surf., B: Biointerfaces* 67: 26–31.
16. Maruyama, H. et al., 2006. The role of NK cells in antitumor activity of dietary fucoidan from Undaria pinnatifida sporophylls (Mekabu). *Planta Med.* 72: 1415–1417.
17. Maruyama, H. et al., 2003. Antitumor activity and immune response of Mekabu fucoidan extracted from Sporophyll of Undaria pinnatifida. *In Vivo* (Athens, Greece) 17: 245–249.
18. Ji, Y.B. et al., 2011. Preliminary study on extracting technique and biological activity of fucoidin in Undaria pinnatifida. *Advan. Mater. Research* (Zuerich, Switzerland) 183–185 (Pt. 2, Environmental Biotechnology and Materials Engineering): 887–890.
19. Wang, J. et al., 2009. Antitumor action of Fucoidan extracted from brown alga. *Shizhen Guoyi Guoyao* 20: 1757–1758.
20. Zhang, W. et al., 2015. Fucoidan from Macrocystis pyrifera has powerful immune-modulatory effects compared to three other fucoidans. *Mar. Drugs* 13: 1084–2104.
21. Vishchuk, O.S. et al., 2011. Sulfated polysaccharides from brown seaweeds Saccharina japonica and Undaria pinnatifida: Isolation, structural characteristics, and antitumor activity. *Carbohydr. Res.* 346: 2769–2776.
22. Vishchuk, O.S. et al., 2013. The fucoidans from brown algae of Far-Eastern seas: Anti-tumor activity and structure-function relationship. *Food Chem.* 141: 1211–1217.

23. Boo, H.J. et al., 2013. The anticancer effect of fucoidan in PC-3 prostate cancer cells. *Mar. Drugs* 11: 2982–2999.

24. Boo, H.J. et al., 2011. Fucoidan from Undaria pinnatifida induces apoptosis in A549 human lung carcinoma cells. *Phytother. Res.* 25: 1082–1086.

25. Yang, L.L. et al., 2013. Fucoidan derived from Undaria pinnatifida induces apoptosis in human hepatocellular carcinoma SMMC-7721 cells via the ROS-mediated mitochondrial pathway. *Mar. Drugs* 11: 1961–1976.

26. Synytsya, A. et al., 2010. Structure and antitumor activity of fucoidan isolated from sporophyll of Korean brown seaweed Undaria pinnatifida. *Carbohydr. Polym.* 81: 41–48.

27. Yang, C. et al., 2008. Effects of molecular weight and hydrolysis conditions on anticancer activity of fucoidans from sporophyll of Undaria pinnatifida. *Intl. J. Biol. Macromol.* 43: 433–437.

28. Mak, W. et al., 2014. Anti-proliferation potential and content of fucoidan extracted from sporophyll of New Zealand Undaria pinnatifida. *Frontiers in Nutr.* 1: 9.

29. Han, Y. et al., 2016. Separation, characterization and anticancer activities of a sulfated polysaccharide from Undaria pinnatifida. *Int. J. Biol. Macromol.* 83: 42–49.

82. UMITORANOO

鼠尾藻　ウミトラノオ

Sargassum thunbergii

Sargassaceae

1. R = B
2. R = A
4. R = C

Umitoranoo is an edible and economic brown seaweed originating from the algae *Sargassum thunbergii*, which is broadly distributed along the shallow marine coast of China, Korea, and Japan. It is an important raw material utilized for the production of alginate, mannitol, polyphenol, and other bioactive substances in chemical, pharmaceutical, and food products. Pharmacological investigations established that umitoranoo possesses antiulcer, hypolipemia, anti-infective, antihypoxia, anticoagulant, neuroprotective, and antihelminthic properties besides antitumor activity.

SCIENTIFIC EVIDENCE OF CANCER-INHIBITORY AND CANCER-PREVENTIVE CONSTITUENTS

1. Polyphenols

Two polyphenols termed STK1 (m.w. $> 1 \times 10^4$) and STK2 (m.w. $< 1 \times 10^4$) were isolated from umitoranoo, showing strong inhibition on human carcinoma cell lines, in which inhibition rates of STK1 in a concentration of 87.5 µg/mL were 90.7% and 89.3% on human A549 lung carcinoma and BEL-7402 hepatoma cell lines, respectively, whereas STK2 reached the similar suppressive potency but in a concentration of 340 µg/mL, implying that the antineoplastic activity of the higher molecular STK1 was more potent than that of the lower molecular STK2.[1]

2. Polysaccharides

Polysaccharide components in the umitoranoo are the major immunoactive inhibitors against carcinoma cells. Daily administration of the polysaccharides by i.p. to mice in 20 mg/kg dose per day for 10 days significantly prolonged the life span of mice-implanted EAC. Interestingly, the surviving mice after the chemotherapy could reject reimplantation of the ascites carcinoma, sarcoma 180, Shionogi carcinoma, and Nakahara–Fukuoka sarcoma *in vivo*. The results indicated that umitoranoo is capable of building up a remarkable immune system against the growth of tumor cells.[2] STP-II (550 KD), a purified fraction from *S. thunbergii* polysaccharides, comprised mainly fucose, xylose, galactose, glucose, and glucuronic acid. STP-II showed higher scavenging activities on hydroxyl radical (76.72% at 0.7 mg/mL) and superoxide radical (95.17% at 2 mg/mL) than vitamin C. STP-II also exhibited the capability of antiproliferation in human Caco-2 colon cancer cells.[3]

Two fucoidans, GIV-A (m.w. 19,000) and GIV-B (m.w. 13,500) prepared from umitoranoo, are L-fucans with 10.4% and 11.2% uronic acid and less than 1.6% and 1.9% protein, respectively, and the two L-fucans contain approximately 28.8% and 34.2% sulfate ester groups in the fucose residues, respectively. Both the fucoidans exerted marked anticancer activity in mice-borne Ehrlich carcinoma with no toxicity and side effects.[3,4] The *in vitro* antitumor activity was found to be closely correlated to its immunopotentiating properties, such as activation of C3 and macrophage and depression of the hepatic microsomal drug-metabolizing system.[5] In addition, GIV-A significantly exerted the antimetastatic effect in the *in vivo* test. After removal of the implanted primary tumor, injection of GIV-A by i.p. inhibited the metastases in mice-borne Lewis lung tumor. During the antimetastatic action, GIV-A depressed the activities of aniline hydroxylase and aminopyrine demethylase in the hepatic microsomal drug-metabolizing system in tumor-bearing mice. Concurrently, the number of peritoneal macrophages was amplified in the lung of the mice, and the binding of C3b to the C3 receptor in peritoneal macrophages was notably enhanced.[5,6] Moreover, cotreatment with GIV-A could markedly augment the inhibitory effect of 5-FU against lung metastases. Simultaneously, GIV-A not only remarkably increased the concentration of 5-FU in the tissues of lung, liver, kidney, spleen, and in blood, but also diminished the 5-FU-induced toxicity, where GIV-A exerted marked abilities to restore the 5-FU-reduced PC-DTH response and to enlarge the indexes of spleen, thymus, and the number of spleen cells.[5] The findings suggest that GIV-A has a promising value as both functional food additive and medicinal supplement for patients in the prevention of cancer metastasis.

In addition, a sulfated polysaccharide (SHP) was isolated from the same genus seaweed *S. henslowianum*. SHP having lower sulfate and uronic acid contents demonstrated marked inhibitory effects on the growth of MKN45 gastric cancer cells and DLD intestinal cancer cells *in vitro*.[7]

3. Steroles

An ethyl acetate extract of *S. thunbergii* in the *in vitro* assay showed excellent cytotoxic effect against human HL-60 leukemia cells at 25 μg/mL concentration and it was cytotoxic to human HT-29 colon cancer and murine B16F10 melanoma cell lines at 100 μg/mL concentration. Treatment of HT-60 cells with the fraction could significantly induce cell shrinkage, cell membrane blubbing, and formation of apoptotic bodies. A standard component was identified to have fucosterol (**1**) by HPLC fingerprinting analysis, which exerted the antitumor activity.[8]

From a closely related seaweed *S. henslowianum*, an alginate component was extracted, which exhibited obvious growth suppressive effect against Ehrlich ascites tumor and sarcoma 180 in mice with the inhibition ratios of 31.76% and 30.43%, respectively.[9] By activity guided fractionation, five anticancer active sterols identified as fucosterol (**1**), 3β,28ζ-dihydroxy-24-ethylcholesta-5,23Z-diene (**2**), 24-ethylcholesta-4,24(28)-diene-3,6-dione (**3**), 24R,28R- and 24S,28S-epoxy-24-ethylcholesterol (**5**), and 24ζ-hydroperoxy-24-vinylcholesterol (**4**), were separated from another similar seaweed *S. carpophyllum*. In the *in vitro* assay, five sterols (**1–5**) remarkably hindered the proliferation of various cancer cell lines. The IC_{50} values were 7.8 and 8.5 μg/mL for **1** and **4** in human HL-60 leukemia cells and 0.7 and 0.8 μg/mL for **2** and **3** in murine P388 leukemia cells, respectively, whereas the IC_{50}s were 4.0, 7.2, 8.8, 10.0, and 10.0 μg/mL for **5** against human MCF-7 (breast), PC3 (prostate), HCT-8 (colon), 1A9 (ovary) cancer cell lines, and HOS osteosarcoma cells, respectively.[10,11]

Conclusion and Suggestion

Umitoranoo has been utilized as a folk medicine and raw material in the chemical industry for many years, though rarely used as a sea vegetable. In recent years, umitoranoo has been explored for its biological activities, especially for its cancer-preventive potential. The bioorganic chemistry studies discovered anticarcinogenic agents, such as polyphenols, sterols, and polysaccharides from umitoranoo. The major cancer inhibitor was found to be the fucoidan-type of polysaccharide, which was effective in suppressing the growth of carcinomas, potentiating the anticancer effects of chemotherapeutic drugs, retarding the metastasis of cancer cells, and lessening the toxicity of anticancer drugs. The polyphenols and sterols isolated from the seaweeds also displayed moderate-to-weak degrees of antiproliferative activities against some cancer cell lines. Due to exerting radical-scavenging and immunoregulating functions, the anticarcinogenic activity of umitaranoo can be considered to also contribute to the antioxidant and immunoaugmenting properties. Consequently, based on its remarkable benefit in lowering cancer incidence, the application of umitoranoo should be encouraged for the development of a novel natural functional food.

REFERENCES

1. Wei, Y.X. et al., 2008. Antitumor activity of polyphenol in Sargassum thunbergii. *Zhongcaoyao* 39: 93–95.
2. Ito, H. et al., 1976. Studies on antitumor activities of Basidiomycetes: influence of the sex of the animal on antitumor activity of the polysaccharide. *Nippon Yakurigaku Zasshi* 72: 77–94.
3. Yuan, X.M. et al., 2015. Extraction optimization, characterization and bioactivities of a major polysaccharide from Sargassum thunbergii. *PLoS One* 10: e0144773/1–e0144773/11.
4. Zhuang, C. et al., 1995. Antitumor active fucoidan from the brown seaweed, Umitoranoo (Sargassum thunbergii). *Biosci. Biotech. Biochem.* 59: 563–567.
5. Zhuang, C. et al., 1994. The host-mediated antitumor polysaccharides. XXV. Antitumor active fucoidan from the brown seaweed, Umitoranoo, Sargassum thunbergii. *Shizuoka Daigaku Nogakubu Kenkyu Hokoku* 43: 61–70.
6. Itoh, H. et al., 1993. Antitumor activity and immunological properties of marine algal polysaccharides, especially fucoidan, prepared from Sargassum thunbergii of Phaeophyceae. *Anticancer Res.* 13: 2045–2052.
7. Shao, P. et al., 2013. In vitro antioxidant and antitumor activities of different sulfated polysaccharides isolated from three algae. *Intl. J. Biol. Macromol.* 62: 155–161.
8. Itoh, H. et al., 1995. Immunological analysis of inhibition of lung metastases by fucoidan (GIV-A) prepared from brown seaweed Sargassum thunbergii. *Anticancer Res.* 15: 1937–1948.
9. Kim, K.N. et al., 2009. In vitro cytotoxic activity of Sargassum thunbergii and Dictyopteris divaricata (Jeju seaweeds) on the HL-60 tumor cell line. *Int. J. Pharmacol.* 5: 298–306.
10. Hou, Z.J. et al., 2001. Research on antitumor activity of alginate from Sargassum henslowianum. *Shipin Kexue* (Beijing) 22: 95–97.
11. Tang, H.F. et al., 2002. Bioactive steroids from the brown alga Sargassum carpophyllum. *J. Asian Nat. Prods. Res.* 4: 95–101.

10 Cancer-Preventive Substances in Microalgae

83. Chlorella/*Chlorella vulgaris, C. pyrenoidosa*

84. Spherical Nostoc/*Nostoc commune*

85. Spirulina/*Spirulina platensis* (= *Arthrospira platensis*)

Microalgae are widely dispersed in freshwater and marine systems and are important for life on the earth because of their ability to perform photosynthesis and production of approximately half of the atmospheric oxygen. Many microalgae species generate unique natural substances such as carotenoids, chlorophyll, fatty acids, antioxidants, vitamins, enzymes, polymers, peptides, sterols, and toxins. The biochemical systems provide basic foodstuff for numerous aquaculture species. In this chapter, three microalgae, (1) Chlorella, (2) spherical Nostoc, and (3) Spirulina, are discussed as a source of both nutritional and functional food because of their benefit in health promotion and body protection. Recent investigations combining bioorganic chemistry and chemical biology reveal these particular microalgae-demonstrated features that promote tumor cell death, inhibition of tumor cell growth, and improve overall human body defense—all of which are useful in the prevention and treatment of cancer and other diseases. Although consumption of these microalgae products is highly recommended, the cultivation of the microalgae at industry scales must be regulated to limit pollution from both toxic microalgae and pathogens and to provide both good quality and good desired products.

83. CHLORELLA

小球藻　クロレラ　클로렐라

Chlorella vulgaris, C. pyrenoidosa

Chlorellaceae

MGDG:
R_1 = linolenoyl or linoeoyl or linoleoyl
    or 7Z,10Z-hexadecadienoyl
R_2 = 7Z,10Z,13Z-hexadecatriencyl,
    or 7Z,10Z-hexadecadienoyl
    or linoleoyl
R_3 = –H

DGDG:
R_1 = linolenoyl or linoleoyl
R_2 = 7Z,10Z,13Z-hexadecatriencyl
    or 7Z,10Z-hexadecadienoyl
R_3 = –gal.

Chlorella, or *Chlorella vulgaris* and *C. pyrenoidosa* (Chlorellaceae), is a blue–green algae. Chlorella may serve as a potential source in food industry because it can provide an inexpensive and nutritional protein supplement to the human diet. Nutritional analysis showed that Chlorella is a rich source of vitamins A, B2, B3, iron, and zinc and a good source of vitamins B1, B6, C, and minerals phosphorus and magnesium. The most important constituents in Chlorella are assigned as chlorophylls-a, -b, and β-carotene. Pharmacological approaches have established multiple biological benefits for Chlorella, including immunoregulating, interferon-simulating, free-radical scavenging, phagocytosis-enhancing, hypolipemic, detoxification, diabetes-preventing, anti atherosclerosis, liver-protecting, cardiovascular-improving, lung-function promoting, and antiaging activities.[1,2] In addition, Chlorella is considered as a source of energy for its photosynthetic efficiency.

Scientific Evidence of Antitumor Activities

Chlorella and its products normally displayed no direct cytotoxicity to either tumor cells or mouse spleen cells *in vitro*, but it exerted an *in vivo* antitumor effect through promotion of host immune responses.[3] The nutritional and functional ingredients in Chlorella, such as amino acids, vitamins, minerals, folic acid, chlorophyll, the active factor Chlorella growth factor (CGF), algae polysaccharides, and nucleic acids, can not only stimulate the production of interferons and the activation of NK cells to improve the human immune system but also boost the cytotoxicity of immune factors to attack cancer cells.[2]

1. Antitumor activities of Chlorella

Both intraperitoneal (i.p.) and oral administrations of autoclaved or heat-extracted substances of *C. pyrenoidosa* every other day significantly prolonged the life duration of mice bearing either MM-2 mammary neoplasm or EL-4 leukemia. With treatment, 73.3%–80% tumor-bearing mice survived over 60 days and 82% mice were protected from sarcoma BP8 grafting.[3,4] When given

10% Chlorella in a basal diet, the number of glutathione S-transferase (GST) placental form-positive foci in the liver of rats were significantly lessened *in vivo*, suggesting that the Chlorella has chemopreventive activity against hepatocarcinogenesis.[5] Rats fed with 3% *C. pyrenoidosa* powder in diet for 14 weeks suppressed N-methyl-N-nitrosourea-triggered mammary carcinogenesis by 61% and lengthened the tumor latency by 12.5 days. This Chlorella powder also diminished the survival of MCF-7 human breast adenocarcinoma cancer cells *in vitro* together with a decrease in mitochondrial membrane potential and increase of ROS generation.[6] A *C. vulgaris* extract showed definite inhibitory and proapoptotic effects in rats bearing hepatoma caused by ethionine (a hepatocarcinogen).[7]

E-25 (a product prepared from *C. vulgaris*) markedly repressed 7,12-dimethylbenz[a]anthracene (DMBA)-caused skin papillomagenesis during pre- and postinitiation stages.[8] Simultaneously, E-25 elevated the levels of sulfhydryl and GST and markedly restrained lipid peroxidation in the tissues of liver and skin.[8,9] A supercritical carbon dioxide (SC–CO_2) extract of *C. vulgaris* at 20–200 μg/mL concentration inhibits human nonsmall lung cancer cell lines (H1299, A549, and H1437) in a dose-dependent manner and at 200 μg/mL effectively reduces the lung cancer cell migration.[10] The SC–CO_2 extract also showed strong antioxidant activities against radical scavenging, ferric-reducing power, and metal-chelating abilities.[10] All the *in vivo* and *in vitro* test results have demonstrated the potentials of Chlorella in anticarcinogenesis, antimetastasis, and chemoprevention.

2. Immunoenhancing activity of Chlorella

The extract in normal mice had no effects on bone marrow and spleen colony forming unit–granulocyte macrophage (CFU–GM), but it could restore the numbers of granulocyte-macrophage progenitor cells (CFU–GM) in the bone marrow and spleen in tumor-bearing mice, thereby significantly prolonging the survival of mice inoculated with the Ehrlich ascites tumor, where the regulation of immunohematopoietic cell activity was mediated by the amplification of spleen mononuclear cell proliferation, colony stimulating activity and NK cell activity, and promotion of IL-2, IFN-γ, and TNF-α production.[11]

SCIENTIFIC EVIDENCE OF ANTITUMOR CONSTITUENTS AND ACTIVITIES

1. Glycoproteins

Glycoproteins are the major anticancer immunity agents in *C. vulgaris*, which are similarly composed of 35%–36.3% protein and 56%–67% polysaccharide with a β-1,6-D-galactopyranose backbone, whose protein moiety sequence has 15 amino acids at its N-terminus. The compositions seem to be essential for the glycoproteins to exert the antitumor immunoenhancing activities. In the lab experiments, the glycoproteins retarded mouse L1210 lymphocytic leukemia cells *in vitro* (IC_{50} of 110 μg/mL) and obviously augmented the survival of tumor-bearing mice.[12,13] Several highly purified antitumor immunoactive glycoproteins such as CVS, ARS-2, and Q2C2 were separated from the unicellular microalga (*C. vulgaris*). The glycoproteins are stable for the extreme treatments of acid, alkali, heat, and carbohydrate degradation but their antitumor activity will disappear after protease digestion.[14–17] However, when these glycol proteins were hydrolyzed by α-amylase, the product (m.w. 4.5×10^4) also displayed antitumor activity against L-1210 leukemia cells *in vitro* and sarcoma 180 *in vivo*.[18]

In both spontaneously and experimentally established metastatic tumor models, CVS by intratumor injection displayed *in vivo* antitumor effect. During the treatment, T-cells (such as CD4 and CD8 T-cells) in lymphoid organs were activated and the recruitment of T-cells was accelerated to the regional lymph nodes that are close to tumor sites, indicating that both CVS-boosted CD4 and CD8 T-cells primarily contributed to the antimetastatic activity. The CVS was also helpful for the inhibition of metastasis and tumor progression in presurgical treatment and for the early recovery of hematopoietic stem cells to alleviate chemotherapy-caused adverse effects.[14–20] ARS-2, which has the same molecular weight (63,100 amu) as CVS, could stimulate spleen-adherent cells from

C3H/HeJ lacking functional TLR4 to produce IL-12 p40. These findings suggested that toll-like receptor (TLR) signaling should partly involve in the anticancer immunity.[15,20] Among the glycoproteins derived from *C. vulgaris*, the most active one was Q2C2 (containing 56.1% carbohydrate and 36.3% protein), which interestingly demonstrated far greater anticancer effect against a rechallenged tumor than against the primarily inoculated Meth-A fibrosarcoma in mice.[17]

2. Polysaccharides

Two distinctive polysaccharides assigned as CPPS-Ia (69658 Da) and CPPS-IIa (109406 Da) were purified from *Chlorella pyrenoidosa*, both of which consist of galactose, rhamnose, mannose, glucose, and an unknown monosaccharide. The predominant monosaccharide was 46.5% galactose in CPPS-Ia and 37.8% rhamnose in CPPS-IIa.[21] Both CPPS-Ia and CPPS-IIa in 200–1000 μg/mL concentrations demonstrated antineoplastic activity against human A549 lung cancer cells *in vitro* in a dose-dependent manner. The highest inhibitory rates of CPPS-Ia and CPPS-IIa were 68.7% and 49.5% at 1000 μg/mL, respectively.[22] From a hot water extract of *C. pyrenoidosa*, an acidic polysaccharide termed chlon-A was purified, which consists of glucuronic acid, glucose, galactose, rhamnose, and arabinose. It exerted the growth inhibitory effect against transplantable Ehrlich ascites tumor and sarcoma 180 in mice with marked life-prolongation rates, and also against IMC maxillary carcinoma, Meth-A fibrosarcoma, B16 melanoma, and Lewis lung cancer with significant anti-growth effect *in vivo*. Moreover, chlon-A was able to enhance the cytotoxicity of mouse macrophages on EL-4 lymphoma cells *in vivo* and to augment the lymphoproliferative effects *in vitro*.[23,24] Furthermore, Chlorella polysaccharides that were obtained by pH6.5 enzymolysis and partly by purification showed some degree of antimigratory effect in human umbilical vein endothelial cells at concentrations of 50 and 100 μg/mL, implying certain antiangiogenic potential.[25]

Interestingly, Reishi (*Ganoderma lucidum*) was found to be able to break the cell wall of *C. pyrenoidosa* to amplify the yield of polysaccharides if Chlorella powder was added in the basic medium of Reishi. The bioconverted polysaccharides by Reishi presented marked immunopotentiating capacity in hepatoma-burdening mice, such as amplifying the number of white blood cells, lymphocyte proliferation, and macrophage function. Predominantly based on immunity, the bioconverted polysaccharides at an optimum dose (0.2 g/kg/day) achieved 76.2% tumor inhibitory rate in a tumor-bearing mouse model.[26]

3. Proteins and peptides

A *C. vulgaris* protein fraction (m.w. ≈ 70 kDa) was obtained by modern separation techniques, which impeded the viability of HepG2 hepatoma cells (IC$_{50}$ of 1.75 μg/mL) and induced cell apoptosis and DNA fragmentation.[27] A peptide fraction was prepared from pepsin hydrolysis of the algae protein waste, which was obtained after the production of *C. vulgaris* essence. The peptide fraction exhibited dose-dependent antiproliferative activity against AGS gastric carcinoma cells *in vitro* and induction of a post-G1 cell-cycle arrest, but it had no cytotoxicity on WI-38 lung fibroblasts cells. A hendecapeptide with an amino acid sequence as VECYGPNRPQF was isolated from this fraction, which showed potent antiproliferative, antioxidant, and NO-production–inhibiting activities.[28] By a similar process, a polypeptide CPAP was prepared from *C. pyrenoidosa*, which exhibited inhibitory activity on human HepG2 hepatoma cells.[29] The micro-/nanoencapsulation of CPAP was further prepared for increasing bioavailability and bioactivity, but the *in vitro* inhibition rates of nonencapsulated, microencapsulated, and nanoencapsulated CPAP in the HepG2 cells were 47.9%, 38%, and 31%, respectively, at the same polypeptide concentrations of 0.4 mg/mL.[29]

4. Glyceroglycolipids

From freshwater cultured *C. vulgaris*, two groups of unique and promising anticancer agents assigned as mono-galactosyl diacylglycerols (MGDG) and digalactosyl diacylglycerols (DGDG) were separated. Due to 7Z,10Z-hexadecadienoic acid content, the MGDG and DGDG molecules played a more potent role in the suppression of tumor promotion than the other isolated glyceroglycolipids.[30]

5. Ergosterols

An *n*-hexane partition fraction obtained from the methanolic extract of *C. vulgaris* displayed marked inhibitory activity against 12-O-tetra-decanoylphorbol-13-acetate (TPA)-induced inflammation in mice. Ergosterol peroxide and several Δ5-sterols and Δ6-sterols were isolated from this fraction. Ergosterol peroxide was found to markedly suppress skin carcinogenesis initiated by DMBA and promoted by TPA in mice.[31]

6. Chlorophyllin

Chlorophyllin, which was isolated from *C. vulgaris*, was demonstrated to have suppressive properties against mutagenicity and genotoxicity elicited by mutagens such as Trp-P-2, 4-nitroquinoline-1-oxide (4NQO) and 3-hydroxy-amino-1-methyl-5H-pyrido[4,3-b]-indole.[32]

7. Carotenoids

Two carotenoid components were separated from freshwater *C. vulgaris* and marine *C. ellipsoidea*, respectively. The carotenoids derived from *C. vulgaris* were almost completely composed of lutein (**1**), whereas the carotenoids from *C. ellipsoidea* were composed of violaxanthin (**2**) with two minor xanthophylls (antheraxanthin and zeaxanthin). The two carotenoids in an *in vitro* system enhanced the cell apoptosis and dose-dependently inhibited the growth of HCT116 cells, yielding IC_{50}s in a range of 40–41 µg/mL. However, the carotenoids of *C. ellipsoidea* was 2.5-fold more potent than the carotenoids of *C. vulgaris* in the proapoptosis of HCT116 cells.[33]

CONCLUSION AND SUGGESTION

Indeed, antitumor and anticarcinogenic studies disclosed the potential usage of Chlorella in the chemotherapy and chemoprevention as a functional food supplement. Eight types of chemical molecules derived from Chlorella displayed different degrees of suppressive activities against the initiation, viability, and proliferation of carcinomas and against some mutagen-elicited carcinogenesis. Of them, the most important and abundant constituents in Chlorella were two kinds of macromolecules: glycoproteins and polysaccharides that play remarkable roles in anticancer immunity and immunoenhancement. The major Chlorella components should be helpful ingredients, which can be utilized as dietary supplement for lessening cancer incidence and amplifying cancer prevention. Indeed, further investigation and development of Chlorella can be considered to be a promising and valuable project in the application of nutraceuticals and pharmaceuticals. Nevertheless, the cultivation of Chlorella in manufactory size must be insured under well-controlled and nonpolluted conditions.

REFERENCES

1. Merchant, R.E. et al., 2001. A review of recent clinical trials of the nutritional supplement Chlorella pyrenoidosa in the treatment of fibromyalgia, hypertension, and ulcerative colitis. *Altern. Ther. Health Med.* 7(3): 79–91.
2. Kotrbáček, V. et al., 2015. The chlorococcalean alga Chlorella in animal nutrition: A review. *J. Applied Phycol.* 27(6): 2173–2180.
3. Miyazawa, Y. et al., 1988. Immunomodulation by an unicellular green algae (Chlorella pyrenoidosa) in tumor-bearing mice. *J. Ethnopharmacol.* 24: 135–146.
4. Vermeil, C. et al., 1976. Experimental role of the unicellular algae Prototheca and Chlorella (Chlorellaceae) in anticancer immunogenesis (murine BP8 sarcoma). *Comptes rendus des seances de la Societe de biologie et de ses filiales* 170: 646–649.
5. Takekoshi, H. et al., 2005. Suppression of glutathione S-transferase placental form-positive foci development in rat hepatocarcinogenesis by Chlorella pyrenoidosa. *Oncol. Reports* 14: 409–414.
6. Kubatka, P. et al., 2015. Antineoplastic effects of Chlorella pyrenoidosa in the breast cancer model. *Nutrition* (NY, NY, US) 31(4): 560–569.
7. Mohd, A.E.S. et al., 2009. Chlorella vulgaris triggers apoptosis in hepatocarcinogenesis-induced rats. *J. Zhejiang Univ. Sci.-B* 10: 14–21.

8. Singh, A. et al., 1999. Inhibitory potential of Chlorella vulgaris (E-25) on mouse skin papillomagenesis and xenobiotic detoxication system. *Anticancer Res.* 19: 1887–1891.

9. Singh, A. et al., 1998. Perinatal influence of Chlorella vulgaris (E-25) on hepatic drug metabolizing enzymes and lipid peroxidation. *Anticancer Res.* 18: 1509–1514.

10. Wang, H.M. et al., 2010. Identification of anti-lung cancer extract from Chlorella vulgaris C-C by antioxidant property using supercritical carbon dioxide extraction. *Process Biochem.* (Amsterdam, Netherlands) 45(12): 1865–1872.

11. a) Justo, G.Z. et al., 2001. Effects of the green algae Chlorella vulgaris on the response of the host hematopoietic system to intraperitoneal Ehrlich ascites tumor transplantation in mice. *Immunopharmacol. Immunotoxicol.* 23: 119–132; b) Ramos, A.L. et al., 2010. Chlorella vulgaris modulates immunomyelopoietic activity and enhances the resistance of tumor-bearing mice. *Nutr. Cancer* 62(8): 1170–1180.

12. Matsueda, S. et al., 1982. Studies on antitumor active glycoprotein from Chlorella vulgaris. I. *Yakugaku Zasshi* 102: 447–451.

13. Matsueda, S. et al., 1983. Studies on antitumor active glycoprotein from Chlorella vulgaris. II. *Science Reports of the Hirosaki Univ.* 30: 127–131.

14. Tanaka, K. et al., 2001. Immunopotentiating effects of a glycoprotein from Chlorella vulgaris strain CK and its characteristics. *Studies in Nat. Prods. Chem.* 25 (*Bioact. Nat. Prods., Part F*): 429–458.

15. Tanaka, K. et al., 1998. A novel glycoprotein obtained from Chlorella vulgaris strain CK22 shows antimetastatic immunopotentiation. *Cancer Immunol. Immunother.* 45: 313–320.

16. Noda, K. et al., 1996. A water-soluble antitumor glycoprotein from Chlorella vulgaris. *Planta Med.* 62: 423–426.

17. Noda, K. et al., 1998. A new type of biological response modifier from Chlorella vulgaris which needs protein moiety to show an antitumor activity. *Phytother. Res.* 12: 309–319.

18. Matsueda, S. et al., 1987. Studies on an antitumor glycoprotein from Chlorella vulgaris. II. Glycoprotein hydrolyzed with hydrolase. *Yakugaku Zasshi* 107: 694–697.

19. Noda, K. et al., 2002. Simple assay for antitumor immunoactive glycoprotein derived from *Chlorella vulgaris* strain CK22 using ELISA. *Phytother. Res.* 16: 581–585.

20. Hasegawa, T. et al., 2002. Toll-like receptor 2 is at least partly involved in the antitumor activity of glycoprotein from Chlorella vulgaris. *Intl. Immuno-pharmacol.* 2: 579–589.

21. Konishi, F. et al., 1996. Protective effect of an acidic glycoprotein obtained from culture of *Chlorella vulgaris* against myelosuppression by 5-fluorouracil. *Cancer Immunol. Immunother.* 42: 268–274.

22. Sheng, J.C. et al., 2007. Preparation, identification and their antitumor activities in vitro of polysaccharides from Chlorella pyrenoidosa. *Food Chem.* 105: 533–539.

23. Komiyama, K. et al., 1986. An acidic polysaccharide, Chlon A, from Chlorella pyrenoidosa. II. Antitumor activity and immunological response. *Chemother.* (Tokyo) 34: 302–307.

24. Umezawa, I. et al., 1982. An acidic polysaccharide, Chlon A. from Chlorella pyrenoidosa. I. Physicochemical and biological properties. *Chemother.* (Tokyo) 30: 1041–1046.

25. Tan, C.Y. et al., 2014. The Preparation and anti-angiogenic activity of Chlorella polysaccharides. *Chinese J. Mar. Drugs* 33(4): 33–38.

26. Yang, C. et al., 2009. Antitumor effect of polysaccharides from ferment liquid of bioconverted Chlorella pyrenoidosa by Ganoderma lucidum. *Zhongguo Niangzao* 5: 83–86; Effects of polysaccharides from ferment liquid of bioconverted Chlorella pyrenoidosa by Ganoderma lucidum on immunological function of tumor-beard mice. *Zhongguo Niangzao* 6: 54–57.

27. Mukti, N.A. et al., 2013. A purified novel protein from the culture media of Chlorella vulgaris inhibits growth and induces cell death in hepatoma HepG2 cells. *Int. Med. J.* 20(2): 140–145.

28. Sheih, I, C. et al., 2010. Anticancer and antioxidant activities of the peptide fraction from algae protein waste. *J. Agricul. Food Chem.* 58: 1202–1207.

29. Wang, X.Q. et al., 2013. Separation, antitumor activities, and encapsulation of polypeptide from Chlorella pyrenoidosa. *Biotechnol. Progr.* 29(3): 681–687.

30. Morimoto, A. et al., 1995. Antitumor-promoting glyceroglycolipids from the green alga, Chlorella vulgaris. *Phytochem.* 40: 1433–1437.

31. Yasukawa, K. et al., 1996. Inhibitory effects of sterols isolated from Chlorella vulgaris on 12-O-tetradecanoylphorbol-13-acetate-induced inflammation and tumor promotion in mouse skin. *Biol. Pharm. Bull.* 19: 573–576.

32. Negishi, T. et al., 1997. Antigenotoxic activity of natural chlorophylls. *Mutation Res.* 376: 97–100.

33. Cha, K.Y. et al., 2008. Antiproliferative effects of carotenoids extracted from Chlorella ellipsoidea and Chlorella vulgaris on human colon cancer cells. *J. Agricul. Food Chem.* 56: 10521–10526.

84. SPHERICAL NOSTOC

葛仙米

Nostoc commune

Nostocaceae

3. $R_1 = R_2 = -CH_3$
4. $R_1 = -OH, R_2 = -CH_3$
5. $R_1 = R_2 = -OH$

Spherical Nostoc originates from the gelatinous colonies of terrestrial cyanobacteria *Nostoc commune* (Nostocaceae) and other algae in the same genus, such as *N. sphaeroides* and *N. pruniforme*. These Nostocs may be collected from various natural habitats for human utilization. The Nostocs, especially *N. commune*, are a health food and folk medicine in many areas, such as Eastern Asia. According to an ancient legend in China, a famous Taoist and pharmaceutist named Ge, Hong (A.D. 283–363) used to collect the Nostocs as his dietary supplements. Hence, spherical Nostoc in China was deemed to be a precious healthy food. The Nostoc (*N. commune*) has been suggested to treat a variety of medical conditions, including inflammation, night blindness, burns, anxiety, and chronic fatigue. Owing to its rich nutrition and remarkable functions, the edible Nostoc species gained increasing attention in recent decades. A variety of bioactive constituents with antitumor, antioxidant, or anti-inflammatory properties have been reported in the scientific journals.[1]

SCIENTIFIC EVIDENCE OF CANCER-INHIBITORY AND CANCER-PREVENTIVE CONSTITUENTS

1. Diterpenoid

Comnostin-B (**1**), an antineoplastic diterpenoid, was isolated from the terrestrial cyanobacterium. In an *in vitro* assay, it demonstrated moderate cytotoxic effect against human KB oral carcinoma cells and human Caco-2 colon cancer cells with ED_{50} values of 0.40 and 0.18 ppm, respectively.[2]

2. Alkaloid

Reduced scytonemin (**2**), isolated from *N. commune*, has been shown to obstruct the growth of human T-lymphoid Jurkat leukemia cells in a dose-dependent manner, the anticancer effect of which was attributable to the induction of autophagic cell death, where the stimulation of ROS plays a critical role for leading to the elicitation of mitochondrial dysfunction and autophagy.[3,4] In an *in vitro* model with murine macrophage RAW264 cells, the anti-inflammatory activity of reduced scytonemin (**2**) was revealed to involve both ROS/PI3K/Akt and p38 MAPK/Nrf2 signaling pathways.[5]

3. Cyclophanes

From the cellular extract of *Nostoc sp.* UIC 10110 cultivation, three cyclophanes designated as merocyclophanes-A (**3**), merocyclophanes-C (**4**), and merocyclophanes-D (**5**) were separated that showed moderate anticancer activities against a panel of three cancer cell lines: (1) MDA-MB-435 (melanoma), (2) MDA-MB-231 (breast adenocarcinoma), and (3) OVCAR3 (ovarian adenocarcinoma) with IC_{50} values of 5.1–9.8 μM for **3**, 1.4–1.6 μM for **4**, and 0.9–2.0 μM for **5**. Of them, the most potent suppressive effects were achieved by merocyclophane-D (**5**) on the MDA-MB-435 and MDA-MB-231 cell lines *in vitro*.[6]

4. Polysaccharides

N. commune polysaccharide (NVPS), a polysaccharide component extracted from *N. commune*, prominently suppressed the proliferation of human MCF-7 (breast) and DLD1 (colon) cancer cell lines *in vitro*, the effect of which was elucidated to be mediated by the induction of intrinsic and extrinsic apoptosis via endoplasmic reticulum stress (ERS)-involved signaling pathways.[7] In an *in vitro* model, Nostoc commune Vauch polysaccharide (NVPS) treatment obviously hindered the migration of NCI-H446 and NCI-H1688 human small cell lung cancer cell lines in association with (1) blocking of epithelial–mesenchymal transition program; (2) suppression of integrin β1/FAK signaling via regulating cell-matrix adhesion; and (3) upregulation of E-cadherin expression and downregulation of *N*-cadherin expression, Vimentin, and MMP-9, leading to interruption of STAT3 nuclear translocation and JAK1 signaling.[8]

5. Proteins

A protein extract was prepared from the blue-green alga and then gradually reacted with ammonium sulfate powder. The protein component was able to effectively restrain the growth of human colon carcinoma cells.[9] Water stress proteins (WSP1) prepared from *N. commune* significantly obstructed the proliferation of four human colon cancer cell lines (DLD1, HCT-116, HT29, and SW480) *in vitro* with IC_{50} values of 0.19, 0.21, 0.39, and 0.41 μg/μL, respectively. Simultaneously, WSP1 induced G1/S cell-cycle arrest and cell apoptosis through a caspase-dependent pathway in the colon cancer cells. The anti-colon cancer activity was further ascertained in nude mice with DLD1 xenograft.[8] Moreover, by promoting cell–cell adhesion and reducing cell–matrix adhesion, the DLD1 cell invasion was deterred by WSP1 treatment. However, it also had the inhibitory effect on a normal human intestinal epithelial FHC cell line (IC_{50} of 0.67 μg/μL).[10]

CONCLUSION AND SUGGESTION

Four types of antitumor constituents have been discovered from spherical Nostoc in chemical biology exploration. Compared with the micromolecules (comnostin-B and reduced-scytonemin), the macromolecules (polysaccharides and water stress proteins) as the major constituents in the Nostoc were more effective in suppressing the proliferation, migration, and invasion of cancer cells and eliciting the cell apoptotic death, especially for small cell lung cancer cells and colon carcinoma cells. Although no experimental report is correlated to its immune activity, these findings clearly provided scientific evidences to support the consumption of spherical Nostoc as a functional food for cancer prevention and therapeutic supplement.

REFERENCES

1. Han, D.X. et al., 2013. Biology and biotechnology of edible Nostoc. Edited by Richmond, A. and Hu, Q. *Handbook of Microalgal Culture* (2nd Ed.), Blackwell Publishing, Oxford, UK, pp. 433–44.
2. Jaki, B. et al., 2000. Novel extracellular diterpenoids with biological activity from the cyanobacterium Nostoc commune. *J. Nat. Prod.* 63: 339–343.
3. Koketsu, M. et al., 2014. Autophagic cell death inducers containing reduced scytonemin. Japanese Kokai Tokkyo Koho JP 2014024813 A 20140206.
4. Itoh, T. et al., 2013. Reduced scytonemin isolated from Nostoc commune induces autophagic cell death in human T-lymphoid cell line Jurkat cells. *Food Chem. Toxicol.* 60: 76–82.
5. Itoh, T. et al., 2014. Reduced scytonemin isolated from Nostoc commune suppresses LPS/IFNγ-induced NO production in murine macrophage RAW264 cells by inducing hemeoxygenase-1 expression via the Nrf2/ARE pathway. *Food Chem. Toxicol.* 69: 330–338.
6. May, D.S. et al., 2017. Merocyclophanes C and D from the cultured freshwater cyanobacterium nostoc sp. (UIC 10110). *J. Nat. Prod.* 80(4): 1073–1080.

7. Guo, M. et al., 2015. Isolation and antitumor efficacy evaluation of a polysaccharide from Nostoc commune Vauch. *Food Funct.* 6: 3035–3044.
8. Guo, S.J. et al., 2015. Water stress proteins from Nostoc commune Vauch. exhibit anti-colon cancer activities in vitro and in vivo. *J. Agricul. Food Chem.* 63(1): 150–159.
9. Li, Z.Y. et al., 2013. Preparation of Nostoc commune protein extract with anticancer activity for preventing and treating large intestine cancer. Faming Zhuanli Shenqing CN 103059112 A 20130424.
10. Guo, S.J. et al., 2015. Effects of water stress proteins from Nostoc commune Vauch. on cell adhesion of human colon cancer. *Shanxi Yike Daxue Xuebao* 46: 416–420, 503.

85. SPIRULINA

螺旋藻　スピルリナ

Spirulina platensis (= *Arthrospira platensis*)

Phormidiaceae

Spirulina, or *Spirulina platensis* (Phormidiaceae), is a kind of cyanobacterium microalgae. Spirulina is a useful nutritional source because it contains high quality and quantity of protein component content (60%–70% of its dry wt.) and an abundance of vitamin B complexes, iron, and manganese, and vitamins E, K, and other minerals such as copper, zinc, and selenium. Thus, Spirulina can provide many nutrients when consumed by humans and other animals. In the pharmacological explorations, Spirulina demonstrated a variety of biological properties, including antioxidant, antimutagenic, anticancer, antiradiation, immunoenhancing, antihyperlipidemia, antithrombosis, anti-allergic, hematopoietic, peptic ulcer healing, cholesterol-reducing, photosensitive, and antiviral activities.[1,2]

SCIENTIFIC EVIDENCE OF ANTITUMORIGENIC ACTIVITY

It is already known that *Spirulina platensis* is capable of exerting remarkable anticancer-related properties such as antioxidant, antiproliferation, immunopromotion, antimutagenic, anti-inflammation, and antiradiation. The biological activities have been demonstrated by extensive lab experiments in the past decades.[1,2]

Anticarcinogenic and anticancer effects: In *in vivo* assays with animal models, Spirulina extracts (SPE) markedly lessened mouse skin papillomagenesis caused by mutagens DMBA and croton oil, impeded benzo[a]pyrene (BAP)-induced mouse forestomach carcinogenesis, and hampered DMBA-induced hamster buccal pouch carcinogenesis.[3,4] The treatment with SPE also hindered dibutyl nitrosamine-elicited rat liver cytotoxicity and retarded the carcinogenesis from 80% to 20%.[5] The water extract of Spirulina in *in vitro* assay showed inhibitory effect against the proliferation of three human pancreatic cancer cell lines (PA-TU-8902, Mia-Paca-2, and BxPC-3) in a dose-dependent manner, wherein the most sensitive cell line was PA-TU-8902 cells at 0.16 mg/mL. In nude mice implanted PA-TU-8902 tumor, the tumor progression was retarded from the third day after oral administration of the water extract.[1] Both 70% ethanol extract and water extract of Spirulina were cytotoxic to human Kasumi-1 acute leukemia and K562 chronic myelogenous leukemia cell lines. By MTT assay, the IC_{50} values were found to be 0.31 mg/mL for Kusumi-1 and 0.40 mg/mL for K562 cell lines for the ethanol extract, cytotoxicity of which is quite comparable with that of cyclophosphamide (an anticancer agent), whereas the IC_{50}s were 9.44 mg/mL for Kusumi-1 and 5.77 mg/mL for K562 cell lines for the water extract.[2] Accordingly, these experimental observations pointed out that the extracts of Spirulina may be used as a source to develop anticancer drugs and cancer-preventive supplements.

Antitumor immunity and immunoregulating effects: Spirulina hot-water extract by oral administration augmented the tumoricidal activity of nature killer (NK) cells through a MyD88 pathway. Combination of this Spirulina extract and Bacillus Calmette-Gudrin cell wall skeleton (BCG–CWS) in the oral treatment leads to synergistic suppression on B16 melanoma *in vivo* together with synergistic amplification of IFN-γ production.[6] The Spirulina extract was also able to amplify phagocytic activity of macrophages and stimulate antibodies and cytokines production. By analyzing blood cells obtained from volunteers after pre- and postoral administration of the hot-water extract, the results recorded that Spirulina extract may act directly on myeloid lineages and NK cells and indirectly on humans, leading to the immunopotentiation.[2,7] Moreover, administration of Spirulina extract also markedly elevated the proportion of peripheral blood CD3+, CD8+, and NKR-P1A+ lymphocyte in rats, enhanced the activities of phase-II enzymes (which are mainly related to detoxification of carcinogens), and augmented the functions of antioxidant enzymes (including superoxide dismutase, glutathione reductase, glutathione peroxidase, catalase, and reduced glutathione) in mouse liver.[4,8] The findings have proved that Spirulina bioactivities in antitumor studies have an immunopotentiating effect deducing a potential for developing adjuvant-based antitumor immunotherapy.

Protective functions: Owing to its remarkable immunity effect, Spirulina is also capable of reducing the genotoxic and toxic side effects caused by chemotherapeutic drugs. By lessening the levels of DNA damage and related gene mRNA expressions, 1% Spirulina powder in a diet significantly impeded the mitomycin-C–elicited genotoxic effect in mouse bone marrow and liver cells during treatment of mice bearing Ehrlich ascites cancer with mitomycin-C.[9] Supplementing the extract or a combination of vitamin C and Spirulina water extract could minimize the lipid peroxidation caused by 5-fluorouracil, cisplatin, and flutamide (anticancer drugs), thereby resulting in protection against hepatotoxicity and/or nephrotoxicity.[10–12] Similarly, dietary Spirulina exerted marked suppression against UVB-induced skin inflammatory responses and skin carcinogenesis through its anti-inflammatory and antioxidant effects, such as lessening of UVB irradiation caused by 8-oxo-7,8-dihydroguanine (8-oxoG) formation in the skin and effectively downregulating the signal pathways of p38 mitogen-activated protein kinase, stress-activated protein, kinase/c-Jun *N*-terminal kinase, and extracellular signal-regulated kinase.[13] An in *vivo* experiment revealed that daily intake of Spirulina extract was significantly able to hinder cadmium-caused nephrotoxicity in rats via inhibition of renal oxidative stress.[14]

Scientific Evidence of Antitumor Constituents and Activities

The antineoplastic constituents in Spirulina were attributed to polysaccharides, biliproteins (a kind of protein complex with covalent bond and bile pigments), and photodithiazine. The two types of macromolecules were capable of decreasing the size and weight of tumor significantly, stimulating the activities of T- and B-lymphocytes markedly and elevating the quantity of antibody prominently. The biliproteins were generally greater than the polysaccharides in the tumor inhibition and immunity enhancement.[15]

1. Polysaccharides

The polysaccharides of Spirulina (PSP) demonstrated 68% and 46% inhibition against the growth of B37 mammary carcinoma and K562 leukemia *in vitro*, respectively, in concentrations of 0.3–1.5 mg/mL, and showed anticancer activity on transplantable sarcoma 180, hepatoma H22, and EAC tumor in mice at a dose of 75 mg/kg/day, resulting in the suppressive rates of 56.9%, 44.7%, and 22.8%, respectively.[16–18] In human HeLa cervical cancer cells, PSP arrested cell cycle at G1 phase and changed the cell morphology, leading to decline of tumor survival rate.[19,20] PSP was also effective in deterring the proliferation of HT-29 (colon), MGC (stomach), Bel7402 and Bel7404 (liver), and 231 (breast) carcinoma cell lines in a dose-dependent manner. Concurrently, the cell apoptosis of colon cancer and hepatoma was triggered by downregulation of Bcl-2 expression, upregulation of Bax and Apaf-1, and activation of caspase-3. When PSP was combined with Ginkgo biloba leaf extract in a ratio of 1:1, the antiproliferative effect on Bel7402 hepatoma, 231 breast cancer, and MGC gastric cancer cell lines could be synergistically amplified.[21–23]

Furthermore, PSP treatment also exerted extensive immunoenhancing effects, such as enlarging the weights of spleen and thymus, amplifying the activity of NK against tumor cells, stimulating splenocyte activity to produce interleukin-2 (IL-2) and raising IL-1, IL-3, granulocyte-macrophage colony-stimulating factor (GM–CSF), and TNF-α levels in the serum. By the PSP treatment, the number of white blood cells (WBC) reduced by cyclophosphamide was recovered and the levels of red cells, white cells in blood, and nucleated cells in bone marrow decreased by ^{60}Co-γ irradiation were elevated back to normal, and the free radicals were effectively scavenged.[16–28] The results confirmed that PSP also possesses chemoprotection-related immunoregulative, radioprotective, and radial-scavenging capabilities besides its antitumor activities. In addition, PSP at 15 mg/L concentration could potentiate the antiproliferative activity of immobilized phycocyanin (a bioactive protein from Spirulina) against SW1990 pancreatic cancer cells.[29] On the basis of remarkable evidences, PSP was suggested to be a potential and valuable adjuvant agent for improving cancer therapy and prevention.

NPSP, a polysaccharide separated from Spirulina, rarely showed the cytotoxicity on the tumor cells but it was able to enhance splenocyte proliferation and increase the activities of cytotoxic T-lymphocytes (CTL) and NK cells in tumor-bearing mice. If NPSP was sulfated, the produced SNPSP exerted marked cytotoxicity toward human SMMC-7721 hepatoma cells *in vitro*. SNPSP at 50 mg/kg dose inhibited the growth of sarcoma 180 cells by 35.42% in mice. Simultaneously, SNPSP prominently potentiated spleen lymphocyte proliferation and NK and CTL cell functions in the tumor-bearing mice.[24] Similarly, Low m.w. NPSP (LNPSP), a polysaccharide with low molecular weight of 10 ku was obtained by hydrochloric acid degradation of spirulinia, and then it was sulfated by chlorosulfonic acid pyridine to afford three sulfated polysaccharides: (1) SLNPSP1, (2) SLNPSP2, and (3) SLNPSP3. *In vitro* assay with SMMC-7721 cells confirmed that the antitumor activity of the SLNPSPs was augmented along with an increase of the sulfur content.[25]

In searching for more biological active agents, several selenium-bound Spirulina polysaccharides (Se–PSPs) were developed. The Se–PSPs, especially Se–PSP2, demonstrated dose-dependent broad antitumor spectra against the proliferation of human SKOV3 (ovary), HepG2 (liver), BGC-803 (stomach), and Tca-8113 (tongue) cancer cell lines.[30] Calcium spirulan (Ca–SP) is a sulfated polysaccharide isolated from Spirulina which is mainly composed of rhamnose with chelating calcium. In the experimental metastasis models, Ca–SP prominently lessened the lung colonization of B16–BL6 melanoma cells and retarded the invasion of HT-1080 fibrosarcoma cells and 26M3.1 colon cancer cells. The antimetastasis effect of Ca–SP was revealed to be correlated with blocking the cancer cell invasion of the basement membrane, blocking cell adhesion, and migration to laminin substrate and protecting heparanase activity.[31,32] Ca–SPIIa and Ca–SPIIb, two other calcium-bound and sulfated Spirulina polysaccharides, were mainly composed of glucose, galactose, rhamnose, fructose, glucuronic acid, mannose, and xylose. Their molar ratios were determined as 6.5:3.3:50.0:38.5:9.6:1.5:1.0 and 7.2:3.5:55.0:40.2:8.5:2.0:1.0 and the sulfate percentages were assigned to be 2.25% and 3.47%, respectively. *In vitro* treatment with 200 µg Ca–SPIIb killed 95% of Ehrlich ascites carcinoma (EAC) cells.[33]

2. Proteins

C-Phycocyanine (C–PC), one of the major light-harvesting biliproteins from Spirulina, is a water-soluble and nontoxic fluorescent protein pigment, which is mainly responsible for the antioxidant, anticancer, immunopotentiating, and anti-inflammatory activities. Treatment with C–PC (50 µM) up to 48 h significantly promoted the apoptosis and diminished the proliferation of human K562 leukemia cells by 49%.[34] In addition, C–PC elicited the apoptosis of human SKOV3 (ovary), SW480 (colon), HEp-2 (larynx), and MCF-7 (breast) cancer cells but exerted weak antiproliferative effect on these cell lines.[35] The potent suppressive effect of C–PC was shown in human SMMC-7721 (liver), ES-2 (ovary), and SPCA-1 (lung) cancer cell lines with IC_{50}s at 3.00, 4.85, and 8.42 µg/mL (in 48 h), respectively.[36] SCF, a supercritical fluid extract of C–PC from *S. platensis*, was cytotoxic to A549 lung cancer cell line (IC_{50} of 26.82 µg/mL).[37] HeLa cervical cancer cells treated by C–PC resulted in cell-cycle arrest and proapoptosis by alteration of the cell characteristic features.[38,39] Trypsinase hydrolysis of C–PC could augment the antitumor potency. At 100 mg/L, the inhibitory rates of C–PC and its hydrolysate were 29.2% and 56.5%, on HeLa cells, respectively.[40]

Moreover, the drug-resistant reversal, drug-enhancing, and anticarcinogenic properties of C–PC were further observed in the explorations. Using 40 and 50 µM C–PC to treat human hepatoma cells for 24 h could lessen by 50% proliferation of both sensitive and resistant HepG2 cells. In the treatment, C–PC elicited the apoptotic death and sub-G0/G1 cell-cycle arrest in doxorubicin-resistant HepG2 cells and enhanced the sensitivity of resistant HepG2 cells to doxorubicin.[41] When combining C–PC with all-*trans* retinoic acid, the growth and development of human A549 lung cancer cells were remarkably prohibited *in vitro* and *in vivo* in a time- and dose-dependent manner.[42] Monotherapy with C–PC impeded 1,2 dimethylhyadrazine (DMH)-induced colon carcinogenesis in rats concomitant with induction of mitochondrial-dependent apoptosis and inhibition of proinflammatory cytokines and angiogenic role. If carried out in a combinational regimen with C–PC and piroxicam (an anti-inflammatory drug) in an anti-inflammatory dose range, more effective chemoprevention would result against the DMH-developed colon carcinogenesis.[43]

Due to its photosensitive characteristics, C–PC has been used in experiments of photodynamic therapies. With the association of lasers (497 or 632.8 nm), treatment with C–PC in 50 µg/mL exhibited incredible photodynamic effect on human Bcap-37 mammary carcinoma cells because C–PC chemically coupled with *N*-(4-azido-benzoyloxy) succinimide to form photoreactive proteins.[44] The photodynamic effects of C–PC were further demonstrated in both *in vitro* and *in vivo* models to kill human MCF-7 (breast), SMMC-7721, and HepG2 (liver) cancers remarkably by cell death promotion.[45–47] The inhibitory rate of UV-immobilized C–PC at 20 µg/mL was observed up to 55% against the proliferation of Bel-7402 hepatoma cells.[48,49] According to another research, the photoimmobilized C–PC also augmented the maturation of cord blood dendritic cells by upregulation of CD86 and CD83 expressions, thereby activating cytokine-induced killer cells (CIK) to attack the Bel-7402 hepatoma cells.[50]

More scientific evidences showed that C–PC is composed of α and β subunits, both of which were purely separated. In human SPC-A-1 lung adenocarcinoma cell line, C–PC β-subunit exhibited more potent suppression of the growth and multiplication of the lung cancer cells than C–PC α-subunit under the same concentration.[51] A selenium-bound phycocyanin (Se–PC) was derived from selenium-enriched *S. platensis*. Compared to C–PC, Se–PC showed stronger abilities of radical scavenging, antiproliferation, and proapoptosis in several antioxidant assays and human cancer assays with A375 melanoma and MCF-7 breast cancer cell lines *in vitro*,[52] inferring that Se–PC may be a promising agent in cancer chemoprevention. In addition, the C–PC treatment also exerted a possible protective role against cisplatin-like chemotherapeutic drug-elicited nephrotoxicity in a mouse model.[53] Overall, these investigations have clearly substantiated the antiproliferative, anticarcinogenic, and proapoptotic properties of C–PC and revealed the possibility of C–PC for overcoming the drug resistance and lowering drug toxicities. The proapoptotic mechanism of C–PC was found to primarily associate with different series of signal transduction in different types of neoplastic cells. The C–PC also presented much potential in combination treatments, photodynamic therapies, and selenium-additive applications.

3. Peptides

The whole protein extract from *S. platensis* can be hydrolyzed by sequential digestion with pepsin, trypsin, and chymotrypsin. Four peptide fractions (Tr1–Tr4) were prepared from the enzymatic hydrolysates. Of them, the most potent antiproliferative effects were observed in Tr2 fraction with IC_{50}s of < 31.25, 36.42, and 48.25 µg/mL on human MCF-7 (breast), HepG2 (liver), and SGC-7901 (stomach) cancer cell lines, respectively. A peptide sequenced as HVLSRAPR exhibited low inhibitory activities on five cancer cell lines (HepG2, MCF-7, SGC-7901, A549, and HT-29). Its best suppression was 62.39% in HT-29 colon cancer cells at 500 µg/mL concentration (IC_{50} of 99.88 µg/mL).[54] Similarly, other peptide fractions (D1–D5) were isolated from the protein hydrolysis that were derived by alcalase/papain digestion in succession. The best antitumor effects were shown by D1 on MCF-7 and HepG2 cells (IC_{50}s of < 31.25 and 49.36 µg/mL, respectively) compared to other fractions. The *in vivo* antitumor activity of D1 was further proved in nude mice transplanted HepG2 hepatoma. At a dose of 200 mg/kg/day, D1 presented its best inhibition up to 39.75% at day 11. Three cancer-suppressive peptides were separated from the fraction and their sequences were identified as AGGASLLLLR, LAGHVGVR, and KFLVLCLR. When KFLVLCLR was further truncated, the produced LCLR peptide showed much improved antiproliferative effect on MCF-7 and HepG2 cells with > 60% inhibitory rate; however, it had weak cytotoxicity (~6%) on L-O2 normal cells at its concentration of 500 µg/mL.[54] Another peptide with YGFVMPRSGLWFR sequence was obtained from papain-digested hydrolysate of the protein extract, whose inhibition was observed on A549 lung cancer and HepG2 hepatoma cell lines (IC_{50} of 104.05 and 188.23 µg/mL, respectively).[55] Three antitumor polypeptide fractions labeled as Y1, Y2, and Y3, which were derived from *S. platensis* proteins by trypsin hydrolysis (38.5% hydrolytic rate), exhibited suppressive effects on human MCF-7 (breast) and HepG2 (liver) cancer cell lines at 1 mg/mL. The greatest inhibitory effects on MCF-7 and HepG2 cells were achieved by Y2 fraction and its inhibitory rates were 97% and 97%, whereas that of 5-FU (an anticancer drug) were 55% and 97%, respectively, at the same concentration of 250 µg/mL.[56] On the basis of better inhibitory activities on cancer cells and low cytotoxicity on normal cells, these polypeptides by enzyme hydrolysis might be useful for producing natural cancer–preventive ingredients in nutraceutical and pharmaceutical industries.

4. Chlorophyll derivatives

Chlorin-E6 (**1**), a stable and water-soluble photosensitizer, was separated from Spirulina. A noncovalent complex of chlorine-E6 (**1**) and *N*-methyl-D-glucosamine exhibited potent *in vitro* and *in vivo* photocytotoxicity against several neoplastic cells (such as CaOv and OV2774 ovarian cancers, PC12 pheochromocytoma, and T36 embryocarcinoma) under light irritation of 650–900 nm.[57,58] According to clinical reports from Russia, chlorin-E6 (**1**) was successfully applied for the treatment of cancer patients.[59] In addition, the structural modification of chlorin-E6 was extensively studied.[60,61] Chlorophyll is a rich component in the Spirulina, which can be employed for chemical preparation of a group of bioactive and photosensitive pheophytin-α derivatives. These derivatives were used in the photodynamic therapies (PDT) for significant promotion of anticancer activities. Treatment with 9-hydroxypheophorbide-α (2, 9-HPbD) plus 665 nm diode laser showed prominent anti-growth effect against human HN3 laryngeal cancer cells *in vitro* and *in vivo*.[62] Due to induction of oxidative stress, 9-HPbD-PDT activated mitochondrial pathway and deterred EGFR expression, leading to the promotion of cell apoptosis and necrosis and suppression of cell migration.[62,63] Similarly, under the PDT, pyropheophorbide-a (3, Ppa) at 0.06 and 0.125 μM concentrations exerted obvious growth inhibition effect on TC-1 and CaSki cervical cancer cells *in vitro* and *in vivo*. Ppa (3) was more phototoxic to TC-1 cells than CaSki cells.[64] Accordingly, the photosensitizers plus PDT with chlorophyll derivatives are a promising modality in the curative and palliative treatment of cancers.

5. Unsaturated fatty acids

γ-Linolenic acid (4) is an important omega-6 polyunsaturated fatty acid in *S. platensis*. γ-Linolenic acid (4) and its methyl ester (5) can be isolated in good yields from the Spirulina. In the *in vitro* assay, γ-linolenic acid (4) and methyl γ-linolenate (5) induced the apoptosis of HepG2 hepatoma cells and A549 lung carcinoma cells, respectively, thereby exerting the antiproliferative effect in a dose- and time-dependent manner. γ-Linolenic acid (4) at a concentration of 250 μM strongly elicited ROS generation and lipid peroxidation.[65,66] The findings implied that the two omega-6 unsaturated fatty acids may be useful in healthcare and functional foods.

Nanoformulation

The algal culture of *S. platensis* (a cold-tolerant strain) has been used to synthesize silver nanoparticles, which in the *in vitro* system showed both antibacterial and anticancer activities. The viability of human Hep2 carcinoma cells could be diminished in a dose-dependent manner and the major role in cancer inhibition was correlated to the cytotoxic effect of silver nanoparticles on cell viability.[67] C-Phycocyanin–carboxymethyl chitosan nanoparticles (C–PC/CMC–NPs) were formulated with an average particle diameter of 118.4 nm. C-Phycocyanin, carboxymethyl chitosan, and C–PC/CMC–NPs were all capable of exerting antiproliferative and proapoptotic effects in HeLa cancer cells by the activation of caspase-3. However, the antitumor effect of C–PC/CMC–NPs was significantly more pronounced owing to an acceptable safety profile of sustained C–PC release.[68]

Toxicities

Spirulina is popularly categorized as a super food for its high nutrition content. Its health benefits for humans are also widely considered to be significant. However, the toxicity and side effects are the most important question for Spirulina consumption. The investigations reported that C-phycocyanine, the major component in Spirulina, is safe for humans owing to its LD_{50} values that are greater than 3 g/kg (p.o.) for rats and mice.[69] Spirulina was also reported having no production of the toxic compounds commonly known as microcystin and cyanotoxin, which have various potential toxicities, causing liver damage, muscle degeneration, shock, and death, especially to children.[69] In Spirulina harvested from wild sources, such as lakes, ponds, and sea, often contamination occurs from other toxins producing blue–green algae, bacteria, and fungi during Spirulina farming. In addition, the environment today is full of toxins from the pollutions of oil, gas, heavy metals, and nuclear isotopes.[70–73] Therefore, the cultivation of Spirulina in large scale must be controlled well under good conditions with no contamination. Multiple quality inspections are necessary before the Spirulina enters the market for human consumption.

CONCLUSION AND SUGGESTION

On the basis of numerous research findings, it is clear now that dietary Spirulina as a food supplement and a medicinal adjuvant would bring incredible health-promoting and body-protecting benefits to humans.[74] A variety of bioactive components discovered from *Spirulina platensis* were identified as proteins, polysaccharides, chlorophyll derivatives, unsaturated fatty acids, and vitamins. The Spirulina proteins, especially phycocyanin (a major protein constituent in Spirulina), are the most important and valuable contributors to a variety of pharmacological properties, including anticancer-related activities (e.g., anti-growth, proapoptosis, immunoregulation, antioxidant, anticarcinogenesis, antiradiation, anti-inflammation, and detoxification). The prominent interactions endowed Spirulina and phycocyanin as a helpful value to play an important role in the prevention and therapy of cancers and other diseases. Consequently, Spirulina and phycocyanin are suitable for amplification of immune system, elimination of cancer initiation, and progression and recovery of self-healing ability, and are also able to enhance chemo- and radiotherapeutic effects, minimize side effects and toxic reactions, and reduce the dosages of chemotherapeutic drugs and radioirritation if used as an adjunctive agent in clinical cancer treatments. Either as a functional food or as a medicinal supplement, Spirulina and phycocyanin demonstrated a great development prospect.

REFERENCES

1. Konickova, R. et al., 2014. Anticancer effects of blue-green alga Spirulina platensis, a natural source of bilirubin-like tetrapyrrolic compounds. *Ann. Hepatol.* 13(2): 273–283.
2. a) Soheili, M. et al., 2011. The potential health benefits of algae and micro algae in medicine: A review on Spirulina platensis. *Current Nutr. Food Sci.* 7(4): 279–285; b) Hernandez, F.Y.F. et al., 2017. Cytotoxic effect of Spirulina platensis extracts on human acute leukemia Kasumi-1 and chronic myelogenous leukemia K562 cell lines. *Asian Pacific J. Tropical Biomed.* 7(1): 14–19.
3. a) Grawish, M.E. et al., 2008. Effects of Spirulina platensis extract on syrian hamster cheek pouch mucosa painted with 7,12-dimethylbenz(a)anthracene. *Oral Oncol.* 44(10): 956–962; b) 2010. Long-term effect of Spirulina platensis extract on DMBA-induced hamster buccal pouch carcinogenesis. *Med. Oncol.* 27(1): 20–28.
4. Dasgupta, T. et al., 2001. Chemomodulation of carcinogen metabolising enzymes, antioxidant profiles and skin and forestomach papillomagenesis by Spirulina platensis. *Mol. Cell. Biochem.* 226: 27–38.
5. Ismail, M.F. et al., Chemoprevention of rat liver toxicity and carcinogenesis by Spirulina. *Int. J. Biol. Sci.* 5(4): 377–387.
6. Akao, Y. et al., 2009. Enhancement of antitumor natural killer cell activation by orally administered Spirulina extract in mice. *Cancer Sci.* 100(8): 1494–1501.
7. Ghaeni, M. et al., 2016. Review for application and medicine effects of Spirulina, microalgae. *J. Advanced Agric. Technol.* 3(2): 114–117.
8. Fujioka, Y. et al., 2002. Effects of extracts from Spirulina on lymphocyte subsets in tumor-inoculated rat. *J. Physical Fitness, Nutr. Immunol.* 12: 3–9.
9. Abou-El Fotoh, M.F. et al., 2013. Role of Spirulina platensis on mitomycin C-induced genotoxicity in Ehrlich ascites carcinoma bearing albino mice: Single-cell gel electrophoresis (comet assay) and semi-quantitative RT-PCR analysis. *Int. J. Current Res.* 5(9): 2636–2640.
10. Ray, S. et al., 2012. Flutamide-induced lipid peroxidation: protective role of water extract of Spirulina platensis. *Int. J. Chem. Tech. Res.* 4(1): 68–73.
11. Ray, S. et al., 2007. In vitro evaluation of protective effects of ascorbic acid and water extract of Spirulina platensis (blue green algae) on 5-fluorouracil-induced lipid peroxidation. *Acta Poloniae Pharm.* 64(4): 335–344.
12. Bhattacharyya, S. et al., 2012. The hepatoprotective potential of Spirulina and vitamin C supplementation in cisplatin toxicity. *Food Funct.* 3(2): 164–119.
13. Yogianti, F. et al., 2014. Inhibitory effects of dietary Spirulina platensis on UVB-induced skin inflammatory responses and carcinogenesis. *J. Investigative Dermatol.* 134(10): 2610–2619.
14. Gaurav, D. et al., 2010. Protective effect of Spirulina platensis on cadmium induced renal toxicity in Wistar rats. *Archiv. Applied Sci. Res.* 2(1): 390–397.

15. Li, B. et al., 2004. Study on the antitumor immune activities of phycocyanin and polysaccharide from Spirulina platensis. *Zhongguo Haiyang Daxue Xuebao, Sci. Edit.* 34: 396–402; Chen, X.M. et al., *Zhongcaoyao* 35: 100.

16. Qu, X.J. et al., 2000. Study on antitumor effects of polysaccharides of Spirulina platensis. *Zhongguo Haiyang Yaowu* 19: 10–14.

17. Gao, X.D. et al., 2000. Antitumor effects of polysaccharide (PSP) from the Spirulina platensis in mice. *J. China Pharm. Univ.* 31: 458–461.

18. Zeng, B.H. et al., 2000. Study on effect of Spirulina platensis polysaccharide on NK cells from acute leukemia patient in vitro. *Zhongguo Haiyang Yaowu* 19: 45–47.

19. Ding, S.Y. et al., 2002. Effects of polysaccharides from Spirulina platensis on the growth of HeLa cells: An in vitro study. *J. Qingdao Univ. Med. College* 38: 346–347.

20. Yu, H. et al., 2003. Effects of polysaccharide from Spirulina platensis on growth of HeLa cells. *Zhongguo Haiyang Yaowu* 22: 26–29.

21. Xu, X.J. et al., 2012. Antitumor function of compound polysaccharides from Spirulina platensis on human HT-29 cell line in vitro. *Shizhen Guoyi Guoyao* 23(9): 2164–2166; Zhang, Z.J. et al., 2009. Antitumor effects of compound PSP on 7402 cells. *Shaanxi Yixue Zazhi* 38(3): 279–281.

22. Qiao, M.X. et al., 2009. Inhibitory effects of compound Spirulina platensis polysaccharide on human gastric carcinoma MGC cells. *Shizhen Guoyi Guoyao* 20(6), 1385–1386; Tang, G.F. et al., 2009. Induction of BEL7404 cell apoptosis with Spirulina polysaccharides. *Guangxi Yike Daxue Xuebao* 26(1): 66–67.

23. a) Kurd, F. et al., 2015. Water soluble polysaccharides from Spirulina platensis: Extraction and in vitro anti-cancer activity. *Int. J. Biol. Macromol.* 74: 498–506; b) Yu, L.Y. et al., 2009. Study on inhibitory effect of compound polysaccharides from Spirulina platensis on human mammary cancer 231 cells. *Anhui Nongye Kexue* 37(3): 928–929, 931.

24. Le, X.T. et al., 2006. Preparation of low molecular weight polysaccharide of Spirulina platensis and antitumor activity of its sulfates ester in vitro. *Pharm. Biotech.* (China) 13: 119–122.

25. Sheng, Y.Q. et al., 2006. Antitumor and immunomodulation effect of polysaccharide from Spirulina platensis and its sulfated derivative. *Pharm. Biotech.* (China) 13: 107–111.

26. Zhang, H.Q. et al., 2001. Chemo- and radio-protective effects of polysaccharide of Spirulina platensis on hemopoietic system of mice and dogs. *Acta Pharmacol. Sinica* 22: 1121–1124.

27. Yu, H. et al., 2003. Immune effects of polysaccharide from Spirulina platensis on the transplanted tumor cells of sarcoma 180 in mice. *Mar. Sci.* 27: 58–60.

28. Liu, X.M. et al., 2002. Effect of polysaccharide from Spirulina platensis on hematopoietic cells proliferation, apoptosis and Bcl-2 expression in mice bearing tumor treated with chemotherapy. *Acta Pharm. Sinica* 37: 616–620.

29. Guan, Y.Q. et al., 2002. Influence of polysaccharide of Spirulina platensis on inhibition activity of immobilized phycocyanin against cancer cell growth. *Acta Nutr. Sinica* 24: 252–255.

30. Shang, J.Y. et al., 2010. Isolation and purification of polysaccharide from Se-enriched Spirulina platensis and their in vitro antitumor activity. *Zhongguo Zhongliu Shengwu Zhiliao Zazhi* 17(6): 630–633.

31. Saiki, I. et al., 2004. Inhibition of tumor invasion and metastasis by calcium spirulan (Ca-SP), a novel sulfated polysaccharide derived from a blue-green alga Spirulina platensis. *Nutr. Sci.* 7: 144–150.

32. Mishima, T. et al., 1998. Inhibition of tumor invasion and metastasis by calcium spirulan (Ca-SP), a novel sulfated polysaccharide derived from a blue-green alga, Spirulina platensis. *Clin. Experim. Metastasis* 16: 541–550.

33. Asker, M.M.S. et al., 2011. Isolation, fractionation and modification of sulfated polysaccharides from Spirulina platensis and their antitumor activity. *BioChem.* (An Indian J.) 5(1): 52–57.

34. Subhashini, J. et al., 2004. Molecular mechanisms in C-Phycocyanin induced apoptosis in human chronic myeloid leukemia cell line-K562. *Biochem. Pharmacol.* 68: 453–462.

35. Pan, R.W. et al., 2015. Spirulina phycocyanin induces differential protein expression and apoptosis in SKOV-3 cells. *Int. J. Biol. Macromol.* 81: 951–959; Ying, J. et al., 2016. Transcriptome analysis of phycocyanin inhibitory effects on SKOV-3 cell proliferation. *Gene* 585(1): 58–64.

36. Yin, L.H. et al., 2011. Orthogonal test design for optimization of suitable conditions to separate C-phycocyanin from Spirulina platensis by high-speed counter-current chromatography using reverse micelle solvent system. *J. Separ. Sci.* 34(11): 1253–1260.

37. Deniz, I. et al., 2016. Supercritical fluid extraction of phycocyanin and investigation of cytotoxicity on human lung cancer cells. *J. Supercritical Fluids* 108: 13–18.

38. Li, B. et al., 2006. Molecular immune mechanism of C-phycocyanin from Spirulina platensis induces apoptosis in HeLa cells in vitro. *Biotechnol. Applied Biochem.* 43: 155–164.

39. Li, B. et al., 2009. Study on the molecular mechanism of, C-phycocyanin from Spirulina platensis induced apoptosis in HeLa cells. *Zhongguo Yaolixue Tongbao* 25(8), 1045–1050.

40. Wang, X.Q. et al., 2008. Study on biological functions of Spirulina platensis phycocyanin and its hydrolysates by trypsinase. *Shipin Kexue* (Beijing, China) 29(10): 433–435.

41. Roy, K.R. et al., 2007. Alteration of mitochondrial membrane potential by Spirulina platensis C-phycocyanin induces apoptosis in the doxorubicin resistant human hepatocellular-carcinoma cell line HepG2. *Biotechnol. Applied Biochem.* 47: 159–167.

42. Li, B. et al., 2015. The synergistic antitumor effects of all-trans retinoic acid and C-phycocyanin on the lung cancer A549 cells in vitro and in vivo. *Eur. J. Pharmacol.* 749: 107–114.

43. Saini, M.K. et al., 2015. Cell cycle regulation and apoptotic cell death in experimental colon carcinogenesis. *Nutr. Cancer* 67(4): 620–636; 2014. Targeting angiogenic pathway for chemoprevention of experimental colon cancer using C-phycocyanin as cyclooxygenase-2 inhibitor. *Biochem. Cell Biol.* 92(3): 206–218; 2012. Piroxicam and C-phycocyanin mediated apoptosis in 1,2-dimethylhydrazine dihydrochloride induced colon carcinogenesis. *Nutr. Cancer* 64(3): 409–418.

44. Chen, X.Q. et al., 2005. Photodynamic effect of three kinds of phycobiliproteins on human mammary cancer line Bcap-37. *J. Zhejiang Univ. Sci. Edit.* 32: 438–441, 447.

45. Li, B. et al., 2010. Apoptotic mechanism of MCF-7 breast cells in vivo and in vitro induced by photodynamic therapy with C-phycocyanin. *Acta Biochim. Biophys. Sin.* (Shanghai). 42(1): 80–89.

46. Wang, Y. et al., 2009. Photodynamic effect of two kinds of phycobiliproteins on human liver cancer cell line SMMC-7721 in vitro. *Shengwu Gongcheng Xuebao* (*Chin. J. Biotechnol.*) 25: 1417–1423.

47. Wang, C.Y. et al., 2012. Photosensitization of phycocyanin extracted from microcystis in human hepatocellular carcinoma cells: Implication of mitochondria-dependent apoptosis. *J. Photochem. Photobiol.* B 117: 70–79.

48. Guan, Y.Q. et al., 2002. Inhibition activity of Spirulina platensis proteins photo-immobilization biomaterial on proliferation of cancer cells. *J. Biomed. Engineering* 19: 1–3.

49. Guan, Y.Q. et al., 2000. Inhibition activity of phycocyanin immobilization biomaterial on proliferation of liver cancer cells 7402. *Lizi Jiaohuan Yu Xifu* 16: 547–552.

50. Zhu, B.S. et al., 2013. Phycocyanine improves the killing function of CBDC-CIK to kill liver cancer. *Practical Oncol. J.* 27: 1–5.

51. Zhang, X. 2010. Isolation of C-PC subunits from Spirulina platensis and inhibitory effect on SPC-A1 cell line. *Zhejiang Daxue Xuebao, Lixueban* 37: 319–323.

52. Chen, T.F. et al., 2008. In vitro antioxidant and antiproliferative activities of selenium-containing phycocyanin from selenium-enriched Spirulina platensis. *J.Agricul. Food Chem.* 56(12): 4352–4358.

53. Lim, B.J. et al., 2012. C-Phycocyanin attenuates cisplatin-induced nephrotoxicity in mice. *Ren. Fail.* 34(7): 892–900.

54. Wang, Z.J. et al., 2017. Isolation and identification of anti-proliferative peptides from Spirulina platensis using three-step hydrolysis. *J. Sci. Food Agricult.* 97(3): 918–922.

55. Wang, Z.J. et al., 2016. Characterization and antitumor activity of protein hydrolysates from Arthrospira platensis (Spirulina platensis) using two-step hydrolysis. *J. Applied Phycol.* 28(6): 3379–3385.

56. Wang, Z.J. et al., 2016. Inhibitory effects of small molecular peptides from Spirulina (Arthrospira) platensis on cancer cell growth. *Food & Funct.* 7(2): 781–788.

57. Abakumova, O.Y. et al., 2000. Novel drug form of chlorin E6. *Proc. SPIE-The Int. Soc. Opt. Eng.* 4059 (Laser Use in Oncology II): 130–138.

58. Nifantiev, N.E. et al., 2003. Preparation of water-soluble porphyrin derivatives as photosensitizers for photodynamic therapy. *U.S.* US 2002–306046 20021127.

59. Reshetnickov, A.V. et al., 2001. Novel photosensitizers for prospective clinical usage and some of their properties. *Proc. SPIE-The Int. Soc. Opt. Eng.* 4156 (Clinical Lasers and Diagnostics): 86–90.

60. Nifantiev, N.E. et al., 2003. *U.S.* US 2002-151764 20020520; 2002. *PCT Int. Appl.* WO 2002-US16992 20020531.

61. Song, P.S. et al., 1993. 10-Hydroxypheophytin a, prepn. thereof, and use as photosensitizer for photodynamic cancer therapeutics. *PCT Intl. Appl.* WO 92-KR67 19921127.

62. Ahn, J.C. et al., 2013. The apoptosis pathway of photodynamic therapy using 9-HpbD-a in AMC-HN3 human head and neck cancer cell line and in vivo. *Gen. Physiol. Biophys.* 32(3): 405–413.

63. He, P.J. et al., 2016. Photosensitizer effect of 9-hydroxypheophorbide α on diode laser-irradiated laryngeal cancer cells: Oxidative stress-directed cell death and migration suppression. *Oncol. Lett.* 12(3): 1889–1895.

64. Chaturvedi, P.K. et al., 2014. Phototoxic effects of pyropheophorbide-a from chlorophyll-a on cervical cancer cells. *J. Porphyrins & Phthalocyanines* 18(3): 182–187.

65. Wang, F. et al., 2015. Anti-neoplastic activity of γ-linolenic acid extract from Spirulina platensis on HepG2 cells and its inhibition effect on platelet aggregation. *Food Agricul. Immunol.* 26(1): 97–108.

66. Jubie, S. et al., 2015. Isolation of methyl gamma linolenate from Spirulina platensis using flash chromatography and its apoptosis inducing effect. *BMC Complem. Altern. Med.*15: 1–8.

67. Namasivayam, S.K.R. et al., 2015. Antibacterial and anticancerous biocompatible silver nanoparticles synthesised from the cold-tolerant strain of Spirulina platensis. *J. Coastal Life Med.* 3(4): 265–272.

68. Lu, C.Y. et al., 2015. Optimized preparation of novel C-phycocyanin-carboxymethyl chitosan nanoparticles and its inhibitory effects on human cervical carcinoma HeLa cells proliferation. *Zhongguo Zhongliu Shengwu Zhiliao Zazhi* 22(1): 34–40.

69. Naidu, K.A. et al., 1999. Toxicity assessment of phycocyanin—A blue colorant from blue green alga Spirulina platensis. *J. Food Biotech.* 13(1): 51–66.

70. Belay, A. 2008. Spirulina (Arthrospira): Production and quality assurance. In: Gershwin, M.E., Belay, A. (Eds.), *Spirulina in Human Nutrition and Health*, CRC Press: London, UK, pp. 1–25.

71. Manali, K.M. et al., 2017. Detection of microcystin producing cyanobacteria in Spirulina dietary supplements using multiplex HRM quantitative PCR. J. Applied Phycol. 29(3): 1279–1286.

72. Elizdath, M.G. et al., Preclinical antitoxic properties of Spirulina (Arthrospira). *Pharm. Boil.* 54(8): 1345–1353.

73. Marles, R.J. et al., 2011. United States pharmacopeia safety evaluation of Spirulina. *Crit. Rev. Food Sci. Nutr.* 51(7): 593–604.

74. Liu, Q. et al., 2016. Medical application of Spirulina platensis derived C-phycocyanin. *Evid.-Based Complem. Altern. Med.* 2016: Article ID: 7803846.

11 Cancer-Preventive Substances in Animal-Based Foods

---

86. Fresh-Water Mussels/*Anodonta woodiana, Cristaria plicata, Hyriopaia cumingii*

87. Marine Mussels/*Mytilus edulis, M. coruscus*

88. Hard Clam/*Meretrix meretrix*

89. Other clams/*Cyclina sinensis, Corbicula fluminea, Ruditapes philippinarum*

90. Sepia Ink/Inks from *Sepiella maindroni, Sepia esculenta, Sepia officinalis*, and *Sepia prabahari*

91. Calamari Ink/Inks from *Loligo chinensis, Ommastrephes bartrami*

92. Sea Cucumber/*Stichopus japonicus* (= *Apostichopus japonicus*), *S. chloronotus*

93. Lollyfish Sea Cucumber/*Holothuria leucospilota, H. scabra*

Most humans eat an omnivorous diet except some vegetarians. Similar to the plant- and fungi-based foods, the animal-based food is also necessary for humans. Intake of meat gives higher biological value protein, energy, and fat compared with plant food sources, and six micronutrients (Vitamin A, vitamin B12, riboflavin, calcium, iron, and zinc). Among the common animal-based foods, several of them not only have nutritional values but also exert functional benefits. Nonetheless, less meat consumption has always been advised by many nutritious books particularly for aged people due to the negative relationship found between meat consumption and some carcinogens. Comparably, fishes and shrimps are greatly suggested to be included in the dietary menu due to the reason that they provide more healthy nutrients apart from proteins and oils. The essential fatty acids such as omega-3 fatty acids are the most important ingredients that are reported to be supportive for lowering incidence of heart and artery diseases, improving brain and nervous system, and preventing carcinogenesis. Such recognitions have been accepted widely for a long time.

Besides the commonly known dietary values, this chapter emphasizes eight unique aquatic animal-based foods. They are mostly consumed by small populations in several locales and demonstrate highly effective functionality in health promotion and cancer prevention besides rich nutritional value. All the scientific evidences regarding the anticarcinogenic, anticancer, and immunoenhancing properties are extensively summarized for these eight foods in this chapter. The consumption of these eight animal-based functional foods, therefore, should be expressly advocated for gaining their remarkable health benefits for body protection and cancer prevention.

86. FRESH-WATER MUSSELS

蚌

Anodonta woodiana, Cristaria plicata, Hyriopaia cumingii

Unionidae

Fresh meat and tears of fresh water mussels are used as a source of delicious food and folk medicine for a long time in their growing areas. The mussels include three kinds of Unionidae animals: (1) *Anodonta woodiana*, (2) *Cristaria plicata*, and (3) *Hyriopaia cumingii*, which commonly inhabit the rivers and lakes of East Asia region. The bivalves are a rich source of vitamin B12 and manganese and a source of vitamin C, iron, selenium, and copper. The best harvesting season is autumn for fresh-water mussels.

Scientific Evidence of Cancer-Inhibitory and Cancer-Preventive Activities

The earlier studies had reported that the extracts derived from mussel meat and mussel tears displayed significant anti-growth effect against mouse ascites hepatoma and Ehrlich ascites tumor *in vivo* with 30%–59.2% tumor tissue reduction.[1] The mussel provides abundant polysaccharide and glycoprotein components, which are responsible for health benefits of mussels. An extract prepared from *A. woodiana* showed marked immunoenhancing antitumor activities *in vivo*, evidenced as amplifying tumoricidal abilities of macrophages and natural killer (NK) cells and enhancing phagocytic activity of macrophages and specific immune activity of T-lymphocyte. Although there is no direct cytotoxicity on L1210 and P388 leukemia cells and HeLaS3 cervical cancer cells *in vitro*, the extract significantly obstructed the cell growth of sarcoma 180, Ehrlich tumor, Lewis lung cancer, B16 melanoma, and P388 leukemia *in vivo* when 25 or 50 mg/kg was administered to tumor-bearing mice for 7 days.[2] From the extract, a glycoprotein fraction (HB) with tumor-inhibitory activity was prepared and further separation of the HB fraction derived three homologous compounds assigned as HB-1a, HB-1b, and HB-1c with molecular weights (m.w.) of 67.0, 67.5, and 66.2 kDa, respectively. The three glycoproteins displayed obvious antiproliferation effect in mice implanted sarcoma 180 or Ehrlich ascites tumor.[3] Furthermore, the HB fraction was prepared with cholesterol and lecithin in a 3–5:1:1–3 proportion to formulation of a liposome. Oral administration of the HB-loaded liposomes in a dose of 400 mg/kg to tumor-bearing mice resulted in suppressive rates of 48.76%–54.38% against sarcoma 180, C26 colon carcinoma, Lewis lung tumor, and B16 melanoma.[4–6] In human QGY hepatoma and MKN-45 gastric carcinoma-inoculated mice, treatment of HB-loaded liposome for 30 days significantly restrained cell growth of the neoplasm without obvious acute toxicological sign.[6]

From the hydrophilic principles of *Cristaria plicata*'s flesh, meat, and liver, a glycoprotein (> 30 kDa) fraction III was separated. It showed a remarkable inhibitory activity on the cell growth of L1210 lymphocytic leukemia *in vitro*, sarcoma 180, and Krebs 2 ascites tumor *in vivo*. The derived fraction III significantly potentiated the activity of NK cells of mice bearing sarcoma 180 to kill the target tumor cells.[7,8] Polysaccharides prepared from *C. plicata* are natural immunomodulators, which were able to stimulate B-lymphocyte multiplication and transformation and to reduce the index of cAMP/cGMP in plasma.[9] A polysaccharide component obtained from *H. cumingii* demonstrated similar antitumor and immunoenhancing properties. Oral administration with the polysaccharide in doses of 50–500 mg per day for 8 days resulted in 34.9%–50.0% growth inhibition in mice against the growth of HepA ascites hepatoma cells via notably repressing the DNA synthesis in HepA cells and upregulating the immunological functions of the thymus gland and spleen in host.[10]

Conclusion and Suggestion

All the above-mentioned encouraging results suggested that the aqueous extract of fresh water mussels and mussel tears can be consumed as a natural anticarcinogenic and immunoregulating food. The studies further demonstrated that the major cancer-preventive contributors in the bivalves were assigned to be glycoproteins and/or polysaccharides. These two macromolecules showed no direct suppression of the proliferation of cancer cells *in vitro* but exerted remarkable immunoenhancing activity and then anti-growth effect against malignant tumors *in vivo*, inferring that their antitumor capacities were found mostly to be contributed by their immunostimulating function. Hence, intake of fresh-water mussels is highly encouraged to amplify body protection and immune system, as both a nutritional and a functional food to be good for cancer prevention.

REFERENCES

1. Zhang, H.Z. et al., 1987. Preclinical study on the antitumor activity of changshenglin. *Shengwu Huaxue yu Shengwu Wuli Jinzhan* 14: 22.
2. Du, L.X. et al., 1991. Antitumor activity and mechanism of Hebang (HB) extract. *Zhongguo Yiyao Gongye Zazhi* 22: 430; 1993. Study on the antitumor activity of HB fraction. *Zhongguo Haiyang Yaowu* 12: 10.
3. Hu, S.G. et al., 1997. Studies on antitumor effective constituent of Anodonta woodiana Leai analysis and characterization of glycoprotein HB-II. *Zhongguo Haiyang Yaowu* 16: 19–21; 23–25.
4. Hu, S.G. et al., 2002. Preparing process and application of clam liposome. Faming Zhuanli Shenqing Gongkai Shuomingshu CN 1329885 A 20020109.
5. Liu, J. et al., 2008. Antitumor activities of liposome-incorporated aqueous extracts of Anodonta woodiana. *Eur. Food Res. Technol.* 227: 919–924.
6. Hu, S.G. et al., 2003. An experiment study on antitumor effect of liposome of effective fraction from Anodonta woodiana in mice. *Zhongguo Haiyang Yaowu* 22: 23–25.
7. Tong, Z.Y. et al., 2003. Experimental study on antitumor effect of extracts from Cristaria plicata. *Zhongguo Haiyang Yaowu* 22: 20–24.
8. Tong, Z.Y. et al., 2002. Comparison of biochemical characters and antitumor activity of Cristaria plicata liver and flesh extracts. *Shengming Kexue Yanjiu* 6: 255–260.
9. Chen, W.X. et al., 2001. Research on immunomodulation function of polysaccharides from Cristaria plicata. *Pharmacol. Clin. Chin. Materia Med.* 27: 17–19.
10. Hu, J.R. et al., 2003. Inhibitive effects of polysaccharide from Hyriopaia cumingii on tumor proliferation. *Chin. J. Modern Appl. Pharmacy.* 20: 13–15.

87. MARINE MUSSELS

Moule   Muscheln   Mejillón

貽貝   ムール貝   홍합

Mytilus edulis, M. coruscus

Mytilidae

Two medium-sized edible marine bivalve mollusks *Mytilus edulis* and *M. coruscus* are commonly harvested from wild sources and aquaculture for many seafood dishes in various cuisines. Although significant seasonal variations influence the compositions of most amino acids, lipid classes, and fatty acids, the two mussels represent a source of health benefiting long chain *n*-3 polyunsaturated fatty acids, vitamins B12 and A, essential amino acids (such as glycine, lysine, threonine, phenylalanine, and arginine), and minerals (such as magnesium, potassium, calcium, and selenium). Accordingly, the marine mussels are always consumed as a nutritional food supplement. Recent chemical biology studies further revealed the biological functions of the mussels, including cancer-inhibitory and cancer-preventive activities.

Scientific Evidence of Cancer-Inhibitory and Cancer-Preventive Activities

1. Hard-shelled mussel (Mytilus coruscus)

Although some small molecular fatty acids such as eiocosadienoic acid (C20:2), eicosapentaenoic acid (C20:5), and docosahexaenoic acid (C22:6) were found in *M. coruscus* cultivated in Korea exerting anti-growth effect against several cancer cell lines together with the induction of cell apoptosis,[1] the major bioactive components in *M. coruscus* were considered to be macromolecules, including polysaccharides and proteins. Mytilus polysaccharide-I (MP-I) was extracted from *M. coruscus* with 2.14% yield, which was mainly composed of glucose. Its *in vitro* antitumor activity was observed against human MKN-45 (stomach), MCF-7 (breast), HO-8910 (ovary), K562 (leukemic), and SMMC-7721 (liver) tumor cell lines in middle (100 μg/mL) and high (500 μg/mL) concentrations. Its *in vivo* antitumor activity was shown in nude mice-implanted MKN-45 carcinoma in doses of 20 and 100 mg/kg/day, cancer inhibition of which in the MP-1–treated groups in a daily dose of 20 mg/kg was noticeably higher than that of 5-FU (an anticancer drug). The mechanism exploration disclosed that downregulation of the NF-κB signal pathway might play an important role in the antitumor activity.[2] MF4 (m.w. of 113,000), a polysaccharide, was also isolated from *M. coruscus*, showing both immunity enhancing and antitumor properties. MF4 in *in vitro* assays markedly motivated the proliferation of T- and B-lymphocytes and in *in vivo* tests deterred the growths of Lewis lung cancer and sarcoma 180 in association with noticeable enhancement of NK cell activity and lymphocyte transformation in mice.[3] Similarly, a crude polysaccharide extract was derived from *M. coruscus* by boiled alkali method. In mouse models, the polysaccharide component was able to amplify splenic lymphocyte transformation efficiency to enhance delayed-type allergy, NK activity, and antibody forming cell activity, and to augment the rates of C-clearance and peritoneal macrophage phagocytizing of chicken red blood cells. It also effectively stimulated the proliferative activities of splenic lymphocyte in tumor-bearing mice.[4] Overall, the observations established *M. coruscus* polysaccharides as having both remarkable immunocompetence and antitumor immunity.

The experiments further discovered that the enzymatic hydrolysis of *M. coruscus* produced the molecular size-lessened agents and amplified the antitumor potencies. Crude *M. coruscus* polysaccharides were prepared from hot-water extraction and papain/trypsin combined enzymic hydrolysis with 23.69% yield, which was effective in scavenging DPPH, superoxide anion and lipid peroxide radicals, and hindering the growth of DU-145 prostate cancer cells (IC$_{50}$ of 2.93 mg/mL in 48 h). From the crude polysaccharides, MT3, a glycosaminoglycan-like polysaccharide (≈18 kDa) was separated, which consisted of mannose, glucosamine, β-D-glucuronic acid, galactose, and fucose. *In vitro* assay showed that MT3 impeded the DU-145 cell proliferation with IC_{50} of 2.71 mg/mL in 48 h,[5] and a similar pepsin-enzymatic hydrolysate of *M. coruscus* exhibited antitumor activity in *in vitro* models with three human cancer cell lines. An anticancer peptide was isolated from the enzymatic hydrolysate of *M. coruscus*, whose sequence was elucidated as Ala–Phe–Asn–Ile–His–Asn–Arg–Asn–Leu–Leu. This peptide effectively elicited the death of PC3 (prostate), breast, and lung carcinoma cells but not normal liver cells, but it showed certain suppressive activity against human PC3 (prostate), MDA-MB-231 (breast), and A549 (lung) neoplastic cell lines with LC_{50}s of 0.94, 1.22, and 1.41 mg/mL, respectively.[6]

2. Blue mussel (Mytilus edulis)

An anticancer peptide component was generated from a trypsin hydrolysis process with the meat of *M. edulis*. In association with retarding Bcl-2 expression, the hydrolytic peptide component induced cell apoptosis, leading to anticancer effect on DU-145 and PC3 prostate cancer cell lines *in vitro*. At 5 mg/mL concentration, the inhibitory rates were 50.23% in DU-145 cells and 41.17% in PC3 cells.[7] In an aquaculture industry in Canada, huge blue mussel waste residues are produced, which are composed of high quality proteins (10%–23% w/w). By enzymatic hydrolysis, a peptide-enriched fraction (50 kDa) was obtained, which contains 56% of proteins/peptides, 3% of lipids, and 6% of minerals on a dry weight basis, and it consists of high levels of threonine, proline, and glycine, low levels of taurine and methionine, and middle levels of other amino acids, presenting a biological activity of interest. At 44 μg/mL concentration, this 50 kDa fraction caused strong mortality of human cancer cell lines, such as 90% for PC3 (prostate), 89% for A549 (lung), 85% for HCT15 (colon), and 81% for BT549 (breast) cells, and at 11 μg/mL concentration, the mortality was 87% for PC3 cells and 76% for A549 cells.[8] Hence, the investigations evidenced that the blue mussel meat and its industry waste are good sources for biofunctional and antitumor peptide mining, and the enzymatic hydrolysis is an important process for increasing promising active ingredients in the nutritional mussels. Moreover, ME-B, a butanol extract from *M. edulis*, showed an ability to elicit differentiation of F9 teratocarcinoma stem cells. Fractionation of ME-B produced a sphingosine fraction labeled as ME–Bu–9d, which was more effective in prompting the F9 cell differentiation via regulation of differentiation-specific genes such as laminin, type-IV collagen, and retinoic acid receptor-β, and induction of morphological changes.[9]

In addition, an ethyl acetate extract and crude polysaccharides isolated from *M. edulis* at its concentration of 10–60/80 μg/mL showed obvious antioxidant properties in free-radical scavenging assays.[10,11] The enhancement of cellular immune functions by polysaccharides was also demonstrated in immunosuppressed mice, activity of which was found to be mediated by moderation of immune-related factors such as upregulation of Th1 cell expression and reversal of cyclophosphamide-caused immunosuppression.[12]

CONCLUSION AND SUGGESTION

On the basis of these scientific findings, the most important component in the two Mytilus mussels could be assigned as polysaccharides that play remarkable roles in the amplification of the body defense and recovery system. The antitumor and anticarcinogenesis-related advantages of Mytilus polysaccharides are fulfilled primarily by immunopotentiating and radical-scavenging actions despite also exerting certain antiproliferative effect directly against cancer cells. Significantly, the studies further revealed that hydrolytic process with enzymes can produce more valuable biofunctional polysaccharides and peptides by degrading the sizes of macromolecules in the mussel meats. In addition, Mytilus mussel contains rich health-beneficial fatty acid ingredients that were also found to be responsible in the cancer-inhibitory effect. Therefore, the marine mussels can be recommended for human diet menu as both nutritional and functional seafood, which can provide a potential approach to prevent carcinogenesis.

REFERENCES

1. Kim, E.K. et al., 2011. Effect of partially purified lipid from the mussel Mytilus coruscus on apoptosis in cancer cells. *J. Kor. Soc. Applied Biol. Chem.* 54(1): 59–65.
2. Zhang, J.P. et al., 2015. Antitumor activity and mechanism of polysaccharide isolated from Mytilus coruscus. *Shanghai Yixue.* 38(1): 57–61; Xu, H.L. et al., 2006. Isolation and purification of water-soluble polysaccharide MP-I from Mytilus coruscus and study on its in vitro antitumor activity. *Dier Junyi Daxue Xuebao.* 27(9): 998–1001.
3. Yi, Y.H. et al., 2005. Mytilus coruscus polysaccharide MF4 with immune enhancing effect and antitumor activity. Faming Zhuanli Shenqing Gongkai Shuomingshu (2005), CN 1583803 A 20050223.
4. Yao, Y. et al., 2005. Extraction of Mytilus coruscus polysaccharides and study on their immunocompetence. *Dier Junyi Daxue Xuebao.* 26(8): 896–899.
5. Zhong, C.C. et al., 2014. Optimized extraction and bioactivity in vitro of polysaccharides from Mytilus coruscus. *Shipin Kexue* (Beijing, China). 35(10): 107–114.
6. Kim, E.K. et al., 2012. Purification of a novel anticancer peptide from enzymatic hydrolysates of Mytilus coruscus. *J. Microbiol. Biotechnol.* 22: 1381–1387.
7. Yang, Y.F. et al., 2011. The anticancer activity of peptide from hydrolysates of Mytilus edulis. *Zhejiang Haiyang Xueyuan Xuebao, Ziran Kexueban.* 30(2): 113–118.
8. Beaulieu, L. et al., 2013. Evidence of antiproliferative activities in blue mussel (Mytilus edulis) by-products. *Marine Drugs.* 11(4): 975–990.
9. Kim, L.L. et al., 1997. Tumor cell differentiation-inducing activity of fractions Stichopus japonicas and marine mullask Mytilus edulis. *J. Kor. Asso. Cancer Prevention.* 1: 73–80.
10. Wu, L.H. et al., 2016. Study on antioxidation activity of Mytilus edulis extracts. *J. Pharm. Res.* 35(6): 325–327.
11. Cheng, S.W. et al., 2010. Study on extraction of polysaccharides from Mytilus edulis and their antioxidant activity in vitro. *Sci. Tech. Food Industry* 31(9): 132–134.
12. Zhang, X. et al., 2011. Effect of crude polysaccharides extracted from Myltilus edulis on the immune factors in immunosuppressed mice. *Acta Nutri. Sinica* 33(5): 497–501.

88. HARD CLAM

文蛤

Meretrix meretrix

Veneridae

Asiatic hard clam, or *Meretrix meretrix* (Veneridae), is one of the bivalvia invertebrates, which broadly grows at the bottom of shallow offshore water around Eastern Asia. This edible shellfish has abundant nutrition and prominent medical properties. Pharmacological investigations have demonstrated that hard clams have multiple health-promoting functions, hypoglycemic, antihyperlipidemic, antimutant, antioxidant, antistress, immunoregulating, detoxification, and antiaging effects besides anticarcinogenesis. The biologically active substances in *M. meretrix* were assigned to be peptides, proteins, enzymes, polysaccharides, essential vitamins (especially vitamin B12) and minerals (such as iron, selenium, magnesium, calcium, copper, and zinc), essential amino acids, and some enzyme inhibitors that are responsible for its nutritional and medicinal properties. As a kind of sea-food diet, the clam is popular in the coastal areas of many places in the world.

Scientific Evidence of Cancer-Inhibitory and Cancer-Preventive Activities

Since an antitumor substance assigned as mercenene was reported from the isolations of clam meat by Schmeer,[1,2] the nutritional clam has been paid more and more attention by scientists. The clam extract was demonstrated to have abilities to prolong the life duration of animals bearing moloney leukemia virus and to restrain the growth of mouse sarcoma 180 *in vivo*.[3] A kind of tablet called HS-72 was made in the late 1980s from hard clam extract, which was used to clinically treat patients with lung carcinoma in China. The results showed that the HS-72 could delay cancer cell growth, improve living quality, and extend the patient's lifetime.[4] Wenge-Jing (an extract of the clam) was effective in lessening the weight of the entity sarcoma 180 and lengthening the life span of mice bearing Ehrlich ascites carcinoma (EAC).[5] The decoction of *M. meretrix* meat was demonstrated to have antimutative and chromosome-protecting activities against chemical mutagen-induced micronuclear increase.[6] In addition, *M. meretrix* ethanol extract was able to strengthen the expressions of T- and B-lymphocytes by 18% and 43%, respectively.[7] In recent years, many bioactive components such as proteins, peptides, glycopeptides, polysaccharides, sterols, taurines, and enzymes have been discovered from *M. meretrix* meat and their properties have been reported in correlation with anticancer, antioxidant, and immunopotentiation.

1. Peptides

In the early studies, mercenene, a polypeptide (m.w. < 10,000), had been reported to have anticancer activity against L1210 leukemia, krebs-2 breast cancer, Bittner mammary tumor, and HeLa cervical carcinoma *in vitro* or *in vivo*.[8] Reinvestigation of mercenene by Chinese scientists further confirmed 89.4% growth-suppressive rate on human SMMC-7721 hepatoma cells together with induction of cell-cycle arrest and apoptosis after treatment with 5.0 µg/mL of mercenene.[9] Several newly purified peptides and polypeptides have been reported exerting obvious inhibitory effects against oxidation and tumor proliferation. By upregulating the growth of thymus and spleen, the polypeptide could improve the host's immunity in a mouse model.[7]

M2 and Mer2: A peptide M2 (18.4 kDa) purified from the clam displayed the growth-inhibitory effect on human BGC-823 gastric cancer cells.[10] A repurified peptide Mer2 (3147 Da) exhibited more effectiveness than M2 on the BGC-823 cell lines. In 4.0 µg/mL concentration, growth inhibitory percentage of Mer2 in BGC-823 cells was about 60%.[11] The marked inhibition from Mer2 was also demonstrated in human HepG2 (liver), HeLa (cervix), A549, SPCA-1 and LTEP-a-2 (lung), and QBC939 (cholangiocellular) carcinoma cell lines *in vitro*, and the HepG2 hepatoma cell line was more sensitive to Mer2 compared to other tested cancer cell lines.[12–14] The anticancer effect was found to accompany with the induction of BGC-823 cell apoptosis, cell skeletal structure of which was obviously destroyed in the Mer2 treatment.[11–15] Simultaneously, M2 and Mer2 were able to activate superoxide dismutase (SOD) and alkaline phosphatase (ALP) and to inactivate tyrosinase, but the activities of small peptide Mer2 were more potent than the large peptide M2.[10,11] The results indicated that the peptides have significant ability for radical scavenging, antioxidant effect of which should closely relate to the anticarcinogenic and anticancer properties.

Mere15: A polypeptide Mere15 (15 kDa) was recently discovered from the separation of the clam meat. In an *in vitro* experiment, Mere15 dose- and time-dependently restrained the growth of human A549 lung adenocarcinoma cells concomitant with the promotion of a G2/M phase arrest and apoptosis, inhibition of tubulin polymerization, and activation of p21.[15] The anticancer activity of Mere15 was further proved in a A549 xenograft nude mice model.[15,16] In addition, the ability of A549 cell adhesion was reduced by 86.74% at a concentration of 12.0 µg/mL of Mere15 and the migration and invasion of A549 cells were lessened by 69.22 and 53.84% after treatment with 15.0 µg/mL of Mere15. During the actions, the secretion of MMPs-2 and -9 were attenuated by 72.0% and 93.24% and MMP-2 and MMP-9 mRNA expression were repressed by 57.54% and 91.22%, respectively.[17] These evidences demonstrate that the anti-growth effect of Mere15 in A549 lung carcinoma cells are primarily mediated by both proapoptotic and antimetastatic pathways.[17] Furthermore, treatment with Mere15 hampered the proliferation of human K562 chronic myelogenous leukemia cells (IC$_{50}$ 38.2 µg/mL). Concurrently, Mere15 concentration-dependently also arrested the cell-cycle progression at the G0/G1 phase and prompted cell apoptosis along with an increase in ROS and loss of mitochondrial membrane potential. The microtubule disassembly of K562 cells could also be triggered by the Mere15 treatment.[18] On the basis of these positive results, Mere15 is considered further to have developing potential for the treatment of various neoplastic diseases in clinics, especially nonsmall cell lung carcinoma and leukemia.

2. Glycopeptide

MGP0405: A kind of glycopeptide (m.w. 9655 Da) was separated from *M. meretrix* and designated as MGP0405, which is stable below 30°C and in neutral solution. MGP0405 is rich in glycine, alanine, valine, methionine, leucine, and isoleucine without tryptophan in its peptide moiety, and it has only single glucose comprising its saccharide moiety. MGP0405 showed moderate anti-growth effect on six human cancer cell lines, such as A549 (lung), HeLa (cervix), HO8910 (ovary), KB (nasopharynx), SMMC-7721 (liver), and BGC (stomach) cells *in vitro*, and on mouse B16 melanoma cells.[17,18] Among these cell lines, KB cells were mostly sensitive to MGP0405. When treated with 200 µg/mL concentration of MGP0405, the inhibitory rate in KB cells was 69% with no apoptosis induction. The *in vivo* antitumor activity of MGP0405 was further confirmed in a mouse model with sarcoma 180. In addition, MGP0405 was demonstrated having antiadhesive and immunoenhancing activities.[19,20]

MGP0501: Another glycopeptide derived from *M. meretrix* was MGP0501 (15,878 Da), which consists of 55.18% saccharide and 44.82% protein. MGP0501 presented temperature tolerance and its best antitumor activity in neutral solution. Its suppressive effect was observed in *in vitro* assay against nine human tumor cell lines and one murine cancer cell with no negative effect on normal spleen lymphocytes. The most potent inhibition for MGP0501 was on B16 melanoma cells and the next most potent inhibition was on five human tumor cell lines, including A549, KB, HeLa, HO8910, and SMMC-7721 cells. The anticancer property of MGP0501 was further proved in murine animal model-implanted sarcoma 180, Heps tumor, and EAC ascites tumor. The MGP0501 treatment in a dose of 6 mg/mL resulted in inhibitory rates of 68.5% and 66.43%, respectively, against sarcoma 180 and Heps tumor in mice. Similar to MGP0405, MGP0501 displayed proapoptotic and antiadhesive activities. The investigation disclosed that MGP0501 was able to specifically augment the activities of GPx and SOD and to decrease the content of MDA in mouse liver as well, implying that the MGP0501 has marked antioxidative function that may relate to its anticancer activity.[21]

Taken together, these findings designated that the glycopeptides are important components to respond to the anticancer and antioxidant nature of the Asiatic hard clam.

3. Protein

A purified antitumor protein named MML (40 kDa) exhibited significant cytotoxic effect on several human cancer cell types, including BEL-7402 hepatoma, MCF-7 breast carcinoma, and HCT-116 colon carcinoma cells, but no such effect on murine normal NIH3T3 fibroblasts and benign human MCF-10A breast cell lines. A nude mice model-transplanted BEL-7402 hepatoma further confirmed the antitumor effect of MML *in vivo*, the cell death inducing effect of which was mediated by the alteration of tumor cell membrane permeability and inhibition of tubulin polymerization without an increase in apoptosis. These positive *in vitro* and *in vivo* results suggested that MML may have potential to be developed as a highly selective and effective anticancer agent for cancer prevention and therapy.[22,23] In addition, three proteins, (1) P1 (18 kD), (2) P2 (28 kD), and (3) P3 (16 kD) isolated from the meat of *M. meretrix* were shown to have catalase (CAT) activity, SOD activity, and inhibitory effect on lipid peroxidation (LPO).[7] The acid- or protease-elicited hydrolysates of the proteins presented potent superoxide radical-scavenging property.[7] The antioxidant response of *M. meretrix* could be amplified synergistically in external examinations.

4. Polysaccharide

Meretrix polysaccharide demonstrated marked antineoplastic and immunoregulating effects. Oral administration of Meretrix polysaccharide at doses of 100 or 200 mg/kg notably diminished the weight of S180 solid carcinoma in mice and prolonged the survival time of mice bearing EAC ascites carcinoma or hepatic carcinoma, but it did not show such effect in L1210 leukemia *in vivo*. During the treatment, the Meretrix polysaccharide notably exerted immunopotentiating effects, such as improving the indexes of thymus and spleen, increasing leukocyte and serum hemolysin production, and enhancing phagocytic power. It could prominently augment the SRBC–DTH and PC–DTH reaction to restore the immune function in mice against cyclophosphamide-caused immunodepression.[24] Oral administration of *M. meretrix* polysaccharides to mice could restore cyclophosphamide-damaged immune system via amelioration of a series of immunological indicators, such as phagocytic power, leukocyte and hemolysin antibody, and amplification of DTH reaction.[7] A water-soluble polysaccharide termed MMPX-B2 (510 kDa) was isolated from *M. meretrix*, which consists of D-glucose and D-galactose residues at a molar ratio of 3.51:1.00 and has a main chain of (1-4)-linked-α-D-glucopyranosyl residues with a few terminal β-D-galactose residues at C-6 position and β-D-galactose residues branched at C-3 position. In *in vitro* immunological tests, it stimulated the murine macrophages to release various cytokines, indicating a remarkable immunopromoting capacity.[25]

5. Sterols

Epidioxysterols are a valuable group of small molecules in the hard clams. From the fractionation of *M. meretrix*, 5α, 8α-epidioxycholest-6-ene-3β-ol (MME) was obtained. By *in vitro* assay, MME (**1**) was found to have cytotoxic effect against three cancer cell lines: (1) human epidermoid carcinoma (KB), (2) Fibrillary sarcoma of uterus (FL), and (3) HepG2 hepatoma with IC_{50} values of 2.0, 3.93, and 2.4 μg/mL, respectively.[26] Studies evidenced that the MME has the ability to inhibit the growth of hepatoma cells and to induce G1-phase cell-cycle arrest in two human hepatoma cell lines (HepG2 and Hep3B), where MME markedly upregulated p53 and p21WAF1/CIP1 expressions in HepG2 cells and upregulated p27KIP1 and p16I NK4A expressions in both HepG2 and Hep3B cells, signifying that the G1-phase arrest mechanism is involved in both p53-dependent and p53-independent pathways. The results proved that this shellfish is one of the functional seafoods for the prevention of liver carcinogenesis and remedy for liver disease and chronic hepatitis.[27] In addition, *M. lusoria* (a close clam species) was specifically cytotoxic to both MCF-7 breast cancer cells and HuH-6KK hepatoblastoma cells.[28] Two epidioxysterols (as stereoisomers) were isolated from an ethyl acetate fraction of *M. lusoria*. Both the epidioxysterols could prompt the apoptosis of human HL-60 leukemia cells via dissipation of mitochondrial membrane potential, release of mitochondrial cytochrome c, and initiation of procaspase-9 and -3 processing. The treatment caused ROS stimulation and a rapid loss of intracellular glutathione content as well, thus exerting the antioxidant effect.[29] Therefore, the two common hard clams are beneficial not only for nutrition but also for cancer chemoprevention.

6. Taurine

Taurine (2-aminoethanesulfonic acid, **1**) is widely distributed in animal tissues and is abundant in the hard clam (3.95–6.52 mg/g), possessing good medical-care function in physiology. The medical values of taurine (**1**) have been found to be involved in anticarcinoma, antioxidation, and antiradical damage potentials, and many health benefits such as antihypertensive, anti-senility, antivirus, and hypoglycemic activities.[30,31]

CONCLUSION AND SUGGESTION

The scientific investigations disclosed that remarkable antitumor and antioxidant activities of the meat of *Meretrix meretrix* are closely attributed to its higher contents of submacro- and macromolecules (such as glycopeptides, peptides, proteins, and polysaccharides) and some micromolecules (such as sterols and taurine). Although showing *in vitro* antiproliferative effect on some carcinoma cell lines, the antitumor property of these submacro- and macromolecules are mostly contributed by their immunopotentiating and antioxidant activities. As major micromolecules, sterols and taurine presented a certain degree of cytotoxic, antiproliferative, proapoptotic, and antioxidant activities. On the basis of these findings, the meat of hard clams can be considered as health-promoting seafood suitable to prevent several types of carcinogenesis, to improve the body defense, and to help in the remedy of some diseases. Hence, the dietary clams are highly recommended as both nutritional and functional foods but it is suggested not to consume clams produced in heavy-metal-polluted areas.

REFERENCES

1. Schmeer, M.R. et al., 1964. Growth-inhibiting agents from Mercenaria extracts: Chemical and biological properties. *Science* 144: 413.
2. Sehmeer, A.C. et al., 1969. Mercenene: An antineoplastic agent extracted from the marine clam, Mercenaria mercenaria. *Natl. Cancer Inst. Monogr.* 31: 581.
3. Xie, H. et al., 2005. Research progress in the pharmaceutical activities of Mercenaria mercenaria. *J. Chengde Petroleum College* 7: 9–12.

4. Ke, L. et al., 1987. Clinical treatment of lung cancer patients with HS-72. *Chinese J. Marine Drugs* 22: 22.
5. Dou, C.G. et al., 1986. Study on anticancer effect of Wenge-Jing. *Res. Reports* 4: 73–75 (in Chinese).
6. Wu, P. et al., 2002. Study on the effect of Wenge on chromosome. *J. Shanghai Fisheries Univ.* 14: 9–12.
7. Xie, W.Y. et al., 2012. Meretrix meretrix: Active components and their bioactivities. *Life Sci. J.* 9(3): 756–762.
8. Schmeer, A.C. et al., 1979. Chemical characterization and biological activity of an anticancer agent of marine origin. *Physiol. Chem. Physics.* 11: 415–424.
9. Leng, B. et al., 2007. Effect of the polypeptides from Meretrix meretrix Linnaeus on proliferation of human hepatocarcinoma SMMC-7721 cells. *J. Xiamen Univ., Nat. Sci.* 46: 593–597.
10. Liu, X.D. et al., 2004. Studies on the physiological activity of a natural peptide from clam (Meretrix meretrix Linnaeus). *J. Xiamen Univ., Nat. Sci.* 43: 432–435.
11. Leng, B. et al., 2005. Inhibitory effects of anticancer peptide from Mercenaria on the BGC-823 cells and several enzymes. *FEBS Lett.* 579: 1187–1190.
12. Fan, C.C. et al., 2009. Antitumor activity of peptide from Meretrix meretrix in vitro. *Tianwan Haixia* 28: 472–476.
13. Kang, J.H. et al., 2009. Effect of peptide from Meretrix meretrix on the human lung adenocarcinoma A549 cells in vitro. *Taiwan Haixia* 28: 477–481.
14. Zhang, J. et al., 2009. Effect of the polypeptides from Meretrix meretrix Linnaeus on proliferation of cervical cancer HeLa cells. *J. Xiamen Univ., Nat. Sci.* 48: 729–732.
15. Wang, C.C et al., 2012. Growth-inhibition effects of a novel antitumor polypeptide from Meretrix meretrix Linnaeus associated with tubulin polymerization. *Zhongguo Shenghua Yaowu Zazhi* 33: 225–228.
16. Wang, C.C. et al., 2012. A novel polypeptide from Meretrix meretrix Linnaeus inhibits the growth of human lung adenocarcinoma. *Experim. Biol. Med.* (London) 237: 442–450.
17. Wang, H. et al., 2013. Mere15, a novel polypeptide from Meretrix meretrix, inhibits adhesion, migration and invasion of human lung cancer A549 cells via down-regulating MMPs. *Pharm. Biol.* (London, U.K.) 51: 145–151.
18. Liu, M. et al., 2012. Induction of apoptosis, G0/G1 phase arrest and microtubule disassembly in K562 leukemia cells by Mere15, a novel polypeptide from Meretrix meretrix Linnaeus. *Mar. Drugs* 10: 2596–2607.
19. Zhang, B. et al., 2006. Studies on stability and anticancer activities of Meretrix meretrix glycopeptide MGP0405. *Yaowu Shengwu Jishu* 13: 24–27, 44.
20. Zhang, B. et al., 2006. Isolation and characterization of glycopeptide MGP0405 from Meretrix meretrix. *Zhongguo Tianran Yaowu* 4: 230–233.
21. Wu, J.L. et al., 2006. The antitumor activity of glycopeptide (MGP0501) from Meretrix meretrix in vitro. *Yaowu Shengwu Jishu* 13: 260–264; 2013. Isolation and characterization of glycopeptide MGP0501 from Meretrix meretrix. *Anjisuan He Shengwu Ziyuan* 35: 41–45.
22. Ning, X.X. et al., 2009. A novel antitumor protein extracted from Meretrix meretrix Linnaeus induces cell death by increasing cell permeability and inhibiting tubulin polymerization. *Intl. J. Oncol.* 35: 805–812.
23. Zhang, Y.Y. et al., 2009. Mechanism of anticancer effect in vitro and in vivo of a novel antitumor protein from Meretrix Meretrix Linnaeus. *Zhongguo Xinyao Zazhi* 18: 1787–1792.
24. Dou, C.G. et al., 1999. Study on antineoplastic and immunoregulation effects of Meretrix polysaccharide. *Zhongguo Haiyang Yaowu* 18: 15–19.
25. Li, L. et al., 2016. Structural and immunological activity characterization of a polysaccharide isolated from Meretrix meretrix Linnaeus. *Mar. Drugs* 14(1): 6.
26. Minh, C.V. et al., 2004. Cytotoxic Constituents of Diadema setosum. *Arch. Pharm. Res.* 27(7): 734–737.
27. Wu, T.H. et al., 2006. Inhibition of cell growth and induction of G1-phase cell cycle arrest in hepatoma cells by steroid extract from Meretrix meretrix. *Cancer Lett.* 232: 199–205.
28. Pan, M.S. et al., 2006. Induction of apoptosis by Meretrix lusoria through reactive oxygen species production, glutathione depletion, and caspase activation in human leukemia cells. *Life Sci.* 79: 1140–1152.
29. Kong, Z.L. et al., 1997. Immune bioactivity in shellfish toward serum-free cultured human cell lines. *Biosci. Biotech. Biochem.* 61: 24–28.
30. Jiang, C.F. et al., 2008. Extraction of taurine from Meretrix meretrix by isoelectric point method and research on taurine's medical-care function. *Liaoning Shiyou Huagong Daxue Xuebao* 28: 30–32.
31. Tan, L.Y. et al., 2000. The bioactivities of taurine and its distribution in ocean organisms. *J. Zhanjiang Ocean Univ.* 20: 75–79.

89. OTHER CLAMS

Palourde   Muschel   Almeja

蛤 アサリ 대합

Cyclina sinensis, Corbicula fluminea, Ruditapes philippinarum

Veneridae or Cyrenidae

There are many other edible hard clams distributed in various places near the sea coast, and they also own a delicious reputation. Of them, two marine bivalve molluscs *Cyclina sinensis* and *Ruditapes philippinarum* (Veneridae) and a freshwater clam *Corbicula fluminea* (Cyrenidae) are consumed as nutritional seafoods as well. The scientific tests demonstrated that the three hard clams that have antitumor potential are similar to a hard clam (*Meretrix meretrix*). These clams are often consumed in both food diet and folk medicine in some Asian regions.

SCIENTIFIC EVIDENCE OF CANCER-INHIBITORY AND CANCER-PREVENTIVE ACTIVITIES

1. Venus hard clam (Cyclina sinensis)

An antioxidative *Cyclina sinensis* polysaccharide (CSPS) was prepared from the meat of the Venus hard clam. *In vivo* administration of CSPS significantly lessened the levels of alanine aminotransferase and aspartate aminotransferase in serum, inhibited the formation of malondialdehyde, and enhanced the activities of liver SOD and glutathione peroxidase in mice with carbon tetrachloride-caused liver injury, resulting in remarkable hepatoprotective activity.[1] From the CSPS, three fractions labeled as CSPS-1 (69 kDa), CSPS-2 (81 kDa), and CSPS-3 (101 kDa) were separated. CSPS, CSPS-1, CSPS-2, and CSPS-3 demonstrated anticarcinogenesis related to moderate H_2O_2 scavenging activity, lipid-peroxidation inhibition effect, and strong Fe^{2+} chelating activity.[1] The CSPS-3 has relatively higher contents of protein, uronic acid, sulfate, and more complicated monosaccharides, displaying strong inhibitory *in vitro* effect on the growth of human BGC-823 gastric cancer cells and potent scavenging activities on superoxide radical and hydroxyl radical *in vitro*.[1,2] CSPS-1 was composed of α-(1-4)-linked glucosyl backbone with branch chains attached to the backbone chain by (1-6)-glycosidic bond.[3] Chemically sulfated CSPS-1 exhibited improved inhibitory activity against the BGC-823 cells *in vitro*.[3] The findings indicated that the clams (*Cyclina sinensis*) have potential in the inhibition of carcinogenesis in liver and stomach due to its notable bioactivities in antioxidation, antiproliferation, and hepatoprotection. In addition, three other peptide fractions that were derived from trypsin-hydrolyzed *C. sinensis* extract also showed inhibitory effects against the cancer cell proliferation.[4]

2. Manila clam (Ruditapes philippinarum)

An aqueous purified extract (PE) was isolated from the clam meat of *R. philippinarum*, which showed prominent tumoricidal activity against human hepatoma SMMC-7721 cells and no cytotoxicity in normal human hepatocyte HL-7702 cells *in vitro* within an experimental concentration range (10–1000 μg/mL). At concentrations of 100 and 1000 μg/mL, PE exerted similar inhibitory effect (74.59% and 77.45%) on the SMMC-7721 cells, and at doses of 125, 250, and 500 mg/kg, PE showed anti-growth activity against solid sarcoma 180 in a dose-dependent manner and promoting effect on concanavalin A-induced T-lymphocyte proliferation. From the PE, two water-soluble homoglucan-protein complexes: (1) PEF1 (2.0×10^6), a protein (26%)-bound and (1-6)-branched (1-4)-α-D-glucan and (2) PEF2 (5.0×10^3), a protein (8.2%)-bound D-glucan with (1-4)-α- and (1-6)-β-linkages were separated and purified. However, the antitumor activities of PEF-1 (34.63%) and PEF-2 (45.58%) were lower than that of PE (74.59%) on the SMMC-7721 cells at the corresponding concentrations.[5] RPOI-1 (**1**), a water-soluble tetrapeptide was isolated from *R. philippinarum* by means of enzymolysis. In 30 mg/mL concentrations for 72 h, RPOI-1 hampered the proliferation of DU-145 human prostate cancer cells by > 90% together with the induction of apoptotic death and cell-cycle arrest at sub-G1 and G2/M phases.[6] Similarly, four more anticancer peptide fractions and a purified peptide with a sequence of Ala–Val–Leu–Val–Asp–Lys–Gln–Cys–Pro–Asp at *N*-terminal were isolated from α-chymotrypsin hydrolysate of *R. philippinarum*. In an *in vitro* assay, the fractions and the peptide displayed potentials to induce apoptosis of several human cancer cells but not normal liver cells. The LC_{50} of the anticancer peptide was 1.29, 1.35, and 1.58 mg/mL on PC3 (prostate), A549 (liver), and MDA-MB-231 (breast) carcinoma cells, respectively.[7]

Accordingly, these findings not only revealed the natural antitumor and immunomodulatory peptides in the clam *R. philippinarum* but also proposed a developing value of antitumor agents from the macromolecules by enzymolysis at industrial scales.

3. Golden Asian clam (Corbicula fluminea)

Corbicula fluminea polysaccharide (CFPS) was a crude polysaccharide fraction extracted from the freshwater clam *C. fluminea*, which showed weak inhibition on the growth of HepG2 hepatoma cells. From the CFPS, two protein-bound polysaccharides: (1) CFPS-1 (283 kDa) and (2) CFPS-2 (22 kDa) were separated with yields of 1.12% and 0.21%, respectively. CFPS-1 contains 10.8% protein and consists of mannose and glucose in a molar ratio of 3.1:12.7 in its saccharide part, whereas CFPS-2 contains 2.4% protein, 8.1% sulfate, and 94.4% sugar. The molar ratio in the saccharide part of CFPS-2 was glucosamine (0.22), galactosamine (0.15), galactose (0.25), fucose (0.86), and glucose (0.68). CFPS-1 weakly deterred the growth of MCF-7 and MDA-MB-231 human breast cancer cells with respective IC_{50}s of 243 and 1142 μg/mL.[8] At 1.25 mg/mL concentration, the inhibitory rates of CFPS-2 were 79.4%, 68.3%, and 56.7%, respectively, on SGC-7901 (stomach), SKOV3 (ovary), and A2780 (ovary) human cancer cell lines but 30.4% and 17.8%, respectively on PC3 (prostate) and HepG2 (liver) cancer cell lines. The IC_{50}s on the SGC-7901, SKOV3, and A2780 cells were about 0.03, 0.16, and 0.36 mg/mL, respectively.[9] Moreover, the obvious antioxidant activity of CFPS-2 was experimentally demonstrated. In 6.0 mg/mL concentration, CFPS-2 exhibited 82.3% radical-scavenging activity.[9]

Collectively, these experiments have evidenced the antioxidant and antitumor activities of CFPS-2 and showed the value of *Corbicula fluminea* meat as a functional food.

CONCLUSION AND SUGGESTION

The scientific investigations disclosed the anticancer, antioxidant, and immunomodulatory potential of three types of clams. The evidences for biological activity in the clam extracts and the major constituents such as protein-bound polysaccharides and polysaccharides in the clam meats indicated that clam consumption may be beneficial to health improvement and helpful to cancer therapy and prevention as a natural bioactive supplement. Interestingly, the enzymolysis of the clam macromolecules derived bioactive peptide components with smaller molecules. The peptides showed more promising suppressive effects against some solid tumor cell lines. Consequently, these discoveries augmented awareness regarding the potential anticancer properties of clams, which should aid in dietary applications for lowering the incidence of carcinogenesis.

REFERENCES

1. Jiang, C.X. et al., 2013. Antioxidant activity and potential hepatoprotective effect of polysaccharides from Cyclina sinensis. *Carbohydr. Polym.* 91: 262–268.
2. Jiang, C.X. et al., 2011. Extraction, preliminary characterization, antioxidant and anticancer activities in vitro of polysaccharides from Cyclina sinensis. *Carbohydr. Polym.* 84: 851–857.
3. Jiang, C.X. et al., 2015. Structural characterization, sulfation and antitumor activity of a polysaccharide fraction from Cyclina sinensis. *Carbohydr. Polym.* 115: 200–206.
4. Yan, H.Q. et al., 2014. Anticancer activity of peptides isolated from hydrolysates of Cyclina sinensis. *Anhui Nongye Kexue* 42(12): 3576–3577, 3579.
5. Zhang, L. et al., 2008. Isolation and characterization of antitumor polysaccharides from the marine mollusk Ruditapes philippinarum. *Eur Food Res. Technol.* 227: 103.
6. Yang, Z.S. et al., 2014. Isolation and purification of oligopeptides from Ruditapes philippinarum and its inhibition on the growth of DU-145 cells in vitro. *Mol. Med. Report.* 11(2): 1063–1068.
7. Kim, E.K. et al., 2013. Purification and characterization of a novel anticancer peptide derived from Ruditapes philippinarum. *Process Biochem.* 48(7): 1086–1090.
8. Liao, N.B. et al., 2016. Protein-bound polysaccharide from Corbicula fluminea inhibits cell growth in MCF-7 and MDA-MB-231 human breast cancer cells. *PlosOne* 11(12): e0167889.
9. Liao, N.B. et al., 2013. Antioxidant and antitumor activity of a polysaccharide from freshwater clam Corbicula fluminea. *Food Funct.* 4: 539–548.

90. SEPIA INK

烏賊墨　セピア墨　세피아 잉크

Inks from *Sepiella maindroni, Sepia esculenta, Sepia officinalis*, and *Sepia prabahari*

Sepiidae

Sepia ink originated from cuttlefishes such as *Sepiella maindroni, Sepia esculenta, Sepia officinalis*, and *Sepia prabahari* (Sepiidae). The sepia ink generated from *S. maindroni* and *S. esculenta* has been employed in the coast of southeast of China as a food source and an herb for 1000 years. Multiple pharmacological properties of sepia ink have been proven by chemical biology approaches, establishing antimicrobial, hematopoietic, antihypertensive, anti-inflammatory, antioxidant, antiretroviral, hemostatic, coagulant-promoting, antiulcerogenic, and immunomodulating properties.[1]

SCIENTIFIC EVIDENCE OF CANCER-INHIBITORY AND CANCER-PREVENTIVE ACTIVITIES

Sepia ink has potential as an anticancer agent based on *in vitro* and *in vivo* studies of various types of tumor cells. After feeding 5% sepia ink (0.5 mL per day) to mice for 5 days, the serum taken from the mice, which was rich in tumor necrosis factor (TNF), exerted tumoricidal effect on mouse L929 fibrosarcoma, human BEL-7402 hepatoma, and AGZY 83a lung carcinoma cell lines *in vitro*.[2] The findings revealed that sepia ink is able to augment TNF production and the TNF-rich sera is able to exert cytotoxicity on human cancer cells.[2,3] Daily administration of sepia ink orally in the same dose for 7 days to tested animals markedly restrained the cell growth of Meth-A sarcoma and sarcoma 180 with inhibitory rates of 93.48% and 73.91%, respectively, associated with a significant enhancement of NK cell activity.[4,5] *In vivo* experiments with nude mice further confirmed the cell growth inhibition against human HHC-15 hepatoma, effect of which was accompanied with 85.6% reduction of α-fetoprotein (AFP) in the mice serum.[6] *In vitro* study in H22 hepatoma cells demonstrated that sepia ink could decrease intracellular Ca^{2+} concentration by 69%–79% and reduced nuclear Ca^{2+}/Mg^{2+}–ATPase activities by 21%–37%. By diminishing the amount of Ca^{2+} transported into nuclei and declining Ca^{2+}-induced c-jun and c-fos expressions, the H22 cell proliferation was finally obstructed. Sepia ink also restrained the activities of tyrosine protein kinase (TPK), cAMP-dependent protein kinase (PKA), and protein kinase C (PKC) in the H22 cells through ras-MAPK signal transduction pathways; however, these enzyme activities were abnormally elevated in the cancer cells.[7-10]

An aqueous crude extract from *S. officinalis* ink showed cytotoxicity on HepG2 hepatoma and U87 glioblastoma cells *in vitro* (respective IC_{50}s of 67 and 25 μg/mL) and anti-growth effect on EAC *in vivo*. The survival time and life span of mice bearing EAC tumor were prolonged by 46.15%. Simultaneously, the levels of AST, ALT, ALP, and liver MDA were significantly lessened and the levels of GSH, SOD, and NO were elevated in the mouse model, inferring the abilities in improving the body condition.[11] However, the cytotoxicity on U87 cells might be due to the presence of tyrosinase.[12] The ink extract of *S. officinalis* also demonstrated antioxidant property in both *in vitro* and *in vivo* experiments.[11] By improving the antioxidant ability of spleen and increasing the levels of erythrocytes, leukocytes, hemoglobin, and bone marrow nucleated cells, *S. officinalis* ink extract protected the hemopoietic system and marrow hemopoiesis from chemotherapeutic injury (such as cyclophosphamine) in mice.[13] More investigations clearly revealed that sepia ink and its extract acted as an immunostimulator, which is capable of significantly augmenting both levels of IL-1 and TNF-α and enhancing the functions of NK cells and macrophages to hamper the cancer cells indirectly in addition to its direct cancer suppression.[3,14] Similarly, the ink of *Sepia prabahari* displayed marked antioxidant and anticancer activities, such as retarding the initiation of lipid oxidation process and deterring the growth of MCF-7 breast cancer cells together with the induction of DNA damage in the tumor cells. However, it is impressive that the melanin-free ink showed better antioxidant and anticancer properties than the crude ink. Although melanin is one of the major components in the sepia ink it is not an important anticancer component.[15]

The present researches have confirmed the cancer-inhibitory potentials of sepia ink, the anticancer activities, which were demonstrated to be mostly attributed to its synergistic capacities such as antiproliferation, antitumor immunity, immunostimulation, antioxidant, and anti-inflammation. The data showed that sepia ink is a functional food that may help human cancer prevention and therapy through diet.

SCIENTIFIC EVIDENCE OF CANCER-INHIBITORY AND CANCER-PREVENTIVE CONSTITUENTS

1. Oligopeptides

Sepia ink oligopeptide (SIO) was a tripeptide (**1**) exracted from *S. esculenta* ink, which exerted antiproliferative effect on human DU-145, PC3, and LNCaP prostate cancer cell lines in a time- and dose-dependent manner. During the treatments, SIO in a dose-dependent manner simultaneously enhanced early-stage apoptosis in the tested cell lines and markedly induced S and G2/M phase cell-cycle arrest in the DU-145 and LNCaP cells and sub-G1 and G0/G1 phase cell-cycle arrest in the PC3 cells.[16] In addition, a peptide derivative was reported to be derived from the ink of *S. esculenta*, which could act as an inhibitor of angiotensin-converting enzyme (ACE).[17]

2. Peptidoglycans

An illexin–peptidoglycan and a peptidoglycan were isolated from the sepia ink. They both showed obvious anti-growth effect against Meth-A sarcoma cells in mice. The illexin–peptidoglycan was a fucose-rich glycoconjugate composed of 57% polysaccharide, 7.8% peptide, and 30% pigment, having a unique structure with equimolar ratios of GlcA, GalNAc, and Fuc, and burdening a unique branched repeating unit, (-3GlcA-β-1-4[GalNAc-α-1-3]-Fuc-α-1-)n.[18–20] The cure rate on Meth-A sarcoma could be 64% by this peptidoglycan treatment *in vivo*.[18–20] The anticancer activity was found to be mainly correlated to the augmented cellular immunity and enhanced phagocytic activity of macrophages *in vivo*, though not directly cytotoxic to Meth-A tumor cells.[18–20] Another peptidoglycan extracted by a different research group from sepia ink was reported to inhibit the proliferation of two types of human prostatic cancer cell lines (DU-145 and PC3) *in vitro*, showing direct cytotoxicity of this peptidoglycan.[21]

Using enzyme hydrolyzation of the sepia ink peptidoglycan with trypsinase, an oligopeptide with *N*-end amino acid sequence of Gln–Pro–Lys (molecular mass of 343.4) was prepared (1.82% yield). It obviously inhibited the proliferation of human DU-145 and PC3 prostate cancer cells and human H1299 nonsmall cell lung cancer cells and stimulated cell apoptosis in both dose- and time-dependent manners. The proapoptotic mechanism of this ink oligopeptide was found to be closely related to downregulation of Bcl-2 expression, enhancement of both p53 and BRCA1 mRNA expressions, and activation of caspase-3 and -9.[22,23]

3. Polysaccharides

SIP (11.3 kDa), a homogeneous heteropolysaccharide, was isolated from the ink of *Sepiella maindroni*. The SIP has a hexasaccharide repeating unit as a backbone consisting of fucose, mannose, and *N*-acetylgalactosamine in a molar ratio of 2:1:2, and has a single branch of glucuronic acid

(GlcA) at the 3-position of the mannose. No cytotoxicity of SIP was found on the tumor cells *in vitro* but it showed strong antimutagenic effect to markedly lessen the frequency of micronucleated cells in polychromatic erythrocytes and reticulocytes induced by cyclophosphamide in tumor-bearing mice.[24] When SIP was sulfated to give SIP–SII that contains 34.7% sulfates, SIP–SII demonstrated remarkable ability to inhibit MMP-2 expression in human SKOV3 ovarian cancer cells and human ECV304 umbilical vein vascular endothelial cells, thereby repressing the invasion and migration of these cells, but it showed only weak inhibition on the tumor cells *in vitro*.[25] In addition, the protein and mRNA expressions of ICAM-1 and bFGF were decreased prominently in human SKOV3 ovarian carcinoma cells and human EA.hy926 vascular endothelial cells, respectively, in the presence of SIP–SII.[25] In mouse model-implanted metastatic B16F10 melanoma cells, SIP–SII at doses of 15 and 30 mg/kg per day markedly restrained the adhesion and angiogenesis of tumor via decreasing ICAM-1 and bFGF expressions, then suppressed the B16F10 cell pulmonary metastasis by 85.9%~88.0%.[26] Therefore, these results evidenced that SIP–SII has a developing potential for preventing the invasion and metastasis of neoplastic cells.

In addition, SEP, a polysaccharide isolated from *S. esculenta* ink, was mainly composed of galactosamine (GalN) and arabinose (Ara) with a small amount of fucose (Fuc) and tiny amounts of mannose (Man), glucosamine (GlcN), glucuronic acid (GlcA), and galacturonic acid (GalA). In a female mouse model, SEP effectively prevented cyclophosphamide (a chemotherapeutic drug)-caused ovarian failure by inhibiting p38 MAPK signaling pathway and activating PI3K/Akt signaling pathway,[27] concluding the capacity of SEP in lessening the toxicity of chemotherapy.

CONCLUSION AND SUGGESTION

In these scientific explorations, the role of sepia ink in the inhibition of cancer-cell viability and proliferation has been established. It is clear now the sepia ink consumption would elicit manifold body protection due to its anticancer-related biological properties, including tumor-inhibitory immunity, antioxidant and radical scavenging, immunoenhancement, direct cancer suppression, detoxification, and anti-inflammation. The major bioactive components in sepia ink were found to be oligopeptides, peptidoglycans, and polysaccharides, which can be responsible for fighting cancer proliferation and invasion and recovering the toxicities caused by malignant diseases and chemotherapeutic drugs. These meaningful results lead to encourage humans to frequently consume the cheap and readily available marine coproduct, sepia ink, as a functional food for lowering the incidences of carcinogenesis and certain other diseases.

REFERENCES

1. Derby, C.D. et al., 2014. Cephalopod ink: Production, chemistry, functions and applications. *Mar. Drugs.* 12(5): 2700–2730.
2. Lü, C.L. et al., 1994. Detection of Sepia ink induced mouse cytotoxic factors. *J. China Med. Univ.* 23: 322–323.
3. Li, C.Y. et al, 1983. Antitumor activity of sea cucumber (Holothuria leucospilota) on mouse sarcoma 180. *Haiyang Yaowu* 3: 27–31.
4. Lü, C.L. et al.,1994. Sepia tumor inhibition in translanted mice. *Practical J. Oncol.* 8: 6.
5. Xie, G.L. et al., 2002. Study of sepia improving natural killer cell activity in mice. *J. China Med. Univ.* 31: 23–24.
6. Huang, M. et al., 2004. Studies on Sepia anticancer activity. *Fujian Zhongyi Xueyuan Xuebao* 14: 23–24.
7. Wang, C.B. et al., 2000. Effect of sepia on intracellular Ca^{2+} concentration, nuclear Ca^{2+}/Mg^{2+}-ATPase activities and c-jun expression in H22 cancer cells. *Weisheng Yanjiu* 29: 96–98.
8. Wang, C.B. et al., 2000. Effects of Sepia on intracellular Ca^{2+} concentration, nuclear Ca^{2+}/Mg^{2+}-ATPase activities and c-fos expression in H22 cancer cells. *J. Shandong Med. Univ.* 38: 420–422.
9. Wang, C.B. et al., 1999. Effect of Sepia on intracellular Ca^{2+}, ATP concentration and mitochondrial Ca^{2+}/Mg^{2+}-ATPase activities in H22 cancer cells. *Zhongguo Haiyang Yaowu* 18: 11–14.

10. Hou, X.Y. et al., 2001. Effects of Sepia on activity of TPK, PKC and PKA in H22 cancer cells. *Zhongguo Haiyang Yaowu* 20: 17–19.

11. Soliman, A.M. 2015. Anti-neoplastic activities of Sepia officinalis ink and coelatura aegyptiaca extracts against Ehrlich ascites carcinoma in Swiss albino mice. *Int. J. Clin. Exp. Pathol.* 8(4): 3543–3555; 2013. In vitro antioxidant, analgesic and cytotoxic activities of *Sepia officinalis* ink and *Coelatura aegyptiaca* extracts. *Afr. J. Pharm. Pharmaol.* 7: 1512–1522.

12. Ellouz, S.C. et al., 2014. Mediterranean cuttlefish sepia officinalis squid ink is cytotoxic but does not inhibit Glioblastoma U87 tumor cells proliferation, with high nutritional values of edible viscera. *Int. J. Basic and Applied Sci.* 3 (2): 146–154.

13. Zhong, J.P. et al., 2009. Protective effects of squid ink extract towards hemopoietic injuries induced by cyclophosphamine. *Mar. Drugs.* 7: 9–18.

14. Zhang, W.W. et al, 2009. Acidic mucopolysaccharide from Holothuria leucospilota has antitumor effect by inhibiting angiogenesis and tumor cell invasion in vivo and in vitro. *Cancer Biol. Therapy* 8: 1489–99.

15. Qian, W.H. et al, 2015. Downregulation of integrins in cancer cells and anti-platelet properties are involved in holothurian glycosamino-glycan-mediated disruption of the interaction of cancer cells and platelets in Hematogenous aetastasis. *J. Vascular Res.* 52: 197–209.

16. Huang, F.F. et al., 2012. Sepia ink oligopeptide induces apoptosis in prostate cancer cell lines via caspase-3 activation and elevation of Bax/Bcl-2 ratio. *Mar. Drugs.* 10: 2153–2165.

17. Kim, S.Y. et al,, 2003. Partial purification and characterization of an angiotensin-converting enzyme inhibitor from squid ink. *Agricul. Chem. Biotechnol.* 46: 122–123.

18. Sasaki, J. et al., 1997. Antitumor activity of squid ink. *J. Nutr. Sci. Vitaminol.* 43: 455–461.

19. Takaya, Y. et al., 1994. An investigation of the antitumor peptidoglycan fraction from squid ink. *Biol. Pharm. Bull.* 17: 846–849.

20. Naraoka, T. et al., 2000. Tyrosinase activity in antitumor compounds of squid ink. *Food Sci. Technol. Res.* 6: 171–175.

21. Zheng, Y.Y. et al., 2012. The peptidoglycan extracted from ink of sepia and the inhibition against the growth of prostatic cancer in vitro. *Shizhen Guoyi Guoyao* 23: 111–113.

22. Ding, G.F. et al., 2011. Sepia ink oligopeptides and its preparation by enzymolysis and application. Faming Zhuanli Shenqing CN 101983968 A 20110309.

23. Ding, G.F. et al., 2011. Anticancer activity of an an oligopeptide isolated from hydrolysates of sepia ink. *Zhongguo Tianran Yaowu* 9: 151–155.

24. Liu, C.H. et al., 2008. Structural characterization and antimutagenic of a novel polysaccharide isolated from Sepiella maindroni. *Food Chem.* 110: 807–813.

25. Wang, S.B. et al., 2008. Inhibition activity of sulfated polysaccharide of Sepiella maindroni ink on matrix metalloproteinase (MMP)-2. *Biomed. Pharmacother.* 62: 297–302.

26. Zong, A.Z. et al., 2013. Antimetastatic and anti-angiogenic activities of sulfated polysaccharide of Sepiella maindroni ink. *Carbohydr. Polym.* 91: 403–409.

27. Liu, H.Z. et al., 2016. Preventive effects of a novel polysaccharide from Sepia esculenta ink on ovarian failure and its action mechanisms in cyclopho sphamide-treated mice. *J. Agr. Food Chem.* 64(28): 5759–5766.

91. CALAMARI INK

魷魚墨 イカ墨 오징어 잉크

Inks from *Loligo chinensis, Ommastrephes bartrami*

Loliginidae and Ommastrephidae

Calamari ink (squid ink) originated from several sleeve fishes such as inshore squid *Loligo chinensis* (Loliginidae) and neon flying squid *Ommastrephes bartrami* (Ommastrephidae). Both squids are one of the common seafood sources in the world. Squid ink is used as an additive for food process and folk medicine in some East Asia regions. Similar to sepia ink, calamari ink showed similar composition of biochemicals, nutrients, and minerals, but their contents are less than in sepia ink. The main constituents in squid ink are found to be melanin and protein–polysaccharide complex.

SCIENTIFIC EVIDENCE OF CANCER-INHIBITORY AND CANCER-PREVENTIVE ACTIVITIES

An ink extract of inshore squid (*L. chinensis*) was reported to induce a variety of precancerous changes, such as esophagus-hyperplasia, leukoplakia vulvae, atrophic gastritis, chronic cervicitis, cervical polyp, rectal polyp, and so on. In recent years, the ink has been found to be useful for the treatment of various carcinomas such as leukemia and solid tumors in esophageal, stomach, liver, lung, rectum, colon, cervix, breast, chorion epithelial, pancreas, nasopharynx, mouth, bladder, lymph, brain, and skin.[1] An extract was prepared from the ink of *L. chinensis* by ultrasound and centrifugation at low temperature. *In vitro* assay evidenced antiproliferative effect of ink extract against human HL-60 (leukemia), HeLa (cervix), and CNE-2Z (nasopharynx) cancer cell lines. The HL-60 cells were the most sensitive cell line to the ink extract in the assay. Administration of the ink extract to tumor-bearing mice by i.p. at a dose of 1.2 g/kg or by i.g. at a dose of 2.4 g/kg for 15 days resulted in a significant anti-growth effect against sarcoma 180 of 70.8% and 69.2% and against H22 hepatoma of 71% and 58%, respectively, without obvious acute toxic reaction.[2]

A polysaccharide component (SIPs) was isolated from squid ink of *Ommastrephes bartrami*. When chemically reacted with pyridine–sulfur–trioxide complex, it yielded sulfated SIP (TBA-1), where the sulfation predominantly occurred at the 4,6-position of GalNAc units. TBA-1 had no obvious *in vitro* effects on the proliferation of human HepG2 hepatoma cells, but it exerted a dose-dependent suppression on the invasion and migration of HepG2 cells. The antiangiogenic activity of TBA-1 was shown in an assay using chick embryo chorioallantoic membrane (CAM). The findings indicated that TBA-1 has a developing potential for inhibition of hepatoma cell proliferation, invasion and metastasis, and blocking of angiogenesis.[3] Moreover, OBP was a polysaccharide extracted from the ink of *O. bartramii*. *In vivo* experiments demonstrated that dietary OBP could enhance intestinal SIgA secretion and the mRNA and protein expression levels of occludin, zonulae occluden (ZO)-1, and E-cadherin and augmented the mRNA expression of tight junction proteins (ZO-2, ZO-3, claudin-2, and cingulin) in the small intestinal epithelium, leading to ameliorate cyclophosphamide-chemotherapy-caused intestinal microflora dysfunction and injury.[4–6] The results have proven the mucosal immunopotentiating property of the squid inks and suggest that the ink used as a functional food is helpful for chemotherapeutic patients and cancer prevention and for therapies of intestinal disorders involving inflammation and infection.

CONCLUSION AND SUGGESTION

Calamari ink (squid ink) is a unique raw material source, which can be developed as a by-product in the marine food industry. Compared to sepia ink, the bioactivities of calamari ink have perhaps been less reported due to less content of bioactive components and less biological potencies. In addition to the polysaccharide, other types of bioactive components in squid ink are still unknown.

Nonetheless, based on its anticancer-related properties such as antitumor immunity, immunostimulation, antioxidant, and so on, the consumption of calamari ink (squid ink) is considered as a functional food and health supplement for cancer prevention and therapy and body defense.

REFERENCES

1. Ma, R.D. et al., 2005. Preparation of Loligo chinensis gray ink extract and its application in medicament and food for preventing and treating human tumors. Faming Zhuanli Shenqing CN 1672691 A 20050928.
2. Su, W.M. et al., 2005. Antitumor effects of extract from the ink of Loligo chinensis. *Chin. J. Mar. Drugs.* 2: 47–50.
3. Chen, S.G. et al., 2010. Sulfation of a squid ink polysaccharide and its inhibitory effect on tumor cell metastasis. *Carbohydr. Polym.* 81: 560–566.
4. Tang, Q.J. et al., 2014. Dietary squid ink polysaccharides ameliorated the intestinal microflora dysfunction in mice undergoing chemotherapy. *Food Funct.* 5: 2529–2535.
5. Zuo, T. et al., 2014. Dietary squid ink polysaccharide could enhance SIgA secretion in chemotherapeutic mice. *Food Funct.* 5: 3189–3196; 2015. The squid ink polysaccharides protect tight junctions and adherens junctions from chemotherapeutic injury in the small intestinal epithelium of mice. *Nutr. Cancer* 67: 364–371.
6. Zuo, T. et al., 2015. Dietary squid ink polysaccharide induces goblet cells to protect small intestine from chemotherapy induced injury. *Food Funct.* 6: 981–986.

92. SEA CUCUMBER

刺參　ナマコ　해삼

Stichopus japonicus, S. chloronotus

Stichopodidae

1. n = 5

3. n = 3

Sea cucumber is an echinoderm from the class Holothuroidea, which is a precious material for cuisines and folk medicine systems in Asia and Middle East communities. The high-value nutrients in sea cucumbers are vitamin A, vitamins B1, B2, B3, and some minerals (such as calcium, magnesium, iron, and zinc). Several sea cucumbers have been reported to have anticancer potential, such as *Stichopus japonicus* (= *Apostichopus japonicus*) and *S. chloronotus*. Pharmacological approaches further established that sea cucumber (*S. japonicus*) possesses immunoregulating, anticoagulant, analgesic, hypolipemic, antiradiation, memory enhancing, antithrombotic, and antifungal effects. In addition, sea cucumber can influence platelet aggregation and smooth muscles.

SCIENTIFIC EVIDENCE OF CANCER-INHIBITORY ACTIVITIES

A hydrolysate extract of sea cucumber *A. japonicus* (SCAJ) can significantly cause tumor cell disintegration and death. In 0.75–1.49 mg/mL concentrations, it noticeably suppressed the growth of human solid carcinoma cell lines of stomach, lung, and liver and mouse tumor cell lines (L929 acrobatma and EMT6 breast adenocarcinoma) *in vitro*. However, the SCAJ hydrolysate extract in lower concentrations of 0.75–5.94 mg/mL weakly promoted cell proliferation of human HeLa cervical cancer and 801 tumor. When the concentration was increased to 11.88 mg/mL, its tumor inhibitory effect was performed on these two cancer cells, indicating that the sensitivity of SCAJ hydrolysate extract toward tumor cells is closely dependent on its concentration.[1]

The investigation further revealed that another sea cucumber *Stichopus chloronotus* (SCSC) is a functional food source for cancer prevention. An aqueous extract of SCSC was effective in suppressing the growth of human C33A cervical carcinoma and A549 nonsmall cell lung carcinoma cell lines with respective IC_{50}s of 10.0 and 28.0 µg/mL. The SCSC extract displayed significant antioxidative activity in scavenging free radicals of linoleic acid and DPPH as well.[2]

SCIENTIFIC EVIDENCE OF CANCER-INHIBITORY CONSTITUENTS

Three types of macromolecules in sea cucumber were found to be major inhibitors of carcinoma cell growth, such as mucopolysaccharides, glycoproteins, and peptides, and small molecules such as triterpenoid saponins and alkene sulfates.

1. Polysaccharides

The acidic mucopolysaccharides (SJAMP) isolated from *S. japonicus* are composed of amidohexose, hexuronic acid, fucose, and sulfate radical (1:1:1:4) with m.w. of 50,000–55,000. SJAMP significantly hindered the growth of murine MA-737 breast cancer, Lewis and T795 lung cancer, Lio-1 lymphosarcoma, melanoma, H22 hepatoma, sarcoma 180, and sarcoma 37 cell lines *in vivo*. The highest inhibitory effect was observed on MA-737 breast carcinoma with the inhibitory rate of 79%–88%.[3–5] If administered before the transplantation of tumor cells, SJAMP exerted not only the reduction of tumor size but also decrease in foci numbers of the cancer-cell metastasis.[3,4] An experiment of TdR incorporation further confirmed that SJAMP obviously lessened DNA synthesis in sarcoma 180 and breast cancer cells, although it promoted DNA synthesis in normal hepatic cells.[6] By decrease in Bcl-2 expression and/or increase in nm23-H1 expression, SJAMP time- and dose-dependently hindered the proliferation of HepG2 and H22 hepatoma cells and promoted cell apoptosis.[7] The HeLa cell-cycle arrest caused by SJAMP treatment was correlated with marked downregulation of PCNA and mdm expression similar to methotrexate (MTX).[8] SJAMP treatment by oral gavage (17.5, 35, 70 mg/kg, and 5 days/week) significantly obstructed diethylnitrosamine (DEN)-prompted hepatoma in rats by lessening both number and volume of nodules and inhibiting tumor growth. The antihepatoma activity of SJAMP was mostly mediated by enhancement of cellular immunity pathways, that is, (1) augmenting NK cell-elicited tumoricidal activity and macrophage phagocytosis; (2) improving spleen and thymus of indexes and function; (3) recovery of CD3+ and CD4+ T-lymphocyte levels and ratio; (4) reducing blood serum AFP expression in liver; and (5) decreasing ALT, AST, GGT, and TNF-α levels in serum and increasing p21 expression and serum IL-2 level[9,10] and by induction of cell-cycle arrest via downregulation of cyclin-D1, CDK4 mRNA, E2F-1s, and PCNA expressions.[11,12] When combined with chemotherapeutic drugs (such as CP, DDP, and 5-FU), SJAMP demonstrated broad-spectrum synergistic effect in HepA and H22 mouse tumor models.[13,14] The additive effect was also observed in combination with SJAMP (40 mg/kg, IP) with cortisone (10 mg/kg) against mouse solid tumors such as MA737, HepA22, U14, S180, L793, and Lewis tumors.[15] In addition, KAMP, a potassium salt of polysulfonic acid mucopolysaccharide derived from *A. japonicus* is stable on boiling in neutral or weak alkaline solutions but it is unstable in weak acid. Due to KAMP-exhibited antitumor activity, its injection has been used in China for clinical treatment of cancer.[16,17]

A. japonicus intestinal polysaccharides (AJIP) exerted dose-dependent inhibitory effect on mouse H22 hepatoma *in vivo*. At daily doses of 200 or 400 mg/kg, the inhibitory rates of AJIP were up to 62.6% and 77.2%, respectively. Besides the antitumor activity, AJIP also markedly promoted the immune functions via augmentation of IL-2 and TNF-α levels and NK cell activity and increase in thymus and spleen indexes.[18] Similarly, SJVP, an acidic polysaccharide was isolated from the viscera of sea cucumber. I.p injection of SJVP in a dose of 40 mg/kg in tumor-bearing mice resulted in 42.2%, 48.5%, and 48.4% inhibitory effects against MA-737 mammary carcinoma, Ehrlich entity cancer, and sarcoma 180, respectively.[10] Furthermore, two types of fucan sulfate were isolated from the body wall of the *A. japonicus*. Its type-A fucan sulfate (9 kDa) consists of a backbone of (1-3)-linked fucosyl residues with a substitution of fucosyl residues at C-4, whereas its type-B fucan sulfate (32 kDa) largely comprised unbranched (1-3)-linked fucosyl residues. Their sulfates are substituted at C-2 and/or C-4 of fucosyl residues. Both types of fucan sulfates were able to hamper osteoclastogenesis *in vitro* more than 95% at a concentration of 50 µg/mL, suggesting fucan sulfates as potent inhibitors of osteoclastogenesis that have potential chemotherapeutic value.[19]

2. Glycoproteins

Glycoproteins (GP) and chondroitin sulfates (CS) isolated from *A. japonicus* also exhibited anticancer and antimutagenic activities. At 5% concentration, the GP exerted strong *in vitro* inhibitory effects on the growth of HT-29 colon carcinoma cells and AZ-521 gastric cancer cells of 89%–95% and 82%–92%, respectively.[20] At a dose of 100 mg/kg, the GP suppressed S180 sarcoma by 64% in mice and prolonged the mice life span by 39%. Besides the cytotoxic activity in the tumor cells, the GP could dose-dependently amplify leukocytes, peritoneal exudate cells, and weights of immune organs. As a result, the antitumor activity of sea cucumber glycoproteins was evidenced to be attributed to the improvement of host immune system.[19] Furthermore, either GP or CS at 5% concentration exerted prominent inhibitory effects against the mutagenicities of aflatoxin B1 (AFB1) by 84%–98% of 3,2′-dimethyl-4-aminobiphenyl (DMAB) by 79%–85%, N-methyl-N′-nitro-N-nitrosoguanidine (MNNG) by 55%–78%, and of 4-nitroquinoline-1-oxide (4-NQO) by 58%–70%.[20–22]

Moreover, HA-3, a water-soluble extract from *S. japonicus*, showed an ability to elicit the differentiation of F9 teratocarcinoma stem cells. HA-3–5 was a mixture of galactose–isoleucine that was derived from the fractionation of HA-3, which was more effective in prompting the F9 cell differentiation via regulation of differentiation-specific genes such as laminin, type-IV collagen and retinoic acid receptor-β, and induction of morphological changes.[23]

3. Peptides

Two low molecular weight peptides (<3 kDa) termed LSCP-1 and LSCP-2 were extracted from the *S. japonicus* by a continuous hydrolyzation technique with trypsin. LSCP-2 showed significant suppressive effect *in vitro* against human SGC-7901 (gastric) and MCF-7 (breast) cancer cell lines, whereas LSCP-1 had significant antitumor activity only on SGC-7901 cells, but the two peptides showed no activity on A549 lung cancer cell line.[24] A3 (6.5 kDa), a peptide was fractionated from the enteron of *A. japonicus*, which showed antiproliferative effect on the A549 cells.[25] By a similar method, a collagen protein with antitumor activity was prepared from the body of *A. japonicus* treated with a complex of proteolytic enzymes, collagen preparation of which could achieve marked *in vivo* anti-growth activity against Ehrlich solid adenocarcinoma and prolonged life duration of the tested mouse.[26]

4. Saponins

Two saponin fractions named pSC-2 and pSC-3 were prepared from 70% ethanolic extract of *S. japonicus*, which exerted remarkable tumor inhibitory activity toward human HeLa (cervix), A549 (lung), SGC-7901 (stomach), and Bel-7402 (liver) cancer cell lines with IC_{50}s in a range of 3.04–4.41 μg/mL. The inhibitory activity, especially for pSC-2, was found to correlate with the apoptosis-promoting ability. The pSC-2 also showed anti-growth effect in a mouse model implanted sarcoma 180 together with the immunoenhancing effect to augment the indexes of thymus and spleen.[27] A saponin named S2 was isolated from the concentrated liquid of *S. japonicus*, which exerted moderate anti-growth effect against sarcoma 180 cells *in vitro* with IC_{50} of 41.04 μg/mL at 44 h.[28] From sea cucumber *S. chloronotus*, stichostatin-1, a lanostane-type saponin was separated, which displayed anticancer effect against P388 leukemia cells *in vitro* in its ED_{50} value of 2.9 μg/mL.[29]

5. Alkene sulfates

Five alkene sulfate compounds were isolated from the intestines of sea cucumber *A. japonicus* and were identified as octyl sulfate (**1**), decyl sulfate (**2**), 2,6-dimethylheptyl sulfate (**3**), (5Z)-dec-5-en-1-yl sulfate (**4**), and (3E)-dec-3-en-1-yl sulfate (**5**). These alkene sulfates in the *in vitro* assay showed cytotoxicities on human A549 lung adenocarcinoma cells and human MG63 osteosarcoma cells. The potent cytotoxicity was exerted by the last four alkenes (**2–5**) on A549 cells and by the last two alkenes (**4** and **5**) on MG63 cells. However, all these alkenes had no cytotoxic activity toward human U251 glioma cells even at a high concentration of 30 mg/mL.[30]

CONCLUSION AND SUGGESTION

As a source of nutritious and luxurious seafood and tonic herb, sea cucumber has been prominently investigated for its chemical biology and anticancer activity. The research findings evidently disclosed that the cancer inhibition-related activities of sea cucumber (edible part) are mostly contributed by its bioactive components, that is, saponins, glycoproteins, polysaccharides, and as enzymatic degradation peptides, although alkene sulfate compounds from the inedible part of sea cucumber are cancer inhibitors as well. The experimental data evidenced these bioactive components markedly to exert their anticancer and anticarcinogenic potentials and their immunoregulating activities toward different types of cancers, leading to moderate-to-weak inhibitory effects against cancer cell initiation, proliferation, and growth. Consequently, the observations strongly support the consumption of sea cucumber as a functional food as it is conducive to cancer prevention and therapy and immunopromotion.

REFERENCES

1. Yin, Z.S. et al., 1990. Study on the pharmacological activities of Sea cucumber (*Stichopus japonicus*). *Zhongyao Yaoli yu Linchuang* 6: 33–35.
2. Althunibat, O.Y. et al., 2009. In vitro antioxidant and antiproliferative activities of three Malaysian sea cucumber species. *Eur. J. Scientific Res.* 37: 376–387.
3. Shen, M. et al., 2001. Investigation of component and pharmacology of Sea cucumber. *Zhongchengyao* 58–61.
4. Zhang, J.F. et al., 2007. Effects of Apostichopus japonicus on antitumor and immune regulation in S180 bearing mice. *J. Ocean Univ. China (Sci. Edit.)* 37: 93–96, 102; 1982. Ma, K.S. et al., *Zhongguo Haiyang Yaowu* (1): 21.
5. Chen, D.D. et al., 2014. Effects of Stichopus japonicus acidic mucopolysaccharide on gene Bcl-2 and Bax expressions in H22-hepatoma-bearing mice. *Qingdao Daxue Yixueyuan Xuebao* 50: 305–308.
6. Wang, Z.L. et al., 1993. Inhibition of DNA synthesis of tumor cell of acidic mucopolysaccharide of Stichopus japonicus (SJAMP) and its metabolism in mice. *Zhongguo Yiyao Gongye Zazhi* 24: 405–408.
7. Lu, Y. et al., 2011. The effects of Stichopus japonicus acid mucopolysaccharide on the apoptosis of the human hepatocellular carcinoma cell line HepG2. *Am. J. Med. Sci.* 339: 141–144.
8. Zhang, X.X. et al., 2008. Effects of Stichopus japonicus acidic mucopolysaccharide on PCNA expression and cell cycling in Henrietta Lacks strain of cancer cells. *Shandong Yiyao* 48: 19–21.
9. Song, Y. et al., 2013. Immunomodulatory effect of Stichopus japonicus acid mucopoly-saccharide on experimental hepatocellular carcinoma in rats. *Molecules.* 18: 7179–7193.
10. Jin, S.J. et al., 2012. Intervention effect of SJAMP on hepatocellular carcinoma rat induced by diethyl-nitrosamine and impact on immune function. *Xiandai Shengwuyixue Jinzhan* 12: 3455–3459.
11. Dai, H.H. et al., 2015. Attenuated and synergized action of Stichopus japonicus acid mucopolysaccharide combined with 5-FU on hepato-carcinoma 22-bearing mouse. *Zhonghua Zhongliu Fangzhi Zazhi* 22: 23–27; 2014. Effect of Stichopus japonicus acidic mucopolysaccharide on cellular proliferation related genes expression in mice bearing neoplasia of H22 hepatoma cells. *Yingyang Xuebao* 36: 263–267; 2014. Immune effect of Stichopus japonicus acid mucopolysaccharide on hepatocarcinoma 22-bearing mouse. *Xiandai Shengwuyixue Jinzhan* 14: 4455–4458; 2014. Antitumor effect of Stichopus japonicus acidic mucopolysaccharide combined with fluorouracil in mice bearing neoplasia of H22 hepatoma cells. *Weisheng Yanjiu* 43: 598–602.
12. Liang, N.N. et al., 2013. Effect of Stichopus japonicus acidic mucopolysaccharide on the cell cycle in rat liver cancer induced by diethyl nitrosamine. *Yingyang Xuebao* 35: 582–586.
13. Zhao, X.M. et al., 2010. Synergistic effect of acid mucopolysaccharides in Stichopus japonicus Selenka on HepA in mice and its mechanism. *Shizhen Guoyi Guoyao* 21: 3062–3063.
14. Fan, H.C. et al., 1983. Study on acidic mucopolysaccharides from the viscera of Sea cucumber. *Zhongguo Haiyang Yaowu* (3): 134–137.
15. Hu, R.J. et al., 1997. The inhibitory effect of SJAMP combined with cortisone on murine solid tumors. *Aizheng* 16: 422–424.
16. Chen, J.D. et al., 1993. Stability of the injection of potassium acidic mucopolysaccharide from Apostichopus japonicus after sterilization. *Zhongguo Haiyang Yaowu* 12: 8–10.
17. Chen, C.T. et al., 1981. Observations on the stability of acid mucopolysaccharide potassium salts from Stichopus japonicus. *Yaoxue Tongbao* 16: 58.
18. Wang, Z.Y. et al., 2012. Effects of Apostichopus japonicus intestinal polysaccharides on immune function and its antitumor activity. *Nongye Shengwu Jishu Xuebao* 20: 560–567.
19. Kariya, Y. et al., 2004. Isolation and partial characterization of fucan sulfates from the body wall of sea cucumber Stichopus japonicus and their ability to inhibit osteoclastogenesis. *Carbohydr. Res.* 339: 1339–1346.

20. Moon, J.H. et al., 1998. Antimutagenic and anticancer effects of glycoprotein and chondroitin sulfates from sea cucumber (Stichopus japonicus). *Han'guk Sikp'um Yongyang Kwahak Hoechi* 27: 350–358.

21. Moon, J.H. et al., 1999. Antitumor effects of glycoproteins extracted from sea cucumber (Stichopus japonicus). *J. Food Sci. Nutr.* 4: 117–121.

22. Su, X.R. et al., 2003. Study on nutritional components and antitumor activity of polysaecharides of sea cucumber. *Yingyang Xuebao* 25: 181–182.

23. Kim, L.L. et al., 1997. Tumor cell differentiation-inducing fractions from Stichopus japonicas and marine mullask Mytilus edulis. *J. Kor. Asso. Cancer Provention* 1: 73–80.

24. Zhou, X.Q. et al., 2012. In vitro antitumor activities of low molecular sea cucumber Stichopus japonicus peptides sequentially hydrolyzed by proteases. *Adv. Mater. Res.* 393–395: 1259–1262.

25. Tan, J. et al., 2012. Isolation and purification of the peptides from Apostichopus japonicus and evaluation of its antibacterial and antitumor activities. *African J. Microbiol. Res.* 6: 7139–7146.

26. Popov, A.M. et al., 2011. Antitumor and anticoagulant activities of collagen protein from the holothurian Apostichopus japonicus modified by proteolytic enzymes. *Russ. J. Marine Biol.* 37: 217–222.

27. Fan, T.J. et al., 2009. Studies on the purification of water-soluble holothurian glycosides from Apostichopus japonicus and their tumor suppressing activity. *Yaoxue Xuebao* 44: 25–31.

28. Su, X.R. et al., 2011. Antitumor activity of polysaccharides and saponin extracted from sea cucumber. *J. Clin. Cell. Immunol.* 2: 100–115.

29. Pettit, G.R. et al., 1976. Antineoplastic agents. XLV. Sea cucumber cytotoxic saponins. *J. Pharm. Sci.* 65: 1558–1559.

30. La, M.P. et al., 2012. Bioactive sulfated alkenes from the sea cucumber Apostichopus japonicus. *Chem. Biodivers.* 9: 1166–1171.

93. LOLLYFISH SEA CUCUMBER

蕩皮參　玉足ナマコ

Holothuria leucospilota, H. scabra

Holothuriidae

1. $R_1 = -A$, $R_2 = -OSO_3Na$, $R_3 = -H$.
2. $R_1 = -B$, $R_2 = -OSO_3Na$, $R_3 = -D$.
3. $R_1 = -C$, $R_2 = -OSO_3Na$, $R_3 = -D$.

Lollyfish sea cucumber, or *Holothuria leucospilota* (Holothuriidae), is utilized as a healthy food source in various cuisines for having a high percentage of protein with less cholesterol as similar as sea cucumber (*Stichopus japonicus*). Pharmacological studies have reported the lollyfish possessing anticoagulant, antioxidant, antithrombus, cytotoxic, immunoregulating, antibacterial, antifungal, and antiviral activities,[1] and the extensive assays further demonstrated that the lollyfish sea cucumber is able to influence platelet aggregation and smooth muscles.[1]

SCIENTIFIC EVIDENCE OF ANTITUMOR CONSTITUENTS AND ACTIVITIES

The antineoplastic property of lollyfish sea cucumber extract was demonstrated in various lab examinations. Three lollyfish toxicins-I, -II and -III were isolated from the lollyfish extract, showing marked cytotoxic effect on the tumor cells, in which activities of toxicins-I and II were stronger than that of vincristine (an anticancer drug) on human cervical cancer cells but were lower than that of vincristine on normal cells. Daily intraperitoneal (i.p.) injection of the extract in a dose of 50 mg/kg for 5 days, or i.p. injection of toxicin-I in a dose of 2 mg/kg for 6 days to mice resulted in 46.7% and 57.7% suppressive effect against the growth of sarcoma 180 cells, respectively.[2,3]

Through bioorganic chemistry approaches, various types of constituents have been isolated from the lollyfish sea cucumber, such as triterpene glycosides (saponins), sterols, phenolics, peptides, chondroitin sulfates, cerebrosides, sulfated/acidic polysaccharides, glycosaminoglycan, and lectins. Of them, two types of constituents, that is, (1) triterpenoid saponins and (2) polysaccharides, were discovered to be truly responsible for the antineoplastic activity of lollyfish.

1. Saponins

A group of sulfated holostane glycosides with cytotoxicities were discovered from *Holothuria* genus sea cucumbers collected in the South China Sea. *In vitro* assay exhibited that holothurin-B, holothurin-B2, and leucospilotaside-D that were separated from *H. leucospilota* markedly restrained the proliferation of human HeLa (cervix), Bel-7402 (liver), and MCF-7 (breast) cancer cell lines.[4] Leucospilotaside-B (**1**) derived from *H. leucospilota* and scabrasides-A (**2**) and -B (**3**) isolated from *H. scabra* displayed significant cytotoxic effect against human HL-60 and Molt-4 (leukemic), A549 (lung), and Bel-7402 (liver) cancer cell lines with IC_{50}s of 0.44–2.62 µg/mL for **1**, 0.05–5.62 µM for **2**, and 0.08–3.40 µM for **3**.[5,6] In the *in vitro* assay, the saponins (**2** and **3**) were more sensitive to the HL-60 and Molt-4 leukemia cells and more active than 10-hydroxy-camptothecine, a chemotherapeutic drug.[5,6] The cytotoxic saponins derived from *H. scabra* such as 24-dehydroechinoside-A, echinosides-A, -B, and holothurins-A, -B were effective to deterring human MKN-45 (stomach) and HCT-116 (colon) carcinoma cell lines, whereas 24-dehydroechinoside-A, echinoside-A, holothurin-A, scabraside-C, and holothurins-A1 were cytotoxic to HL-60 and Molt-4 leukocythemia cells and A549 lung cancer cells, *in vitro*.[7,8] The most potent cytotoxic effects in the assay were achieved by scabraside-C (IC_{50}s 0.05 and 0.09 µM) and holothurins-A1 (IC_{50}s 0.25 and 0.08 µM) in the Molt-4 and A549 cell lines, respectively.[8]

The marked growth inhibitive effect on the tumor cells was also achieved by similar saponins derived from other *Holothuria* sea cucumbers. Hillasides-A–C and holothuria-A (from *H. hilla*) displayed marked cytotoxicities against eight human tumor cell lines (A549, MCF-7, IA9, CAKI-1, PC3, KB, KB-VIN, and HCT-8) with IC_{50} data in a range of 0.1–3.8 µg/mL. Among the cell lines, hillaside-C was sensitive to human CAKI-1 kidney cancer cells and next to human IA9 ovarian cancer cells, whereas hillasides-A and -B were highly cytotoxic to IA9 cells.[9,10] Impatienside-A and bivittoside-D (from *H. impatiens*) exhibited cytotoxicities on seven human cancer cell lines (HCT-116, HT-29, A549, HepG2, DU145 MCF-7, and KB) *in vitro* with IC_{50}s of 0.37–2.75 µg/mL, wherein the most sensitive cell lines to both the saponins were HCT-116 (colon) and A549 (lung) human cancer cells.[11] Five cytotoxic saponins separated from *H. fuscocinerea* were identified as fuscocinerosides-A–C, holothurin-A, and pervicoside-C. Fuscocineroside-C was the most potent one against human HL-60 leukemia and Bel-7402 hepatoma cells in the *in vitro* test.[12]

2. Polysaccharides

Several polysaccharides isolated from *H. leucospilota* have been found to possess remarkable suppressive activities toward the growth of cancer cells. A sulfate-rich acidic polysaccharide termed HL-P was prepared from the dried body wall of the sea cucumber, which consists of galactosamine, glucuronic acid, fucose, and sulfate with a molar ratio of 10:9.4:8.4:36. HL-P as a powerful inhibitor of thrombin exerted significant anti-growth effect against several types of tumor cells in mice. When HL-P was administrated in a dose of 50 mg/kg i.p. to mice-borne tumor, the cell growth inhibitory rates were shown as 68.1% on MA737 mammary cancer, 35.2% on Lewis lung carcinoma, 38% on sarcoma 180, and 43.3% on B16 melanoma.[13] HS, an acidic mucopolysaccharide derived from the fresh lollyfish, presented interesting activity by blocking some steps in the cancer cell metastasis cascade. At its cytotoxic doses, HS was able to restrain the growth of B16F10 melanoma cells and proliferation of HUVEC *in vitro*, and significantly obstruct VEGF-induced capillary-like tube networks in a dose-dependent manner. By treatment with HS, the growth, migratory, and invasive abilities of B16F10 cells were suppressed *in vitro* and *in vivo* via lessening of Matrigel-embedded Boyden chamber and MMPs-2, -9, and VEGF protein levels. In addition, HS in doses of 5.2–26 mg/kg markedly obstructed the lung metastasis of tumors in a mouse model in a dose-dependent fashion. These data established that the antimetastatic properties of HS were attributed to its anti-invasive effect via inactivation of MMPs and to its antiangiogenic effect via blocking of VEGF function.[14] Similarly, holothurian glycosaminoglycan (hGAG), a sulfated polysaccharide extracted from lollyfish sea cucumber, was highly efficacious against the tumor hematogenous metastasis in human MDA-MB-231 breast cancer cells, effect of which was mediated by decreasing platelet–cancer cell complex formation and both levels of β1 and β3 integrins, downregulation of MMPs-2 and -9 expressions, and upregulation of TIMP-1 expression.[15]

CONCLUSION AND SUGGESTION

The scientific investigations have corroborated that the presence of appreciable amounts of bioactive constituents, especially sulfated holostane-type saponins and polysaccharides, endowed lollyfish sea cucumber (*Holothuria leucospilota*) to have a biological capacity for the suppression of cancer cells and carcinogenesis. The cytotoxicities of Holothuria saponins were observed all in *in vitro* models, but the cytotoxic effects of Holothuria saponins are probably correlated to their hemolytic activity.[16] Thus, it is better to confirm their anticancer activities by using *in vivo* assay system. The sulfated and acidic polysaccharides are abundant in lollyfish sea cucumber, and can be considered the major anticancer agents in *Holothuria leucospilota*. These polysaccharides demonstrated multiple inhibitory effects against cell growth, invasion, and metastasis of some types of carcinomas and against the angiogenesis in tumor tissue. In addition to the anticancer properties, sea cucumber also exhibited various pharmacological activities and nutritional values. Accordingly, it is confirmed that Holothuria sea cucumbers may be applied as functional foods and nontoxic remedies of supplementary therapy for prevention and treatment of carcinomas and various other diseases.

REFERENCES

1. Bordbar, S. et al., 2011. High-value components and bioactives from sea cucumbers for functional foods—A review. *Mar. Drugs.* 9(10): 1761–1805.
2. Liao, H.N. et al., 1995. Advances in marine antitumor substances. *Progr. Biotechnol.* 15: 8–14; Li, C.Y. et al, 1982. *Haiyang Yaowu* 2: 23–24.
3. Li, C.Y. et al., 1983. Antitumor activity of sea cucumber (Holothuria leucospilota) on mouse sarcoma 180. *Haiyang Yaowu* 27–31.
4. Han, H. et al., 2012. Cytotoxic triterpene glycosides from sea cucumber Holothuria leucospilota. *Chinese Pharm. J.* 47: 1194–1198.
5. Han, H. et al., 2010. A novel sulfated holostane glycoside from sea cucumber Holothuria leucospilota. *Chem. Biodivers.* 7: 1764–1769.
6. Han, H. et al., 2009. Two new cytotoxic triterpene glycosides from the sea cucumber *Holothuria scabra*. *Planta Med.* 75: 1608–1612.
7. Yan, B. et al., 2005. Study on bioactive triterpene glucosides of sea cucumber Holothunia scabra Jaeger. *Acta J. Sec. Mil. Med. Univ.* 26: 626–631.
8. Han, H. et al., 2010. Cytotoxicitic triterpene glycosides from sea cucumber Holothunia scabra Jaeger. *Chin. J. Med. Chem.* 20: 290–297.
9. Wu, J. et al., 2006. Structure and cytotoxicity of a new lanostane-type triterpene glycoside from the sea cucumber Holothuria hilla. *Chem. Biodivers.* 3: 1249–1254.
10. Wu, J. et al., 2007. Hillasides A and B, two new cytotoxic triterpene glycosides from the sea cucumber Holothuria hilla Lesson. *J. Asian Nat. Prod. Res.* 9: 609–618.
11. Sun, P. et al., 2007. A new cytotoxic lanostane-type triterpene glycoside from the sea cucumber Holothuria impatiens. *Chem. Biodivers.* 4: 450–457.
12. Zhang, S.Y. et al., 2006. Bioactive triterpene glycosides from the sea cucumber Holothuria fuscocinerea. *J. Nat. Prod.* 69: 1492–1495.
13. Fan, H.C. et al., 1981. Acidic polysaccharides from Holothuria leucospilota. *Yaoxue Tongbao* 16: 631.
14. Zhang, W.W. et al., 2009. Acidic mucopolysaccharide from Holothuria leucospilota has antitumor effect by inhibiting angiogenesis and tumor cell invasion in vivo and in vitro. *Cancer Biol. Therapy* 8: 1489–1499.
15. Qian, W.H. et al., 2015. Downregulation of integrins in cancer cells and anti-platelet properties are involved in holothurian glycosamino-glycan-mediated disruption of the interaction of cancer cells and platelets in hematogenous aetastasis. *J. Vascular Res.* 52: 197–209.
16. Soltani, M. et al., 2014. Hemolytic and cytotoxic properties of saponin purified from Holothuria leucospilota sea cucumber. *Reports of Biochem. Mol. Biol.* 3(1): 1–8.

Index of Latin Names for Functional Comestibles

Index of English Names for Functional Comestibles

Index of Acronyms